Sunscreens for Skin of Color

Renita Rajan

Sunscreens for Skin of Color

Springer

Renita Rajan
RENDER Skin and Hair Clinic
Chennai, Tamil Nadu, India

ISBN 978-981-97-3197-8 ISBN 978-981-97-3195-4 (eBook)
https://doi.org/10.1007/978-981-97-3195-4

This Springer imprint is published by the registered company Springer Nature Singapore Pte Ltd.
The registered company address is: 152 Beach Road, #21-01/04 Gateway East, Singapore 189721, Singapore

To Nylah and Karthik, for completing me.
To my team at RENDER and CHOSEN, for being the wind beneath my wings.

Foreword

Sun and sunlight are essential for life. Photosynthesis does not happen in the absence of sunlight. Sunlight has many beneficial effects such as its role in the synthesis of vitamin D. However, exposure to sunlight can also have deleterious effects, and to dermatologists, this deleterious effect is of great importance. Sunlight consists of many waves of importance to the dermatologist: the ultraviolet, the visible light, and the infrared light. All these lights can either aggravate the given condition or induce certain diseases such as idiopathic polymorphic light eruptions.

Since it has multiple side effects, such as skin cancers, darkening of the skin, and aging of the skin, human beings need to protect themselves from sunlight. Protection can be behavioural alterations such as avoiding sunlight, wearing suitable clothing, and sun protective glasses. However, physical protection is not a practical option for all the areas of the body at all times of the day. Sunscreens have become one of the major cosmetic and therapeutic agents to protect areas of the skin which are not protected by clothing and other measures.

'Use the proper sunscreen' may sound like a practical approach, but in practice, finding the right sunscreen and applying it at required intervals and in the sufficient quantity required call for a better understanding of the sunscreen. Since dermatologists have to advice regarding the use of sunscreen, it is desirable that dermatologist understands the different types of sunscreens, the type of chemicals present in the sunscreen, the cost incurred by using the formulation, the degree of protection offered, and lastly the unwanted side effects of the sunscreen.

This book on sunscreen by Dr. Renita is out to address this issue. The author has spent a lot of time understanding the technicalities and the intricacies of sunscreens and has successfully provided us with an easily understandable, readable book. To understand, ease of reading is essential. W. Somerset Maugham wrote that anything that is difficult to understand will be left unread. This book is divided into multiple chapters addressing almost all aspects of sunscreens, and at the beginning of each chapter, the relevant information the reader is likely to gather is briefly outlined. This accomplished, the author has proceeded to discuss each aspect in detail and has quoted relevant references as and when required.

If you are a dermatologist and you want to prescribe sunscreens based on facts which you can explain to the patient, this is the book for you. If you are formulating sunscreen, this book will ensure that you deliver the right formulations. If you are a student of dermatology, this book will lay the foundation for what you need to learn about sun protection.

Professor, Department of Dermatology
Kalinga Institute of Medical Sciences,
Bhubaneswar, Odisha, India

Chakravarthi R. Srinivas

Foreword

An Introduction to "Sunscreens for Skin of Colour"

Sunscreens for Skin of Colour is a comprehensive and meticulously crafted book authored by a highly experienced physician. Spanning 12 informative chapters, this book delves into every aspect of sunscreens, making it an indispensable resource for dermatologists, researchers, healthcare providers, and anyone keen on understanding the science and application of sun protection.

This book begins with an in-depth exploration of photobiology. The author explains the mechanisms of UV-induced skin damage, such as DNA mutations, photoaging, and the body's natural defence responses like melanin production.

One of the key highlights of this book is its detailed examination of technological advancements in sunscreen formulations. The author traces the evolution of sunscreens from their rudimentary beginnings to sophisticated modern products that offer broad-spectrum protection. This section covers the science behind various active ingredients, including organic (chemical) filters like avobenzone and oxybenzone and inorganic (physical) filters such as zinc oxide and titanium dioxide. This book also discusses innovations such as nanoparticle technology and enhanced stability for prolonged efficacy.

A critical aspect covered in this book is the interplay between sunscreen use and vitamin D synthesis. The author provides evidence-based guidelines to balance sun protection with maintaining adequate vitamin D levels. Practical advice on safe sun exposure, dietary sources of vitamin D, and supplementation is offered.

Dedicated chapters address the unique needs of children and individuals with skin of colour. Children's skin is more susceptible to UV damage, requiring special formulations that are both effective and gentle. For those with darker skin tones, this book explores the specific challenges and considerations, such as hyperpigmentation and sunscreen residue. The author provides tailored recommendations to ensure comprehensive sun protection for these groups.

The relationship between sunscreen uses and skin cancer prevention is a significant focus. The author discusses how regular sunscreen use can reduce the risk of skin cancers, including melanoma, squamous cell carcinoma, and basal cell carcinoma, by preventing UV-induced DNA damage. This book emphasizes the importance of proper and consistent sunscreen application for effective protection.

A unique aspect of this book is its thorough discussion on phototyping in skin of colour. The author explores how different skin types react to sunlight and the role of visible light and infrared radiation in pigmentation and skin health. This section is particularly valuable for understanding the comprehensive impact of sun exposure beyond UV radiation.

Drawing on her extensive experience in clinical practice and research, the author combines scientific rigor with practical advice, making *Sunscreens for Skin of Colour* both informative and accessible. Each chapter is well-referenced, ensuring readers have access to the latest scientific findings and recommendations.

In conclusion, *Sunscreens for Skin of Colour* is an essential resource that covers all facets of sunscreen science and application. Its thorough approach ensures readers gain a deep understanding of sun protection, the latest technological advancements, and practical guidance for diverse populations, making it a definitive guide for safeguarding skin health.

Laxmisha Chandrashekar
Professor, Department of Dermatology
Jawaharlal Institute of Postgraduate
Medical Education and Research (JIPMER),
Puducherry, India

Preface

I have long been fascinated by the story of melanin in skin of colour. And what follows melanin is invariably, pigmentation, which is a big concern again, in skin of colour. And in understanding pigmentation, the role of sun exposure is a fascinating area to explore. And when the cause is apparent, mitigation in the form of sunscreens in this context is a central part of the treatment plan that any dermatologist extends to their patients who come in with complaints of pigmentation.

As a specialist and national and regional Key Opinion Leader (KOL) for laser technologies for pigmentation, the use of sunscreens in preventing further pigmentation after in clinic treatments, such as a postinflammatory hyperpigmentation, so common in the population I serve, was my initial point of getting to know sunscreens. Over time, the effect of sunscreens in maintenance treatment and even as stand-alone care such as in the amelioration of pigmentary conditions like melasma ensured that sunscreens were an important part of my counselling and prescription.

Over the last 5 years, the sunscreen domain has undergone several paradigm shifts, many of them notably influenced by the reach of social media and connectivity world over. Myths, myth busters, influencers and influences, trends, and trend makers, all worked together to enhance the acceptability of sunscreens as a personal care product, admittedly more effectively than what dermatologists have been able to over the years. Benzene detection in sunscreens, systemic absorption of sunscreens, sunscreens in our immediate environment, recent approvals of sunscreen filters and bans as well, all are now matters in the public domain. And when these questions find their way into the dermatologist's consultation, distorted en route by some level of media led misinformation, I hope this book is able to equip the physician with the correct answers.

I have tried my best to include the most relevant clinical information with practical impact for clinical decision-making across different subsets of patients. The output is also tempered by my experience in formulating sunscreens as a certified cosmetic chemist, where revolutionary formulation concepts are ushering in higher levels of safety and durability in sunscreen products than ever before. The field of sunscreen science is fast evolving, and it is hoped that the outcome of this book would be to empower the reader to learn the art of learning about sunscreens.

This book is written for postgraduate students of dermatology and for undergraduate students with an interest in dermatology. It is also meant for practising dermatologists who are looking to upgrade practical knowledge on this key personal care product. The awareness of sunscreen use, atleast in India, has been taken forward as much by dermatologists as has been by skin care influencers and beauty gurus. To that understanding, this book has been specifically worked on for enhanced readability, even for those without a formal medical background.

The flow of the content has been planned as a narrative, starting from an understanding of melanin and its protective behaviour in skin of colour. We then move on to understanding the impact of light, across all of the solar domains, with particular emphasis on skin of colour and stop to briefly explore the role of sunscreens in preventing skin cancer. The story continues on to the types and kinds of sunscreens, old and new, and concludes with understanding the clinical considerations around sunscreens, chapters of interest for practising clinicians, presented in crisp vignettes. Keeping in mind that this book will be used by postgraduates, brief reviews of the various filters, recent advances, and capsule summaries for quick reading and even quicker revisions are included.

My purpose in writing this book would be fulfilled if the insights shared here are used practically in every day clinical consultations. Melanin and its primary ramification in terms of hyperpigmentation is a force to be reckoned with in clinical practice, and sunscreens may well be the most clinically relevant and widely used self-care product in SOC.

Hope that this book is enjoyed as it is read.

A reader first and then an author.

Chennai, Tamil Nadu, India Renita Rajan

Acknowledgements

Sunscreens have always fascinated me over the years, and writing a book about them, specifically for our skin types, has been a joyous exercise.

As with all worthy endeavours, the outcome of this book is owed to the support and contributions of some very kind people, acknowledged below.

Dr. C. R. Srinivas is a pioneer and an inspiration to anyone working in the field of sunscreen sciences in India, and I am grateful for his foreword that graces this book.

I consider myself lucky to have been a student of Dr. Laxmisha Chandrasekhar, and I am delighted that he has graciously agreed to contribute to the foreword of this book. I extend my gratitude to Dr. Renu George and Dr. Susanne Abraham, my teachers, for the learnings that have guided me far beyond my residency.

It was a pleasure working with Raman and Dr. Naren of Springer Nature, who turned a casual conversation into this project and guided it to completion through Neeraja and her team.

I am especially thankful to Dr. Anuba for her assistance during the final editing process and to Faizal and Inba for their support with the images.

Saravanan, Divya Shah, and Vibha Parekh of Abbott Healthcare are owed much gratitude for their support in providing reference articles, which was an immense help in completing the manuscript.

I am deeply indebted to Kavi and my team of consultants at RENDER Clinic: Dr. Subashini, Dr. Divya, Dr. Ragavi, and Dr. Vanathi, whose support and coordination have been instrumental for completing this project.

The R&D department at Silphion Research and Dr. Pavithra have played a crucial role in my understanding of sunscreen science, formulation chemistry, and cutaneous photobiology, and I am deeply grateful for the journey and the opportunity to explore sunscreen agents up close. A special note of thanks goes to Tamil Priya and Killivalavan for their work on the sunscreen science project.

All of my clinical knowledge, expertise, and experience in this domain have been driven by the encouragement and feedback from my beloved clientele over the years. For this, I am forever grateful.

Above all, I am grateful to my family for their sacrifices in allowing me the space and time to pursue my goals, including this book.

I hope that readers will find our collective efforts in the form of this book useful and enriching to their practice.

Contents

Chapter 1
Melanin: The Original Sunscreen

Abbreviations

ACTH	Adrenocorticotropic hormone
CAGR	Compounded annual growth rate
CPD	Cyclobutane pyrimidine dimers
DHI	5,6-dihydroxyindole
EDN3	Endothelin 3
EVs	Extracellular vesicles
MART-1	Melanoma-associated antigen recognized by T cells
MC1R	Melanocortin 1 receptor
MITF	Microphthalmia-associated transcription factor
MSH	Melanocyte-stimulating hormone
POMC	Proopiomelanocortin
PPD	Persistent pigment darkening
SOC	Skin of colour
TRP	Tyrosinase-related protein
UVR	Ultraviolet radiation

Key Objectives

- Melanin in the skin can be considered to be the original sunscreen, having been developed in humans as a multistep evolutionary response, over a million years ago. These events seem to have been modulated by evolutionary pressure from mechanisms related to the synthesis of vitamin D and to conserving folate, resulting in human races with varying levels and distribution of two specific types of melanin.
- Eumelanin and pheomelanin behave remarkably differently, with the former acting as a cytoprotector and the latter, a pro-oxidant.
- The density of melanocytes is the same across all ethnicities. However, the melanocyte distribution over the body areas differs, but still remains consistent across ethnicities.

R. Rajan, *Sunscreens for Skin of Color*,
https://doi.org/10.1007/978-981-97-3195-4_1

Across the world, topical protection with sunscreens has come to be established as one of the principal means of protecting the skin against the short- and long-term consequences of solar radiation. Sunscreens are one of the most commonly used personal care products today, world over. The sun protection market is estimated at $11.52 billion in 2024, with an anticipated compounded annual growth rate (CAGR) of 4.14% for the next 5 years, reaching an estimate of $24.4 billion in 2029 [1, 2]. It is interesting to know that this demand is significantly driven by geographical regions with skin of colour, typically Africa [3], Latin America (LATAM) [4], and Asia Pacific (APAC) [5] with respective compounded annual growth rates (CAGRs) for this period, pegged at 7.96%, 7.82%, and 6.01%, compared to 2.21% and 2.12%, for Europe [6] and North America [7], respectively.

The post-pandemic increase in personal care use, witnessed a sharp rise in the sun care market, with a specifically steeper gradient of increase for sun protection related products, 7.10% [8] and 6.01%, compared to overall skin care at 2.60% [9] and 3.41% [10], particularly in the Indian and Asia Pacific segments, respectively. The growth is potentially a result of an increase in awareness in the last decade powered by social media, though the overall sunscreen market penetration is significantly low compared to face and body products in skin of colour (SOC) markets [10–12].

UV and sunlight affect skin of colour in ways that are unique and different from those in lighter skin types. Specifically, there is a disproportionate impact in terms of pigmentation, while for photocarcinogenesis in darker skin types, melanin provides immense protection [13]. The rising usage of sunscreens reflects the increased awareness of solar pigmentation and the benefits of sun protection on cutaneous ageing in SOC.

To understand the potential utility of sunscreens in SOC, we must begin by getting to know a pigment that has divided the world into races, groups, started wars, caused massive human division, and now, through the intermixing of ethnicities, is unifying the world again—melanin. Loosely speaking, sunscreens can be considered to provide a surrogate support to the central role that melanin plays, in protecting the skin from the sun's light.

1.1 Melanin in Human Evolution

The discussion on SOC needs a strong understanding of the concepts of race and ethnicity. While the term ethnic encompasses concepts of culture and/or language, race denotes genetic similarities among a group of individuals. Both race and ethnicity, along with geography and other exposomal factors such as nutrition and facultative pigmentation, influence the course of this discussion.

The human races today are differentiated by a very distinct feature—skin pigmentation [14]. Pigmentary evolution itself, however, was preceded by several other remarkable changes in the integument. The human skin as we know it today is considered functionally naked, with very limited areas of hair distribution compared to other primates. This loss of hair may have been necessitated by natural selection when the species found itself with the need for better heat dissipation due to increased physical activity, in hot environments roughly around 1.2–2 million years ago [15, 16].

Around this time, the sweat gland system evolved to facilitate heat loss by evaporation, and the epidermal skin barrier function was enhanced by the evolution of keratinization and surface differentiation genes. The loss of fur, and therefore of some level of sun protection, necessitated the acquisition of another form of photoprotection, namely, skin pigmentation.

Research suggests that the initial complexion of the early man was light brown, as he/she/they lived in the sheltered forests of South Africa. In due course of migration, the races that moved out into the open plains of equatorial Africa with higher levels of ultraviolet radiation (UVR), evolved to have larger melanosomes with a higher melanin concentration in those organelles, reflected in the black skin colour. Those races which migrated to northern Africa, Europe, and Asia with lesser UVR, evolved to develop melanocytes with smaller melanosomes and less melanin content [17]. McEvoy et al. created a speculative tree model suggesting a list of genetic changes that may have accompanied specific skin lightening or skin darkening changes in different races, Fig. 1.1.

The events of skin lightening may have been necessary to utilize the decreasing quantities of UVR more effectively for synthesis of vitamin D, a secosteroid neurohormone central to a number of vital physiological processes, as the races migrated to higher latitudes. The need for a balance between UVR stimulated vitamin D synthesis and the prevention of photolysis of folate with implications for physiology and fertility, seems to have significantly influenced cutaneous pigmentation over years of human migration [18].

Specifically for melanin, the adaptive evolution of the MC1R locus with resultant persistence of dense, constitutional skin pigmentation, marked the ability of the earliest modern humans, *Homo sapiens,* to live and reproduce successfully, in equatorial regions receiving the highest amounts of sunlight. It is supposed that the photolability of folate may have exerted significant evolutionary pressure on skin pigmentation. Folate is essential for fertility and thermoregulation—key functions for an evolving race and the ability of melanin to protect against UVR-induced folate degradation may have conferred an advantage for higher constitutional pigmentation [19].

Similarly, for races migrating out of Africa for better food and survival prospects, the inability to synthesize adequate levels of vitamin D in the skin may have induced, over multiple levels of mutations, a reduction in constitutive skin pigmentation, contributing to racial differences seen in current times [15]. Vitamin D is a key hormone for regulation of bone health and reproductive fitness and is considered highly important for species propagation. However, this is hotly debated by Hanel et al., who suggest that there was just a single skin lightening mutation in Caucasian ancestry and point the origin to a single carrier in the Middle East, who lived as recently as 22,000–28,000 years ago [16]. Still, most of the currently available evidence points to progressive genetic changes in geographically divergent

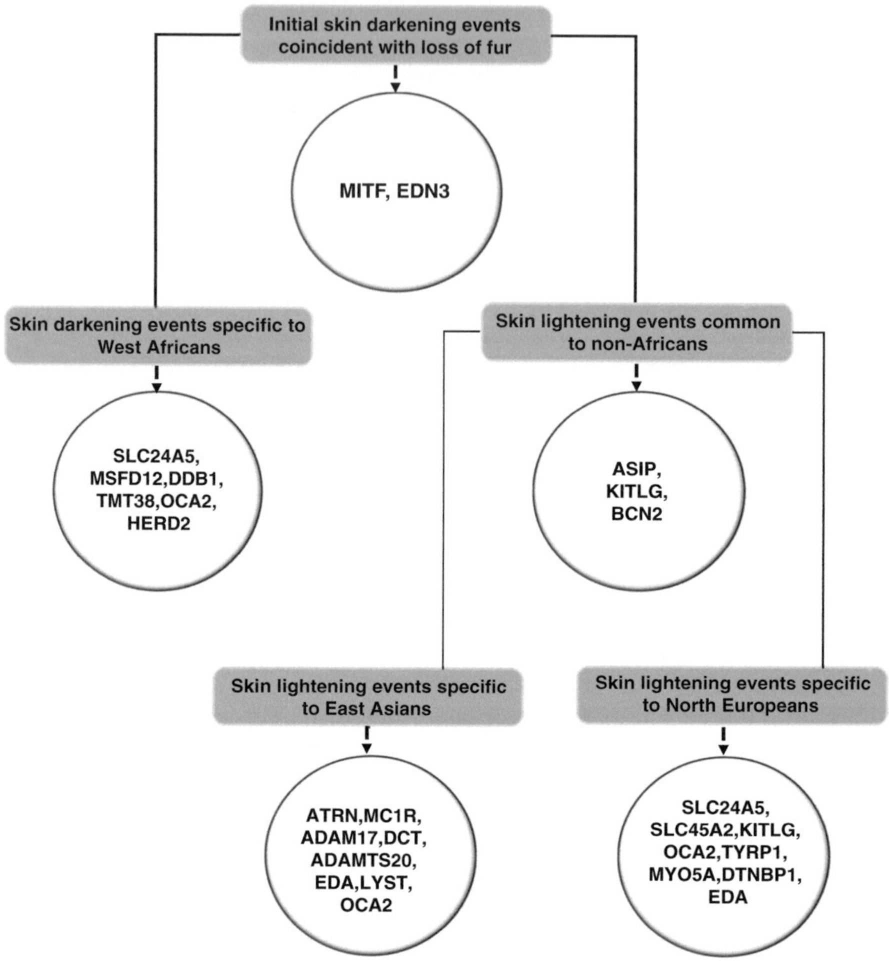

Fig. 1.1 Image of skin lightening and skin darkening events in humans, adapted from a speculative evolutionary tree model for human skin pigmentation in three populations. (By Del Bino et al. [20], an open access article distributed under the terms and conditions of the Creative Commons Attribution (CC BY) licence (http://creativecommons.org/licenses/by/4.0/). [20])

sub-populations, potentially both predating and following population divergence [18]. The East Asian and Northern European cohorts are considered to have evolved as a single group from a common African ancestor, following mutations in the MITF and EDN3, and then proceeded to undergo subsequent respective mutations for each. Continuation of the original pigment genetic makeup, as the West Africa phenotype, also witnessed genetic events specific to this group [18, 20].

While we do know at present that skin pigmentation tends to be darker in equatorial and tropical regions which receive the maximum UVR, it is not uncommon to see significant intra racial variations in the colour of the skin, hair, and the iris [20].

Today, five races are identified broadly [14]:

Caucasoid: Europeans, Middle Eastern people and Indians
Negroid: African Negroes, African Americans, and African Carribeans
Mongoloid: East Asiatics, Indonesians, Polynesians, Micronesians, Amerindians, Eskimos
Australoid: Aborigines, Melanesians, Papuans, Tribal people of India, Negritos
Capoid: Kung San African tribals

However, multiple sub-races exist, with differences within these subgroups, and today, the concept of ethnicity is used almost interchangeably with that of race. Jayasinghe et al. put forward a global map of the ethnicities at the end of the twentieth century from multiple data sources, Fig. 1.2 [21].

Darker races differ significantly in their ability to protect against and recover from sun damage as compared to lighter skin types, creating striking differences in critical outcomes such as photoaging, photocarcinogenesis, and skin hyperpigmentation. The key player that drives this distinction is a highly intriguing pigment called melanin. Melanin, and to a lesser extent haemoglobin, bilirubin, and carotenoids regulate skin colour [17, 22, 23]. In addition, facultative features such as skin thickness, tanning, and photoaging are also known to modulate the skin colour [23]. Human constitutive skin pigmentation is regulated by a number of melanocyte related and extrinsic genes, modified by the evolutionary process as adaptations to

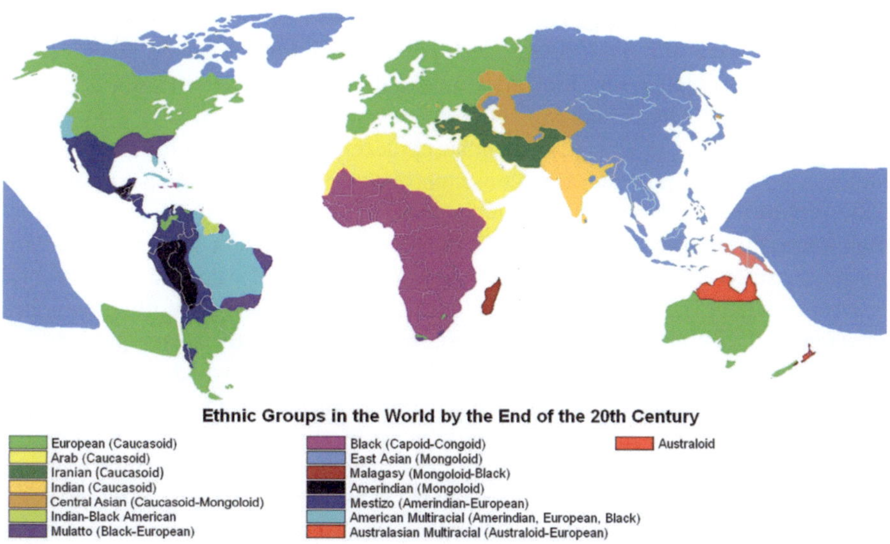

Fig. 1.2 Global distribution of ethnic groups in the world, by the end of the twentieth century, according to CIA world factbook, US census, Francisco Lizcano UNAM works, craniofacial anthropometry works, in the twentieth century, and other data sources. (Obtained with permission from Jayasinghe and Jayasinghe [21])

UVR in different environmental conditions and geographic locations, as discussed above. The number of melanocytes in the basal layer and the metabolic activity of these cells, the stage and activity of melanosomes within melanocytes, and the type and overall distribution of the melanosomes at various levels within the epidermis all play a role in determining the final perceived skin colour [24].

1.2 Melanin Synthesis and Function

Melanin is produced within lysosome family organelles called melanosomes, in specialized, neural crest derived cells called melanocytes located in the basal layer of the epidermis. These melanocytes are present among keratinocytes in the human skin in a ratio of around 1:30–1:40, together forming the epidermal melanin unit [20, 25]. In the basal layer, the ratio of keratinocytes to melanocytes is 10:1. The significant presence of melanocytes acts as a formidable solar barrier, with epidermal melanin protecting the epidermis and the dermis by absorbing UVR [26].

Melanocytes are located in the region of the dermo epidermal junction and transfer melanin to the keratinocytes through long dendrites. Inherently resistant to apoptosis, melanocytes survive longer than the keratinocytes that surround them and are known to proliferate mainly in response to injury. Despite their limited ability to proliferate, the longevity of these cells makes them prone to accumulate cellular damage and mutations over time, in response to repeated UV exposure [26].

Melanin exists in one of two forms, black/brown coloured eumelanin and the cysteine derivative, the reddish/yellowish pheomelanin, both derived from a common precursor, tyrosine, Fig. 1.3 [16]. Eumelanin is the main determinant of constitutive skin colour, across races and ethnicities, and correlates directly with overall melanin content in the skin [27]. Human epidermis contains approximately 74% eumelanin and 26% pheomelanin, consistently across skin types in unexposed skin [28]. At photo exposed sites, there is an increase of insoluble DHI—eumelanin [14]. Both derivatives from dopachrome, DHICA is said to have a higher antioxidant profile, the structures of DHI and DHICA are shown in Figs. 1.4 and 1.5, respectively.

Also called dark melanin [29], eumelanin is a more effective UV filter than pheomelanin and its concentration in the epidermis is considered a strong predictor of protection from skin cancer. In darker skin types, eumelanin, which is more photostable, is seen to be richly present within melanosomes in all the layers of the epidermis, and especially in the stratum corneum. In contrast, in lighter skin types, melanosomes with lower eumelanin content undergo degradation, and 'melanin dust', a breakdown product of the more photo unstable pheomelanin, is found in the epidermis, predominantly in the basal and suprabasal locations. Overall, dark skin contains more melanin than light skin by a factor of 4–6 [30].

Cysteine, which imparts the reddish-yellow colour to pheomelanin, contains sulfhydryl bonds which are prone to oxidation, and this contributes to the lower photo stability of pheomelanin compared to eumelanin and probably drives the pro-oxidant behaviour of pheomelanin [19]. Applied research tools are now able to

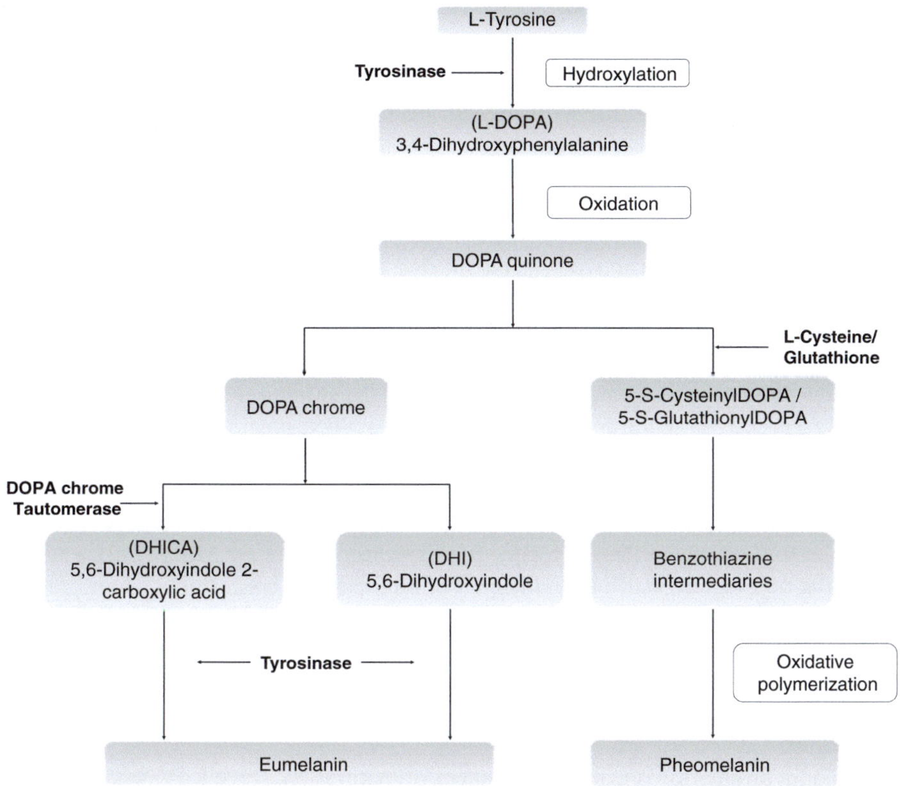

Fig. 1.3 The biochemical pathway of melanin synthesis [27, 30, 53]

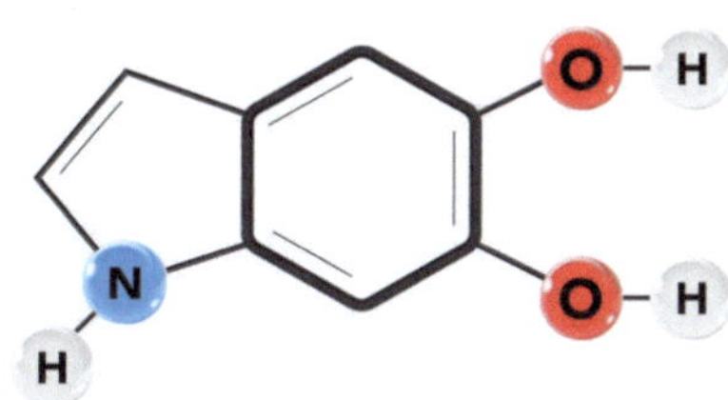

Fig. 1.4 Structure of 5,6-dihydroxyindole (DHI)

quantify the levels of eumelanin and pheomelanin in skin, using inverse skin reflectance pigmentation analysis, and early results indicate that this approach could be used to quantify response to pigmentation and skin whitening treatments [31, 32]. It would also imply that such measurements could highlight either a lack of eumelanin or a predominant presence of pheomelanin, to understand potential for skin cancer risk. However, across all skin types, pheomelanin contributes to a very small proportion of epidermal melanin [33].

Where eumelanin functions as a free radical scavenger and is therefore considered photoprotective, pheomelanin may act as an endogenous photosensitizer

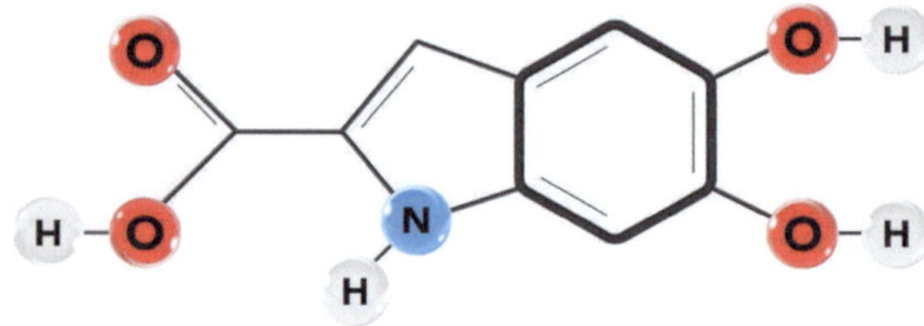

Fig. 1.5 Structure of 5,6-dihydroxyindole-2-carboxylic acid (DHICA) [54]

capable of generating reactive oxygen species and is hence considered phototoxic [22, 34]. This pro-oxidant behaviour of pheomelanin can be attributed to a depletion of glutathione, the predominant cellular antioxidant in the process of pheomelanin production, a reduction in antioxidant enzymes like catalases with increasing pheomelanin content in the skin, and the presence of the sulphur moiety in pheomelanin creating a proclivity to the generation of reactive oxygen species [19]. In the absence of eumelanin, such as in cells expressing the melanoma activating $BRAF^{v600E}$ mutation, the pro-oxidant effect of pheomelanin results in the spontaneous generation of melanomas, even in the absence of exposure to UVR or external carcinogenic stimuli, at least in animal studies [35, 36]. In this seminal work by Mitra et al., a status of having no melanin at all, as in the case of albino mice, conferred a better protection against melanoma risk, as compared to having pheomelanin, due to the inherent ability of the latter to generate oxidative stress [36]. Considering that eumelanin is protective and behaves as a free radical quencher and pheomelanin has pro-oxidant properties, the presence of pheomelanin can be said to be worse than even a lack of eumelanin.

Melanin production occurs in four stages of maturation, stage I–IV, with progressively increasing melanization with each step. The isolated synthesis of melanin within the melanosomes shields the rest of the cell from the toxic effects of the quinoid pigment intermediaries, Fig. 1.6.

Stage I melanosomes are spheroid to round organelles within which a matrix derived from the endoplasmic reticulum begins to assemble. These melanosomes are located around the nucleus of the melanocyte.

Stage II melanosomes are ovoid in shape, where, by now the internal matrix is knit into longitudinally arranged fibres, to receive the melanin in stage III.

Stage III melanosomes are characterized by maximum tyrosinase activity, and the early deposition of melanin on the matrix striations.

Stage IV melanosomes are fully packed with melanin on the matrix and are therefore opaque and show no demonstrable tyrosinase activity [37].

These melanin granules then go on to form perinuclear and supranuclear caps to shield the genomic DNA in the nucleus of the keratinocyte from solar radiation [19, 38]. Supranuclear cap formation seems to be mediated by the important photoreceptor Opsin 3 in the skin. Opsin 3 acts through calcium dependent G protein-coupled receptor signalling pathways, to upregulate specific cellular dynein and dynactin proteins, to eventually cause polarization of melanin to a supranuclear location on stimulation by light [39, 40]. Opsin 3 is known to be specifically stimulated by UVA, to form these supranuclear caps, evocatively called as microparasols,

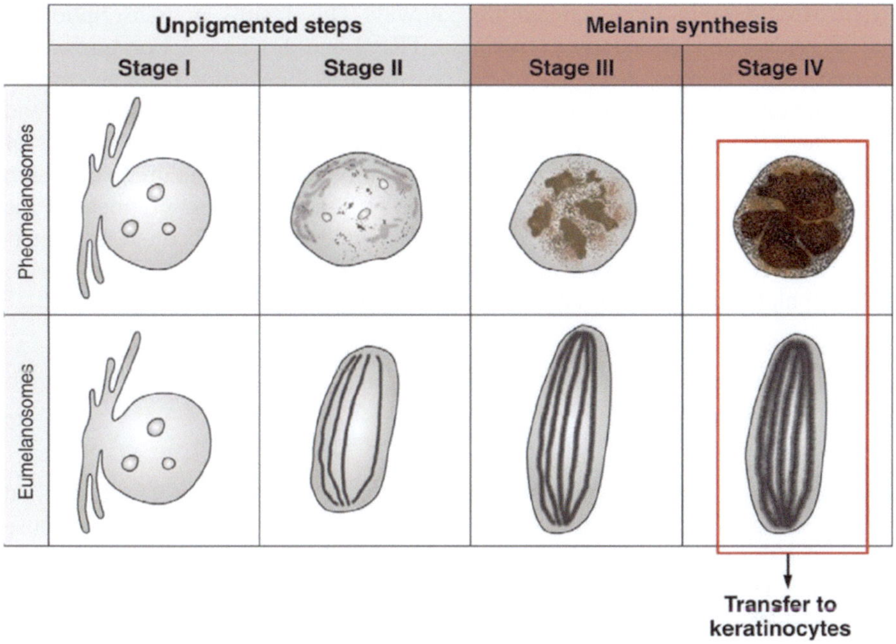

Fig. 1.6 Stages in the development of pheo- and eumelanosomes (Obtained with permission from D'Alba and Shawkey [37]). Between stages I and II, pre-melanosomal protein (PMEL) fibrils form a well-defined scaffolding of protein sheets. In stages III and IV, melanin synthesis takes place. In pheomelanosomes, PMEL is downregulated; thus, there is no protein scaffolding. Mature melanosomes in epidermis are then transferred to keratinocytes [37]

mini-umbrellas, by researchers [39], however, melanin polarization may also be seen without UVR stimulation [40]. In 1957, Staricco and Pinkus first described melanin in its supranuclear location in the basal cells as akin to an octopus surrounding an object with its tentacles [41]. These keratinocyte umbrellas are said to protect against the generation of cyclobutane pyrimidine dimers (CPDs) and 6–4 photoproducts [40]. Considering the absorption spectrum of human melanin across the solar spectrum, these supranuclear caps play an important role in protecting the nucleus [42].

Skin pigmentation is regulated by the highly polymorphic MC1R gene, with its multiple alleles resulting in the huge variation of human skin colour, as we see every day [19]. Though close to 17 genes are likely involved in a complex polygenic interaction, the prominent role of MC1R in skin pigmentation is well established [20, 30]. The distribution of melanocytes is identified by melanosomal protein markers such as the well characterized enzyme tyrosinase, tyrosinase-related protein 1 (TYRP1), dopachrome tautomerase, Glycoprotein gp100, Melan A protein or MART-1 and microphthalmia-associated transcription factor (MITF). MITF orchestrates the final expression of melanin in the cell. On stimulation, three agonist hormones, α-Melanocyte-stimulating hormone (MSH), Adrenocorticotropic hormone (ACTH), and Proopiomelanocortin (POMC), activate the MC1R gene, through the cyclic AMP-protein kinase signalling pathway. This results in transcription of MITF, leading to expression of tyrosinase, TRP 1 and 2, which act on tyrosine to convert it into melanin. While the role of tyrosinase as the starting point and principal driver of melanin production is well established, less is known about TRP 1 and 2. So far, TRP 1 is considered to shift the ratio towards eumelanin [43]. Loss of function of the MC1R gene due to somatic mutations leads to impaired eumelanin production and a predisposition to melanoma [19]. The microenvironment of the melanosome, in particular, the pH, plays a role in modulating skin colour. In lighter-skinned individuals, the pH is acidic with lower tyrosinase activity, and in darker skin, the higher, neutral pH is associated with increased tyrosinase activity [20].

1.3 Melanin Transfer

Both keratinocytes and melanocytes are actively involved in the transfer of formed melanin. Stage IV mature melanosomes are transferred to keratinocytes in response to cellular signals from the keratinocytes, by actin dependent, bidirectional transport through microtubules, Fig. 1.7 [44]. More recently, other mechanisms have also been considered, including the heterophagocytosis of melanocyte dendrites by keratinocytes, release of melanosome loaded vesicles by melanocytes in the extracellular space, keratinocyte endocytosis of the melanin core released by melanocytes in the extracellular space, direct fusion with keratinocyte membrane and transfer using specialized nanotubes or filopodia [44]. Waster et al. demonstrated that a significant proportion of UVR-induced transfer of melanin to keratinocytes occurs through melanin containing extracellular vesicles (EVs) derived from melanocytes. On UV exposure, melanocytes shed melanosomes, as extracellular vesicles. The shedding response is mediated more by UVA as compared to UVB, and occurs within minutes of exposure, with the release of small EVs called ectosomes. Larger sized enlargeosomes are also secreted, in time. Distribution of these melanosome packages into the extracellular space appears to be a response to increase overall melanin density in the epidermis, with melanocytes able to generate extracellular vesicles 100 times more than keratinocytes. This could explain the persistence of pigmentation in persistent pigment darkening (PPD), where the overall content of melanin in keratinocytes is increased, though neomelanogenesis also occurs [30].

Once within the keratinocyte, the melanosomes undergo differential processing and distribution in light- and dark-skinned individuals. The melanosomes are present predominantly in keratinocytes in the basal layer of fair-skinned individuals, in comparison to basal and suprabasal location of melanosomes in keratinocytes in dark epidermis. Apart from the distribution, there is also a difference in melanosome turnover. Persistence of melanin or reduction in melanin content within keratinocytes is regulated by autophagy within the cell, with higher levels of lysosomal activity seen in lighter-skinned epidermal keratinocytes, compared to dark skin derived keratinocytes, with resultant decrease in melanin content in the former. On

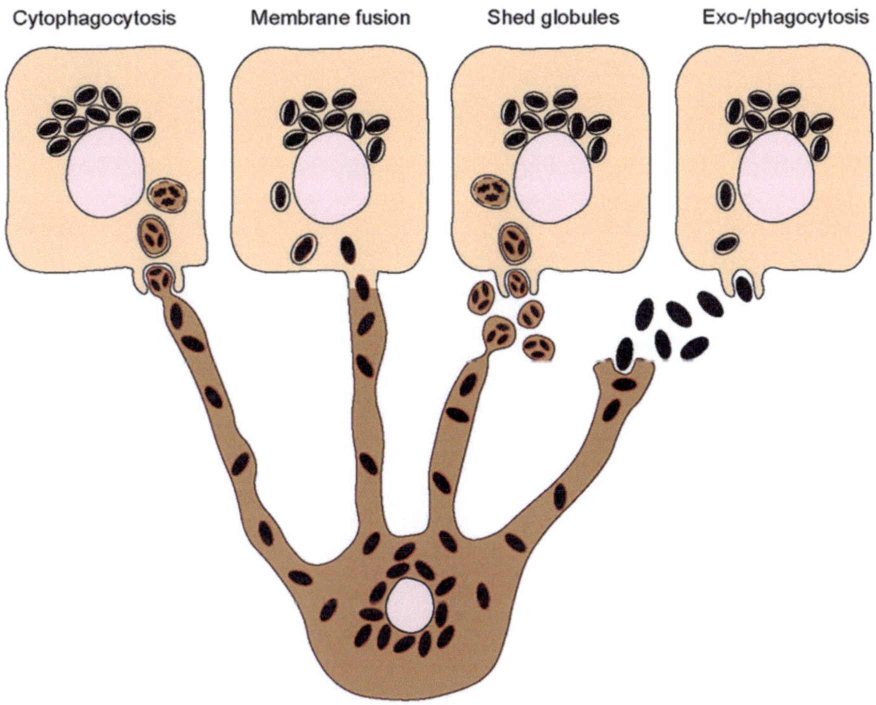

Fig. 1.7 The mechanisms of melanosome transfer from melanocytes to keratinocytes (Obtained from Bento-Lopes et al. [40], an open access article distributed under the terms and conditions of the Creative Commons Attribution (CC BY) license (https://creativecommons.org/licenses/by/4.0/)). Melanin transfer from melanocytes to keratinocytes. Four different models have been proposed to explain the mechanism(s) of melanin transfer from melanocytes (dark-coloured) to keratinocytes (light-coloured), including the cytophagocytosis of melanocyte dendrites by keratinocytes; the direct fusion of melanocyte and keratinocyte membranes; the shedding of melanosome-laden globules by melanocytes; and the coupled exocytosis/phagocytosis of the melanin core. Despite the evidence published using different models, recent studies using human and mouse cell lines, as well as more complex models such as reconstructed human skins/epidermis and skin biopsies, have supported the transfer of melanin in globules or as melanocores [40]

the other hand, persistence of melanin due to reduced autophagy results in the formation of pigmented lesions, such as solar lentigos.

1.4 Melanocyte Distribution in Human Skin

In 1954 [45], Szabo calculated the average number of melanocytes in the human epidermis to be about 1000/sq.mm, with regional variations, going up to 2000/sq.mm in potentially sun exposed areas such as the forearm skin or head [46]. At 400, the lowest number of melanocytes was noted in the abdomen, and the highest

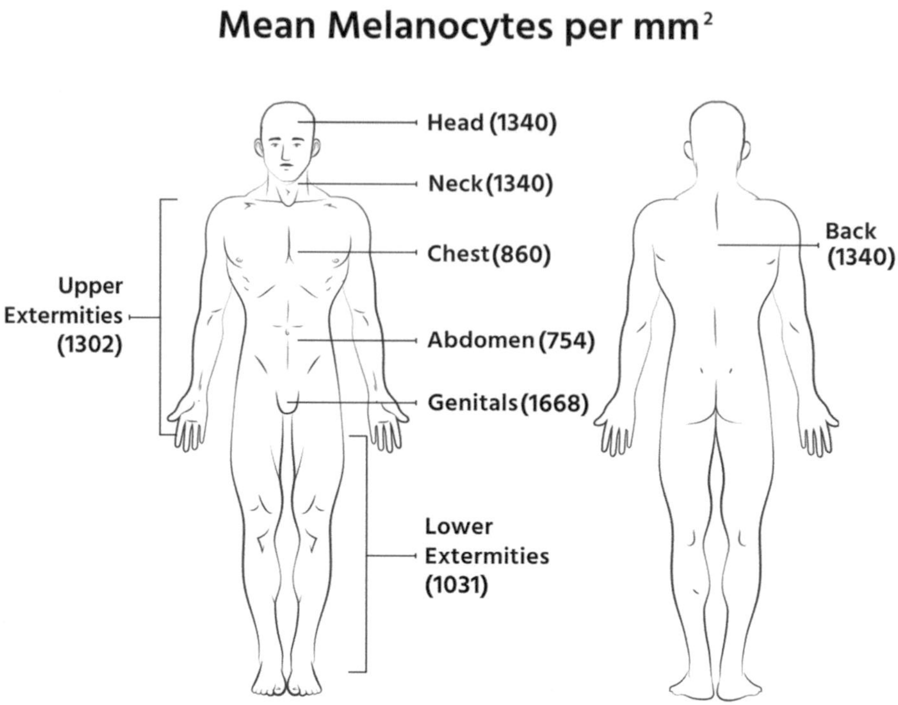

Fig. 1.8 The distribution of melanocytes across various anatomical sites, cell count per sq.mm, based on the work done by Starrico et al. [41]

in the genital regions at 2784/sq.mm. Staricco and Pinkus, who characterized the number of melanocytes in coloured and white skin, confirmed that melanocyte density was similar by race, varying by anatomic site. The melanocyte cell count per sq.mm, based on the work of these authors is depicted in Fig. 1.8 [41]. In certain anatomical locations like the palms, the melanocyte density is about only 10–20% that of other areas in the body.

Since then, more researchers have confirmed that this number of melanocytes remains the same or similar, across races, in corresponding anatomical sites [30, 47, 48]. It is the difference in the amount and type of melanin produced by these melanocytes, and the distribution of such melanin in the epidermis that determines the differences in constitutional pigmentation visually perceived as a variety of skin hues across different races, and histopathologically evident on Masson Fontana staining [49]. The average melanin content and the ratio between the two types of melanin across ethnicities have been documented by Visscher et al., Fig. 1.9 [50].

Two morphologies of melanocytes were identified by Starrico and Pinkus. In areas like the abdomen, the melanocyte was found to have two main dendrites from which other smaller branches took off. In areas with high melanocyte density, such as the face, the cells appeared stellate. The dendrites arising from these melanocytes are depicted as surrounding the basal cell layers as if in a network outlining the cell.

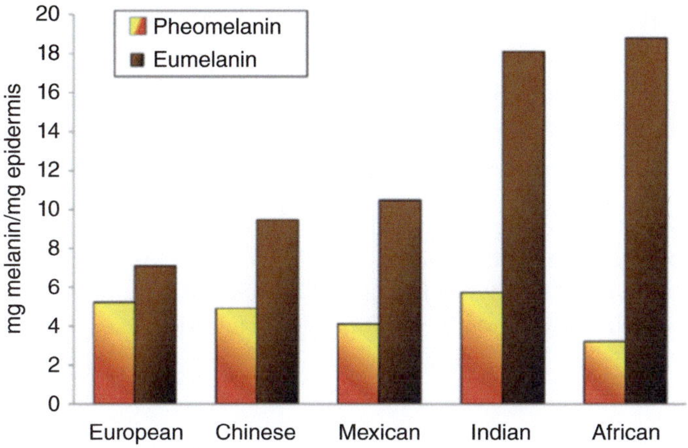

Fig. 1.9 Average melanin content of individuals in various geographical locations, melanin levels for European, Chinese, Mexican, Indian, and African people. Lightness (sun protected) was highest for Europeans and lowest for Africans. Indian skin was significantly darker than European, Chinese, and Mexican skin. L* was significantly and inversely correlated with levels of eumelanin and total melanin overall and for all groups (correlation coefficients, 0.77–0.89 for both total melanin and eumelanin). Although significant, L* was inversely correlated with pheomelanin levels with lower correlations (0.23 overall ranging from 0.53 to 0.83). (Obtained with permission from Visscher [50])

A higher number of larger dendrites was noted in SOC specimens. The authors also found that the presence of melanocytes was uniform along the basal layer, and the increased perception of melanocytes near the dermal ridges as compared to the valleys was more an optical phenomenon than a physical crowding of melanocytes in the rete ridges [41]. Furthermore, early work by Miller-Millingza and Staricco found that melanocyte numbers decreased in response to UV radiation, along with an increase in melanocyte size [51]. This has since been confirmed by more recent and more sophisticated research. Comparing responses to UVB irradiation between cultured melanocytes from light-skinned and dark-skinned individuals, Lopez et al. found that dark melanocytes exhibited more differentiation and less proliferation, characterized by an increase in cell size, dendricity, and increased expression of melanogenic genes. In contrast, melanocytes from light-skinned individuals showed the converse—more proliferation and less differentiation, with an overall decrease in melanogenesis. This differential behaviour on UVB exposure is considered to be one of the key protective mechanisms whereby SOC tolerates sun exposure better, without a significant risk for carcinogenesis [52].

In the coming chapter, we will explore the interaction between solar light and the skin in general, with at least the majority of these interactions modulated by melanin in the skin.

1.5 Chapter Summary

Melanin is a key determinant of the photoprotective mechanisms, operant in skin of colour. Originating as an evolutionary need, the ratio of the two main melanins in the human skin, and their distribution in the epidermis, and the differential response to sun exposure, all underlie the importance of this pigment in determining the susceptibility to, or protection from, photo-induced outcomes such as photocarcinogenesis, photoaging, and photopigmentation. The melanocyte concentration in SOC is the same as in other skin types for a given anatomical area, but the melanin content differs significantly driven by the functioning melanocyte.

References

1. Sun Protection - Worldwide | Statista Market Forecast [Internet]. [cited 2024 Mar 2]. Available from: https://www.statista.com/outlook/cmo/beauty-personal-care/skin-care/sun-protection/worldwide
2. Ginzburg AL, Blackburn RS, Santillan C, Truong L, Tanguay RL, Hutchison JE. Zinc oxide-induced changes to sunscreen ingredient efficacy and toxicity under UV irradiation. Photochem Photobiol Sci [Internet]. 2021 Oct 1 [cited 2024 Mar 11];20(10):1273–85. Available from: https://pubmed.ncbi.nlm.nih.gov/34647278/
3. Sun Protection - Africa | Statista Market Forecast [Internet]. [cited 2024 Mar 2]. Available from: https://www.statista.com/outlook/cmo/beauty-personal-care/skin-care/sun-protection/africa
4. Sun Protection - LATAM | Statista Market Forecast [Internet]. [cited 2024 Mar 2]. Available from: https://www.statista.com/outlook/cmo/beauty-personal-care/skin-care/sun-protection/latam
5. Sun Protection - APAC | Statista Market Forecast [Internet]. [cited 2024 Mar 2]. Available from: https://www.statista.com/outlook/cmo/beauty-personal-care/skin-care/sun-protection/apac
6. Sun Protection - Europe | Statista Market Forecast [Internet]. [cited 2024 Mar 2]. Available from: https://www.statista.com/outlook/cmo/beauty-personal-care/skin-care/sun-protection/europe
7. Sun Protection - North America | Statista Market Forecast [Internet]. [cited 2024 Mar 2]. Available from: https://www.statista.com/outlook/cmo/beauty-personal-care/skin-care/sun-protection/north-america
8. Sun Protection - India | Statista Market Forecast [Internet]. [cited 2024 Mar 2]. Available from: https://www.statista.com/outlook/cmo/beauty-personal-care/skin-care/sun-protection/india
9. Skin Care - India | Statista Market Forecast [Internet]. [cited 2024 Mar 2]. Available from: https://www.statista.com/outlook/cmo/beauty-personal-care/skin-care/india
10. Skin Care - APAC | Statista Market Forecast [Internet]. [cited 2024 Mar 2]. Available from: https://www.statista.com/outlook/cmo/beauty-personal-care/skin-care/apac
11. Skin Care - LATAM | Statista Market Forecast [Internet]. [cited 2024 Mar 2]. Available from: https://www.statista.com/outlook/cmo/beauty-personal-care/skin-care/latam
12. Skin Care - Africa | Statista Market Forecast [Internet]. [cited 2024 Mar 2]. Available from: https://www.statista.com/outlook/cmo/beauty-personal-care/skin-care/africa
13. Cole Y, Ilyas AM, Ilyas EN. Availability of adequate photoprotection for skin of color. Cureus. 2023;15(8):e42794.
14. Rawlings AV. Ethnic skin types: are there differences in skin structure and function? Int J Cosmet Sci [Internet]. 2006 Apr [cited 2024 Mar 2];28(2):79–93. Available from: https://pubmed.ncbi.nlm.nih.gov/18492142/

15. Jablonski NG, Chaplin G. The colours of humanity: the evolution of pigmentation in the human lineage. Philos Trans R Soc B Biol Sci [Internet]. 2017 [cited 2024 Mar 2];372(1724). Available from: https://royalsocietypublishing.org/doi/10.1098/rstb.2016.0349
16. Hanel A, Carlberg C. Skin colour and vitamin D: an update. Exp Dermatol [Internet]. 2020 Sep 1 [cited 2024 Mar 2];29(9):864–75. Available from: https://pubmed.ncbi.nlm.nih.gov/32621306/
17. Menke HE. Pigment disorders and pigment manipulations. In: The melanin millennium: skin color as 21st century international discourse [Internet]. 2013 Aug 1 [cited 2024 Mar 2];183–205. Available from: https://link.springer.com/chapter/10.1007/978-94-007-4608-4_12
18. McEvoy B, Beleza S, Shriver MD. The genetic architecture of normal variation in human pigmentation: an evolutionary perspective and model. Hum Mol Genet [Internet]. 2006 Oct 15 [cited 2024 Mar 2];15 Spec No 2(SUPPL. 2). Available from: https://pubmed.ncbi.nlm.nih.gov/16987881/
19. Swope VB, Abdel-Malek ZA. MC1R: front and center in the bright side of dark eumelanin and DNA repair. Int J Mol Sci [Internet]. 2018 [cited 2024 Mar 11];19(9). Available from: https://pubmed.ncbi.nlm.nih.gov/30205559/
20. Del Bino S, Duval C, Bernerd F. Clinical and biological characterization of skin pigmentation diversity and its consequences on UV impact. Int J Mol Sci [Internet]. 2018 Sep 8 [cited 2024 Mar 2];19(9). Available from: https://www.ncbi.nlm.nih.gov/pmc/articles/PMC6163216/
21. Jayasinghe DY, Jayasinghe CL. An investigation into adult human height distributions using kernel density estimation. Sankhya B Indian J Stat [Internet]. 2022 May 1 [cited 2024 Mar 2];84(1):79–105. Available from: https://ideas.repec.org/a/spr/sankhb/v84y2022i1d10.1007_s13571-020-00243-w.html
22. Gupta V, Sharma VK. Skin typing: Fitzpatrick grading and others. Clin Dermatol [Internet]. 2019 Sep 1 [cited 2024 Mar 2];37(5):430–6. Available from: https://pubmed.ncbi.nlm.nih.gov/31896400/
23. Ly BCK, Dyer EB, Feig JL, Chien AL, Del Bino S. Research techniques made simple: cutaneous colorimetry: a reliable technique for objective skin color measurement. J Invest Dermatol [Internet]. 2020 Jan 1 [cited 2024 Mar 2];140(1):3–12.e1. Available from: https://www.researchgate.net/publication/338303610_Research_Techniques_Made_Simple_Cutaneous_Colorimetry_A_Reliable_Technique_for_Objective_Skin_Color_Measurement
24. Addor FAS anna, Barcaui CB, Gomes EE, Lupi O, Marçon CR, Miot HA. Sunscreen lotions in the dermatological prescription: review of concepts and controversies. An Bras Dermatol [Internet]. 2022 Mar 1 [cited 2024 Apr 2];97(2):204–22. Available from: https://pubmed.ncbi.nlm.nih.gov/35039207/
25. Piętowska Z, Nowicka D, Szepietowski JC. Understanding Melasma-how can pharmacology and cosmetology procedures and prevention help to achieve optimal treatment results? A narrative review. Int J Environ Res Public Health [Internet]. 2022 Oct 1 [cited 2024 Mar 2];19(19). Available from: https://pubmed.ncbi.nlm.nih.gov/36231404/
26. Lefèvre-Utile A, Braun C, Haftek M, Aubin F. Five functional aspects of the epidermal barrier. Int J Mol Sci [Internet]. 2021 Nov 1 [cited 2024 Mar 2];22(21):11676. Available from: /pmc/articles/PMC8583944/.
27. (PDF) Biochemical aspects of mammalian melanocytes and the emerging role of melanocyte stem cells in dermatological therapies [Internet]. [cited 2024 Mar 2]. Available from: https://www.researchgate.net/publication/322592409_Biochemical_aspects_of_mammalian_melanocytes_and_the_emerging_role_of_melanocyte_stem_cells_in_dermatological_therapies
28. Del Bino S, Ito S, Sok J, Nakanishi Y, Bastien P, Wakamatsu K, et al. Chemical analysis of constitutive pigmentation of human epidermis reveals constant eumelanin to pheomelanin ratio. Pigment Cell Melanoma Res [Internet]. 2015 Nov 1 [cited 2024 Mar 2];28(6):707–17. Available from: https://onlinelibrary.wiley.com/doi/full/10.1111/pcmr.12410
29. Kanellis VG. A review of melanin sensor devices. Biophys Rev [Internet]. 2019 Dec 1 [cited 2024 Mar 2];11(6):843–9. Available from: https://link.springer.com/article/10.1007/s12551-019-00581-8

30. Fajuyigbe D, Young AR. The impact of skin colour on human photobiological responses. Pigment Cell Melanoma Res [Internet]. 2016 Nov 1 [cited 2024 Mar 2];29(6):607–18. Available from: https://pubmed.ncbi.nlm.nih.gov/27454804/
31. Kongshoj B, Thorleifsson A, Wulf HC. Pheomelanin and eumelanin in human skin determined by high-performance liquid chromatography and its relation to in vivo reflectance measurements. Photodermatol Photoimmunol Photomed [Internet]. 2006 Jun [cited 2024 Mar 2];22(3):141–7. Available from: https://pubmed.ncbi.nlm.nih.gov/16719868/
32. Hani AFM, Baba R, Shamsuddin N, Nugroho H. Determination of melanin types and relative concentrations: an observational study using a non-invasive inverse skin reflectance analysis. Int J Cosmet Sci. 2014;36(5):451–8.
33. Alaluf S, Atkins D, Barrett K, Blount M, Carter N, Heath A. Ethnic variation in melanin content and composition in photoexposed and photoprotected human skin. Pigment Cell Res [Internet]. 2002 [cited 2024 Mar 8];15(2):112–8. Available from: https://pubmed.ncbi.nlm.nih.gov/11936268/
34. Ito S, Wakamatsu K, Sarna T. Photodegradation of eumelanin and pheomelanin and its pathophysiological implications. Photochem Photobiol [Internet]. 2018 May 1 [cited 2024 Mar 3];94(3):409–20. Available from: https://onlinelibrary.wiley.com/doi/full/10.1111/php.12837
35. Morgan AM, Lo J, Fisher DE. How does pheomelanin synthesis contribute to melanomagenesis?: Two distinct mechanisms could explain the carcinogenicity of pheomelanin synthesis. Bioessays [Internet]. 2013 Aug [cited 2024 Mar 2];35(8):672–6. Available from: https://pubmed.ncbi.nlm.nih.gov/23650156/
36. Mitra D, Luo X, Morgan A, Wang J, Hoang MP, Lo J, et al. An ultraviolet-radiation-independent pathway to melanoma carcinogenesis in the red hair/fair skin background. Nature 2012 491:7424 [Internet]. 2012 Oct 31 [cited 2024 Mar 2];491(7424):449–53. Available from: https://www.nature.com/articles/nature11624
37. D'Alba L, Shawkey MD. Melanosomes: biogenesis, properties, and evolution of an ancient organelle. Physiol Rev [Internet]. 2019 Jan 1 [cited 2024 Mar 8];99(1):1–19. Available from: https://journals.physiology.org/doi/10.1152/physrev.00059.2017
38. Solano F. Photoprotection and skin pigmentation: melanin-related molecules and some other new agents obtained from natural sources. Molecules [Internet]. 2020 [cited 2024 Mar 2];25(7). Available from: https://pubmed.ncbi.nlm.nih.gov/32230973/
39. Lan Y, Zeng W, Wang Y, Dong X, Shen X, Gu Y, et al. Opsin 3 mediates UVA-induced keratinocyte supranuclear melanin cap formation. Commun Biol [Internet]. 2023 Dec 1 [cited 2024 Mar 2];6(1). Available from: https://pubmed.ncbi.nlm.nih.gov/36869204/
40. Bento-Lopes L, Cabaço LC, Charneca J, Neto M V., Seabra MC, Barral DC. Melanin's journey from melanocytes to keratinocytes: uncovering the molecular mechanisms of melanin transfer and processing. Int J Mol Sci [Internet]. 2023 Jul 1 [cited 2024 Mar 2];24(14). Available from: https://pubmed.ncbi.nlm.nih.gov/37511054/
41. Staricco RJ, Pinkus H. Quantitative and qualitative data on the pigment cells of adult human epidermis. J Invest Dermatol [Internet]. 1957 [cited 2024 Mar 2];28(1):33–45. Available from: https://pubmed.ncbi.nlm.nih.gov/13416674/
42. Kollias N, Baqer AH. Absorption mechanisms of human melanin in the visible, 400–720 nm. J Invest Dermatol. 1987;89(4):384–8.
43. Gillbro JM, Olsson MJ. The melanogenesis and mechanisms of skin-lightening agents—existing and new approaches. Int J Cosmet Sci [Internet]. 2011 Jun 1 [cited 2024 Mar 2];33(3):210–21. Available from: https://onlinelibrary.wiley.com/doi/full/10.1111/j.1468-2494.2010.00616.x
44. Wäster P, Eriksson I, Vainikka L, Rosdahl I, Öllinger K. Extracellular vesicles are transferred from melanocytes to keratinocytes after UVA irradiation. Scientific Reports 2016 6:1 [Internet]. 2016 Jun 13 [cited 2024 Mar 2];6(1):1–13. Available from: https://www.nature.com/articles/srep27890
45. SZABO G. The number of melanocytes in human epidermis. Br Med J. 1954;1(4869): 1016–7. https://doi.org/10.1136/bmj.1.4869.1016

46. Brenner M, Hearing VJ. The protective role of melanin against UV damage in human skin. Photochem Photobiol [Internet]. 2008 May [cited 2024 Mar 2];84(3):539. Available from: https://www.ncbi.nlm.nih.gov/pmc/articles/PMC2671032/
47. Yamaguchi Y, Beer JZ, Hearing VJ. Melanin mediated apoptosis of epidermal cells damaged by ultraviolet radiation: factors influencing the incidence of skin cancer. Arch Dermatol Res [Internet]. 2008 Apr [cited 2024 Mar 2];300 Suppl 1(SUPPL. 1). Available from: https://pubmed.ncbi.nlm.nih.gov/17985102/
48. Fajuyigbe D, Douki T, van Dijk A, Sarkany RPE, Young AR. Dark cyclobutane pyrimidine dimers are formed in the epidermis of Fitzpatrick skin types I/II and VI in vivo after exposure to solar-simulated radiation. Pigment Cell Melanoma Res [Internet]. 2021 May 1 [cited 2024 Mar 3];34(3):575–84. Available from: https://pubmed.ncbi.nlm.nih.gov/33369222/
49. Coelho SG, Choi W, Brenner M, Miyamura Y, Yamaguchi Y, Wolber R, et al. Short- and long-term effects of ultraviolet radiation on the pigmentation of human skin. The journal of investigative dermatology Symposium proceedings /the Society for Investigative Dermatology, Inc [and] European Society for Dermatological Research [Internet]. 2009 [cited 2024 Mar 2];14(1):32. Available from: https://www.ncbi.nlm.nih.gov/pmc/articles/PMC2799903/
50. Visscher MO. Skin color and pigmentation in ethnic skin. Facial Plast Surg Clin North Am [Internet]. 2017 Feb 1 [cited 2024 Apr 7];25(1):119–25. Available from: https://pubmed.ncbi.nlm.nih.gov/27888889/
51. Miller-Milinska A, Staricco RC. Preliminary and short report Quantitative response of the melanocytes to ultraviolet light*. J Invest Dermatol. 1963;41:7–8.
52. López S, Alonso S, García de Galdeano A, Smith-Zubiaga I. Melanocytes from dark and light skin respond differently after ultraviolet B irradiation: effect of keratinocyte-conditioned medium. Photodermatol Photoimmunol Photomed [Internet]. 2015 May 1 [cited 2024 Mar 3];31(3):149–58. Available from: https://onlinelibrary.wiley.com/doi/full/10.1111/phpp.12169
53. The simplified scheme of the melanin synthesis in melanocytes during... | Download Scientific Diagram [Internet]. [cited 2024 Mar 2]. Available from: https://www.researchgate.net/figure/The-simplified-scheme-of-the-melanin-synthesis-in-melanocytes-during-melanogenesis-The_fig 2_236622051.
54. Watt A, Bothma JP, Meredith P, Watt AAR. The supramolecular structure of melanin the supramolecular structure of melanin †. 2014 [cited 2024 Mar 8]; Available from: http://pubs.rsc.org

Chapter 2
Interaction of Solar Radiation with the Human Skin

Abbreviations

ACTH	Adrenocorticotropic hormone
BCC	Basal cell carcinoma
CFL	Compact fluorescent lamp
COLIA 1	Collagen type I **α**-1
CPD	Cyclobutane pyrimidine dimers
DT	Delayed tanning
DWAT	Deeper subcutaneous white adipose tissue layer
EDGL	Electronic device generated light
HEVL	High energy visible light
HEVR	High energy visible radiation
IL	Interleukin
IPD	Immediate pigment darkening
IR	Infrared
LED	Light emitting diode
LLP	Long lasting pigmentation
LOS	Lipid oxygen species
LWI	Long wave index
MAA	Mycosporine like amino acids
MC1R	Melanocortin 1 receptor
MED	Minimal erythemal dose
MI	Melanin index
MITF	Microphthalmia-associated transcription factor
MMD	Minimal melanogenic dose
m-MITF	Mitochondrial-microphthalmia associated transcription factor
MMP	Matrix metalloproteinases
MMP	Matrix metalloproteinases
MPPD	Minimal persistent pigment dose
MSH	Melanocyte-stimulating hormone
mTORC1	Mammalian target of rapamycin1

R. Rajan, *Sunscreens for Skin of Color*,
https://doi.org/10.1007/978-981-97-3195-4_2

OPN-3	Opsin- 3
PIH	Postinflammatory hyperpigmentation
POMC	Proopiomelanocortin
PPD	Persistent pigment darkening
ROS	Reactive oxygen species
SCC	Squamous cell carcinoma
SED	Standard erythemal dose
SOC	Skin of colour
SPF	Sun protection factor
SPT	Skin phototype
SSR	Solar simulated radiation
SWAT	Superficially located dermal white adipose tissue
UV	Ultra violet
UVR	Ultraviolet radiation
VL	Visible light

Key Objectives

- The components of the solar spectrum noted to cause significant impact on the skin, include the ultraviolet, visible, and infrared wavelengths. They impact the skin in unique ways, depending on the depth of their penetration into the skin.
- Within the ultraviolet spectrum, UVB has been long associated with skin cancer, with recent evidence implicating UVA as well in cutaneous photocarcinogenesis. With UVA, the UVA2 subcomponent has a photobiological behaviour similar to that of UVB, and the UVA1 spectrum behaves more like the visible spectrum. Visible light has been proven to have a dominant role in photopigmentation, and disproportionately so in skin of colour. Infrared radiation, which penetrates into the hypodermis, has implications for both photopigmentation and photoageing.
- Recently, exposomal factors such as EDGL (electronic device generated light) have been noted to behave similar to HEVL in causing cutaneous pigmentation. Skin concerns, like acne, have also been noted to be worsened with exposomal factors like UVR, in addition to the well-established domain of photoageing.
- UVR, in particular, and solar radiation in general, influence the peripheral clocks located in skin cells such as melanocytes and keratinocytes to influence skin health and carcinogenesis.

Of the sunlight that reaches the earth's surface, 2–5.4% is ultraviolet (UV) radiation, with infrared rays contributing up to 66%, and the remainder being visible light (VL) [1–4]. UV radiation has been well established to be a mutagen, a tumour initiator, and promoter of carcinogenesis [5]. While intermittent and intense UV exposure contributes to precursor skin changes, and eventually lesions of basal cell carcinoma (BCC) and squamous cell carcinoma (SCC), prolonged and persistent exposure has been considered to initiate and promote melanoma skin cancer [6]. This is presumed to be due to the higher threshold for melanocytes to undergo apoptosis, even after severe damage resulting from UV exposure. Therefore, with subsequent exposures to intense UV, and progressive cellular impact, melanocytes accumulate the damage, which triggers melanomagenesis, in the absence of adequate repair or apoptosis [4].

The importance of sunscreen as a prominent personal care product is largely driven by the ability of solar light to cause photocarcinogenesis, and more recently photoageing and pigmentation. Until recently, most of these deleterious effects of sunlight were thought to be due to the UV segment of the spectrum, which has resulted in a huge body of research on the impact of UV rays on the skin.

Located between gamma rays and visible light energy in the solar spectrum, ultraviolet radiation is divided into UVA, UVB, and UVC subcomponents. UVA forms 95% of the ultraviolet radiation in natural sunlight, with the higher energy UVB forming only 5%. UVA is further partitioned into UVA1 and UVA2, since the photobiological effects of UVA2 are closer to that of UVB, than UVA1 as shown in Fig. 2.1 [7]. Visible light is the only part of the solar spectrum, that is, well, visible to the naked eye! [4].

The atmospheric ozone layer absorbs all of the UVC, at 100–280 nm, and about 90% of UVB [8], leaving only a small fraction of UVB and all of the UVA rays present in the ambient sunlight to reach the earth surface [8, 9]. UVB forms about 5% of the UVR that reaches earth, i.e., in a ratio of 1:20 to UV [5, 9, 10]. In terms of absolute energy, this translates to about 40 Wm^2 of UVA, and less than 3 Wm^2 of UVB, pertaining to locations in Europe [11]. The ratio varies across the day, depending on the position of the sun in the sky, as the UVB diminishes in proportion during the early mornings and the late evenings. The ratio UVB:UVA at 1:20 was found to be a constant at solar elevations more than 60 degrees, based on observations by Kollias et al. reporting from Kuwait City, 29 degree North [10]. Interestingly, in a

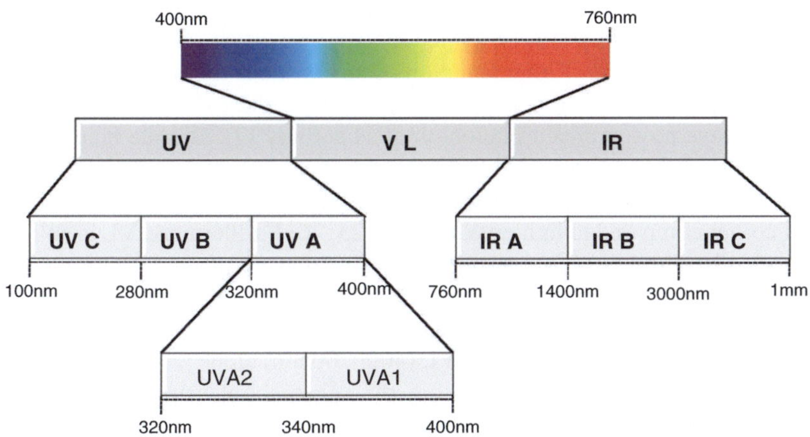

Fig. 2.1 Subcomponents of the solar spectrum. The visible light (VL) spectrum extends from 400 to 700 nm. UV (ultraviolet) rays occupy the zone between 100 and 400 nm, with UVB between 280 and 320 nm and UVA from 320 to 400 nm. UVA is further divided into UVA2 from 320 to 340 nm, and UVA1 from 340 to 400 nm. The infrared (IR) spectrum spans from 760 nm to 1 mm, and is further subdivided into IR A, B, and C

South Indian city, closer to the Equator at 11 degree north, the ratio of UVA: UVB was found to be 1:500 to 1:600 during early hours and late evening and 1:200 during mid-day [9, 12].

UVA is less energetic than UVB and is itself more energetic than visible light. Around three times the magnitude of UVA radiation is required to induce a similar level of skin damage as UVB, which is 1000 times more erythmogenic than UV [8]. Regardless of such variations in energy, all of the UV spectrum from 100 to 400 nm is considered carcinogenic by the International Agency for Research on Cancer, IARC affiliated to the World Health Organization [13].

The UV rays penetrate to different depths in the skin [14], Fig. 2.2. UVB is almost completely absorbed by the melanin in the epidermis, while UVA penetrates deeper into the upper dermis. Longer wavelength components such as the visible light rays and the infrared rays penetrate deeper, further into the dermis and into the upper subcutis [15, 16]. The stratum corneum absorbs about 70% of the incident UVB, while 20% reaches the epidermis and the small remainder fraction is able to reach the uppermost layers of the dermis. About 1/3rd of UVA reaches the deep dermis, the rest being absorbed by the epidermis, and therefore UVA is the principal driver of dermal changes in photoageing [4]. The dose of UV radiation received by the skin varies by anatomical site, depending on the activity engaged in. For most outdoor activities, the cheek receives an average of 15–47%, while the dorsum of the hand receives a much higher dose, 23–71%, of the ambient UVR [11].

Different subcomponents of the solar spectrum have different effects, depending on the interaction with skin based on the depth of penetration [2, 4, 13, 16–18], as illustrated in Table 2.1 and Fig. 2.3 [19–24]. UVA2 has a photobiological behaviour closer to UVB than to UVA1, while UVA1 has overlapping effects with the high energy visible light (HEVL) portion of visible light. UVA1 also demonstrates an additive effect for pigmentation when combined with HEVL [24]. On irradiation, UVA2 induces erythema followed by pigmentation in skin types I and II, while with higher skin types III and IV, pigmentation occurs without visible erythema [19].

Visible light represents roughly about half of the solar radiation and was earlier thought to have no significant photobiological activity [7]. Despite being lower in energy, visible light is responsible for 50% of the free radical generation of the solar spectrum, contributing to photoageing and pigmentation with differential effects on skin of colour compared to lighter skin types [25, 26] Furthermore, VL is able to act synergistically with UVA1 and promote the development of pigmentation and erythema in SOC [26, 27]. Kohli et al. found the pigmentation induced by irradiation in the UVA1+ VL spectrum (370–700 nm) to be darker and more persistent than pigmentation induced by exposure to VL (400–700 nm) alone [27] Furthermore, the photobiological behaviour differs within the sub-spectral components of visible light. The blue-violet end of the visible light spectrum, the HEVL zone, has been identified as having significant photobiological activity with a propensity to stimulate pigmentation. High energy visible radiation (HEVR) or HEVL extends from wavelengths of 380 nm up to 450 nm in the blue light region. Overall, HEVL contributes to increased oxidative damage, persistent skin pigmentation, alters skin hydration and has been postulated to even cause DNA damage [26, 28]. Jo et al.

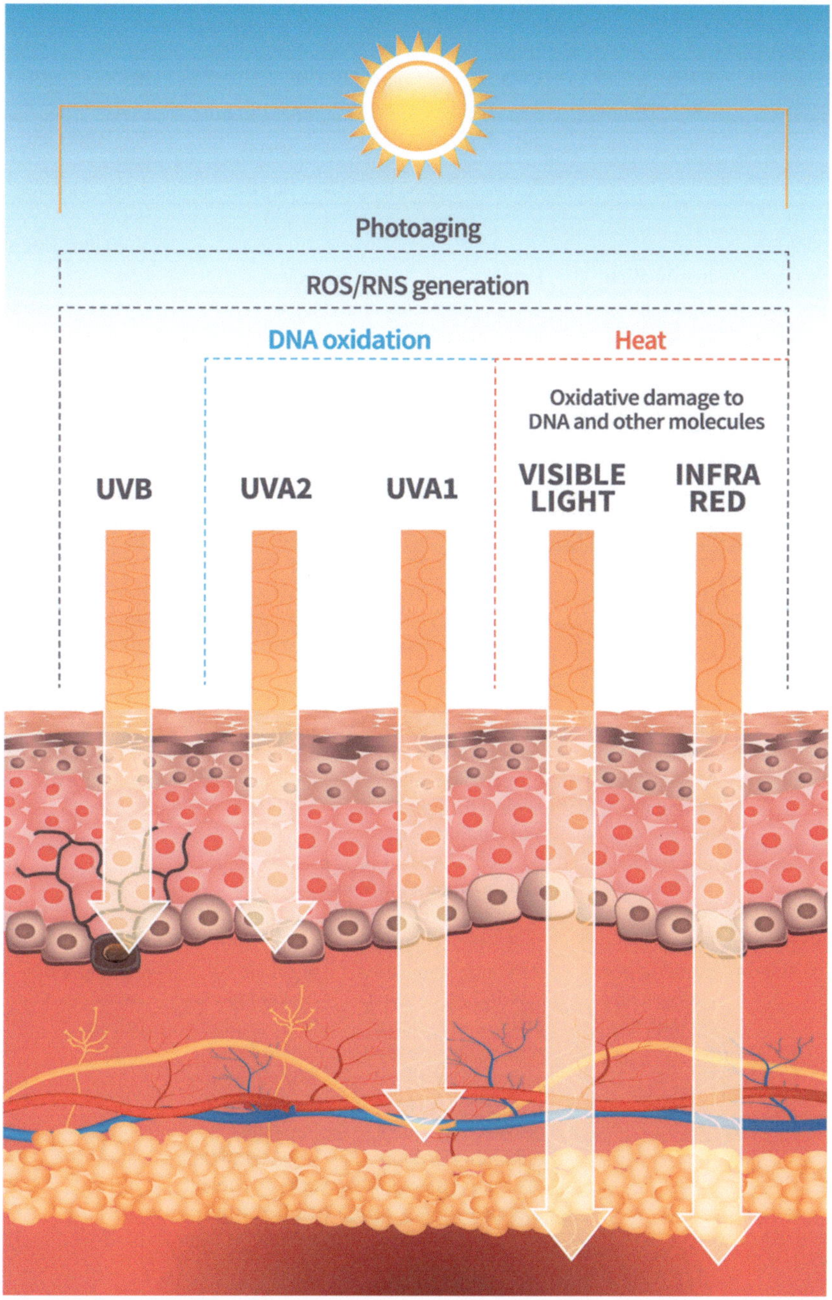

Fig. 2.2 The solar spectrum is composed of various wavelengths, which penetrate into skin at different levels. The longer the wavelength the deeper the rays penetrate the skin. Each wavelength has both different and overlapping effects. UV ultraviolet radiation, ROS reactive oxygen species, RNS reactive nitrogen species. (Obtained with permission from Krutmann et al. [14])

Table 2.1 Effects of solar radiation on the skin

Properties [2, 4, 19–24]	UVB	UVA	VL	IR
Wavelength	280–320 nm	320–340 nm (UVA2) 340–400 nm (UVA1)	400–760 nm	IRA— 760–1400 nm IRB— 1400–3000 nm IRC 3000 nm–1 mm
Energy	Intermediate	Low	Low	Low
Skin Penetration	Up to the epidermis	UVA2 penetrates up to the epidermis UVA 1 penetrates into the dermis	Up to hypodermis	Up to hypodermis
Depth of penetration in microns	100	450	750	1000–5000
Proportion in ambient light	0.3–0.5%	5.1–6%	38.9–62.7%	31.9–40%
Filtered by glass	99–100% filtration by glass	Passes through glass. Above wavelengths of 380 nm, filtered by films and laminated glass	Passes through glass.	Mostly does not pass through glass, but a greenhouse effect is possible due to the heat generated
Erythema post-irradiation	Erythema, resolving in 1–3 days in Skin of colour (SOC), and in 1–2 weeks in lighter skin types	Biphasic erythema response with an immediate peak lasting for up to 4 h, and another phase between 6 and 24 h, may be monophasic in some cases.	Immediate erythema, fading within 2 h	Erythema with perception of heat, resolving in 1 h
Pigmentation on irradiation	Pigmentation is possible after sunburn and erythema	Immediate pigment darkening that fades within 2 h, delayed tanning may occur with melanogenesis after 3–5 days and may progress to persistent pigment darkening or long lasting pigmentation	Immediate pigment darkening and delayed pigment darkening lasting up to a few weeks. Persistent pigmentation is also possible in higher skin types.	Known to worsen pigmentary conditions like melasma

analysed products claiming blue light protection and found that pigmentation induced by blue light at a wavelength of 456 nm was lesser for products containing titanium dioxide mineral filter, compared to those with organic UV filters [29].

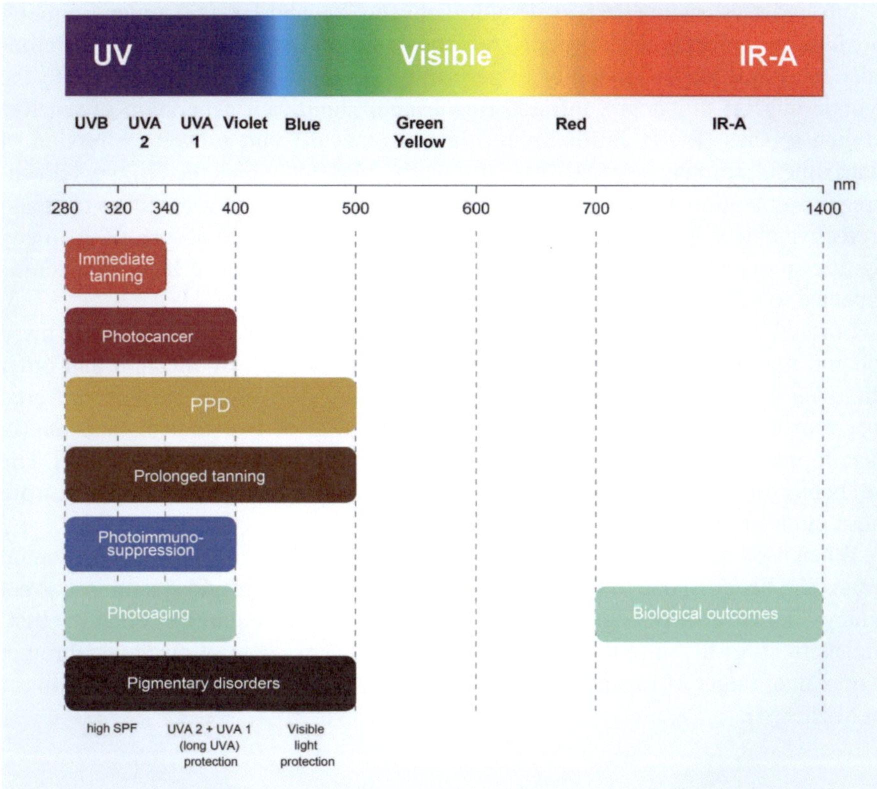

Fig. 2.3 Schematic representation of the effects on the skin of different types of solar radiation. IR-A infrared-A (780 nm–1.4 µm), PPD persistent pigmentary darkening. (From an open access article obtained under the Creative commons license (http://creativecommons.org/licenses/by/4.0/), from Addor et al. [119])

Similarly, emerging data for photocarcinogenesis based on animal studies implicates blue light but not red or green light [30].

Visible light penetrates deep into the dermis, with the longer ends of the spectrum even able to reach the hypodermis. Given intact skin, filtration of 99% of UVB light is expected to occur at a depth of 100 µm into the skin, approximately at the level of the superficial papillary dermis. For UVA, this depth is 450 microns, at the upper reticular dermis. For lighter skin types, the depth of penetration of visible light is up to a maximum of 750 µm. By this model, 99% of visible light would be expected to be filtered out at around 3 mm. If we were to calculate the thickness of the dermis at 2–3 mm, then some part of visible light, especially the longer wavelengths, likely reach the hypodermis, after passing through the dermis. At this depth, the damage to the skin structures from this spectrum is considered to be significant, even if on the whole, VL is a less energetic component of light compared to UVR [31].

Infrared rays occupy the wavelengths between 700 and 100,000 nm or 1 mm. Of the three components of IR rays, IR-A in the spectrum from 700 to 1400 nm is clinically relevant, due to its ability to penetrate deeply into the dermis and into the hypodermis. At this depth, infrared rays trigger significant generation of reactive oxygen species (ROS). Furthermore, they also set off unregulated expression of matrix metalloproteinases (MMP), particularly, MMP-9, which then triggers downstream degradation of collagen, along with reduced neocollagenesis. Since the main protective chromophore of the skin, namely melanin, does not absorb IR-A to any significant extent, a direct mitochondrial damage resulting out of IR-A exposure is expected to drive the dermal damage [15].

Infrared light penetrates the hypodermis. The penetration ability of each of these spectral ranges is subject to effective filtering out of light by melanin and other photodefence mechanisms present in the skin. Along with visible light, the infrared spectrum has also been implicated in the generation of free radicals and matrix metalloproteinases 1 and 9, resulting in premature photoageing of the skin [31]. The cutaneous pigmentation induced by VL and IR are spectroscopically different from those induced by UVA [32].

When used in medical applications, controlled delivery of IR may have potential antiageing benefits, due to the stimulation of collagen I and II and elastin. A correct synergy between wavelength, intensity, and irradiation is required to elicit the beneficial effects of IR, since this spectrum is also capable for promoting ageing through mammalian target of rapamycin 1 (mTORC1) activation in addition to the impact on MMPs [4].

2.1 Direct DNA Damage

UV exposure damages epidermal DNA in several ways [33]. DNA absorbs UV rays acting as a photophore, maximally in the UVC range, but also in most of the UVB spectrum and in some parts of the UVA spectrum. Since most of the UVC is filtered before it reaches the earth's surface, UVB is mostly responsible for the direct DNA damage.

The impact of UV photons on cutaneous cell DNA initiates the formation of thymine and cytosine dimers, namely, thymine-thymine (T=T), cytosine-cytosine (C=C), thymine-cytosine (T=C), and cytosine-thymine (C=T). The generation of these cyclobutane pyrimidine dimers (CPDs), particularly of subtype CC, results in C-->T and CC--> TT dimers, and when replicated in an adequate frequency, these signature mutations may develop into UV hotspots.

Normally, cellular repair mechanisms led by the p53 tumour suppressor gene shift such cells into apoptosis, however, with mutations in p53 itself, and solar-induced immunosuppression, DNA damaged cells survive, escape cellular repair and damage control mechanisms, and go on to produce tumours and skin cancer [33, 34]. Simply put, an incorrect and inadequate repair of the photoproducts resulting in abnormal base pair combinations, triggers mutations, typified by CPD [35].

Direct interaction of the DNA with UV rays also leads to the generation of 6,4 photoadducts which are usually neutralized more rapidly by cellular repair mechanisms compared to CPDs. However, when such repair systems are overwhelmed by excessive exposure, photocarcinogenesis is initiated [36]. Furthermore, with ageing, the natural cellular repair mechanisms for managing solar light-induced CPDs and 6–4 photoproducts become less efficient [36]. Hemminki et al. demonstrated the persistence of these UV-induced dimers for up to 3 weeks post-irradiation in volunteers with a higher level of damage as noted in type I skin compared to skin type IV, indicating better repair mechanisms in the latter [37].

Indirectly, molecules like melanin, porphyrin, tryptophan, and riboflavin, which are endogenously present in the cellular milieu, act as photophores that are excited on interaction with incident UV light. When they return to their resting state, they generate energy which may cause DNA damage as above or generate reactive oxygen species [38].

UVB shoulders the blame for much of the direct DNA damage, due to its higher energy, plus its site of action at the basal epidermis, a zone of high cell turnover [38]. Compared to an immediate, though direct DNA damage from UVB, where UVA is involved, the damage to DNA seems to continue even hours after exposure to UV radiation, characterized by continuous generation of CPDs and free radical damage to melanin [36].

Longer exposure to UVA, say for more than 3 h has been implicated in the development of CPD similar to UVB exposure. These CPDs attributable to UVA exposure, and which continue to be generated even after cessation of UV exposure, latently, are called dark CPDs [38]. In fact, these CPDs are considered to be the most relevant marker of UVA-induced DNA damage in the skin [39]. Occurring due to the interaction of UV generated reactive oxygen and nitrogen species and skin melanin, these dark dimers are considered distinct from those generated by UVB [40], which occur at the time of UV radiation called 'light CPD'. Such 'dark CPD', when occurring in significant quantities overwhelm cellular repair mechanisms, eventually resulting in somatic mutations that culminate in carcinogenesis [38]. Furthermore, CPDs induced by UVA radiation are suspected to persist longer due to less robust activation of cell cycle arrest pathways, due to the depth of penetration of these rays [35]. With its ability to penetrate deeper, UVA plays a role in photoageing in addition to photocarcinogenesis [6, 33, 34, 41]. Based on the most research until recently, UVB was considered responsible for the photocarcinogenesis burden of sunlight. However, UVA is the larger part of the ambient light that reaches the skin surface, constituting 95% of incident UVR, and has recently been proven to promote photocarcinogenesis. UVA irradiation was demonstrated to cause DNA single strand breaks 40 times higher in melanocytes from lighter skin types as compared to dark skin, suggesting a role for UVA in melanomagenesis [42, 43]. Therefore, current sunscreens must go beyond erythema management and UVB protection and address coverage of the UVA spectrum.

Skin of colour seems to be significantly better protected against UVR-induced DNA damage. Fajuyigbe et al. demonstrated that the occurrence of both light and dark CPDs were absent in the areas of high melanin concentration, such as the basal layer of type VI skin [44]. The authors noted that since the cellular repair dynamics of CPDs post-UV exposure was similar in lighter and darker skin types in their study, a higher melanin concentration seems to confer some protection against CPD generation in the first place. As noted above, UVA-induced DNA strand breaks were more common in lighter-skinned individuals [42, 43]. Skin pigmentation is the most important photoprotective factor, since melanin has, in addition to its UV absorbing properties, antioxidant and free radical scavenging abilities [45].

This protective effect is due to eumelanin as pheomelanin seen in lighter skin types is known to be a pro-oxidant with a demonstrated absence of an ability to protect against generation of CPDs. Therefore, eumelanin in higher skin types remains central to the lower incidence of UV driven DNA damage in keratinocytes [44]. Furthermore, it has also been found that the repair mechanisms of DNA damage are more efficient in SOC compared to lighter skin types [46]. Lopez et al. described an inherent difference in melanocyte behaviour on exposure to UVB, between melanin rich skin and lighter skin. The former showed an increase in melanogenesis, resulting from increased cellular differentiation. Melanocytes from lighter skin showed proliferative behaviour without any effective increase in melanogenesis signalling a lack of protection against potential UVB-induced damage [47]. The average melanin content in the skin.

With the other parts of the spectrum, typically VL and IR, the potential for DNA damage is unclear. Interestingly, infrared rays have been known to protect against UV-induced DNA damage. Specifically, IR-A irradiation was known to reduce subsequent UVB-induced apoptosis and DNA damage in keratinocytes in animal studies. A similar protective effect due to IR was also noted in human fibroblast cultures, with sustained benefits. Visible light has not been considered to cause DNA damage thus far [4, 19]. Duteil et al. compared the effects of blue-violet light to UVB radiation and noted that the typical markers of UVB-induced cutaneous damage, such as keratinocyte necrosis or p53 expression, and markers of oxidative stress, such as 8-oxoguanine expression, were not seen significantly with blue-violet light [7]. However, recent animal studies have suggested a potential role for the blue segment of the visible light spectrum 380–500 nm, with a peak irradiance at 479 nm, in photocarcinogenesis in mice exposed to 12 h of blue light every day for a year. An effect of photoageing was also observed in these mice, with a decreased expression of dermal collagen compared to animals exposed to red light (600–700 nm), and green light (500–560 nm) [30].

Despite an overall good reputation thus far, on DNA damage, when it comes to free radical damage, however, visible light is heavily implicated, contributing to over 50% of all light-induced generation of free radicals [21]. The contribution of the infrared spectrum is also significant, with IR-A, 700–1400 nm capable of generating ROS in the skin. The other IR components, IR-B (1400–3000 nm) and IR-C (3000 nm–1 mm) are not known to have any meaningful skin penetration [15].

2.2 Free Radical Generation

UVR produces its deleterious effects on the skin, acting principally through direct DNA damage but also through the generation of reactive oxygen species and downstream free radicals [11, 48, 49]. Reactive oxygen species (ROS) refers to highly reactive oxygen molecules which are capable of creating structural damage to cellular organelles and DNA [38]. The entire spectrum of light, from UV to VL to IR, is capable of generating free radicals in the skin [21], with even electronic gadget related light demonstrated to induce oxidative damage in human fibroblasts [50]. The peak generation of free radicals, reactive oxygen species and reactive nitrogen species, occurs at around 355 nm in the UVA zone, whereas the much-studied erythema response occurs in the lower wavelength zone of 290–310 nm, Fig. 2.4 [21].

Visible light rays, even though said to reside outside of the deleterious light spectrum [45], accounts for 50% of free radical generation, though UV rays are most efficient at producing ROS [15, 47]. Also, visible light is 15 times more abundant in ambient sunlight at sea level, compared to UVA [51], which is present more abundantly than UVB. Therefore, even though the energy levels progressively decline from the UVB through UVA to the visible light spectrum, the overall amount of

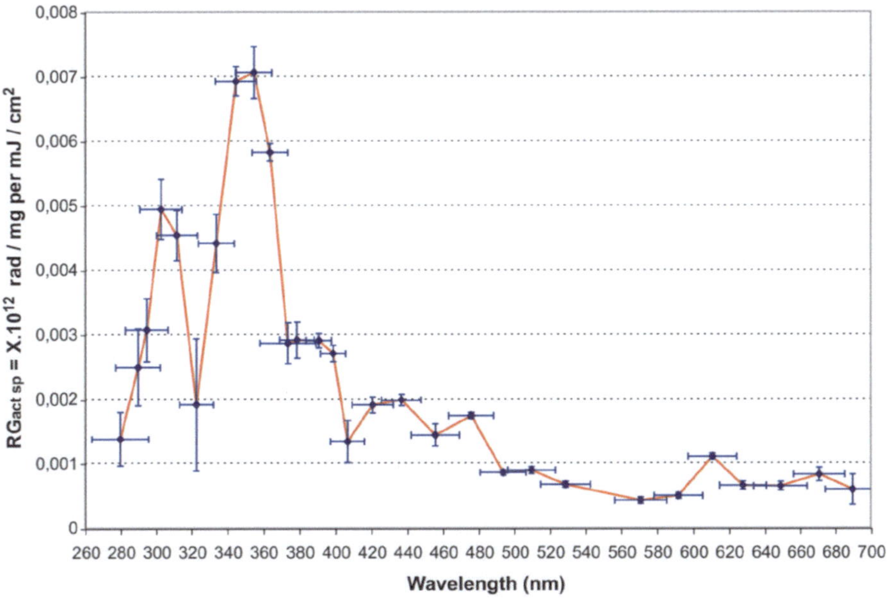

Fig. 2.4 Image showing wavelength dependent generation of free radicals in human skin, with a peak action around 355 nm in the UVA spectrum. Action spectrum–wavelength dependence for free radical generation RG act sp = X.10^{12} radicals/mg skin per mJ/cm^2 and per nm, horizontal bars represent the spectral bandpass value of pairs of adjacent cut-off filters, vertical bars represent the standard error associated with RG (radical generation) measurement. (Reproduced with permission from Zastrow et al. [21])

radiation makes visible light an important component to be photoprotected from. UVA induces photodegradation in incident cells with the generation of free radicals, superoxide anions, and singlet oxygen species which are then quenched by melanin, which undergoes oxidation itself in the process.

For the infrared spectrum from 700 to 1600 nm, free radical generation is related to an increase in skin temperature on sun exposure [21, 49]. IR exposure at a temperature of 39 °C was found to be associated with free radical generation, while no oxidative damage was noted at IR radiation at 37 °C [19, 21].

Zastrow et al. demonstrated the generation of free radicals in the skin from the UVB zone of 280 nm all the way to 1600 nm in the near-infrared region. They also differentiated between free radicals generated by the UV radiation as short lived ROS—reactive oxygen species, and long persisting lipid peroxidation products, lipid oxygen species (LOS) [51, 52]. The ratio of ROS to LOS may play a role in determining whether an exposure to UV produces an easily quenched, short lived burst of free radical generation in the ROS domain or contributes to the generation of longer lasting LOS photoadducts with potential for carcinogenesis and photoageing [49].

Incident visible light is able to generate reactive oxygen species resulting in the release of inflammatory cytokines and stimulation of matrix metalloproteinases in human epidermal equivalents, potentially contributing to skin ageing [26]. VL has also been implicated in solar dermatoses like cutaneous porphyrias and urticaria, and pigmentary conditions like melasma and postinflammatory hyperpigmentation. Acting synergistically with UVA1, VL produces erythema in the lighter skin types, and pigmentation without erythema [50], and rarely with erythema [53], in higher phototypes.

ROS generation is also known to occur due to electronic device generated light (EDGL), a new exposomal factor in the Digital Age.

2.3 Erythema Responses to Sunlight

Erythema has been the hallmark response of UV radiation and has been the main endpoint in sunscreen science, until recently. Even now, for the user, sunscreen efficacy is nearly synonymous with sun protection factor (SPF) rating, a metric which was developed to measure sun protection using the surrogate marker of solar-induced erythema. Erythema or skin redness is an inflammatory reaction of the skin, occurring as a function of skin phototype, and is accompanied by warmth and skin tenderness. While the erythema response is almost immediate in lighter skin types, a delayed erythema response is possible in all skin types, though difficult to appreciate clinically in darker skin. Of all the solar subcomponents, UVB is the most erythemogenic, being 1000 fold more likely to induce skin redness than UVA. A biphasic erythema response to UVA has been known to occur. Here again, immediate erythema was common only in the lighter phototypes. UV-induced erythema may also be modulated by the duration of exposure in addition to the dose, and also by prior sun exposure [19]. Further sunscreen use may also blunt the erythema response, as a photoadaptation response [34]. Visible light-induced erythema, paradoxically, is seen more commonly in higher skin types, as first demonstrated by [51]. Here, melanin acts as a chromophore, which gets heated by incident VL and then goes on to produce erythema, with higher melanin loads in darker skin generating more thermal output. The impact of heat is significantly higher with IR, where irradiation is associated with erythema and thermal pain on the skin. With increased levels of radiation, and overheating of tissues, vasodilatation leading to circulatory failure may also result [19].

Key differences exist between erythema responses across skin types, with significant relevance for skin of colour. The SPF of Black epidermis is four times that of White epidermis, 13.4 vs. 3.4. Furthermore, the time taken to achieve one minimal erythemal dose (MED) is almost three times longer at 45 min, in skin type IV, compared to skin type I or II where 1 MED is achieved within 15 min. During this interval though, type IV skin received one MPPD—Minimal Persistent Pigment Dose, equivalent to 15 J/cm^2 of UVA. In other words, for every dose of MED, only one third of MPPD is received by lower skin types, compared to a ratio of 1:1 for higher skin types [54, 55].

Welti et al. observed that the MED dose for UVA did not correlate as clearly with skin type, unlike MED–UVB, which increased with higher skin type. This agrees with the lesser role of UVA in causing erythema. The MED–UVA was reduced, though in people with photodermatitis than in those without, indicating a lower threshold for UVA-induced erythema in compromised skin [56]. MED—UVB is influenced both by geographical location as well as by ethnicity. Reporting from Malaysia, Wong et al. noted that UVB–MED results among Asian populations vary significantly from those of Americans and the Spanish, even within the same phototype. Considering the wide repertoire of ethnicities within the umbrella term of Asian, intra-group variations are the norm. In Wong's study, the UVB–MED results in Malaysians were found to be closer to that reported from Singapore and Taiwan, despite wide variations within phototypes [57]. Such variability could also arise from the presence of overlap in ethnicities residing in these countries, and the unreliability of Fitzpatrick skin typing in Asian skin. MEDs in different skin types, based on data from a few locations across the world, have been summarized [55, 57–61] in Fig. 2.5. Echoing this, Leeutaphong reported the lack of utility of Fitzpatrick phototypes in assessing sensitivity to UV, in Thai people. Neither skin type, constitutional pigmentation nor facultative pigmentation was found to reliably predict the sensitivity to UVB in Thai [58], in contrast to Wong et al., demonstrating a good correlation between facultative and constitutive skin colour with MED–UVB and Minimal melanogenic dose (MMD)–UVB. Unlike the Thai study, skin lightness measured with L*, skin erythema, and pigmentation were found to predict a cutaneous response to UVR [57].

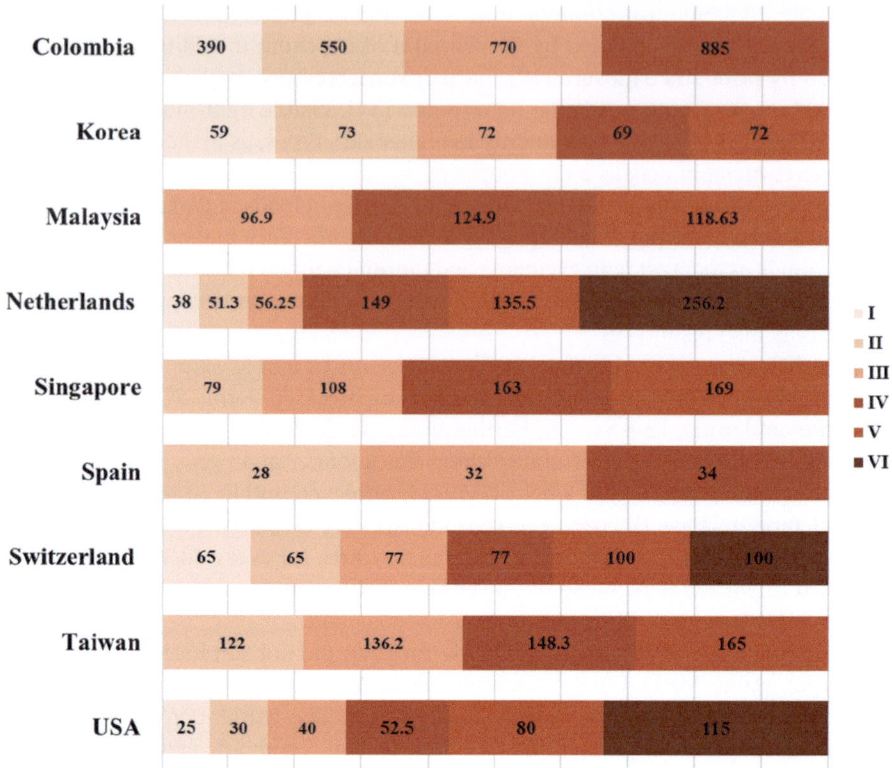

Fig. 2.5 Minimal erythemal dose (mJ/sq.cm) reported by Fitzpatrick type in several geographical locations, across the globe [55, 57–61]

2.4 Pigment Responses

UV-induced changes on the skin have been more extensively studied as compared to HEVL or IR-induced pigmentary changes. However, this photobiological response is highly important to individuals with SOC.

The tanning induced by UV has a few phases: immediate pigment darkening, persistent pigment darkening, and delayed tanning [40, 62, 63].

Immediate pigment darkening attributed mostly to UVA exposure [39] occurs loosely similar to the chromatophore response in animals like chameleons. Also known as immediate transient pigmentation [64], the skin darkening occurs due to a simple redistribution of preformed melanin to the sun facing aspect of the keratinocytes, and the photooxidation of such melanin, the Meirowsky phenomenon, giving the skin a greyish hue [65].

The onset of this pigmentation begins within a few minutes of sun exposure and can last for hours [66], triggered by energy as low as approximately 1 J/cm^2 [67]. Mahmoud et al. demonstrated the ability of the UVA1 spectral band to produce immediate pigment darkening, in skin types IV–VI, without any erythema response [51]. The darkening was evident at a minimum threshold dose of 5 J/cm^2. At doses higher than 5 J/cm^2, the response may transition into one of persistent pigment darkening [68]. There was no difference in melanocyte number or melanin content between radiated and nonirradiated sites, confirming that IPD results from oxidative darkening of preformed melanin.

In contrast to the grey-black hue of immediate pigment darkening, persistent pigment darkening is noticed as a brown to tan hue [40]. PPD is reliably noticed from 2 to 3 h after exposure to the light source. This pigmentation lasting for days is considered to be predominantly driven by UVA and does not involve significant synthesis of new melanin, though some melanin synthesis is possible depending on the dose of UVA and at doses of more than 10 J/cm^2, PPD can be expected to be persist significantly. Histopathologically, PPD is characterized by the migration of melanosomes towards the upper layers of the epidermis, and increased melanosome transfer to keratinocytes [40, 63].

Immediate pigment darkening may also be induced by visible light [68]. Reporting on volunteers with skin types IV and V from Bangalore in India, Ramasubramaniam et al. suggested that the IPD induced by VL is similar to that induced by UV, acting through similar transient melanin precursor species generated by irradiation, and which go on to produce the clinically visible immediate pigment darkening [68]. However, compared to VL, UV was found to be 25 times more efficient at inducing persistent pigmentation [68], in contrast to Mahmoud et al., who found that pigmentation induced by VL was darker and more persistent than UVA1-induced pigmentation [50]. Ramasubramaniam et al. used natural sunlight as the light source, Mahmoud et al. used artificial sources of visible light at a fourfold higher intensity than the former [19, 51, 68].

Immediate pigment darkening and persistent pigment darkening are considered a biphasic response, collectively grouped under immediate tanning, which is not thought to be photoprotective, where driven predominantly by UVA [67]. In contrast, UVB even with a single exposure is said to induce melanogenesis, to aid in subsequent protection against the sun. The erythema typically noted with UVB radiation can be followed through with a delayed pigment response, depending on dosage and duration [40].

Delayed tanning happens due to neomelanogenesis, resulting from UVR-induced increased synthesis and activity of tyrosinase. Erythemogenic or repeated suberythemogenic exposures to UVA, also stimulates delayed pigmentation [64]. UVB-induced sunburn results in an eventual, delayed tanning. Over time, repeated exposure to UVB causes upregulation of genes involved in the pigmentation pathway. Direct DNA damage induced by UVB leads to increased p53 expression with resultant transcription of the pro-opiomelanocortin (POMC) gene [69]. This results in the production of α-MSH, adrenal corticotropin hormone (ACTH) and the opioid peptide β-endorphin. In paracrine fashion, MC1R becomes stimulated, with increased expression of mitochondrial-microphthalmia associated transcription factor (m-MITF) and melanin synthesis. Subsequently, the melanin is transferred to keratinocytes, specifically to a supranuclear location for photoprotection. A similar response to UVA has not been established as yet [40, 67]. Though delayed tanning is considered as a distinct entity, there is significant overlap and ambiguity about the relative contributions of the different segments of the UV spectrum [67]. This is a potential result of renewed research efforts in this area of high consumer interest, resulting in uncovering of newer aspects and mechanisms of cutaneous photopigmentation. Overall, the delayed tanning response is characterized by a small, less than 2X fold increase in skin melanin, in contrast to the significant skin darkening observed clinically. This is due to the changes in particle size and distribution that magnify the perceived skin colour in addition to melanin synthesis itself [40]. A certain level of pre-exposure seems to aid the process of photopigmentation [19, 45]. Interestingly, the expression of POMC increases with age [70].

Compared to UVB-induced tanning, UVA-induced tanning seems to persist longer, lasting for months and sometimes, more than a year. This may be related to the level of melanization induced by UVA and UVB, each with a different depth of penetration into the skin. UVA-induced pigmentary changes occur at a deeper location in the stratum basale of the epidermis, while the more superficial UVB-induced pigmentation is lost within a month due to routine epidermal turnover [64].

A relatively recent addition here is the concept of LLP or long lasting pigmentation [63]. Tan lines, as visibly apparent to people, occur as an extended pigmentary response to intense periods of sun exposure. Coelho et al. noted that LLP is proportionate to the UV dose, with a two MED dose eliciting LLP significantly higher than with a one MED dose. LLP was noted in 40–70% of subjects who received more than a two MED dose of UV, but this study did not find a relationship between constitutive pigmentation based on melanin index, and LLP [71]. The authors suggest that based on duration, exposed individuals can be classified into one of the three groups—those that do not develop this phenomenon, those who develop the pigmentation within 9 months, and those in whom the pigmentation is sustained for 9 months or more, typified as LLP. The authors found that minimal melanogenic dose (MMD) and MED were the best predictors for LLP, while advancing age was identified to potentially increase LLP. Interestingly, skin melanin content and phototype were not found to significantly influence the development of LLP. Pigmentation tends to be more persistent if for some reason, the surface epidermis does not shed off or exfoliate over time, and also if there is continued ongoing sun exposure which keeps the melanogenic system activated. While pigmentation has some benefits in terms of ongoing protection against sun exposure, persistent pigmentation is undesirable, both from the perspective of solar-induced pigmentary disorders in skin of colour, and the potential for uncontrolled pigment cell proliferation and melanomagenesis in lighter skin at risk [71]. In fact, persistence of hyperpigmentation in LLP may not be related to an increase in the number or proliferative activity of melanocytes, but to an impaired removal of melanin from keratinocytes. UV-induced attenuation of hemidesmosomes at the basal layer, leads to impaired melanin removal resulting in a hyperpigmented basal epithelium with increased interdigitation, which may evolve into age spots, and in susceptible individuals, has the potential to progress to malignancy [72].

2.5 Does Tanning Increase Subsequent Protection Against UV Damage?

Tanning is facultative pigmentation when sun exposure leads to skin darkening above the constitutive baseline pigmentation. It is a photoadapative response leading to melanin redistribution and eventually, increased melanin synthesis in the skin as a response to UV-induced stress, with melanocortins in the skin playing a regulatory role [73, 74].

Immediate pigment darkening, which simply involves redistribution of existing melanosomes towards the surface of the keratinocyte, is considered to have limited potential for further skin protection from solar radiation. In contrast, neomelanogenesis, as occurs in delayed pigment darkening, may be more relevant as an adaptive and potentially protective response. This increased melanin content in the epidermis is thought to gradually offer some level of protection against continued sun exposure over time [49].

Increased stratum corneum thickening and increased pigmentation are seen as forms of natural sun protection that develops with sun exposure. Through this mechanism, sun exposure during the summer-spring months in the Northern hemisphere is said to afford an increased level of sun protection, by a factor of 2 [75]. Among Asian ethnicities, the MED-UVB of Taiwanese was found to approach that of Singaporeans who live closer to the Equator. This is likely due to the effect of summer season on the study, considering sun exposure promotes hardening and creates some level of photoprotection against further UV exposure. Skin hardening typically requires 4–6 weeks of sun exposure to reflect as an increase in sun tolerance, in photosensitive individuals. The ability of hardening to protect against photocarcinogenesis has not been established [57, 76]. Reduction of intensity of tan-recovery from a tan strongly depends on avoidance of further sun exposure, and unimpaired keratinocyte desquamation [71].

The long-term effects of visible light have not been completely characterized as yet [51], though we now know that it has been possible to elicit cutaneous pigmentation without the involvement of UV, but only with VL and IR spectrum (390–1700 nm) [32]. Over the years, the importance of visible light in the development of pigmentary conditions common in SOC has become well established. The effect of visible light on pigmentation seems to be heavily influenced by skin type.

VL appears to contribute to all the temporal components of a tan—IPD, PPD, and DPD. Porges et al. demonstrated that higher energies, 80–120 J/cm^2, were required to elicit delayed tanning (DT) compared to a threshold of 40–80 J/cm^2 for IPD, in an elegant experiment evaluating the impact of wavelengths between 385 and 700 nm generated by a solar simulator [53].

Darkening of skin was proportionate to incident energy.

Within the visible light spectrum, blue light also called as high energy visible light in the spectrum between 400 and 500 nm, has been proven to cause pigmentation and photoageing responses in vivo and in vitro [77]. Specifically, the pigmentary response to blue light was more pronounced in higher skin types, and in this group, found to be more sustained than the pigmentation induced by UVA [45, 51]. Mahmoud et al. compared the effects on UVA1 and VL on melanocompetent higher phototype individuals. They found that the chromaticity of the pigmentation induced by light in the UVA spectrum between 340 and 400 nm was found to be grey initially, turning brown after a day, in high phototype volunteers, compared to the brownish pigmentation observed right from when the skin was exposed to visible light between 400 and 700 nm in lighter skin. Also, while UVA1 elicited no erythema, VL was shown to induce skin erythema, immediately and persisting for up to 2 h after irradiation. This erythema response was noted only in volunteers with higher phototypes. This study used light sources with filtered out infrared rays to avoid the confounding factor of erythema induced by heating. Therefore, it is remarkable that the development of redness here was attributed to the heating of melanin pigment on absorption of visible light. Since such heat is a function of melanin concentration, a similar response was not seen in lighter-skinned study subjects with lesser constitutive pigmentation. Considering the abundance of VL versus UVA, the authors calculate that 1 h of ambient sun exposure may deliver about 300 J/cm^2 of visible light compared to 20 J/cm^2 of UVA for the same period of exposure, confirming that visible light may contribute to significant pigmentation in SOC. The colour of the UV-induced IPD was found to be grey compared to the brownish pigmentation induced by VL [51]. However, a later study noted that the IPD was of the same darkish brown colour with both VL and UV in skin types IV and V [68].

Impact of visible light on skin pigmentation was also confirmed in a study by Campiche et al., who used individual typology angle (ITA) cutoffs to quantify blue light-induced pigmentation responses. The investigators found that persistent pigment darkening was easily induced by monochromatic blue light exposure, and lasted up to 2 months, where follow-up was concluded. Notably, antioxidants like niacinamide and microalgal extracts were found to be of benefit in mitigating blue light-induced skin pigmentation and redness, respectively. Also of interest, the b value increased over the course of the study. The b value indicates yellowing of the skin, probably a result of light-induced protein carbonylation, as occurs in photoageing. Visible light causes darker skin types to tan more easily compared to lighter skin types, however, the high melanin content in darker skin may also make it difficult to appreciate erythema in higher phototypes [77].

In contrast to UV light where the immediate pigment darkening phenomenon is evident within a few minutes of sun exposure, with visible light, multiple exposures seem to be required for significant pigmentation. This pigmentation depends to some extent on constitutive pigmentation as well as on the dosage of exposure [45].

It is still not completely resolved as to whether the process of pigmentation induction by visible light is accompanied by cytotoxic changes and free radical generation, to the same extent noted during UV irradiation of the skin. Notably, visible light was not known to cause thymine dimer formation, a change typical for UVR. This remained true even for higher doses of visible light. However, Liebel et al. showed that exposure to visible light increases the generation of reactive oxygen species, matrix metalloproteinases, and inflammatory cytokines in the epidermis, which were amenable to mitigation by the use of antioxidants [31].

Specifically blue light damage to the skin is thought to be mediated by reactive oxygen species generation much like the other solar components and the nitrous oxide (NO) pathway [78]. On the other end of the spectrum, exposure to red light wavelengths was not found to cause any pigmentation [7]. Rather, red light photobiomodulation has been found to reduce pigmentation severity in melasma, notably in darker skin types V and VI [79, 80]. The pigmentation induced by the blue-violet spectrum of light was found to be more prominent than that by the shorter UVB spectrum as well as by the longer wavelengths around red light [7].

Based on these findings, Duteil et al. hypothesized that a mechanism distinct from ROS generation, and p53 stimulation, such as seen with UVB-induced pigmentation, may be operative in the case of HEVL related pigmentation, with relevance for clinical hyperpigmentation conditions such as melisma [7, 70]. Regazzetti et al. identified a direct pathway of melanocyte stimulation by blue light acting through the opsin receptor, Opsin-3 (OPN-3). OPN-3 proteins in the epidermal melanocytes are directly stimulated by VL wavelengths to stimulate melanogenesis in the process of tanning [81]. Stimulation of the opsin pathway causes an increased calcium flux into melanocytes, with resultant increased transcription of MITF-1 leading to melanin synthesis. Sustained pigmentation is maintained by the generation of multimeric tyrosinase-/tyrosinase-related protein complexes, formed in response to blue light exposure. In other words, melanocytes in the skin are able to 'see' blue light using the OPN-3 opsin sensors, behaving similarly to retinal cells, and in response, stimulate significant and persistent pigmentation [69]. Figure 2.6. Specific attenuation of this effect through the use of iron oxides in sunscreens has been found to be effective in reducing short VL-induced pigmentation in melasma [82].

Research comparing the impact of progressively increasing wavelengths from 334 to 549 nm found that wavelengths above 470 nm did not induce measurable immediate pigment darkening compared to the shorter wavelengths [83]. ROS generation was also found to tail off above 582 nm, in dermal fibroblasts exposed to the same dose of 150 J/cm^2 at different wavelengths [77]. de Galvez et al. suggest that wavelengths above 480 nm may not be associated with the deleterious effects of photoageing and hyperpigmentation seen with shorter wavelengths between 415 and 465 nm [65].

Evaluating for the various coloured subcomponents of the visible light spectrum, in terms of the ability to cause skin pigmentation, Marionnett et al. found that the blue light at 400–500 nm contributed to a major part of visible light-induced pigmentation at 71% with blue-violet zone between 400 and 450 nm, accounting for 47%; green light 500–600 nm accounted for 37% of the pigmentation 24 h after exposure, but lasting up to 6 weeks. The red spectrum was not associated with any significant pigmentation [24].

Visible light is responsible for 50% of the free radical generation of the solar spectrum [26], contributing to photoageing.

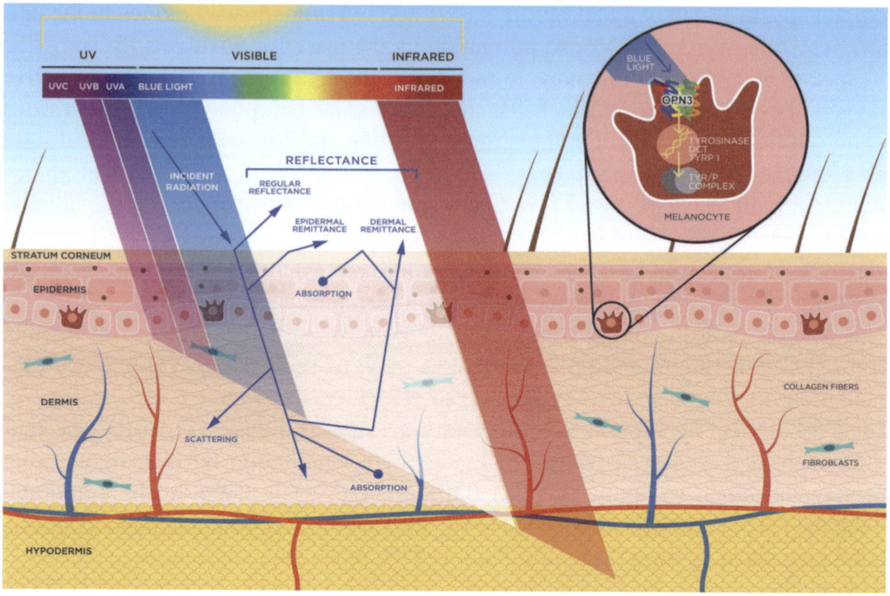

Fig. 2.6 Schematic representing optical pathways (reflectance, absorbance, and scattering) and relative penetration depth of UV and visible light for 99% reduction (2 log10 reduction) in incident intensity (Data extrapolated from the study by Anderson and Parrish [1981]) (Obtained with permission from Lim et al. [83]). Blue light directly activates the OPN3 (Opsin 3) receptor at the surface of melanocytes that further induces the transcription of melanocytic enzymes but also stabilizes tyrosinase (TYRP) activity by promoting its complex with DCT (dopachrome tautomerase), leading to prolonged melanogenesis (see insert, upper right) [83]

Is Blue Light from Gadgets Harmful to Skin?

The irradiance of the blue light emitted from gadgets is about 1/100th to 1/1000th that of the blue light in the solar spectrum [84]. A meta-analysis concluded that gadget emitted blue light may not be adequate to incite clinically significant skin pigmentation [85]. However, it must be noted that blue light constitutes 30% of the light emitted by gadgets, and up to 40% of the radiation emitted by indoor lighting, and up to 25% of sunlight. While the energy of the blue light emitted by artificial devices is significantly lower than that of solar blue light, the cumulative effect of solar and gadget emitted blue light needs to considered as potentially impactful for people predisposed to skin pigmentation [65], especially with increasing exposure to blue light from devices [90]. Pigmentation induced by the blue-violet HEVL spectrum, typically what spectrum is emitted by electronic gadgets, has been shown to persist for months [7].

2.6 Dermal and Hypodermal Changes with Solar Radiation

At the level of the dermis, the principal active components of sunlight are UVA, VL, and IR.

UV radiation stimulates collagen degradation acting through MMPs. Elastase is also stimulated leading to defective elastin formation with decreased integrity of the dermal extracellular matrix [4]. Visible light is also able to induce MMP formation, mediated through ROS generation, resulting in collagen degradation [4, 69].

Infrared energy, which is known to penetrate well into this region promotes the increased expression of matrix metalloproteinases 1, 3, and 12, leading to collagen and protein degradation in the dermal extracellular matrix, acting through cellular mitochondria and cytochrome C oxidase. IR-induced increase in MMP and decrease in collagen type I α-1 (COLIA1) expression leads to increased collagen breakdown coupled with reduced synthesis, destroying existing fibre networks in the dermis, and manifesting clinically as wrinkles and loss of skin elasticity [4, 15].

Despite most work related to photoageing, focusing predominantly on the epidermis and the dermis, skin adipose tissue also participates in the photoageing process. The superficially located dermal white adipose tissue (SWAT) acts a 'fat bridge' between the reticular dermis and the deeper subcutaneous white adipose tissue (DWAT) layer. Significant exposure to UVR causes a reduction in the thickness of the DWAT layer, resulting in skin fibrosis, and ultimately, skin coarseness and wrinkling. Changes may also be noticed in the SWAT which shows lesser accumulation of free fatty acids and triglycerides on sun exposed skin compared to sun protected areas, probably triggered by the diffusion of soluble inflammatory cytokines like IL-1, IL-8, and monocyte chemotactic protein-3 into the SWAT. The cumulative result is skin atrophy and wrinkle formation, due to thinner and coarser skin adipose tissue [86].

2.7 The Solar Exposome

The exposome concept as relates to human health was put forth by Christopher Wild in the year 2005 [87], soon after the successful Human Genome Project. The Human Genome Project has just laid open the detailed genetic code of our species, and research focused on working out disease predispositions driven by the genome.

The exposome, here defined as the sum of all the exposures right from in utero through the entire length of life, is proposed as an important complement to the genome, in the final manifestation of a trait or a disease. While most of the disease processes have previously been looked at from the point of view of genetic susceptibility of an individual, exposome science looks at measuring the external exposures as intently as an individual's genome which drives predispositions in the first place. Recently, Krutmann et al. proposed a set of exposome factors that underlie cutaneous ageing, Fig. 2.7.

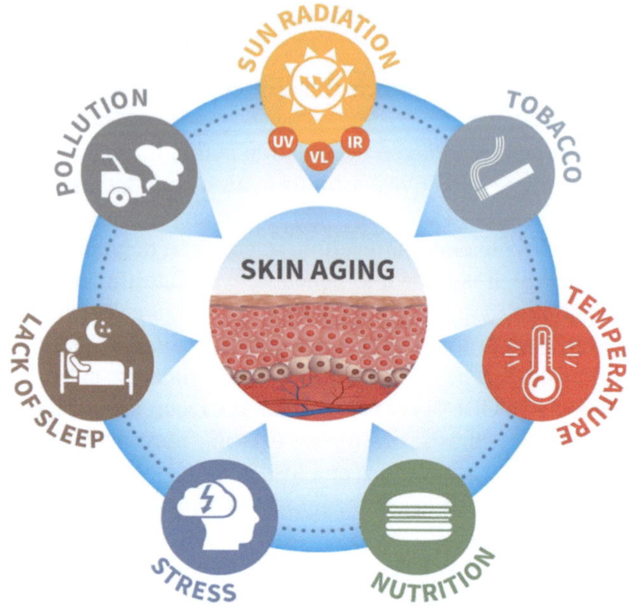

Fig. 2.7 Skin ageing exposome factors have been identified to potentiate skin ageing. Exposure to sun, pollution and tobacco are now well known to trigger molecular processes that damage the skin structure, leading to the aged skin appearance. Other, less well studied factors are recognized as potentiators for skin ageing. These factors have been shown to act either separately or by interacting with each other and potentiating the process. (Obtained with permission from Krutmann et al. [14])

Exposome factors leading to skin stress can be acute or chronic and can be defined as any disturbance of homeostasis of skin functions due to environmental agents like solar radiation, meteorological factors, pollution or tobacco smoke, and internal agents like unhealthy diet, hormonal changes, impaired sleep hygiene, and psychosocial stress [81, 88].

Acute sun exposure is an exposome factor that produces significant changes in the skin, from stimulation of pigmentation and DNA damage to the generation of oxidative stress, inflammation, immunosuppression, necrotic changes in keratinocytes (sunburn cells), breakdown of barrier function, alteration of osmolyte homeostasis, and the cutaneous microbiome. Acting together with pollutants, typically particulate matter, UVR depletes tissue antioxidants and increases tissue peroxidation [81].

The use of sunscreens to protect against a very evident exposomal component like solar radiation offers a great way to manipulate skin health, right from preventing photocarcinogenesis all the way to aspirational health goals like antiageing.

Moving from the solar exposome to the sunscreen exposome: While the sun's rays have been postulated as a primary exposome, the most common tool used for photoprotection, namely sunscreens, have been driving an exposome research of their own, from endocrine disruption attributable to some UV filters to coral bleaching due to certain others.

The exposome concept is highly exciting, as it appears to provide researchers with actionable areas to positively manipulate outcomes driven by genomic predispositions. However, the exposome concept is only as strong as the input driven by environmental epidemiology which is only emerging now, with increased research interest in SOC [89].

Electronic device generated light (EDGL) is the newest light exposome that is considered relevant today. In the present Digital Age, light pollution, defined as the presence of unwanted, inappropriate, or excessive artificial lighting, is a ubiquitous problem [90].

EDGL emitted by devices, which produce bright white light for easy reading, includes light in the wavelengths between 400 and 500 nm, falling into the HEVL spectrum. HEVL, in the wavelengths from 400 to 490 nm, negatively impacts the skin leading to increased generation of ROS, induction of cell apoptosis and necrosis, increased cutaneous vascularity, hyperpigmentation and premature ageing [4].

When used at a distance of less than 1 cm from the screen, EDGL was found to stimulate the generation of ROS in skin fibroblasts. Specifically, the wavelengths emitted by these devices were found to be of the HEVL and IR wavelengths, but not UV [91]. Whether EDGL has any significant impact on the skin at the standard reading distances recommended by the device manufacturers remains to be explored.

EDGL was also found to impact the cutaneous microbiome. Exposure to blue light from smartphones was shown to increase the growth of *Staphylococcus* aureus, a bacterium implicated in acne and similar inflammatory conditions. However, the distance from the smartphone in this study was 2–3 mm [90]. Smartphone and tablet exposure was also known to increase the generation of free radicals, up to 80% more than controls [50].

However, even without a UV component, EDGL is capable of eliciting pigmentation, due to the HEVL wavelengths. Duteil et al. demonstrated that compared to UV, HEVL-induced pigmentation was more persistent, lasting for even up to 3 months [7].

Indoor ambient lighting in the form of LEDs and CFLs also contributes significantly to light-induced skin damage. CFLs can emit light in the UVB, UVA, VL, and IR spectrum, and necessitate the use of sunscreens when CFLs are used extensively in indoor environments, particularly in the case of photosensitive individuals. LED indoor lighting may be a better option for people with photodermatoses compared to CFL, with the latter capable of generating more erythema on exposure at close quarters [92]. However, LED light sources have also been known to cause photodermatosis like solar urticaria [93]. Sun exposure is listed as one of the aggravating factors in the acne exposome [94–96].

2.8 Circadian Rhythm, the Skin and UVR

The day and night rhythm, also known as the circadian rhythm, is a 24-hour cycle, aligned on the sunset and sunrise, that modulates the physiological processes of all life on the planet. Though centrally located in the suprachiasmatic nucleus of the anterior hypothalamus, the circadian system involves modulation of peripheral tissues through neuronal and hormonal pathways, in response to environmental stimuli, predominantly by light incident on the retina. Interestingly, the skin is able to act independently of the central control of the circadian mechanism acting through core clock derived genes in the skin, which respond to light exposure, undergoing upregulation or downregulation. Autonomous clocks have been identified in keratinocytes, melanocytes, fibroblasts, mast cells, and hair follicle cells in human skin [97, 98]. Independently oscillating clock systems are thought to exist in the skin, namely the interfollicular epidermal clock, the hair follicle clock, dermal and adipose clocks, immune, vascular and neuronal clocks, and clocks of the pigment cell system of the skin.

The minimal erythema dose has been found to vary across different points in the circadian rhythm, implying an impact on the peripheral cutaneous clocks from UV exposure [99]. This independent clock system influenced by UVB appears to be disturbed in the process of cutaneous photocarcinogenesis and appears to be related to Vitamin D receptor signalling in the skin [100, 101]. While dysregulation of cutaneous clocks has been considered as capable of inducing cutaneous carcinogenesis, studies from nurses in night shift work have only found a reduction in skin cancer rates [97, 102].

Certain time periods over the day and night have been found to have differing levels of DNA repair. Accordingly, DNA repair happens mostly during the night and the early morning hours, and during the mid-day, the DNA repair of human skin is the lowest. Interestingly, this provides opportunities to develop skin care cosmeceuticals that can precisely sync with the cutaneous circadian rhythm. So, a daytime routine would predominantly be based on sunscreens which reduce the UVR dose to the skin, along with photostable antioxidants that promote DNA repair by UVR that endures despite sunscreen use. In the second half of the day, where the barrier permeability is the highest, night creams have both a higher chance of penetration and an avenue for enhanced DNA repair. It is also likely that the increased barrier permeability and moisture loss at night increases the chance for irritation from potentially harsh skin care products. The decreased DNA repair that occurs in the day may also reflect decreased overall cell proliferation in the skin, a factor determined by the interfollicular epidermal clock. The rhythmicity of natural circadian clock related skin repair mechanisms may be suppressed or altered by UV irradiation [97]. Physiological functions impacted by the circadian clock were summarized by Matsui et al., allowing an understanding of timing of product use in routine clinical recommendations, Fig. 2.8.

Clock genes triggered by light play a role in cutaneous ageing, and UV irradiation has been known to disrupt clock rhythm. Chronic disruption of sleep cycles and

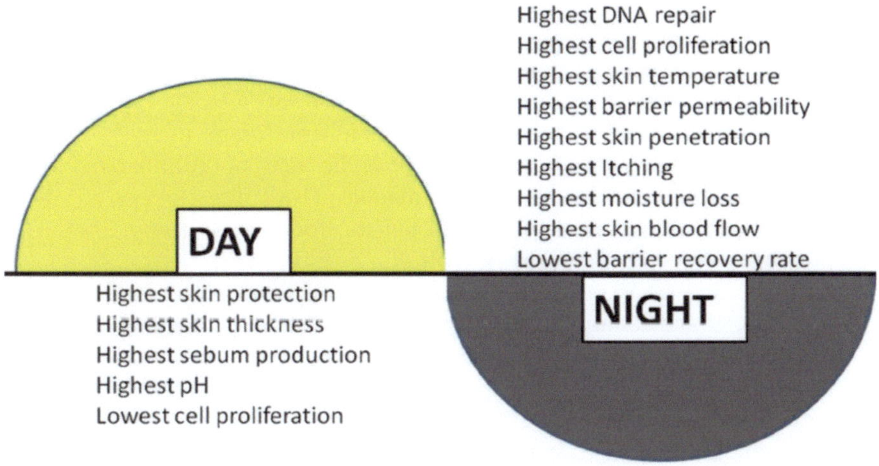

Fig. 2.8 The oscillation of human skin properties as they cycle through the day and night. For example, sebum production has been shown to be higher during the daytime that at night. Higher values for itch and moisture loss occur during the evening. Obtained from Matsui et al. [96], an open access article under the terms and conditions of the Creative Commons Attribution (CC-BY) license (http://creativecommons.org/licenses/by/4.0/) [96, 101]

shortened sleep time have been known to promote both ageing-induced hair loss and cutaneous ageing [97, 102]. Increased generation and accumulation of free radicals due to circadian rhythm disruption contribute to this ageing [97, 102].

Key Differences Between Lighter Skin Types and Skin of Colour

- Skin phototype (SPT) VI is said to have an MED that is 2–10 times higher than that of the lighter skin types I–III [103]. In more early studies in the 70s, the ratio of MED was pegged even higher at 33:1, for dark African skin to Caucasian skin, despite no differences in melanocyte number [104].
- The minimal erythema dose for skin type I is low, starting at 150 J/m^2, while the MED for skin type VI may go up to 600 J/m^2 [105]. Expressing this as standard erythemal dose (SED), this would translate to 1.5 SED for skin type I, to 6 SED for skin type VI, where 1 SED is equivalent to 100 J/m^2.
- Melanosomes are large and distributed singly in darker skin, while they are small, and contained within melanosome complexes in lighter skin types. More specifically, at sizes below 0.35 microns, the melanosomes were found to be present in membrane bound complexes [104]. The rate of degradation of melanosomes in keratinocytes of higher skin types is slower compared to that in keratinocytes in light skin. Darker skin is noted to have more, larger melanosomes, which are found to be dispersed evenly and

individually across all the layers of the epidermis [55]. The largest melanosomes were found to be present in those of Africa ancestry followed by those with Indian, Mexican, Chinese, and European ethnicities [106].

- More melanosomes in darker skin make it more prone to injury post-trauma and inflammation, explaining the higher rates of postinflammatory hyperpigmentation (PIH) in these individuals [106]. The chances of pigmentation with ablative laser resurfacing was found to be nearly 100% in skin type VI, compared to 20–30% in skin type III [107].
- SPF of skin type V and VI was found to be four times higher than that of skin type II, indicating an ability to filter out 75% of UVB, naturally! [108]
- The epidermal melanin barrier in light-skinned phototypes allows filters out only 76% of UVB and 45% of UVA, compared to an efficient filtering out of 92.6% of UVB and 82.5% of UVA in dark-skinned individuals [43].
- Pigmentation responses to HEVL are higher in SOC [7, 45].
- SOC has an increased contrast gloss of the skin [109].
- Photoageing in lighter skin types occurs with skin wrinkling and sagging, while uneven skin tone and focal hyperpigmentation is more common in SOC [55].
- Barrier integrity is higher in darker skin types due to increased structural integrity of the stratum corneum, compared to Asian skin, even within SOC [55].
- Melanocytes from light-skinned individuals show increased proliferative activity on UVB exposure. In contrast, SOC melanocytes exhibit protective differentiation resulting in increased melanogenesis [47].
- Differences in the skin also exist deeper to the epidermis, influenced by geographical ancestry. African skin was noted to have a thicker epidermis, a more convoluted dermoepidermal junction with deeper rete ridges compared to Eurasian and Far East Asian skin. African skin was also richer in fibrillar collagens, fibrillin rich microfibrils and fibulin-5, but contained lesser elastin. These differences underlie unique patterns of skin response to exposomal factors as well as to intrinsic influencers and certain dermatological conditions, between different ethnicities [110].

The differences in response to light in SOC mainly attributed to the density and distribution of melanin in pigmented skin since the presence of melanocytes is the same across phototypes for similar anatomical locations. Rijken et al. demonstrated the effects of similar physical doses of solar simulated radiation and evaluated the differences observed. They found that most of the solar simulated radiation (SSR) induced changes in White skin, such as dermal and epidermal DNA damage, increased cellular infiltrate with infiltrating neutrophils in the dermis, and infiltration of IL-10 positive cells into the epidermis, along with increased keratinocyte activation, and higher levels of elastase and matrix metalloproteinases, were not present in irradiated black skin. In the latter, there was evidence of DNA damage in the suprabasal layer of the epidermis, but the basal layer itself was found to be well protected [110]. One of the main observations is that the depth of DNA damage following sun exposure has been shown to vary between skin types here.

In a similar experiment by Fisher et al., photoadducts were noted in both the epidermis and the upper dermis of lighter skin, following SSR, while this damage was limited to the upper epidermis in darker skin. To address this, a higher level of sunscreen protection is recommended, specifically in terms of DNA protection. The DNA protection factor which measures the ability of a sunscreen to prevent the generation of cyclobutane pyrimidine dimers (CPD) and oxidized DNA bases on sun exposure, in protected versus unprotected skin, is recommended to be higher by a factor of 60, for lighter skin to achieve a similar level of protection, as in melanin rich darker skin [39, 111]. The Sun Protection Factor for DNA (DNA-SPF) is calculated by using specific DNA repair enzymes, and it is defined as the capacity for inhibiting the generation of CPD and oxidized DNA bases compared with unprotected control samples.

In addition to skin lightness as a concept of fairness, gloss as a skin attribute is widely prized among individuals with SOC, driven in some part due to social media promotions of 'glass skin'. Skin reflectance and its contrast to underlying skin tone, is considered as a sign of skin health. Ethnically, this contrast gloss was noted to be higher among South African and Indian women compared to Japanese, Chinese, and French women, by Voegeli et al. [109].

It is not new that behavioural constructs drive the skin care market. However, this is happening at an unprecedented level due to the combination of two major factors—social media and the selfie camera. The latter, made available due to the front facing camera technology, enables the use of image modifying filters which may enhance or change the skin tone, skin colour, facial features, eye colour to name a few. The availability of a social platform provides an audience for people to share these enhanced images for self-gratification, as measured by increased social acceptability in the form of engagement—likes, shares or equivalents. Expectations related to skin colour, skin ageing now have to be met with by the natural life cycle of the human organism, in a potentially losing battle [11].

2.9 Skin Colour Variability in India

Demography and migration, natural selection, and sexual selection are thought to play a major role in determining skin colour of populations.

In India, where skin colour is extremely varied among the different regions and ethnicities, Iliescu et al. found that social factors and population structure were more strongly implicated in determining skin colour compared to natural selection [112]. Considering that India has been inhabited since the Pleistocene era, the impact of several migration, admixtures, and population churn due to natural and political events, on skin colour in various states of India, is significant. The range of the melanin index, used in this study as one of the primary metrics, was found to be very high compared to melanin indices in other parts of the world. Within India, the range was 48.8 (30.1–78.9). For all of Europe, the range of the melanin index was less than 20 units. This wide range of skin colour was true not just for the entirety of the studied geographical locations within India (Andhra Pradesh, Telangana, Tamil Nadu, Uttar Pradesh, and Bihar), but even for intrapopulation assessments, the range of the melanin index was 30, compared to 10, within European populations. Ancestry, social status, endogamy, sexual selection for lighter skin, ongoing migratory patterns were factors noted to have a higher impact on skin colour, compared to UVR levels in the region, which could explain only 16% of the variation in skin colour. Furthermore, specific skin genotypes were not reliably associated with the corresponding skin colour phenotypes [112]. While this study is specific to India in many domains, these observations may eventually be applicable to the global scenario, thanks to advances in travel, changing social structures and geopolitical shifts which have made the intermixing of races very common now, than earlier in world history. In agreement, earlier work by Jonnalagadda et al. also noted a lack of a significant role for natural selection on skin colour, and a stronger impact of social hierarchy and endogamy on skin pigmentation based on data obtained from subjects in Maharashtra, central India [113]. Addition of a social class criterion significantly impacted the correlation between skin pigmentation phenotypes and genetic markers [114]. A more recent study from four North Indian states proposed factors like endogamy, unilateral sexual selection indicating a male preference for lighter than average-skinned women, culture driven clothing practices, to explain the observed gender impact on melanin and erythema indices [115]. Furthermore, the study observed an association between erythema index and geographical location and altitude, considering the terrain of the study location in Northern India along the foothills of the Himalayan Mountain range. The study subjects were required to be residents in the region for at least two generations, to ensure that the skin colour was representative of ethnic groups [115]. A larger impact of latitude on melanin index was observed by Sarkar et al., with higher melanin index at lower latitudes compared to other Indian regions further away from the equator, contributing to about 19% of the variance in skin colour. Chromosomal markers were found to have some association with phenotypes, contributing 17% to the observed variance in phenotypic skin colour [116].

Overall, it seems to be that social structure, endogamy, and cultural constructs have played a significant role in shaping the population structure of India, when it comes to skin colour, as denoted by the melanin index.

2.10 Cutaneous Microbiome and Photoprotection

The skin hosts a billion bacteria per square centimetre on its surface, usually living in homeostasis, and acting as a second cutaneous barrier to external agents. Multiple factors influence the balance between pathogens and beneficial commensals [20], including UV exposure, nutrition, skin pH, skin hygiene practices, temperature fluctuations, exposure to chemicals, pollution, stress levels, an intact skin barrier, and the health of the host [98]. For example, exposure to pollution in general and polycyclic aromatic hydrocarbons in particular, causes dysregulation of this ecosystem, with increased skin surface levels of Propionibacterium and Malassezia proportional to exposure to pollutants. The skin–gut axis also has feedback loops on the quantity and quality of the skin microbiota. The role of UVR is more nuanced. In conditions like atopic dermatitis, UVB therapy shifts the equation against the superantigen Staphylococcus aureus and promotes disease amelioration [20]. UVR exposure causes both immunosuppression, and protective alterations of cutaneous flora. Exposure to UVA and UVB was known to induce the increase of Cyanobacteria, as a protective mechanism as these organisms are known to possess an intrinsic resistance to UVR, through defence mechanisms including the production of antioxidant enzymes like superoxide dismutase and mycosporine like amino acids (MAA) which have UV absorbing abilities [117]. Interestingly, sunscreens have been known to preserve the cutaneous microbiome on UV exposure [118].

The existence and impact of a skin-gut axis in human health is well established. Recently, the effect of UVR on the gut microbiome has elicited significant interest [118]. Acting directly, or through the regulation of vitamin D synthesis in the skin, UVR exposure has been shown to have a significant impact on the gut flora. Neuroendocrine factors including cytokines, enkephalins, corticotropin releasing hormones, urocortins, and bioactive peptides with potential impact on multiple organ systems are known to be stimulated by UV exposure on skin [20]. Thus, it seems that the skin is capable of influencing gut health. The converse has always been known to be true. To illustrate, oral supplementation with probiotic lactobacillus johnsonii La1 strains was found to favourably influence the recovery from UV-induced immunosuppression, providing a systemic channel for photoprotection [118]. Probiotics are also commonly used in topical cosmetics. The use of probiotics in sunscreens for photoprotection is a recent concept.

2.11 Chapter Summary

Solar radiation exerts its effect on human skin, best understood as differential effects created by the various subcomponents of sunlight, specifically, UVR, VL, and IR. Depending on the depth of penetration and the mechanisms of injury triggered by each of these sub-spectra, the clinical outcomes vary from tanning to persistent pigmentation and from photoageing to photocarcinogenesis. Understanding the individual contributions of these wavelengths, especially in SOC, helps us elucidate the role of sunscreens in this population, more specifically and realistically.

References

1. (PDF) Assessment of anti-bacterial effect, anti-odour effect, UV-protection factor and xrd on formic acid treated modal and cotton fabric [Internet]. [cited 2024 Mar 3]. Available from: https://www.researchgate.net/publication/333419423_Assessment_of_anti-bacterial_effect_anti-_odoureffect_uv-protection_factor_and_xrd_on_formic_acid_treated_modal_and_cotton_fabric
2. Pizano-Andrade JC, Vargas-Guerrero B, Gurrola-Díaz CM, Vargas-Radillo JJ, Ruiz-López MA. Natural products and their mechanisms in potential photoprotection of the skin. J Biosci [Internet]. 2022 Dec 1 [cited 2024 Mar 3];47(4):1–14. Available from: https://link.springer.com/article/10.1007/s12038-022-00314-2
3. Green A, Williams G, Neale R, Hart V, Leslie D, Parsons P, et al. Daily sunscreen application and betacarotene supplementation in prevention of basal-cell and squamous-cell carcinomas of the skin: a randomised controlled trial. Lancet [Internet]. 1999 Aug 28 [cited 2024 Mar 3];354(9180):723–9. Available from: https://pubmed.ncbi.nlm.nih.gov/10475183/
4. Furukawa JY, Martinez RM, Morocho-Jácome AL, Castillo-Gómez TS, Pereda-Contreras VJ, Rosado C, et al. Skin impacts from exposure to ultraviolet, visible, infrared, and artificial lights–a review. J Cosmet Laser Ther. 2021;23(1–2):1–7.
5. Serpone N. Sunscreens and their usefulness: have we made any progress in the last two decades? Photochem Photobiol Sci. 2021 20:2 [Internet]. 2021 Feb 18 [cited 2024 Mar 3];20(2):189–244. Available from: https://link.springer.com/article/10.1007/s43630-021-00013-1
6. Maier T, Korting HC. Sunscreens—which and what for? Skin Pharmacol Physiol [Internet]. 2005 Nov [cited 2024 Mar 3];18(6):253–62. Available from: https://pubmed.ncbi.nlm.nih.gov/16113595/
7. Duteil L, Cardot-Leccia N, Queille-Roussel C, Maubert Y, Harmelin Y, Boukari F, et al. Differences in visible light-induced pigmentation according to wavelengths: a clinical and histological study in comparison with UVB exposure. Pigment Cell Melanoma Res [Internet]. 2014 [cited 2024 Mar 3];27(5):822–6. Available from: https://pubmed.ncbi.nlm.nih.gov/24888214/
8. Rai R, Shanmuga S, Srinivas CR. Update on photoprotection. Indian J Dermatol [Internet]. 2012 Sep [cited 2024 Mar 3];57(5):335–42. Available from: https://pubmed.ncbi.nlm.nih.gov/23112351/
9. Hedayat K, Nasrollahi SA, Firooz A, Rastegar H, Dadgarnejad M. Comparison of UVA protection factor measurement protocols. Clin Cosmet Investig Dermatol [Internet]. 2020 [cited 2024 Mar 3];13:351. Available from: /pmc/articles/PMC7244352/
10. Kollias N, Ruvolo E, Sayre RM. The value of the ratio of UVA to UVB in sunlight. Photochem Photobiol [Internet]. 2011 Nov 1 [cited 2024 Mar 3];87(6):1474–5. Available from: https://onlinelibrary.wiley.com/doi/full/10.1111/j.1751-1097.2011.00980.x
11. Matts PJ, Nash JF. Sunscreens—another endangered species? Int J Cosmet Sci [Internet]. 2023 Oct 1 [cited 2024 Mar 3];45 Suppl 1(S1):20–32. Available from: https://pubmed.ncbi.nlm.nih.gov/37799079/
12. Balasaraswathy P, Kumar U, Srinivas C, Nair S. UVA and UVB in sunlight, optimal utilization of UV rays in Sunlight for phototherapy. Indian J Dermatol Venereol Leprol [Internet]. 2002 Jul 1 [cited 2024 Mar 3];68(4):198. Available from: https://ijdvl.com/uva-and-uvb-in-sunlight-optimal-utilization-of-uv-rays-in-sunlight-for-phototherapy/
13. Marionnet C, de Dormael R, Marat X, Roudot A, Gizard J, Planel E, et al. Sunscreens with the new MCE filter cover the whole UV spectrum: improved UVA1 photoprotection in vitro and in a randomized controlled trial. JID Innov [Internet]. 2021 Jan 1 [cited 2024 Mar 3];2(1). Available from: https://pubmed.ncbi.nlm.nih.gov/35072138/
14. Krutmann J, Bouloc A, Sore G, Bernard BA, Passeron T. The skin aging exposome. J Dermatol Sci [Internet]. 2017 Mar 1 [cited 2024 Apr 7];85(3):152–61. Available from: https://pubmed.ncbi.nlm.nih.gov/27720464/

15. Egambaram OP, Kesavan Pillai S, Ray SS. Materials science challenges in skin UV protection: a review. Photochem Photobiol [Internet]. 2020 Jul 1 [cited 2024 Mar 3];96(4):779–97. Available from: https://pubmed.ncbi.nlm.nih.gov/31886889/
16. Stiefel C, Schwack W. Photoprotection in changing times—UV filter efficacy and safety, sensitization processes and regulatory aspects. Int J Cosmet Sci [Internet]. 2015 Feb 1 [cited 2024 Mar 3];37(1):2–30. Available from: https://onlinelibrary.wiley.com/doi/full/10.1111/ics.12165
17. Shetty N, Schalka S, Lim HW, Mohammad TF. The effects of UV filters on health and the environment. Photochem Photobiol Sci [Internet]. 2023 Oct 1 [cited 2024 Mar 3];22(10):2463–71. Available from: https://pubmed.ncbi.nlm.nih.gov/37344707/
18. Amaro-Ortiz A, Yan B, D'Orazio JA. Ultraviolet radiation, aging and the skin: prevention of damage by topical cAMP manipulation. Molecules [Internet]. 2014 [cited 2024 Mar 3];19(5):6202. Available from: https://www.ncbi.nlm.nih.gov/pmc/articles/PMC4344124/
19. Sklar LR, Almutawa F, Lim HW, Hamzavi I. Effects of ultraviolet radiation, visible light, and infrared radiation on erythema and pigmentation: a review. Photochem Photobiol Sci [Internet]. 2013 [cited 2024 Mar 3];12(1):54–64. Available from: https://pubmed.ncbi.nlm.nih.gov/23111621/
20. Rai S, Rai G, Kumar A. Eco-evolutionary impact of ultraviolet radiation (UVR) exposure on microorganisms, with a special focus on our skin microbiome. Microbiol Res [Internet]. 2022 Jul 1 [cited 2024 Mar 3];260. Available from: https://pubmed.ncbi.nlm.nih.gov/35483310/
21. Zastrow L, Groth N, Klein F, Kockott D, Lademann J, Renneberg R, et al. The missing link--light-induced (280-1,600 nm) free radical formation in human skin. Skin Pharmacol Physiol [Internet]. 2009 Jan [cited 2024 Mar 3];22(1):31–44. Available from: https://pubmed.ncbi.nlm.nih.gov/19122479/
22. Ash C, Dubec M, Donne K, Bashford T. Effect of wavelength and beam width on penetration in light-tissue interaction using computational methods. Lasers Med Sci [Internet]. 2017 Nov 1 [cited 2024 Mar 3];32(8):1909. Available from: https://pubmed.ncbi.nlm.nih.gov/28900751/
23. Parisi A V., Turnbull DJ, Kimlin MG. Influence of solar UVA on erythemal irradiances. Phys Med Biol [Internet]. 2006 Jun 21 [cited 2024 Mar 3];51(12):3241–9. Available from: https://pubmed.ncbi.nlm.nih.gov/16757874/
24. Marionnet C, Piffaut V, Sasai J, Jouni H, Nouveau S, Roudot A, et al. A precise analysis of the relative contribution of UVA1 and visible light colour domains in solar light-induced skin pigmentation. J Eur Acad Dermatol Venereol [Internet]. 2023 Apr 1 [cited 2024 Mar 3];37 Suppl 4(S4):3–11. Available from: https://pubmed.ncbi.nlm.nih.gov/36994912/
25. Pantelic MN, Wong N, Kwa M, Lim HW. Ultraviolet filters in the United States and European Union: a review of safety and implications for the future of US sunscreens. J Am Acad Dermatol [Internet]. 2023 Mar 1 [cited 2024 Mar 3];88(3):632–46. Available from: https://pubmed.ncbi.nlm.nih.gov/36442641/
26. Ezekwe N, Maghfour J, Kohli I. Visible light and the skin. Photochem Photobiol [Internet]. 2022 Nov 1 [cited 2024 Mar 3];98(6):1264–9. Available from: https://onlinelibrary.wiley.com/doi/full/10.1111/php.13634
27. Kohli I, Nahhas AF, Braunberger TL, Chaowattanapanit S, Mohammad TF, Nicholson CL, et al. Spectral characteristics of visible light-induced pigmentation and visible light protection factor. Photodermatol Photoimmunol Photomed [Internet]. 2019 Nov 1 [cited 2024 Mar 3];35(6):393–9. Available from: https://pubmed.ncbi.nlm.nih.gov/31152612/
28. Aguilera J, Gracia-Cazaña T, Gilaberte Y. New developments in sunscreens. Photochem Photobiol Sci [Internet]. 2023 Oct 1 [cited 2024 Mar 3];22(10):2473–82. Available from: https://pubmed.ncbi.nlm.nih.gov/37543534/
29. Hiramoto K, Kubo S, Tsuji K, Sugiyama D, Hamano H. Induction of skin cancer by long-term blue light irradiation. Biomedicines [Internet]. 2023 Aug 1 [cited 2024 Mar 3];11(8). Available from: https://www.ncbi.nlm.nih.gov/pmc/articles/PMC10452187/

30. Liebel F, Kaur S, Ruvolo E, Kollias N, Southall MD. Irradiation of skin with visible light induces reactive oxygen species and matrix-degrading enzymes. J Invest Dermatol [Internet]. 2012 [cited 2024 Mar 3];132(7):1901–7. Available from: https://pubmed.ncbi.nlm.nih.gov/22318388/
31. Kollias N, Baqer A. An experimental study of the changes in pigmentation in human skin in vivo with visible and near infrared light. Photochem Photobiol [Internet]. 1984 [cited 2024 Mar 3];39(5):651–9. Available from: https://pubmed.ncbi.nlm.nih.gov/6739557/
32. Cutaneous photoprotection: a review of the current status and evolving strategies—PubMed [Internet]. [cited 2024 Mar 26]. Available from: https://pubmed.ncbi.nlm.nih.gov/32226337/
33. González S, Aguilera J, Berman B, Calzavara-Pinton P, Gilaberte Y, Goh CL, et al. Expert Recommendations on the evaluation of sunscreen efficacy and the beneficial role of non-filtering ingredients. Front Med (Lausanne). 2022;9:790207.
34. Reichrath J, Lehmann B, Carlberg C, Varani J, Zouboulis CC. Vitamins as hormones. Horm Metab Res [Internet]. 2007 Feb [cited 2024 Mar 3];39(2):71–84. Available from: https://pubmed.ncbi.nlm.nih.gov/17326003/
35. Berry EG, Bezecny J, Acton M, Sulmonetti TP, Anderson DM, Beckham HW, et al. Slip versus slop: a head-to-head comparison of UV-protective clothing to sunscreen. Cancers (Basel) [Internet]. 2022 Feb 1 [cited 2024 Mar 3];14(3):542. Available from: https://www.mdpi.com/2072-6694/14/3/542/htm
36. Bykov VJ, Sheehan JM, Hemminki K, Young AR. In situ repair of cyclobutane pyrimidine dimers and 6–4 photoproducts in human skin exposed to solar simulating radiation. J Invest Dermatol. 1999;112(3):326–31.
37. Swope VB, Abdel-Malek ZA. MC1R: front and center in the bright side of dark eumelanin and DNA repair. Int J Mol Sci [Internet]. 2018 Sep 8 [cited 2024 Mar 11];19(9). Available from: https://www.ncbi.nlm.nih.gov/pmc/articles/PMC6163888/
38. Schuch AP, Lago JC, Yagura T, Menck CFM. DNA dosimetry assessment for sunscreen genotoxic photoprotection. PLoS One [Internet]. 2012 Jun 29 [cited 2024 Mar 3];7(6). Available from: https://pubmed.ncbi.nlm.nih.gov/22768281/
39. Ito S, Wakamatsu K, Sarna T. Photodegradation of eumelanin and pheomelanin and its pathophysiological implications. Photochem Photobiol [Internet]. 2018 May 1 [cited 2024 Mar 3];94(3):409–20. Available from: https://onlinelibrary.wiley.com/doi/full/10.1111/php.12837
40. Jesus A, Sousa E, Cruz MT, Cidade H, Lobo JMS, Almeida IF. UV filters: challenges and prospects. Pharmaceuticals [Internet]. 2022 Mar 1 [cited 2024 Mar 3];15(3). Available from: https://www.ncbi.nlm.nih.gov/pmc/articles/PMC8955451/
41. Wenczl E, Van Der Schans GP, Roza L, Kolb RM, Timmerman AJ, Smit NPM, et al. (Pheo) melanin photosensitizes UVA-induced DNA damage in cultured human melanocytes. J Invest Dermatol [Internet]. 1998 [cited 2024 Mar 3];111(4):678–82. Available from: https://pubmed.ncbi.nlm.nih.gov/9764853/
42. Brenner M, Hearing VJ. The protective role of melanin against UV damage in human skin. Photochem Photobiol [Internet]. 2008 May [cited 2024 Mar 2];84(3):539. Available from: /pmc/articles/PMC2671032/
43. Fajuyigbe D, Douki T, van Dijk A, Sarkany RPE, Young AR. Dark cyclobutane pyrimidine dimers are formed in the epidermis of Fitzpatrick skin types I/II and VI in vivo after exposure to solar-simulated radiation. Pigment Cell Melanoma Res [Internet]. 2021 May 1 [cited 2024 Mar 3];34(3):575–84. Available from: https://pubmed.ncbi.nlm.nih.gov/33369222/
44. Randhawa M, Seo IS, Liebel F, Southall MD, Kollias N, Ruvolo E. Visible light induces melanogenesis in human skin through a photoadaptive response. PLoS One [Internet]. 2015 Jun 29 [cited 2024 Mar 3];10(6). Available from: https://pubmed.ncbi.nlm.nih.gov/26121474/
45. Sheehan JM, Cragg N, Chadwick CA, Potten CS, Young AR. Repeated ultraviolet exposure affords the same protection against DNA photodamage and erythema in human skin types II and IV but is associated with faster DNA repair in skin type IV. J Invest Dermatol [Internet]. 2002 [cited 2024 Mar 3];118(5):825–9. Available from: https://pubmed.ncbi.nlm.nih.gov/11982760/

46. López S, Alonso S, García de Galdeano A, Smith-Zubiaga I. Melanocytes from dark and light skin respond differently after ultraviolet B irradiation: effect of keratinocyte-conditioned medium. Photodermatol Photoimmunol Photomed [Internet]. 2015 May 1 [cited 2024 Mar 3];31(3):149–58. Available from: https://onlinelibrary.wiley.com/doi/full/10.1111/phpp.12169
47. Zastrow L, Meinke MC, Albrecht S, Patzelt A, Lademann J. From UV protection to protection in the whole spectral range of the solar radiation: new aspects of sunscreen development. Adv Exp Med Biol [Internet]. 2017 [cited 2024 Mar 3];996:311–8. Available from: https://pubmed.ncbi.nlm.nih.gov/29124711/
48. Herrling T, Jung K, Fuchs J. Measurements of UV-generated free radicals/reactive oxygen species (ROS) in skin. Spectrochim Acta A Mol Biomol Spectrosc [Internet]. 2006 Mar 13 [cited 2024 Mar 3];63(4):840–5. Available from: https://pubmed.ncbi.nlm.nih.gov/16543118/
49. Herrling T, Jung K. The Radical Status Factor (RSF): a novel metric to characterize skin products. Int J Cosmet Sci [Internet]. 2012 [cited 2024 Mar 3];34(4):285–90. Available from: https://pubmed.ncbi.nlm.nih.gov/22563768/
50. Mahmoud BH, Ruvolo E, Hexsel CL, Liu Y, Owen MR, Kollias N, et al. Impact of long-wavelength UVA and visible light on melanocompetent skin. J Invest Dermatol [Internet]. 2010 Aug [cited 2024 Mar 3];130(8):2092–7. Available from: https://pubmed.ncbi.nlm.nih.gov/20410914/
51. Zastrow L, Doucet O, Ferrero L, Groth N, Klein F, Kockott D, et al. Free radical threshold value: a new universal body constant. Skin Pharmacol Physiol [Internet]. 2015 Aug 20 [cited 2024 Mar 3];28(5):264–8. Available from: https://pubmed.ncbi.nlm.nih.gov/26227304/
52. Lohan SB, Ivanov D, Schüler N, Berger B, Zastrow L, Lademann J, et al. Switching from healthy to unhealthy oxidative stress—does the radical type can be used as an indicator? Free Radic Biol Med. 2021;162:401–11.
53. Tsai J, Chien AL. Photoprotection for skin of color. Am J Clin Dermatol [Internet]. 2022 Mar 1 [cited 2024 Mar 3];23(2):195. Available from: https://www.ncbi.nlm.nih.gov/pmc/articles/PMC8766623/
54. Rawlings A V. Ethnic skin types: are there differences in skin structure and function?1. Int J Cosmet Sci [Internet]. 2006 Apr 1 [cited 2024 Mar 3];28(2):79–93. Available from: https://onlinelibrary.wiley.com/doi/full/10.1111/j.1467-2494.2006.00302.x
55. Welti M, Ramelyte E, Dummer R, Imhof L. Evaluation of the minimal erythema dose for UVB and UVA in context of skin phototype and nature of photodermatosis. Photodermatol Photoimmunol Photomed [Internet]. 2020 May 1 [cited 2024 Mar 3];36(3):200–7. Available from: https://pubmed.ncbi.nlm.nih.gov/32027041/
56. Wong LC, Jamil A, Md Nor N. The effect of pre-phototest sun exposure on minimal erythema dose and minimal melanogenic dose among skin phototypes III, IV and V. Photodermatol Photoimmunol Photomed [Internet]. 2018 Nov 1 [cited 2024 Mar 3];34(6):400–4. Available from: https://pubmed.ncbi.nlm.nih.gov/29953669/
57. Leenutaphong V. Relationship between skin color and cutaneous response to ultraviolet radiation in Thai. Photodermatol Photoimmunol Photomed [Internet]. 1995 [cited 2024 Mar 3];11(5–6):198–203. Available from: https://pubmed.ncbi.nlm.nih.gov/8738714/
58. Valbuena Mesa MC, Nova Villanueva JA, Sánchez Vanegas G. minimal erythema dose: correlation with Fitzpatrick skin type and concordance between methods of erythema assessment in a patient sample in Colombia. Actas Dermosifiliogr [Internet]. 2020 Jun [cited 2024 Mar 4];111(5):390–7. Available from: https://pubmed.ncbi.nlm.nih.gov/32408973/
59. [Determination of the minimal erythema dosage and natural photoprotection of the skin in the population]—PubMed [Internet]. [cited 2024 Mar 4]. Available from: https://pubmed.ncbi.nlm.nih.gov/10103166/
60. Ferriols AP, Aguilera J, Aguilera P, De Argila D, Barnadas MA, De Cabo X, et al. Determination of minimal erythema dose and anomalous reactions to UVA radiation by skin phototype. Actas Dermosifiliogr [Internet]. 2014 [cited 2024 Mar 4];105(8):780–8. Available from: https://pubmed.ncbi.nlm.nih.gov/24996228/

61. Westerhof W, Estevez-Uscanga O, Meens J, Kammeyer A, Durocq M, Cario I. The relation between constitutional skin color and photosensitivity estimated from UV-induced erythema and pigmentation dose-response curves. J Invest Dermatol [Internet]. 1990 [cited 2024 Mar 4];94(6):812–6. Available from: https://pubmed.ncbi.nlm.nih.gov/2355184/
62. Coelho SG, Choi W, Brenner M, Miyamura Y, Yamaguchi Y, Wolber R, et al. Short- and long-term effects of ultraviolet radiation on the pigmentation of human skin. The journal of investigative dermatology Symposium proceedings/the Society for Investigative Dermatology, Inc [and] European Society for Dermatological Research [Internet]. 2009 [cited 2024 Mar 2];14(1):32. Available from: https://www.ncbi.nlm.nih.gov/pmc/articles/PMC2799903/
63. Moyal D. Prevention of ultraviolet-induced skin pigmentation. Photodermatol Photoimmunol Photomed [Internet]. 2004 Oct [cited 2024 Mar 4];20(5):243–7. Available from: https://pubmed.ncbi.nlm.nih.gov/15379874/
64. de Gálvez EN, Aguilera J, Solis A, de Gálvez MV, de Andrés JR, Herrera-Ceballos E, et al. The potential role of UV and blue light from the sun, artificial lighting, and electronic devices in melanogenesis and oxidative stress. J Photochem Photobiol B [Internet]. 2022 Mar 1 [cited 2024 Mar 4];228. Available from: https://pubmed.ncbi.nlm.nih.gov/35189578/
65. Immediate pigment darkening: description, kinetic and biological function—PubMed [Internet]. [cited 2024 Mar 4]. Available from: https://pubmed.ncbi.nlm.nih.gov/10066954/
66. Yardman-Frank JM, Fisher DE. Skin pigmentation and its control: from ultraviolet radiation to stem cells. Exp Dermatol [Internet]. 2021 Apr 1 [cited 2024 Mar 4];30(4):560–71. Available from: https://pubmed.ncbi.nlm.nih.gov/33320376/
67. Ramasubramaniam R, Roy A, Sharma B, Nagalakshmi S. Are there mechanistic differences between ultraviolet and visible radiation induced skin pigmentation? Photochem Photobiol Sci [Internet]. 2011 [cited 2024 Mar 4];10(12):1887–93. Available from: https://pubmed.ncbi.nlm.nih.gov/21993454/
68. Regazzetti C, Sormani L, Debayle D, Bernerd F, Tulic MK, De Donatis GM, et al. Melanocytes sense blue light and regulate pigmentation through opsin-3. J Invest Dermatol [Internet]. 2018 Jan 1 [cited 2024 Mar 4];138(1):171–8. Available from: https://pubmed.ncbi.nlm.nih.gov/28842328/
69. Kang HY, Lee JW, Papaccio F, Bellei B, Picardo M. Alterations of the pigmentation system in the aging process. Pigment Cell Melanoma Res [Internet]. 2021 Jul 1 [cited 2024 Mar 5];34(4):800–813. Available from: https://onlinelibrary.wiley.com/doi/full/10.1111/pcmr.12994
70. Coelho SG, Zhou Y, Bushar HF, Miller SA, Zmudzka BZ, Hearing VJ, et al. Long-Lasting Pigmentation (LLP) of Human Skin, a New Look at an Overlooked Response to UV. Pigment Cell Melanoma Res [Internet]. 2009 Apr [cited 2024 Mar 4];22(2):238. Available from: /pmc/articles/PMC2709973/
71. Coelho SG, Valencia JC, Yin L, Smuda C, Mahns A, Kolbe L, et al. UV exposure modulates hemidesmosome plasticity, contributing to long-term pigmentation in human skin. J Pathol [Internet]. 2015 May 1 [cited 2024 Mar 4];236(1):17–29. Available from: https://pubmed.ncbi.nlm.nih.gov/25488118/
72. Jablonski NG, Chaplin G. The colours of humanity: the evolution of pigmentation in the human lineage. Philos Trans R Soc B Biol Sci [Internet]. 2017 [cited 2024 Mar 2];372(1724). Available from: https://royalsocietypublishing.org/doi/10.1098/rstb.2016.0349
73. Lawrence KP, Sarkany RPE, Acker S, Herzog B, Young AR. A new visible light absorbing organic filter offers superior protection against pigmentation by wavelengths at the UVR-visible boundary region. J Photochem Photobiol B. 2022;227:112372.
74. Wulf HC, Sandby-Møller J, Kobayasi T, Gniadecki R. Skin aging and natural photoprotection. Micron [Internet]. 2004 [cited 2024 Mar 4];35(3):185–91. Available from: https://pubmed.ncbi.nlm.nih.gov/15036273/
75. Li YW, Chu CY. The minimal erythema dose of broadband ultraviolet B in Taiwanese. J Formos Med Assoc [Internet]. 2007 [cited 2024 Mar 4];106(11):975–8. Available from: https://pubmed.ncbi.nlm.nih.gov/18063522/

76. Campiche R, Curpen SJ, Lutchmanen-Kolanthan V, Gougeon S, Cherel M, Laurent G, et al. Pigmentation effects of blue light irradiation on skin and how to protect against them. Int J Cosmet Sci [Internet]. 2020 Aug 1 [cited 2024 Mar 4];42(4):399–406. Available from: https://onlinelibrary.wiley.com/doi/full/10.1111/ics.12637
77. Kumari J, Das K, Babaei M, Rokni GR, Goldust M. The impact of blue light and digital screens on the skin. J Cosmet Dermatol [Internet]. 2023 Apr 1 [cited 2024 Mar 4];22(4):1185–90. Available from: https://pubmed.ncbi.nlm.nih.gov/36594795/
78. Mpofana N, Abrahamse H. The management of melasma on skin types V and VI using light emitting diode treatment. Photomed Laser Surg [Internet]. 2018 Oct 1 [cited 2024 Mar 4];36(10):522–9. Available from: https://pubmed.ncbi.nlm.nih.gov/30227084/
79. Oh CT, Kwon TR, Choi EJ, Kim SR, Seok J, Mun SK, et al. Inhibitory effect of 660-nm LED on melanin synthesis in in vitro and in vivo. Photodermatol Photoimmunol Photomed [Internet]. 2017 Jan 1 [cited 2024 Mar 4];33(1):49–57. Available from: https://pubmed.ncbi.nlm.nih.gov/27696509/
80. Passeron T, Zouboulis CC, Tan J, Andersen ML, Katta R, Lyu X, et al. Adult skin acute stress responses to short-term environmental and internal aggression from exposome factors. J Eur Acad Dermatol Venereol [Internet]. 2021 Oct 1 [cited 2024 Mar 4];35(10):1963–1975. Available from: https://pubmed.ncbi.nlm.nih.gov/34077579/
81. Espósito ACC, Cassiano DP, da Silva CN, Lima PB, Dias JAF, Hassun K, et al. Update on Melasma-part I: pathogenesis. Dermatol Ther (Heidelb) [Internet]. 2022 Sep 1 [cited 2024 Mar 4];12(9):1967–88. Available from: https://pubmed.ncbi.nlm.nih.gov/35904706/
82. Rosen CF, Jacques SL, Stuart ME, Gange RW. Immediate pigment darkening: visual and reflectance spectrophotometric analysis of action spectrum. Photochem Photobiol [Internet]. 1990 May 1 [cited 2024 Mar 4];51(5):583–8. Available from: https://onlinelibrary.wiley.com/doi/full/10.1111/j.1751-1097.1990.tb01969.x
83. Lim HW, Kohli I, Granger C, Trullàs C, Piquero-Casals J, Narda M, et al. Photoprotection of the skin from visible light–induced pigmentation: current testing methods and proposed harmonization. J Invest Dermatol [Internet]. 2021 Nov 1 [cited 2024 Mar 23];141(11):2569–76. Available from: https://pubmed.ncbi.nlm.nih.gov/34112516/
84. Ceresnie MS, Patel J, Lim HW, Kohli I. The cutaneous effects of blue light from electronic devices: a systematic review with health hazard identification. Photochem Photobiol Sci [Internet]. 2023 Feb 1 [cited 2024 Mar 4];22(2):457–64. Available from: https://pubmed.ncbi.nlm.nih.gov/36245016/
85. Bhatia N, Mesinkovska NA, Samolitis N, Soon S, Steele T, Enright KM. Knowledge, perceptions and photoprotective behaviors against the damaging effects of direct, indirect, and blue light: there are no “cheat days.” J Clin Aesthet Dermatol [Internet]. 2022 Aug 1 [cited 2024 Mar 4];15(8):E61. Available from: https://www.ncbi.nlm.nih.gov/pmc/articles/PMC9436221/
86. Wild CP. Complementing the genome with an “exposome”: the outstanding challenge of environmental exposure measurement in molecular epidemiology. Cancer Epidemiol Biomarkers Prev [Internet]. 2005 Aug [cited 2024 Mar 4];14(8):1847–50. Available from: https://pubmed.ncbi.nlm.nih.gov/16103423/
87. Peters A, Hoek G, Katsouyanni K. Understanding the link between environmental exposures and health: does the exposome promise too much? J Epidemiol Community Health (1978) [Internet]. 2012 Feb [cited 2024 Mar 4];66(2):103–5. Available from: https://pubmed.ncbi.nlm.nih.gov/22080817/
88. Cassiano DP, Espósito ACC, da Silva CN, Lima PB, Dias JAF, Hassun K, et al. Update on melasma-part II: treatment. Dermatol Ther (Heidelb) [Internet]. 2022 Sep 1 [cited 2024 Mar 14];12(9):1989–2012. Available from: https://pubmed.ncbi.nlm.nih.gov/35906506/
89. Light pollution—Wikipedia [Internet]. [cited 2024 Mar 4]. Available from: https://en.wikipedia.org/wiki/Light_pollution
90. Exposure to visible light emitted from smartphones and tablets increases the proliferation of staphylococcus aureus: can this be linked to acne?—PubMed [Internet]. [cited 2024 Mar 4]. Available from: https://pubmed.ncbi.nlm.nih.gov/28580338/

91. Austin E, Huang A, Adar T, Wang E, Jagdeo J. Electronic device generated light increases reactive oxygen species in human fibroblasts. Lasers Surg Med [Internet]. 2018 Aug 1 [cited 2024 Mar 3];50(6):689–95. Available from: https://pubmed.ncbi.nlm.nih.gov/29399830/
92. Montaudié H, Lacour JP, Rostain G, Duteil L, Passeron T. Solar urticaria to visible light triggered by light-emitting diode therapy. J Am Acad Dermatol [Internet]. 2014 Sep 1 [cited 2024 Mar 4];71(3):e74–5. Available from: http://www.jaad.org/article/S0190962214010494/fulltext
93. Piquero-Casals J, Morgado-Carrasco D, Rozas-Muñoz E, Mir-Bonafé JF, Trullàs C, Jourdan E, et al. Sun exposure, a relevant exposome factor in acne patients and how photoprotection can improve outcomes. J Cosmet Dermatol [Internet]. 2023 Jun 1 [cited 2024 Mar 4];22(6):1919–28. Available from: https://pubmed.ncbi.nlm.nih.gov/36946555/
94. Dreno B, Shourick J, Kerob D, Bouloc A, Taïeb C. The role of exposome in acne: results from an international patient survey. J Eur Acad Dermatol Venereol [Internet]. 2020 May 1 [cited 2024 Mar 4];34(5):1057–64. Available from: https://pubmed.ncbi.nlm.nih.gov/31785166/
95. Dréno B, Bettoli V, Araviiskaia E, Sanchez Viera M, Bouloc A. The influence of exposome on acne. J Eur Acad Dermatol Venereol [Internet]. 2018 May 1 [cited 2024 Mar 4];32(5):812–9. Available from: https://pubmed.ncbi.nlm.nih.gov/29377341/
96. Matsui MS, Pelle E, Dong K, Pernodet N. Biological Rhythms in the Skin. Int J Mol Sci [Internet]. 2016 Jun 1 [cited 2024 Mar 4];17(6):801. Available from: https://www.ncbi.nlm.nih.gov/pmc/articles/PMC4926335/
97. Plikus M V., Van Spyk EN, Pham K, Geyfman M, Kumar V, Takahashi JS, et al. The circadian clock in skin: implications for adult stem cells, tissue regeneration, cancer, aging, and immunity. J Biol Rhythms [Internet]. 2015 Jun 4 [cited 2024 Mar 4];30(3):163–82. Available from: https://pubmed.ncbi.nlm.nih.gov/25589491/
98. Damiani G, Pacifico A, Scoditti E, di Gregorio S, Del Fabbro M, Cozzolino C, et al. Circadian oscillations of minimal erythema dose (MED) are also influenced by diet in patients with psoriasis: a chronomedical study. Dermatol Ther (Heidelb) [Internet]. 2023 Oct 1 [cited 2024 Mar 4];13(10):2229–46. Available from: https://pubmed.ncbi.nlm.nih.gov/37573289/
99. Lamnis L, Christofi C, Stark A, Palm H, Roemer K, Vogt T, et al. Differential regulation of circadian clock genes by UV-B radiation and 1,25-dihydroxyvitamin D: a pilot study during different stages of skin photocarcinogenesis. Nutrients [Internet]. 2024 Jan 1 [cited 2024 Mar 4];16(2). Available from: https://pubmed.ncbi.nlm.nih.gov/38257148/
100. Sun Y, Wang P, Li H, Dai J. BMAL1 and CLOCK proteins in regulating UVB-induced apoptosis and DNA damage responses in human keratinocytes. J Cell Physiol [Internet]. 2018 Dec 1 [cited 2024 Mar 4];233(12):9563–74. Available from: https://pubmed.ncbi.nlm.nih.gov/29943823/
101. Heckman CJ, Kloss JD, Feskanich D, Culnan E, Schernhammer ES. Associations among rotating night shift work, sleep and skin cancer in Nurses' Health Study II participants. Occup Environ Med [Internet]. 2017 Mar 1 [cited 2024 Mar 4];74(3):169–75. Available from: https://pubmed.ncbi.nlm.nih.gov/27663986/
102. Fajuyigbe D, Young AR. The impact of skin colour on human photobiological responses. Pigment Cell Melanoma Res [Internet]. 2016 Nov 1 [cited 2024 Mar 2];29(6):607–618. Available from: https://pubmed.ncbi.nlm.nih.gov/27454804/
103. Skin color, melanin, and erythema—PubMed [Internet]. [cited 2024 Mar 4]. Available from: https://pubmed.ncbi.nlm.nih.gov/4745289/
104. Diffey BL, Jansen CT, Urbach F, Wulf HC, Morison WL. The standard erythema dose: a new photobiological concept. Photodermatol Photoimmunol Photomed [Internet]. 1997 [cited 2024 Mar 4];13(1–2):64–6. Available from: https://pubmed.ncbi.nlm.nih.gov/9361131/
105. Alaluf S, Atkins D, Barrett K, Blount M, Carter N, Heath A. Ethnic variation in melanin content and composition in photoexposed and photoprotected human skin. Pigment Cell Res [Internet]. 2002 [cited 2024 Mar 8];15(2):112–8. Available from: https://pubmed.ncbi.nlm.nih.gov/11936268/

106. Goldman MP. Universal classification of skin type. Simplified Facial Rejuvenation [Internet]. 2008 [cited 2024 Mar 5];47–50. Available from: https://link.springer.com/chapter/10.1007/978-3-540-71097-4_3
107. MA P, DL F. Photobiology of melanin pigmentation: dose/response of skin to sunlight and its contents. J Am Acad Dermatol [Internet]. 1983 [cited 2024 Mar 4];9(5):724–33. Available from: https://pubmed.ncbi.nlm.nih.gov/6358278/
108. Voegeli R, Campiche R, Biassin R, Rawlings A V., Shackelford TK, Fink B. Predictors of female age, health and attractiveness perception from skin feature analysis of digital portraits in five ethnic groups. Int J Cosmet Sci [Internet]. 2023 Oct 1 [cited 2024 Mar 5];45(5):672–687. Available from: https://pubmed.ncbi.nlm.nih.gov/37338195/
109. Langton AK, Sherratt MJ, Sellers WI, Griffiths CEM, Watson REB. Geographical ancestry is a key determinant of epidermal morphology and dermal composition. Br J Dermatol [Internet]. 2014 Aug 1 [cited 2024 Mar 5];171(2):274–82. Available from: https://pubmed.ncbi.nlm.nih.gov/24484315/
110. Rijken F, Bruijnzeel PLB, Van Weelden H, Kiekens RCM. Responses of black and white skin to solar-simulating radiation: differences in DNA photodamage, infiltrating neutrophils, proteolytic enzymes induced, keratinocyte activation, and IL-10 expression. J Invest Dermatol. 2004;122(6):1448–55.
111. Iliescu FM, Chaplin G, Rai N, Jacobs GS, Basu Mallick C, Mishra A, et al. The influences of genes, the environment, and social factors on the evolution of skin color diversity in India. Am J Hum Biol [Internet]. 2018 Sep 1 [cited 2024 Mar 5];30(5). Available from: https://pubmed.ncbi.nlm.nih.gov/30099804/
112. Jonnalagadda M, Ozarkar S, Ashma R, Kulkarni S. Skin pigmentation variation among populations of West Maharashtra, India. Am J Hum Biol [Internet]. 2016 Jan 1 [cited 2024 Mar 5];28(1):36–43. Available from: https://pubmed.ncbi.nlm.nih.gov/26126512/
113. Jonnalagadda M, Norton H, Ozarkar S, Kulkarni S, Ashma R. Association of genetic variants with skin pigmentation phenotype among populations of west Maharashtra, India. Am J Hum Biol [Internet]. 2016 Sep 10 [cited 2024 Mar 5];28(5):610–8. Available from: https://pubmed.ncbi.nlm.nih.gov/26918427/
114. Dabas P, Nayak B, Khajuria H, Jain S, Dutt S, Saraswathy K. A cross-sectional assessment of quantitative epidermal melanin and erythema indices among North Indians. Indian Dermatol Online J [Internet]. 2023 May 1 [cited 2024 Mar 5];14(3):366–70. Available from: https://pubmed.ncbi.nlm.nih.gov/37266078/
115. Sarkar A, Nandineni MR. Association of common genetic variants with human skin color variation in Indian populations. Am J Hum Biol [Internet]. 2018 Jan 1 [cited 2024 Mar 5];30(1). Available from: https://pubmed.ncbi.nlm.nih.gov/28984396/
116. Souak D, Barreau M, Courtois A, André V, Poc CD, Feuilloley MGJ, et al. Challenging cosmetic innovation: the skin microbiota and probiotics protect the skin from UV-induced damage. Microorganisms [Internet]. 2021 May 1 [cited 2024 Mar 5];9(5). Available from: https://pubmed.ncbi.nlm.nih.gov/33925587/
117. Conteville LC, Vicente ACP. Skin exposure to sunlight: a factor modulating the human gut microbiome composition. Gut Microbes [Internet]. 2020 Sep 2 [cited 2024 Mar 5];11(5):1135. Available from: https://www.ncbi.nlm.nih.gov/pmc/articles/PMC7524261/
118. Guéniche A, David P, Philippe B, Stephanie B, Elif B, Isabelle CH. Probiotics for photoprotection. Dermatoendocrinol [Internet]. 2009 Sep [cited 2024 Mar 5];1(5):275–9. Available from: https://pubmed.ncbi.nlm.nih.gov/20808516/
119. Addor FAS anna, Barcaui CB, Gomes EE, Lupi O, Marçon CR, Miot HA. Sunscreen lotions in the dermatological prescription: review of concepts and controversies. An Bras Dermatol [Internet]. 2022 Mar 1 [cited 2024 Apr 2];97(2):204–22. Available from: https://pubmed.ncbi.nlm.nih.gov/35039207/

Chapter 3
Phototyping in Skin of Colour

Abbreviations

FST	Fitzpatrick skin types
HDRS	Hybrid diffuse reflectance spectroscopy
ITA	Individual typology angle
JST	Japanese skin type
LES	Lancer ethnicity score
MED	Minimal erythemal dose
MMD	Minimal melanogenic dose
PIH	Postinflammatory hyperpigmentation
SOC	Skin of colour
SPF	Sun protection factor

Key Objectives

- Skin phototyping in SOC has been a challenge due to the ability to detect erythema as a measure of photoreactivity.
- Several skin colour classification systems have been proposed to suit regional needs.
- Simple matching using visual aids like the Felix von Luschen colour charts are helpful for simple and quick skin colour assessments.
- The ITA metric based on the CIELAB colour space system provides an objective way to assess skin colour across all skin types and ethnicities.
- Existing sunscreen testing guidelines. Overcoming this limitation, the newer HDRS methodologies offer the scope to provide non-invasive, inclusive sunscreen testing and development for SOC.

The human race is said to have developed skin pigmentation, roughly about 2 million years ago [1]. Around this time, hominids lost body hair to dissipate heat better, and skin pigmentation was required to protect the skin against sun exposure. Majority of research in skin of colour pertains to non-white races in countries such

R. Rajan, *Sunscreens for Skin of Color*,
https://doi.org/10.1007/978-981-97-3195-4_3

as the USA, where up to 50% of population is expected to be of non-European origin by 2050, and therefore be considered under the umbrella term of skin of colour (SOC) [2–5]. Even within Asia, the majority of sunscreen work and development has been mostly in the Far East, involving individuals with lighter skin colour. Only in recent times, characterization of sun protection and sunscreen use for dermatological conditions for skin of colour has been more focused upon, by studies from the Indian subcontinent [6–9]. Still, for specific populations like children, there is no data on the utility of sunscreens in skin of colour.

Skin phototyping is the established way of understanding the differential behaviour of ethnic human skin in relation to sun exposure, pigmentation, and ageing and has been in vogue for close to 50 years now. Skin colour and melanin content has been the foundational difference, however, the reactivity of the skin to sun exposure was the parameter around which skin typing has evolved, until recently.

The Fitzpatrick skin types (FST) introduced in 1975 classified human skin as under 6 phototypes, based on the ability of the skin to develop erythema on sun exposure, Table 3.1 [10]. Originally, the scale was just for 4 phototypes, and phototypes 5 and 6 denoting darker skin types were added later, in 1988 [4, 11]. Over time, this classification would come to be used extensively in multiple applications ranging from the development of sunscreens and dosing iterations for phototherapy [12]. Furthermore, skin phototyping has been central to understanding the potential for postinflammatory hyperpigmentation (PIH) with laser devices, and for developing the treatment guidelines thereof [13]. Though the phototyping has since been modified to suit ethnic skin types [4, 12], most of the academic pursuit related to sunscreens have only been based on the phototypes originally described by Fitzpatrick. This development of modified Fitzpatrick scales to suit ethnic skin types is the result of the acknowledgement that even skin of colour is photoreactive, despite the elevated melanin levels [14, 15]. In India, skin types have huge variability given that the country has been a melting pot of cultures for thousands of years [16]. Accordingly, the modified Fitzpatrick grading proposed by Sharma et al. is an attempt to capture these variations more inclusively than the original Fitzpatrick scale [12].

Table 3.1 Fitzpatrick skin type classification [25]

Skin type	Description
I	White skin. Always burns, never tans.
II	Fair skin. Always burns, tans with difficulty.
III	Average skin colour. Sometimes mild burn, tan about average.
IV	Light-brown skin. Rarely burns. Tans easily.
V	Brown skin. Never burns. Tans very easily
VI	Black skin. Heavily pigmented. Never burns, tans very easily.

These modifications of skin type by ethnicity are very useful, considering that in darker skin types, the subjective ability to match the skin colour to the type is limited by the rigid colour palette available in the Fitzpatrick system. To illustrate, Sharma et al. noted that one third of their cohort changed their choice from dark-brown or black to brownish black, when given the option for a more accurate way of expressing their skin tone [12]. Furthermore, the ability to articulate the skin's reactivity to sun is not always uniform across study participants and are less accurate than the corresponding inputs by trained personnel [17, 18]. This is a real problem in skin of colour, where erythema cannot be reliably seen, and the sensation of heat may be more related to a perception of burn than skin redness itself, especially in tropical climates. Self-reporting of skin colour has been found to be more accurate than self-reporting of erythemal sensitivity, in an African cohort [19].

Much earlier though, in 1986, the Kawada Skin Classification system was introduced in Japan, based on the same parameter as the FST, but for specific use by the Japanese. The JST— Japanese skin types were found to correlate with MED; however, the minimal melanogenic dose (MMD) was not found to decrease with increasing skin types. Further for all JST types, the minimal melanogenic dose was more than the minimal erythema dose, leading the researchers to conclude that the exposure to UV induced a predominantly erythemogenic response than a melanogenic response in the Japanese [20–22]. Interestingly, the measured SPF of the same sunscreen was found to vary between JST skin types I and III, highlighting racial differences in skin reactivity to UV, even among lighter skin types [22, 23].

The Lancer ethnicity score (LES) was introduced in 1998, where a score based on ethnicity is calculated for each of the four grandparents, and then divided by 4, to arrive at the LES for the individual, Table 3.2. While this score may be useful for select indications such as to predict potential for PIH before chemical peels and laser surgeries, it does not have a wider practical applicability [4, 5, 24]. The inclusion of hair type in this grading has also been debated [25].

Goldman World Classification of Skin Types [25] was proposed as an attempt to qualify the risk of hyperpigmentation, which is variable even among members of the same ethnicity, Table 3.3. Accordingly, five racial groups are identified, and within these groups, subgroups—pale, tan, and deep tan, are characterized to indicate a progressively increasing chance of postinflammatory hyperpigmentation [25].

Fanous et al., proposed a classification to assess and identify potential post-procedure complications in SOC, as direct attributes of race and ethnicity, where skin response to lasers or procedures are considered to be genetically programmed. As shown in Fig. 3.1, six groups are identified, the Nordics originating from northern Europe, Europeans from mid Europe, Mediterranean from Southern Europe, northern most Africa, and western middle Asia, the Indo -Pakistanis from upper-middle Africa, western lower Asia, Africans from middle and lower Africa and the last group, Asians from central and east Asia. While this classification may serve as a broad guideline to identify individuals with SOC at risk of PIH, variation in response to sunlight expressed in MED, is possible even within each race [26–29].

Even assessment by trained personnel has significant interobserver variability, and so, more objective measurements of skin colour, such as hybrid diffuse

Table 3.2 Lancer ethnicity scale [25]

Geography	Fitzpatrick skin type	LES skin type
African background		
Central East, West African	V	5
Eritrean and ethiopian	V	5
North Africa, Middle East	V	5
Arabian background		
Sephardic Jewish	III	4
Asian background		
Chinese, Korean, Japanese, Thai, Vietnamese	IV	4
Filipino, Polynesian	IV	4
European background		
Ashkenazi Jewish	II	3
Cetlic	I	1
Central Eastern European	III	2
Nordic	I–II	1
Northern European(general)	I	1–2
Southern European, Mediterranean	III	3–4
Latin/Central/South American background		
Central/ South American Indian	IV	4
North American background		
Native American (including Inuit)	II	3

Obtained with permission from Goldman [25]

Table 3.3 World classification of skin type [25]

European/Caucasian—white	(a) Pale, cannot tan, burns easily, no postinflammatory pigmentation (b) Tan, rarely burns, rarely develops postinflammatory pigmentation (c) Deep tan, never burns, develops postinflammatory pigmentation
Arabian/Mediterranean/Hispanic—light brown	(a) Pale, cannot tan, burns easily, no postinflammatory pigmentation (b) Tan, rarely burns, rarely develops postinflammatory pigmentation (c) Deep tan, never burns, develops postinflammatory pigmentation
Asian—yellow	(a) Pale, cannot tan, burns easily, no postinflammatory pigmentation (b) Tan, rarely burns, rarely develops postinflammatory pigmentation (c) Deep tan, never burns, develops postinflammatory pigmentation
Indian—brown	(a) Pale, cannot tan, burns easily, no postinflammatory pigmentation (b) Tan, rarely burns, rarely develops postinflammatory pigmentation (c) Deep tan, never burns, develops postinflammatory pigmentation
African—black	(a) Pale, cannot tan, burns easily, no postinflammatory pigmentation (b) Tan, rarely burns, rarely develops postinflammatory pigmentation (c) Deep tan, never burns, develops postinflammatory pigmentation

Obtained with permission from Goldman [25]

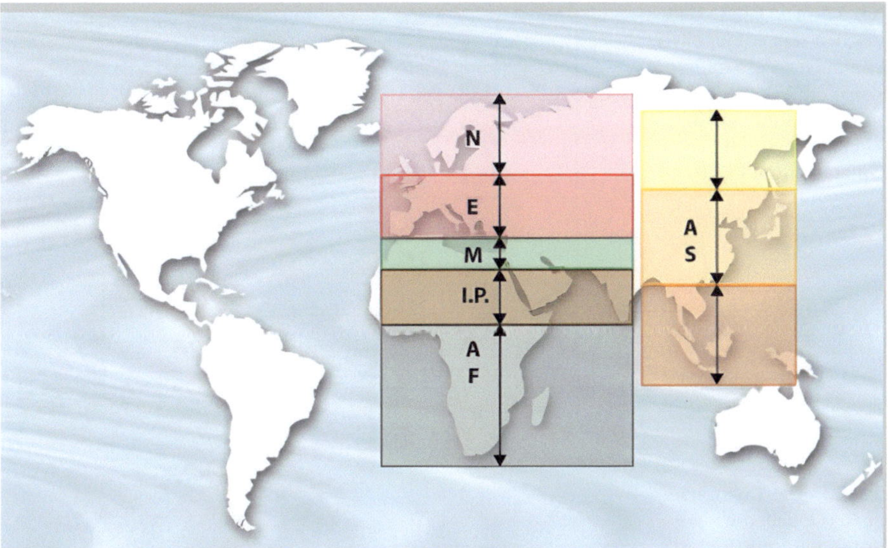

Fig. 3.1 The new genetico-racial classification of skin colour and features runs in a north-to-south direction, vertically across Europe and Africa, and in a parallel vertical direction across Asia. In Europe and Africa, the following roots are found: N Nordic (pink), E European (red), M Mediterranean (green), I.P. Indo-Pakistani (brown), AF African (grey). In Asia, the Asian (AS) roots are found: northern Asian (yellow), central Asian (light orange), and southern Asian (dark orange) (Obtained with permission from Fanous et al. [29])

reflectance spectroscopy (HDRS) and ITA typing, may soon replace subjective phototyping. These technologies are currently, but not widely, available and provide good repeatability and do not involve a need for UV exposure to assess skin reactivity.

The Willis and Earle scale includes measures of skin colour, propensity to pigmentary conditions and reaction to UV light, in people of African descent [30].

Scales that behave more like visual aids have been useful in increasing objectivity and have been responsible for taking skin colour identification out of the research lab and into consumer centric practical applications such as the development of colour cosmetics. Still, their clinical utility remains relevant. These user-friendly measurement scales like the Felix von Luschen skin colour chart, Fig. 3.2 [31, 32], Taylor hyperpigmentation scale using hue cards, Fig. 3.3 [33], and the colour bar method suggested by Ho and Robinson, Fig. 3.4 [34] have been demonstrated to correlate with melanin index and with ITA, they can be reliably used in everyday clinical practice as needed.

The Taylor hue cards, developed in 2006, have among the widest range of colour matching options, with 15 plastic cards, each with ten colour shades, conceived as a scale for identifying progressive levels of hyperpigmentation, or recovery from the same. Each of the hue bands is provided with a circular aperture in the centre, allowing the card to be directly placed on the skin, to select the shade with the best colour match. While noted to have significant inter and intraindividual variation, the Taylor hue cards have been considered as easy for routine use [33].

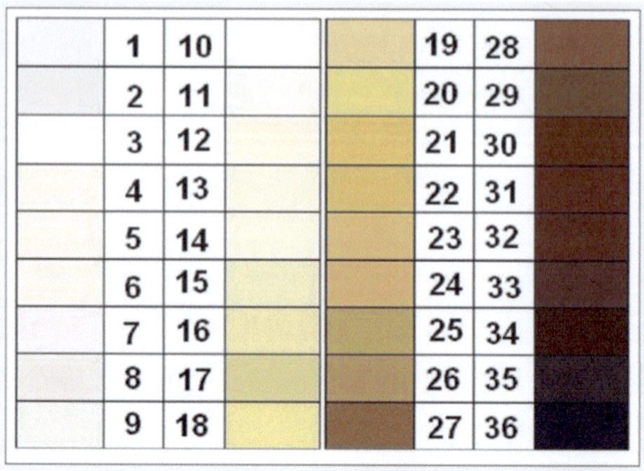

Fig. 3.2 The Felix von Luschen skin colour chart is an open access tool hosted on Wikimedia commons, for assessing skin colour visually. (Obtained from [32])

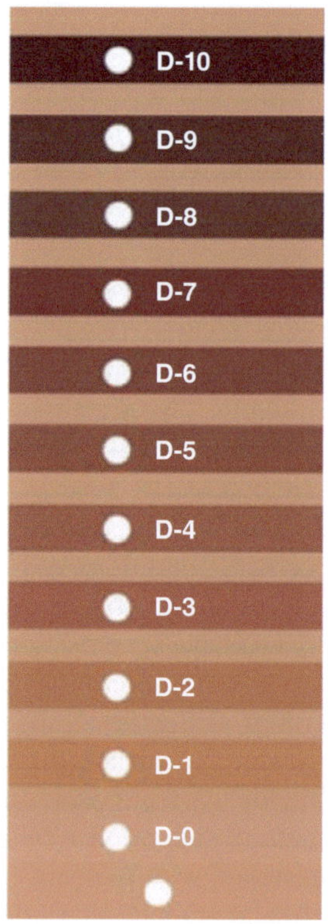

Fig. 3.3 The Taylor hue cards. (Obtained with permission from Taylor et al. [33])

The visual nature of these colour charts may be more accurate than questionnaire based assessments, in addition to being economical and quick [35]. The Roberts hyperpigmentation scale is designed to identify the potential for PIH, based on clinical examination, past medical history, and ancestry. It is considered to provide a bedside opportunity for discussion of post procedure complications like hyperpigmentation and scarring, which are unique to SOC, which are known to recur with subsequent procedures [3, 4].

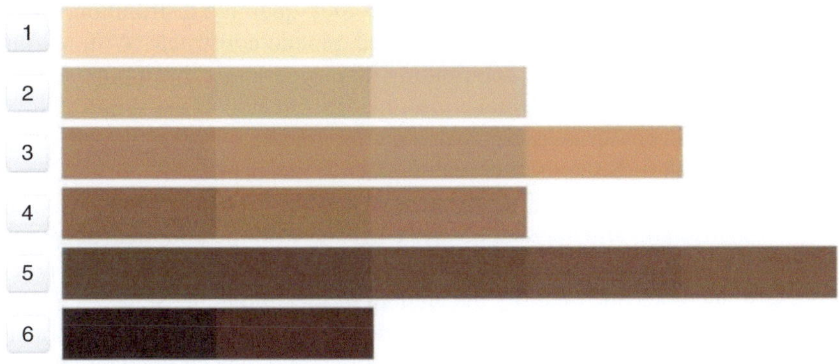

Fig. 3.4 Ho and Robinson colour bar tool, Color bar survey item. The participant selected the colour bar that most closely matched the skin tone on the inside part of their upper arm. (Obtained with permission from Ho and Robinson [34])

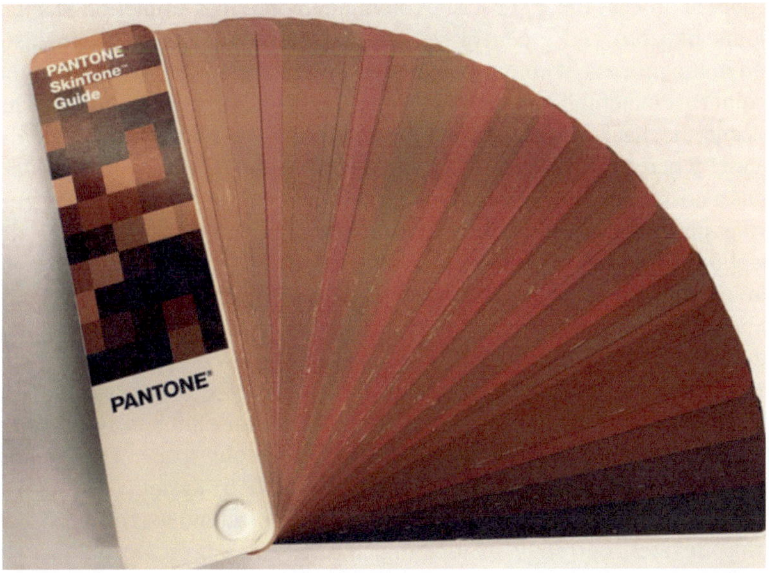

Fig. 3.5 Handheld Pantone SkinTone Guide (Obtained from Hoffman et al. [36]. An open-access article distributed under the terms of the Creative Commons Attribution-Non Commercial-No Derivatives License 4.0 (CCBY-NC-ND) [36]

The Pantone skin tone guide has been used in reconstructive medicine to provide guidance on colour matches for skin transplantation [36]. Considered comprehensive and easy to use, this guide has been used by prosthetics manufacturers for colour matching. It is a handheld tool with 110 colour swatches showing a progressive variation in lightness and undertone, to realistically represent human skin tones, Fig. 3.5. More recently, machine learning techniques have been developed around this scale to classify facial skin colour for colour cosmetics [37].

Constitutive skin colour is defined by the colour, quantity, distribution, and type of epidermal melanin, based on predetermined genetic constructs. With mixing of races, the value of ancestry in determining skin type and skin photoreactivity is questionable. Furthermore, external exposomal factors act on the skin to influence the facultative skin colour, together with other internal factors like endocrinological influences [33]. Though the most common practice has been to slot people into different phototypes based on the skin's reactivity to the sun, skin colour as visually perceived is different, and may not always correlate with the photoreactivity anticipated for that colour. So, the most ideal way would be to quantify skin colour using colorimetric methods and quantify the amount of melanin in the skin.

Colour perception by the human eye depends upon absorption of the incident wavelengths by the photoreceptor cells in the brain and then subsequent interpretation of the same by the optical cortex of the brain. Two principles are at play here—the trichromatic colour theory and the opponent process theory. The trichromatic colour theory explains colour perception as a component of the three primary colours, Red, Blue, and Green and their perception by the retinal cones in the eye. The opponent process theory describes colour perception as a function of antagonistic colours like red and green or yellow and blue. Both these mechanisms are involved in the process of colour perception, for example, when evaluating the ability to point to a matching colour when assessing skin colour using colour bars [33]. These same mechanisms are also responsible for the phenomenon of the dreaded white cast, where the sunscreen reflects the white light in its totality, making it appear as a cosmetically unappealing Kabuki mask. To state it simply, the colour of the chromophore perceived by the eye is the wavelength that is not absorbed by the chromophore, within the spectrum of visible light.

More reproducible and reliable methods like colorimetry and reflectance spectrophotometry which can measure constitutional pigmentation can significantly alleviate the lack of objectivity that is seen with both phototyping and self-reported colour matching. These technologies have also been used robustly to validate the modifications of the phototyping scales to suit different ethnicities and depend on colour organization systems such as the CIELAB colour space. The Commission Internationale de l'Eclairage (CIE) recognizes the L*a*b* system as a standard reference for measuring skin colour, and this system is used in most of the skin colour measuring devices, currently in use, Fig. 3.6. L* measures the lightness of the colour, a* measures the intensity of the colour in the red/green spectrum, and b*, the colour intensity in the yellow/blue spectrum [38]. In skin colorimetry, the L value correlates to the skin pigmentation level and is scored as a grey scale, from 0 denoting black colour to white, denoted by a value of 100. The values of a* correlate with erythema and b* with yellowness of the skin.

The colorimetric devices measure the intensity of light reflected from the skin. Significant differences in skin colour typing have been noted when using the L*a*b* system across different races. Skin colour was measured at four body sites, using a spectrophotometer and represented as L*a*b* values for comparison across four ethnic groups—Caucasian, Chinest, Kurdish, and Thai. Comparing across ethnic groups, yellowness denoted by b* was found to be higher in Asian women of Thai

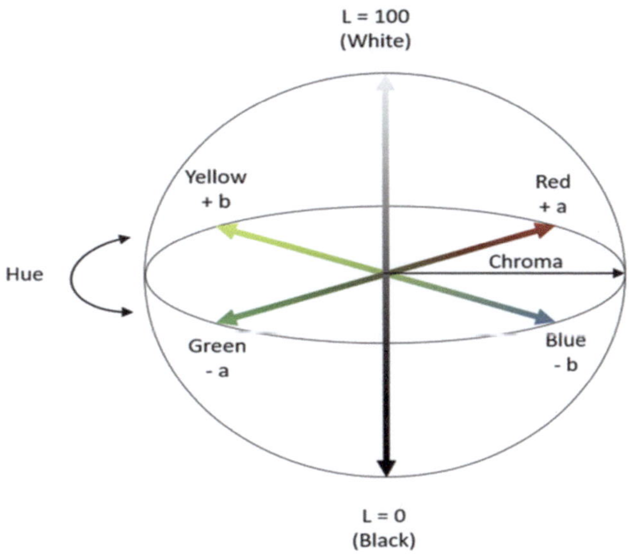

Fig. 3.6 The CIELAB colour space diagram [37]. The CIELAB colour space diagram. The CIELAB, or CIE L* a* b*, colour system represents quantitative relationship of colours on three axes: L*value indicates lightness, and a* and b* are chromaticity coordinates. On the colour space diagram, L* is represented on a vertical axis with values from 0 (black) to 100 (white). The a* value indicates red-green component of a color, where þa* (positive) and a* (negative) indicate red and green values, respectively. The yellow and blue components are represented on the b* axis as þb* (positive) and b* (negative) values, respectively. At the centre of the plane is neutral or achromatic. The distance from the central axis represents the chroma (C*) or saturation of the colour. The angle on the chromaticity axes represents the hue (ho). The L*, a*, and b* values can be transcribed to dermatological parameters. The L* value correlates with the level of pigmentation of the skin. The a* value correlates with erythema. The b* value correlates with pigmentation and tanning. CIE, Commission Internationale de l'Eclairage. (Obtained from Ly et al. [38])

ethnicity compared to Caucasian women, by Xiao et al. Yellowness was also identified to be the most distinct attribute between the groups. Intragroup variation was highest within the Caucasian group and least among the Chinese [39].

Voegeli's group noted that L* and a* values were lower in Indian and South African women, compared to Chinese, Japanese, and French women, with French women showing the least b* value. Overall, b* and L* values seem to correlate most with ethnic variations while redness, a*, may be influenced by anatomical location, but also by environmental factors such as cold and altitude [40–42]. Lightness, L* value needs to be interpreted in context of site and facultative pigmentation [39].

Working on a method to arrive at the best colour match for skin graft specimens, Huang et al. found that the L* value was proportionate to the product of epidermal melanocyte ratio and the melanin index. While the correlation of the lightness value to the melanin index was significant, adding the proportion of melanocytes to the equation increased the significance of the correlation. Accordingly, the L value as measured by the spectrophotometer can be used as a guide to achieve precise colour match for skin grafting applications in patients with burns or vitiligo [43].

The individual typology angle, Fig. 3.7, was introduced to acknowledge the fluidity of melanin distribution cutoffs across different ethnicities [44]. This system provides the ability to localize individual ITA readings to discrete values within a

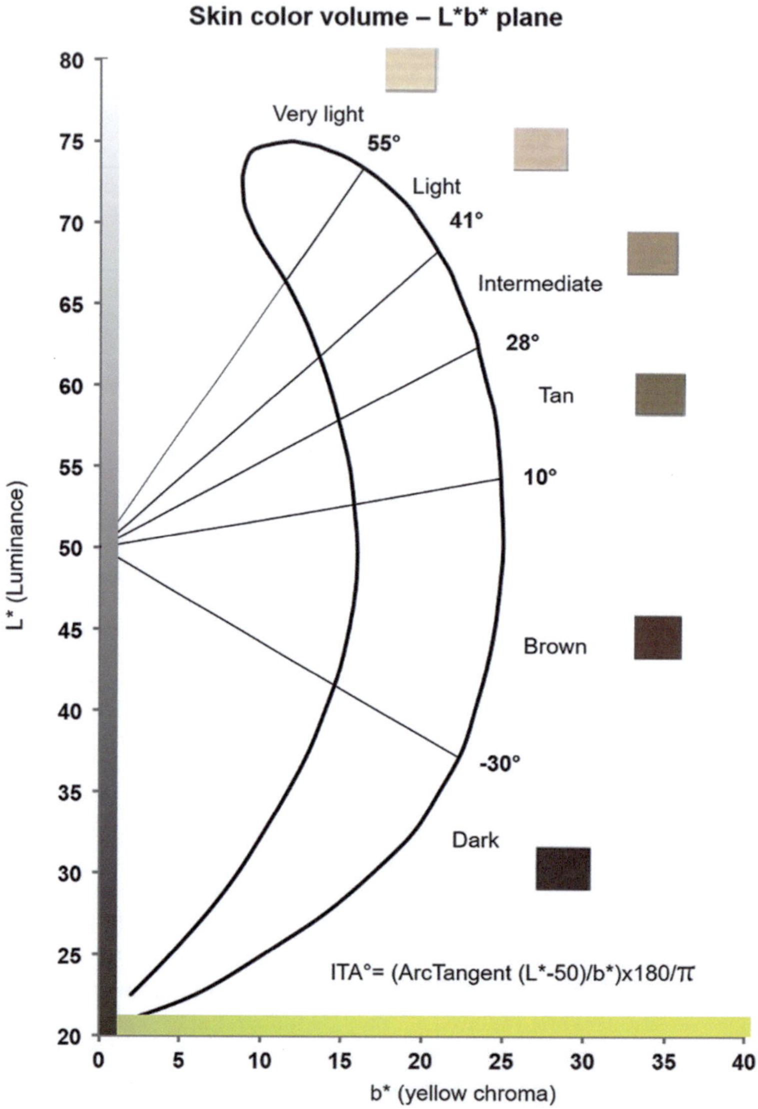

Fig. 3.7 Skin colour volume allows for objective quantification and classification of skin colour into six groups: very light, light, intermediate, tan, brown, and dark [44, 45]. The skin colour volume aligns the colorimetric 1976 CIE L*a*b* parameters with the ITA value. The L* (luminance) value of the skin colour is represented on the vertical axis and the b* (yellow-blue) component is on the horizontal axis. The ITA of the corresponding skin colour can be obtained from the L* and b* values according to the formula. The colour swatches are representative average skin colours for each colour group that match the L'Oréal Skin Colour Chart [46]. CIE Commission Internationale de l'Eclairage, ITA individual typology angle. (Obtained from Ly et al. [38])

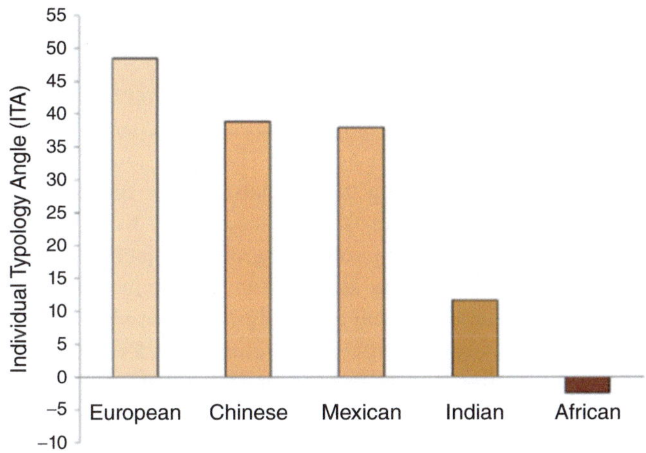

Fig. 3.8 ITA values for European, Chinese, Mexican, Indian, and African people. Lightness (sun protected) was highest for Europeans and lowest for Africans. Indian skin was significantly darker than European, Chinese, and Mexican skin. L* was significantly and inversely correlated with levels of eumelanin and total melanin overall and for all groups (correlation coefficients, 0.77 to 0.89 for both total melanin and eumelanin). Although significant, L* was inversely correlated with pheomelanin levels with lower correlations (0.23 overall ranging from 0.53 to 0.83). (Obtained with permission from Visscher [49])

continuous numerical scale. ITA may be considered to be a better foundational metric compared to ethnicity and race, for the purpose of establishing biophysical standards across different populations. This would ensure more objectivity and reproducibility, while having a better practical value for today's world with changing ethnic boundaries [47]. ITA across different populations were compared by Visscher et al., Fig. 3.8.

Though for sunscreen testing, the subject selection juxtaposes the Fitzpatrick skin phototypes and the ITA scales, these metrics are very distinct and not interchangeable [48]. The ITA measures a physical factor—namely constitutive pigmentation, while the phototypes measure the biological responsiveness of that factor to photo stimulation [10]. But they may be comparable with further research that provides ITA cutoffs drawn from more studies in larger groups of subjects representing multiple ethnicities and varied geographies. Since a sunburn is only an aspect of the skin damage brought on by sun exposure, and since even sub-MED UV doses can also cause skin damage, Fitzpatrick phototypes may be considered as correlating with SPF values. On the other hand, ITA may be more suited to understand the melanin response to various stimuli and may be crucial to understanding pigmentary changes in skin of colour, including photo pigmentation as a component of ageing.

Sunscreen testing at this point in time is not available for individuals with lower ITA angles, implying those of a higher skin type, and a higher melanin content. The advent of colorimetry and reflectance spectroscopic measures should usher in an era of greater inclusivity both in terms of quantitative understanding of pigmentary problems as well as generating protective solutions in terms of better sunscreen testing leading to improved sunscreen products for SOC.

3.1 Chapter Summary

Prototyping in skin of colour explores the evolution of skin typing systems over the years. While noting historical biases in research, this chapter highlights recent efforts to address the dermatological needs of skin of colour (SOC) populations. Skin typing methodologies, including the Fitzpatrick scale and alternative classifications, are discussed alongside user-friendly assessment tools. Advancements in colorimetry and reflectance spectrophotometry offer objective measures of skin colour, where the individual typology angle (ITA) and the melanin indices as measurements of skin pigmentation, signal a paradigm shift of skin testing away from subjective and/or reactive methodologies. This chapter underscores the importance of inclusive sunscreen testing and development to meet the diverse needs of SOC individuals.

References

1. Hanel A, Carlberg C. Skin colour and vitamin D: an update. Exp Dermatol [Internet]. 2020 Sep 1 [cited 2024 Mar 2];29(9):864–875. Available from: https://pubmed.ncbi.nlm.nih.gov/32621306/
2. Race and ethnicity in the United States—Wikipedia [Internet]. [cited 2024 Mar 5]. Available from: https://en.wikipedia.org/wiki/Race_and_ethnicity_in_the_United_States
3. The Roberts skin type classification system—PubMed [Internet]. [cited 2024 Mar 5]. Available from: https://pubmed.ncbi.nlm.nih.gov/18505137/
4. Roberts WE. Skin type classification systems old and new. Dermatol Clin [Internet]. 2009 Oct [cited 2024 Mar 5];27(4):529–33. Available from: https://pubmed.ncbi.nlm.nih.gov/19850202/
5. Ware OR, Dawson JE, Shinohara MM, Taylor SC. Skin of color Racial limitations of Fitzpatrick skin type. 2020;105(2):77.
6. Ankad BS, Behera B, Lallas A, Akay BN, Bhat YJ, Chauhan P, et al. International Dermoscopy Society (IDS) criteria for skin tumors: validation for skin of color through a Delphi expert consensus by the "imaging in skin of color" IDS Task Force. Dermatol Pract Concept [Internet]. 2023 Jan 1 [cited 2024 Mar 5];13(1). Available from: https://pubmed.ncbi.nlm.nih.gov/36892378/
7. A Clinical, Dermoscopic, and histopathological analysis of common acquired melanocytic nevi in skin of color—PubMed [Internet]. [cited 2024 Mar 5]. Available from: https://pubmed.ncbi.nlm.nih.gov/36312828/
8. Hongal AA, Aithal SS, Revathi TN. Facial Angiofibroma Severity Index: a beneficial tool to evaluate the treatment response in the skin of colour. Indian J Dermatol Venereol Leprol [Internet]. 2023 Jan 1 [cited 2024 Mar 5];89(1):130–2. Available from: https://pubmed.ncbi.nlm.nih.gov/36331837/
9. Jindal R, Chauhan P, Sethi S. Dermoscopy of the diverse spectrum of cutaneous tuberculosis in the skin of color. Dermatol Pract Concept [Internet]. 2022 Oct 1 [cited 2024 Mar 5];12(4):2022203. Available from: https://www.ncbi.nlm.nih.gov/pmc/articles/PMC9681234/
10. Osto M, Hamzavi IH, Lim HW, Kohli I. Individual typology angle and Fitzpatrick skin phototypes are not equivalent in photodermatology. Photochem Photobiol [Internet]. 2022 Jan 1 [cited 2024 Mar 5];98(1):127–9. Available from: https://pubmed.ncbi.nlm.nih.gov/34796498/
11. Fitzpatrick TB. The validity and practicality of sun-reactive skin types I through VI. Arch Dermatol [Internet]. 1988 Jun 1 [cited 2024 Mar 5];124(6):869–71. Available from: https://pubmed.ncbi.nlm.nih.gov/3377516/

12. Sharma VK, Gupta V, Jangid BL, Pathak M. Modification of the Fitzpatrick system of skin phototype classification for the Indian population, and its correlation with narrowband diffuse reflectance spectrophotometry. Clin Exp Dermatol [Internet]. 2018 Apr 1 [cited 2024 Mar 6];43(3):274–80. Available from: https://pubmed.ncbi.nlm.nih.gov/29318654/
13. Sharma AN, Patel BC. Laser Fitzpatrick skin type recommendations. StatPearls [Internet]. 2023 Mar 6 [cited 2024 Mar 6]; Available from: https://www.ncbi.nlm.nih.gov/books/NBK557626/
14. Mahmoud BH, Ruvolo E, Hexsel CL, Liu Y, Owen MR, Kollias N, et al. Impact of long-wavelength UVA and visible light on melanocompetent skin. J Invest Dermatol [Internet]. 2010 Aug [cited 2024 Mar 3];130(8):2092–7. Available from: https://pubmed.ncbi.nlm.nih.gov/20410914/
15. Fajuyigbe D, Young AR. The impact of skin colour on human photobiological responses. Pigment Cell Melanoma Res [Internet]. 2016 Nov 1 [cited 2024 Mar 2];29(6):607–618. Available from: https://pubmed.ncbi.nlm.nih.gov/27454804/
16. Iliescu FM, Chaplin G, Rai N, Jacobs GS, Basu Mallick C, Mishra A, et al. The influences of genes, the environment, and social factors on the evolution of skin color diversity in India. Am J Hum Biol [Internet]. 2018 Sep 1 [cited 2024 Mar 5];30(5). Available from: https://pubmed.ncbi.nlm.nih.gov/30099804/
17. Eilers S, Bach DQ, Gaber R, Blatt H, Guevara Y, Nitsche K, et al. Accuracy of self-report in assessing Fitzpatrick skin phototypes I through VI. JAMA Dermatol [Internet]. 2013 Nov [cited 2024 Mar 6];149(11):1289–94. Available from: https://pubmed.ncbi.nlm.nih.gov/24048361/
18. Reeder AI, Hammond VA, Gray AR. Questionnaire items to assess skin color and erythemal sensitivity: reliability, validity, and "the dark shift." Cancer Epidemiol Biomarkers Prev [Internet]. 2010 May [cited 2024 Mar 6];19(5):1167–73. Available from: https://pubmed.ncbi.nlm.nih.gov/20447914/
19. Wright CY, Wilkes M, du Plessis JL, Reeder AI. Self-reported skin colour and erythemal sensitivity vs. objectively measured constitutive skin colour in an African population with predominantly dark skin. Photodermatol Photoimmunol Photomed [Internet]. 2015 Nov 1 [cited 2024 Mar 6];31(6):315–24. Available from: https://pubmed.ncbi.nlm.nih.gov/26147690/
20. UVB-induced erythema, delayed tanning, and UVA-induced immediate tanning in Japanese skin—PubMed [Internet]. [cited 2024 Mar 6]. Available from: https://pubmed.ncbi.nlm.nih.gov/3588352/
21. Kawada A, Hiruma M, Noda T, Kukita A. Skin typing, sun exposure, and sunscreen use in a population of Japanese. J Dermatol [Internet]. 1989 [cited 2024 Mar 6];16(3):187–90. Available from: https://pubmed.ncbi.nlm.nih.gov/2794220/
22. Kawada A. Risk and preventive factors for skin phototype. J Dermatol Sci [Internet]. 2000; [cited 2024 Mar 6];23(SUPPL. 1). Available from: https://pubmed.ncbi.nlm.nih.gov/10764988/
23. Kawada A, Noda T, Hiruma M, Ishibashi A, Arai S. The relationship of sun protection factor to minimal erythema dose, Japanese skin type, and skin color. J Dermatol [Internet]. 1993 [cited 2024 Mar 6];20(8):514–6. Available from: https://pubmed.ncbi.nlm.nih.gov/8245315/
24. Bashour M. Risk factors for epithelial erosions in laser in situ keratomileusis. J Cataract Refract Surg [Internet]. 2002 Oct [cited 2024 Mar 6];28(10):1780–8. Available from: https://pubmed.ncbi.nlm.nih.gov/12388028/
25. Goldman MP. Universal classification of skin type. Simplified Facial Rejuvenation [Internet]. 2008 [cited 2024 Mar 5];47–50. Available from: https://link.springer.com/chapter/10.1007/978-3-540-71097-4_3
26. Fanous N. A new patient classification for laser resurfacing and peels: predicting responses, risks, and results. Aesthetic Plast Surg [Internet]. 2002 Mar [cited 2024 Mar 6];26(2):99–104. Available from: https://pubmed.ncbi.nlm.nih.gov/12016493/
27. Fanous N, Yoskovitch A. New classification scheme for laser resurfacing and chemical peels. Modifications for the different ethnic groups. Facial Plastic Surgery Clinics [Internet]. 2002 Nov [cited 2024 Mar 6];10(4):405–13. Available from: https://pubmed.ncbi.nlm.nih.gov/15062301/

28. Côté V, Fanous N. The new “genetico-racial” skin classification: maximizing the safety of skin treatments for Asians. Facial Plast Surg Clin North Am [Internet]. 2010 Feb [cited 2024 Mar 6];18(1):99–104. Available from: https://pubmed.ncbi.nlm.nih.gov/20206093/
29. Fanous N, Côté V, Fanous A. The new Genetico-Racial Skin Classification: how to maximize the safety of any peel or laser treatment on any Asian, Caucasian or Black patient. Can J Plast Surg [Internet]. 2011 [cited 2024 Mar 6];19(1):9. Available from: https://www.ncbi.nlm.nih.gov/pmc/articles/PMC3086503/
30. A new skin classification system relevant to people of African descent [Internet]. [cited 2024 Mar 6]. Available from: https://www.researchgate.net/publication/286988450_A_new_skin_classification_system_relevant_to_people_of_African_descent
31. Treesirichod A, Chansakulporn S, Wattanapan P. Correlation between skin color evaluation by skin color scale chart and narrowband reflectance spectrophotometer. Indian J Dermatol [Internet]. 2014 [cited 2024 Mar 6];59(4):339–42. Available from: https://pubmed.ncbi.nlm.nih.gov/25071249/
32. File:Felix von Luschan Skin Color Chart.JPG—Wikimedia Commons [Internet]. [cited 2024 Apr 7]. Available from: https://commons.wikimedia.org/wiki/File:Felix_von_Luschan_Skin_Color_Chart.JPG
33. The Taylor Hyperpigmentation Scale: a new visual assessment tool for the evaluation of skin color and pigmentation—PubMed [Internet]. [cited 2024 Mar 6]. Available from: https://pubmed.ncbi.nlm.nih.gov/16315565/
34. Ho BK, Robinson JK. Color bar tool for skin type self-identification: a cross-sectional study. J Am Acad Dermatol [Internet]. 2015 Aug 1 [cited 2024 Mar 6];73(2):312–313.e1. Available from: https://pubmed.ncbi.nlm.nih.gov/26183973/
35. Gupta V, Sharma VK. Skin typing: Fitzpatrick grading and others. Clin Dermatol [Internet]. 2019 Sep 1 [cited 2024 Mar 2];37(5):430–6. Available from: https://pubmed.ncbi.nlm.nih.gov/31896400/
36. Hoffman AF, Park JJ, Berman ZP, Alfonso AR, Diep GK, Mills E, et al. Establishing a clinically applicable methodology for skin color matching in vascularized composite allotransplantation. Plast Reconstr Surg Glob Open [Internet]. 2020 [cited 2024 Mar 6];8(2). Available from: https://www.ncbi.nlm.nih.gov/pmc/articles/PMC7159949/
37. Zhu W, Sang P, He Y. Facial skin colour classification using machine learning and hyperspectral imaging data. IET Image Process [Internet]. 2022 Feb 1 [cited 2024 Mar 6];16(2):509–20. Available from: https://onlinelibrary.wiley.com/doi/full/10.1049/ipr2.12366
38. Ly BCK, Dyer EB, Feig JL, Chien AL, Del Bino S. Research techniques made simple: cutaneous colorimetry: a reliable technique for objective skin color measurement. Journal of Investigative Dermatology [Internet]. 2020 Jan 1 [cited 2024 Mar 2];140(1):3–12.e1. Available from: https://www.researchgate.net/publication/338303610_Research_Techniques_Made_Simple_Cutaneous_Colorimetry_A_Reliable_Technique_for_Objective_Skin_Color_Measurement
39. Xiao K, Yates JM, Zardawi F, Sueeprasan S, Liao N, Gill L, et al. Characterising the variations in ethnic skin colours: a new calibrated data base for human skin. Skin Res Technol [Internet]. 2017 Feb 1 [cited 2024 Mar 6];23(1):21–9. Available from: https://pubmed.ncbi.nlm.nih.gov/27273806/
40. Dabas P, Nayak B, Khajuria H, Jain S, Dutt S, Saraswathy K. A cross-sectional assessment of quantitative epidermal melanin and erythema indices among North Indians. Indian Dermatol Online J [Internet]. 2023 May 1 [cited 2024 Mar 5];14(3):366–70. Available from: https://pubmed.ncbi.nlm.nih.gov/37266078/
41. Weatherall IL, Coombs BD. Skin color measurements in terms of CIELAB color space values. J Invest Dermatol [Internet]. 1992 [cited 2024 Mar 6];99(4):468–73. Available from: https://pubmed.ncbi.nlm.nih.gov/1402005/
42. Voegeli R, Campiche R, Biassin R, Rawlings A V., Shackelford TK, Fink B. Predictors of female age, health and attractiveness perception from skin feature analysis of digital portraits in

five ethnic groups. Int J Cosmet Sci [Internet]. 2023 Oct 1 [cited 2024 Mar 5];45(5):672–687. Available from: https://pubmed.ncbi.nlm.nih.gov/37338195/

43. Huang WS, Wang YW, Hung KC, Hsieh PS, Fu KY, Dai LG, et al. High correlation between skin color based on CIELAB color space, epidermal melanocyte ratio, and melanocyte melanin content. PeerJ [Internet]. 2018; [cited 2024 Mar 6];2018(5). Available from: https://www.ncbi.nlm.nih.gov/pmc/articles/PMC5971097/
44. Chardon A, Cretois I, Hourseau C. Skin colour typology and suntanning pathways. Int J Cosmet Sci [Internet]. 1991 [cited 2024 Apr 7];13(4):191–208. Available from: https://pubmed.ncbi.nlm.nih.gov/19291061/
45. Del Bino S, Ito S, Sok J, Nakanishi Y, Bastien P, Wakamatsu K, Bernerd F. Chemical analysis of constitutive pigmentation of human epidermis reveals constant eumelanin to pheomelanin ratio. Pigment Cell Melanoma Res. 2015;28:707–17. https://doi.org/10.1111/pcmr.12410
46. de Rigal J, Abella ML, Giron F, Caisey L, Lefebvre MA. Development and validation of a new Skin Color Chart. Skin Res Technol. 2007 Feb;13(1):101–9. https://doi.org/10.1111/j.1600-0846.2007.00223.x. PMID: 17250540
47. Rawlings A V. Ethnic skin types: are there differences in skin structure and function? Int J Cosmet Sci [Internet]. 2006 Apr [cited 2024 Mar 2];28(2):79–93. Available from: https://pubmed.ncbi.nlm.nih.gov/18492142/
48. Zou W, Ramanathan R, Urban S, Sinclair C, King K, Tinker R, et al. Sunscreen testing: a critical perspective and future roadmap. TrAC Trends Anal Chem [Internet]. 2022 Dec 1 [cited 2024 Mar 20];157:1–19. Available from: https://researchrepository.rmit.edu.au/esploro/outputs/9922155909201341
49. Visscher MO. Skin color and pigmentation in ethnic skin. Facial Plast Surg Clin North Am [Internet]. 2017 Feb 1 [cited 2024 Apr 7];25(1):119–25. Available from: https://pubmed.ncbi.nlm.nih.gov/27888889/

Chapter 4
Sunscreens and Skin Cancer: An Update

Abbreviations

AAR	Age-adjusted rates
BCC	Basal cell carcinoma
CPD	Cyclobutane pyrimidine dimers
EORTC	European Organisation for Research and Treatment of Cancer
IARC	International Agency for Research on Cancer
NBUVB	Narrowband ultraviolet B
NMSC	Nonmelanoma skin cancer
PAH	Polycyclic aromatic hydrocarbons
PUVA	Psoralen and ultraviolet A therapy
SCC	Squamous cell carcinoma
SOC	Skin of colour
UV	Ultraviolet
UVR	Ultraviolet radiation
VL	Visible Light
WHO	World Health Organization

Key Objectives

- Globally, the burden of disease attributable to skin cancer, is on the rise. However, the contribution of SOC towards this burden remains significantly lesser compared to lighter skin types.
- The Nambour trials are a key evidence to understanding the role of sunscreens in cancer prevention and trace the contribution of sunscreens to cancer prevention over time.
- However, larger reviews do not find a protective benefit for sunscreen use, and some studies highlight the increased occurrence of melanoma in sunscreen users. Many factors ranging from sunscreen formulations to product labelling to consumer behaviour play a role in this perception of a lack of sunscreen efficacy against cancer occurrence.

R. Rajan, *Sunscreens for Skin of Color*,
https://doi.org/10.1007/978-981-97-3195-4_4

- Sunscreen usage in SOC for the purpose of prevention of skin cancer is unclear. The high melanin content in the skin which acts as a natural sunscreen, the low incidence of skin cancer in SOC, and the unique clinical presentation of melanomas in this population all point to a smaller role for sunscreens in cancer prevention in SOC, as compared to that in lighter phototypes.

Sun exposure is considered as the single largest contributor to skin cancer development [1]. The connection between sun exposure and skin cancer was established as early as 1927 for basal cell carcinoma (BCC) and squamous cell carcinoma (SCC) and by 1955 for melanoma [2].

Skin cancers have been historically less prevalent in Indian skin types in particular and in skin of colour (SOC) in general [3, 4]. Between ethnicities, skin cancer accounted for 35–45% of all neoplasms in Caucasians compared to 2–4% in Asians and even lesser 1–2% in Blacks [5]. Specifically in the region of the Americas, skin cancers accounted for 65.8% and 79.2% of all skin cancers in females and males, respectively, with the corresponding number for Europe being 79.6% and 71.3% [6].

Melanoma skin cancers occur much less commonly in SOC populations, with an incidence rate of 1% in the South Asian region, compared to 54% in Australasia and 21% in North America. The World Health Organization (WHO) data notes that the incidence of melanoma and non-melanoma skin cancers has increased by five folds in the last 3 decades [7]. This is despite widespread awareness about sun avoidance and sunscreen use. Specifically, for India, the melanoma incidence rate is 0.5% [8]. Compared to melanoma skin cancers, keratinocyte neoplasms, namely basal cell carcinoma and squamous cell carcinoma are more common in ethnicities with higher skin types, but even here, the overall skin cancer risk is much lower compared to lighter skin types [9, 10].

A recent comparison of skin cancers in India versus the Western population noted that the age-adjusted rate (AAR) for all skin cancers was significantly lower in India as anticipated. The maximum AAR per 100,000 population for melanoma skin cancers in India was 1.62 in males, compared to the global maximum of 36.9. Among females, the figures were 1.21 and 31.7, respectively. For non-melanoma skin cancers, the Indian AAR among males was 6.2 vs 3.49 in females, with the corresponding global numbers being 225.4 and 68.6, respectively [6].

Within India, the highest occurrence of skin cancer in men was noted in the North Eastern region, for both melanoma and nonmelanoma cancers. Even among females, the North Eastern region was the main contributor to nonmelanoma skin cancer, while AAR of melanoma skin cancers was highest for females in the Northern region, despite the possibility of a referral bias in the latter case. In certain countries which have different ethnicities even within a defined geography like Singapore, which is home to distinct Asian ethnicities, the occurrence of melanoma is higher within lighter skinned Chinese compared to darker skinned Indians [11]. Very recently, the WHO published the estimates of nonmelanoma skin cancer among 183 countries, between 2000 and 2019 with a focus on occupational UV exposure, and listed sun exposure as the third largest cause of occupational exposure to carcinogenesis. Interestingly, this report noted that the burden of disease for nonmelanoma skin cancer (NMSC) was higher among people in the African Region, the Regions of the Americas, and the Western Pacific Region. A further characterization of the different ethnicities that bear the NMSC burden within these geographical regions would provide a better understanding of the sun protection abilities of dark skin, which has until now been considered a key factor in cancer prevention [12].

The overall lower risk of skin cancer is attributed to the increased melanin content in the epidermis of SOC. Larger melanosomes with a higher melanin content in SOC, distributed more evenly across the entire epidermis, likely contribute to reducing the development of skin cancer by filtering out ultraviolet radiation, twice as much as is possible in other skin types [5, 13]. The photoprotection benefit may have been necessitated by the climatic conditions along the pathway of the human evolution story, where humans adapted to living in high ultraviolet radiation (UVR) equatorial regions. A need to conserve vitamin D and folate in populations migrating 'out of Africa' resulted in lighter skin with a lesser ability to protect against UVR [14]. Broadly speaking, the risk of photocarcinogenesis is brought down in skin of colour due to three reasons: more robust prevention of DNA damage in the lower epidermis as compared to lighter skin types, more advantageous rates of repair of any incurred DNA damage, and a better equipped mechanism to remove UV damaged cells by apoptosis in melanin rich skin [15]. An inverse relationship exists between the amount of melanin in the skin and the generation of signature UV-induced photoproducts, the cyclobutane pyrimidine dimers (CPDs) [16].

This difference between skin cancer manifestations in SOC versus other populations can also be illustrated by etiopathogenesis. Figure 4.1 [17] lists the most common risk factors for skin cancer. The risk factors for nonmelanoma skin cancers, globally, include environmental causes like UVR, indoor tanning, psoralen and ultraviolet A (PUVA) therapy and ionizing radiation, chemical exposures such as arsenic and polycyclic aromatic hydrocarbon (PAH), skin type, chronic cutaneous inflammation, immunosuppression, and a family history of cancer. However, only some of these factors seem relevant to the Indian scenario [6]. In regions of India where basal cell carcinomas are reported to occur more commonly than the national average, interaction of the biological effects of UVB with those resulting from the high levels of arsenic in ground water is implicated as a significant factor for carcinogenesis [10]. Arsenic susceptibility is understood to be genetically influenced. Additionally, the 'arsenic belts' in India in the North and Northeastern regions, are also the higher latitude and altitude areas inhabited by people of lighter phototypes. The interplay of these predisposing factors may play a role in the increased occurrence of skin cancers observed in this region compared to the rest of India. For squamous cell carcinoma in SOC, scarring and inflammation, immunological imbalances, and viral infections are all significant risk factors [5]. Specifically, long-standing inflammatory conditions such as lupus erythematosus, lichen planus, chronic ulcers, and scars are relevant for malignant transformation into squamous cell carcinomas in the Indian population. For melanoma skin cancers, the globally relevant risk factors include more than 5 sunburns, fair phototype, genetic

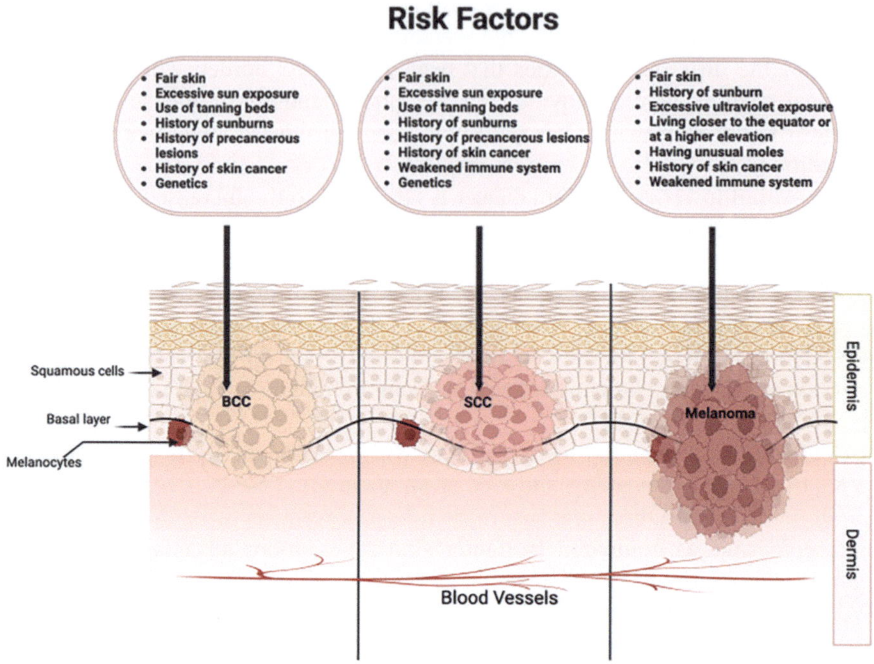

Fig. 4.1 Risk factors for the most common types of skin cancer. BCC basal cell carcinoma, SCC squamous cell carcinoma [17] (Obtained from Tow et al. [17]. An open access article distributed under the terms and conditions of the Creative Commons Attribution (CC BY) license (https://creativecommons.org/licenses/by/4.0/))

predisposition as evidenced by a family history of skin cancer, and immunosuppression. However, in the Indian population, only the fair skin type was likely relevant.

Though PUVA therapy has been considered in the past as a significant risk factor for skin cancers even in the Indian population [6], a 10-year data analysis in Fitzpatrick skin types IV and V by Ravindran et al. concluded that the risk of developing cutaneous malignancy was negligible [18]. The follow-up duration in this study was 3 years for patients who had received PUVA and 6.5 years for those who had been treated with NBUVB. This is also supported by a recent international review, which concluded that phototherapy-related exposure was not a risk for keratinocyte cancers in SOC. Rather than as a general assumption of UV exposure leading to keratinocyte cancer, the authors opine that the type of UV exposure, such as sun exposure versus phototherapy, has a differential impact on the occurrence of keratinocyte cancers in SOC. Even for factors related to UV exposure outside of phototherapy, such as geographical location and occupation, the small positive associations for keratinocyte malignancies observed in East Asian communities may be a function of the constituent ethnicities within these populations [18, 19].

Is Phototherapy a Risk Factor for Skin Cancer?
Globally, PUVA has been considered a risk factor for skin cancer. Speaking for SOC, a recent Indian study has found no evidence of skin cancer in patients who received PUVA or NBUVB, followed-up for 3 and 6.5 years, respectively [18, 20]. While this duration of follow-up may be adequate to assess the risk for SCC, melanomas and BCC may take longer to develop and may require longer follow-up. Looking at the melanoma risk in a large cohort of patients with vitiligo who received NBUVB therapy, Chia et al. found that there was no melanoma occurrence over a follow-up period of 9 years. Also, the absolute number of skin malignancies was low in this group from Singapore, though in patients with psoriasis, phototherapy was noted to increase the risk of malignancy proportionate to the cumulative and maximal doses and to concomitant use of systemic treatments. However, Lin et al. noted that in Taiwanese with skin types III–IV, the duration of phototherapy did not worsen outcomes in terms of cutaneous malignancies in patients receiving NBUVB for psoriasis [21]. Similarly, in patients undergoing phototherapy for psoriasis, vitiligo, and mycosis fungoides, Mimouni et al. reporting out of Israel found no association between the number of treatment sessions and the risk of skin cancer [22]. Remarkably, in this study with a follow-up period of 13 years, age and fair skin type were the only risk factors, highlighting the protective effect of melanin in SOC. To conclude, more studies in SOC, with adequate follow-up periods and with considerations on the effect of concurrent immunosuppression influences, will dictate whether phototherapy is not a significant factor even in the long run, as established in a recent review [23].

As with other aspects of skin typing, using the ITA over FST, and addition of other features like colour of the eyes, hair colour, tanning ability, and reactivity to sunlight, may add some advantages to identifying SOC individuals for whom sunlight may be a potential factor for photocarcinogenesis [13].

Historically, short bouts of intense sun exposure have been considered adequate to initiate melanoma skin cancers, while chronic cumulative sun damage is said to influence the occurrence of nonmelanoma skin cancers, typically squamous cell carcinomas [13, 24]. However, the lines are blurred. Basal cell carcinoma is associated with early life exposure to both chronic and intense intermittent sun exposure [25]. Between basal and squamous cell carcinomas, the latter are considered to be more solar radiation dependent [26], with even a single episode of sunburn in childhood being associated with the occurrence of solar keratosis [27]. However, it is also considered that basal cell carcinomas that arise in the highly mitotically active basal layer may have a lower threshold to malignant transformation of cells leading to tumour initiation, compared to the superficial epidermal cells which give rise to squamous cell carcinomas. Interventions such as sunscreen use are understood to be more useful for the latter, due to the longer promotion phase, while an earlier age of sun protection behaviour is required for a meaningful level of prevention of BCC [26].

Specifically for melanoma skin cancers, the occurrence has been understood to be UV dose-dependent, with a linearly increasing risk for malignancy for an increasing number of sunburns, representing intense but intermittent sun exposure over a lifetime [24]. More recently, this was challenged in an elegant study that showed that cumulative, continuous sun exposure over a lifetime also influences the occurrence of cutaneous melanoma, with specific relevance to darker skin types [28]. However, the historically low overall incidence of melanomas in darker skin types runs counter to this observation considering the high level of UVR exposure in latitudes closer to the equator and no relatable increase in melanomas in SOC. This standpoint is also endorsed by a recent systematic review by Lopes et al., which concludes that UV exposure may not be a significant risk factor for the development of cutaneous melanoma in skin of colour [23]. This is further strengthened by the fact that the UV signature mutations are less exhibited in melanomas that occur in persons with SOC [13]. Regardless, melanoma in skin of colour has a poorer prognosis, with a lower melanoma specific survival comparatively [13], often presenting at a later stage, due in some part to a lesser index of suspicion. If the difference in incidence of skin cancers in the tropics despite the high UV index is striking, then the phenotypic characteristics are even more interestingly distinct in SOC. To start with, in melanoma in skin of colour, the involvement of non-sun exposed areas is significant [13, 29]. Typically, melanoma in SOC is commonly known to involve the palmar, plantar, subungual, and mucosal surfaces [11], areas that are not associated with sun exposure. The specific subtype, the acral melanoma which occurs on the palms and the soles, accounts for 2–3% of all melanomas in the light-skinned population while contributing to more than 50% of all melanomas recorded in SOC populations. Detected at a later stage, and with a poorer survival rate compared to cutaneous melanoma, acral melanoma is considered one of the deadliest types of melanomas [30]. Understanding this significance, the 2023 WHO classification of tumours classifies melanomas into those arising in sun-exposed areas and those occurring in sun-protected areas [31].

Clearly, the pathways for cutaneous carcinogenesis differ significantly across populations. Sunscreens have been considered one of the most important tools for the prevention of cutaneous malignancies, with widespread use. However, it is still not conclusively clear if sunscreens actually protect against skin cancer [32].

4.1 Do Sunscreens Protect Against Skin Cancer?

All wavelengths in the UV spectrum are considered carcinogenic. This was the conclusion put out by the International Agency for Research on Cancer (IARC) at a consensus gathering of 20 scientists from 9 countries in 2009 [33]. Therefore, sunscreen coverage has to be, essentially, broad spectrum, covering UVA, UVB, and UVC ranges, from wavelengths 100 to 400 nm.

The first evidence for the efficacy of sunscreens in photoprotection against cancer was provided by the Nambour study, published in 1999. Specifically, the

Nambour study found sunscreens to be of potential benefit in reducing the incidence of squamous cell cancers in the group randomized to sunscreen use over sun-exposed parts. And this effect was observed, not just during the study, but in a follow-up period of 8 years after the conclusion of the initial 4.5 year study. However, this benefit was not significant for basal cell carcinoma, even though these malignancies were found to decrease in the sunscreen group compared to the no sunscreen group [34, 35]. A case control study using an SPF 17 sunscreen compared to a base cream without UV filters found that the incidence of solar keratosis decreased in those who used sunscreens versus those who were given the cream base, in whom there was an increase in lesions during the course of one summer in Australia. Additionally, sunscreen use was noted to induce the remission of existing lesions and prevent new lesion formation, in a dose–response relationship, with positive benefits related to higher quantities of sunscreen used [36].

For melanoma, no consensus has been reached regarding the utility of sunscreens for prevention [37, 38]. According to a review by the International Agency for Research on Cancer, more studies showed an increased risk of melanoma with sunscreen use, compared to those which demonstrated a preventive benefit for sunscreen use. However, counter views exist. A meta-analysis found heterogeneous outcomes for the risk of melanoma in ever versus never use of sunscreen, using data pooled from 28 studies, which included one randomized controlled trial, the Nambour cohort [38], which showed a protective benefit.

Several underlying factors likely contribute to this paradoxical effect. Many of these studies were performed at a time when sunscreen efficacy was not as robust as the current day, in addition to issues around stability and the spectrum of protection. Considering that the initial photocarcinogenesis focus was strongly on UVB, sunscreen products did not provide adequate UVA protection. The concept of UVA testing was introduced only in the 1980s and in that decade, only 1% of sunscreens were found to contain UV filters with efficacy in the UVA spectrum [39]. Though this number increased to 35% in the 1990s, even recently comparing between sunscreens in Europe and the USA, Diffey found that compared to the former, lesser UVA coverage was obtained from sunscreens available in the USA [33]. However, the role of UVA in the development of melanoma and nonmelanoma skin cancers has been established conclusively in recent years [32]. Sunscreen formulations with predominantly UVB coverage and insufficient UVA protection were found to be associated with a higher risk of melanoma, at latitudes higher than 40 degrees [40], with a protective effect for latitudes lesser than 40 degrees. Current, newer formulations which focus on broad-spectrum coverage as a mandatory requirement may reduce the risk for vulnerable populations. Even among broad-spectrum sunscreens, lack of an adequate level of UVA protection failed to protect against UV-induced immune suppression, as denoted by delayed-type hypersensitivity, underscoring the role of UVA in photo-immunomodulation [41]. Further, sunscreens that protect only in the UVB zone have been shown to perform in dependence of the time of the day and the latitude, with reduced protection at temperate latitudes compared to broad-spectrum sunscreens. However, in this study, the SPF protection was very low at a value of 6, which may not have been adequate to protect against the end point of erythema [32]. Some researchers suggest that sunscreen use in latitudes above 40 degree north, providing only UVB coverage, may have contributed to increased skin cancer, due to the lack of UVA protection [40]. Overall, current research concludes that only sunscreens with broad-spectrum UV coverage, specifically covering UVA and UVB, are capable of mitigating the biological damage produced by UV irradiation [42]. Sunscreens with high sun protection factor (SPF) and UVA protection factor (UVA-PF) credentials are capable of providing proportionately higher levels of protection against irradiation [43].

The photoinstability of sunscreens, especially when more than one UV filter was used, is a potential factor contributing to the perceived lack of sunscreen efficacy. Avobenzone, the only chemical filter approved for UVA coverage in the USA, is in wide use globally. In New Zealand, up to 70% of sunscreen products contain avobenzone as the UVA blocker [44]. The cancer protective effect of such sunscreen products used in the past remains doubtful, due to the notorious lack of stability of avobenzone in sunscreen formulations. To illustrate, sunscreen formulations containing avobenzone and octinoxate was used as the intervention in the Nambour study, which showed a modest protection for SCC, though not for BCC. This combination has since been shown to have some level of photoinstability, where octinoxate exhibited photolysis in the presence of avobenzone [45]. Subsequently, however, multiple innovations to increase the photostability of UV filters have been brought into practice, such as the addition of octocrylene, avoidance of irrational combinations which increase photoinstability and/or promote free radical generation. These make currently available sunscreens potentially more efficacious in preventing cutaneous carcinogenesis. Further, this area continues to be in focus for essential reasons, with recent and emerging research identifying UV filter combinations which are potentially counterproductive to sunscreen product efficacy [46, 47], enabling the development of safer and more effective sunscreens.

Higher SPF sunscreens proven to provide better UV attenuation have only been available in the market for the past 2–3 decades [48]. Most of the earlier studies in the 1980s and 1990s, including the Nambour study at 15 SPF, have employed lower SPF formulations [35, 49]. A higher SPF sunscreen has the advantage of higher sun protection and longer durability on the skin which may offset the disadvantage of lesser product use by the consumer [50]. This factor has the potential to make a positive case for sunscreens against skin cancer development.

Next, the latency period to develop melanomas from the time of initial sun exposure is very long, about 10–50 years, which also plays a role in undermining any possible protective effect of sunscreens in melanoma prevention [24].

Further, using erythema as a surrogate marker for UV-induced skin damage leading to carcinogenesis has proved troublesome for lighter skinned individuals. Early sunscreens were aimed at reducing UVB led damage and therefore at reducing erythema. Erythema is driven by nitric oxide, which acts as a natural warning system indicating skin damage. In the absence of erythema as a visible end point for excessive sun exposure while using sunscreens, individuals stayed longer in the sun still being exposed to the remaining components of solar radiation. This suppression of the inbuilt warning sign of redness may have provided a false sense of security to individuals, who stay out in the sun longer and receive more UVR, at least some of which reaches the target zones in the skin [51]. This resulted in a paradoxical increase in skin cancers, where users of sunscreen reported higher rates of cutaneous malignancy than those who did not. This view is also supported by the outcomes of the EORTC (European Organisation for Research and Treatment of Cancer) melanoma case control study which concluded that sunscreens were not protective against cancer. This trial also found tanning sunscreens which contain agents such as psoralens that induce skin pigmentation probably anticipating higher UV protection to be actually associated with an increased melanoma risk [52]. The paradox seems to also be driven by climate conditions as illustrated by the difference in cutaneous melanoma incidence in Atlantic Canada. Comparing provinces with higher incidence of cutaneous melanomas to those with lower levels, Alli et al. found that though people practised sun protection behaviour and were more sun aware in the former group, they also received higher levels of UV exposure. In contrast, despite a less common use of sunscreens and sun protective clothing, people living in provinces with lower sun exposure had a resultant lesser incidence of melanoma. Here the level of UV exposure contributed to the sunscreen paradox, than erythema (or its lack) driven human behaviour alone, where increased sunscreen use can still be associated with increased sun exposure [53].

SPF labelling on a product may have also played a role. The SPF label on a sunscreen was found to influence personal exposure time in the sun [32].

Challenges in Demonstrating the Utility of Sunscreens for Skin Cancer Prevention

1. Lack of UVA coverage in sunscreens used in the past
2. Photoinstability of sunscreen filters used in sunscreen efficacy studies
3. Lower SPF sunscreens used as an intervention in past studies
4. Long latency period to the development of skin cancers, particularly basal cell carcinoma
5. Reliance on erythema as a visual end point to denote sunburn, leading to unintended increase in sun exposure
6. False sense of security afforded by SPF labelling on a product, which at best indicates protection only from the UVB spectrum.

As of now, the clear benefit of sunscreen use in all skin types and for all types of skin cancer has not been established conclusively [17, 54]. While benefits for SCC exist in some studies as above, longer term studies are required for BCC and melanoma, with study outcomes specifically focused to demonstrate a benefit for sunscreens in preventing cancer in melanin rich skin or a lack thereof. Even though UVA has been identified as a risk factor for photocarcinogenesis, and the newer sunscreen filters approved in Europe, though not in the USA, potentially reduce overall UV load on the skin, there are no studies at this point to demonstrate that increasing spectrum coverage reduces skin cancer risk [55]. Diffey noted that sunscreens approved in the USA allowed three times as much UVR to reach the skin as did European sunscreens, comparing select brands. But given the lack of data, these wide-spectrum sunscreens may or may not essentially reduce cancer risk, and the uncertainty would be considered to remain, until future studies if and when feasible shed more light on this issue. However, there is reason to believe that the newer sunscreen formulation developments are in the right direction, though it may take longer for tangible benefits to be seen [56].

Overall, the argument in favour of sunscreen usage for protection against cancer is enunciated by Weinberg as one of understanding causality. UVB is a known cause for the development of melanomas and sunscreens are proven to reduce the quantum of UVB that reaches the skin and therefore potentially play a protective role against skin malignancies [40]. This standpoint may be said to be similar to a meta-analysis of 9067 patients which pooled together from 11 trials and found that sunscreen use was not associated with an increased melanoma risk. The authors suggested that subject selection and uncontrolled confounding may have been factors that portray sunscreens as associated with increased risk of melanoma. However, the study was unable to show a protective impact for topical sunscreen use and development of malignant melanoma, suggesting that sunscreens be used for reduction of exposure to the risk factor, namely UV, from a causality point of view [57].

So, it is safe to conclude that sunscreens have been found to be beneficial as only one among several interventions required to reduce cancer incidence [58, 59], even though it is the most commonly used tool for sun protection and as a cancer prevention self-care act [60]. The question that we are now faced with is this: If the overall cancer risk is low and 2 of the major types of skin cancer, namely melanoma and squamous cell carcinomas, have factors other than sun exposure as the main trigger [5], what then is the role of sunscreens in skin of colour?

Nambour Trial and Outcomes

The Nambour Trial remains the largest body of evidence for sunscreen use for prevention of photocarcinogenesis, even if the quantum of protection was not significant for all types of cancers.

The Nambour sunscreen trial is the most cited randomized controlled trial to demonstrate the protectiveness of sunscreens against skin cancer. A brief discussion of the sun protection studies carried out in the residents of Nambour community, in Queensland, Australia, is shared below by publication timeline.

1994: The Nambour Trial, or the Nambour Skin Cancer and Actinic Eye Disease Prevention Trial, was registered to be conducted as a randomized trial, to evaluate the role of sunscreens and/or beta-carotene supplementation in the prevention of skin cancers, over a follow-up period of 4.5 years in 1626 participants residing in Nambour, Queensland, Australia. Occurrence of pre-malignant solar keratosis lesions, actinic eye disease, and photoageing were other outcome measurements for the trial [49].

1998: In the same community, the history of even a single episode of sunburn was shown to be significant for the prevalence of solar keratosis [27].

1999: The Nambour study was published, having been successfully run for a study period of 4.5 years. It found that sunscreen usage did not have a significant protective effect against basal cell carcinoma. The occurrence of squamous cell carcinomas was lesser by 25% in the regular sunscreen users group, compared to discretionary sunscreen use, though the difference did not reach significance. However, in sites of actual sunscreen usage, the total tumour incidence rate was significantly lesser in the sunscreen group compared to the no sunscreen arm, for squamous cell carcinoma, while this advantage could not be seen for basal cell carcinoma. The study used a single daily application of an octinoxate–avobenzone sunscreen, with an SPF rating of 16, with reapplication advised only if there was prolonged sun exposure, bathing, or heavy sweating. The control group used sunscreen, on a discretionary or recreational basis [26].

2002: Behavioural outcomes related to the amount of sunscreen use also came to light in the Nambour community trials. It was found that most commonly people used less than half the sunscreen amount that is needed to achieve labelled SPF [61]. Study participants were found to use an average of 0.79 mg/cm^2 compared to the 2 mg/cm^2 standard that was used in sunscreen SPF testing at the time. This insight from real world usage may have influenced the current day testing standards, where volumes less than 2 mg/cm^2 are used in the various ISO protocols. (Going by recent guidelines however, the FDA 2011 recommends in vitro sunscreen testing at 0.75 mg/cm^2 and ISO 24443 standard uses a quantity of 1.3 mg/cm^2—see section on SPF testing.) [62]

2003: The update on the ability of sunscreens and/or beta-carotene supplementation to prevent solar keratosis was published, with sunscreen usage showing a nonsignificant reduction in lesion counts in those who were randomized to use sunscreens daily, regularly, versus those who used sunscreens at their own discretion, mostly for recreational use. Beta-carotene supplementation failed to demonstrate any protective effect against the development of solar keratosis in this trial [63]. Given that actinic keratosis is now considered as in situ squamous cell carcinoma, compared to their earlier status of precursor lesions [64], the use of sunscreens may still be considered to have a beneficial effect (see Box—on challenges).

2005: Given that skin cancers are not a finite, single occurrence, the utility of sunscreens in reducing the risk for subsequent BCCs was evaluated in the Nambour cohort. While sunscreen usage was not found to be significantly protective against the occurrence of a BCC for the first time ever, sunscreen use was found to lower the risk of subsequent BCC, though this reduction was not statistically significant [65].

2006: One of the most important outcomes of the Nambour Trial was human behavioural change that led to regular use of sunscreen in study participants who were in the regular sunscreen group, compared to the discretionary sunscreen use group. After the conclusion of the study period that lasted through 4.5 years, participants were followed up on sunscreen use behaviour. Though the overall usage was low, the highest usage rates being 20% on the face and 15% on the forearms for the regular sunscreen use group, the difference was significant between the two groups [66]. Since protection from sunscreens is only temporary, related to the duration of usage, habit formation is very important to achieve meaningful sun protection benefits.

2011: A 10-year follow-up of the Nambour cohort found that long-term sunscreen use may prevent invasive melanomas. However, the reduction in incidence of melanoma overall was only found to just approach significance [35].

2012: Sunscreen use was not found to affect vitamin D levels in this cohort, as were other protective measures like using a hat, sunglasses, or umbrella or wearing long sleeved clothes. Seeking shade was found to be associated with lower vitamin D levels, especially when not spending time outdoors, otherwise. This observation concluded that it is possible to practise sun safe behaviour without significant impact on vitamin D levels [67].

2013: The last study from the Nambour Trial evaluated skin ageing due to sun exposure. A subgroup of individuals aged 55 years or less was randomly drawn from the trial registry, and signs of ageing were compared between the regular sunscreen group and the discretionary sunscreen group. The study found that there was no detectable increase in skin ageing during the study period of 4.5 years in those who had been randomized to the daily sunscreen group, inferring that regular sunscreen usage has the potential to retard skin ageing in healthy individuals. Beta-carotene supplementation provided no benefit for skin ageing, very much like its lack of protective effect against skin cancers.

To summarize, the risk of skin cancer in SOC is largely mitigated, due to the presence of higher amounts of melanin in darker versus lighter skin. Fundamentally, the increased density of melanin in pigmented skin reduces the level of UVR-induced damage of the cellular DNA in the lower epidermal keratinocytes and melanocytes. Any damage that still happens is repaired more effectively, along with a more efficient removal of UV damaged, potentially precancerous cells, through apoptosis. Overall, melanin in the skin works as an efficient sunscreen for dark skin [15, 68].

4.2 Chapter Summary

Sunscreens are popularly considered as the first line of protection against skin cancer, by the vast majority of users. The role of sunscreens in protecting against UVR is well established; however, the translation of this effect in reducing clinical burden of skin cancer remains unclear. This may be, in some part, due to the lesser product efficacy of early sunscreens such as were used in these studies. The ability of newer, more efficient sunscreens with better spectral homeostasis, to prevent skin cancer, remains to be established. For SOC, the inherent protection afforded by the higher melanin content in the skin is a key factor in the lower skin cancer rates, compared to lighter skin types. Further, specific melanoma types as common in this population occur in sun-protected regions, making the role of sunscreen use for cancer prevention, unclear at present. For lighter skinned phototypes, the series of trials done at Nambour, Australia, remains a key way of understanding the protective impact of sunscreens on skin cancer. Despite clear and conclusive quantification of protection, from the point of causality alone, sunscreens still remain an important tool in preventing UV-induced skin cancer.

References

1. Young AR. The adverse consequences of not using sunscreens. Int J Cosmet Sci [Internet]. 2023 Oct 1 [cited 2024 Mar 11];45 Suppl 1(S1):11–9. Available from: https://pubmed.ncbi.nlm.nih.gov/37799076/
2. Armstrong BK, Kricker A, English DR. Sun exposure and skin cancer. Australas J Dermatol [Internet]. 1997 [cited 2024 Mar 11];38 Suppl 1:S1–6. Available from: https://pubmed.ncbi.nlm.nih.gov/10994463/
3. Leiter U, Keim U, Garbe C. Epidemiology of skin cancer: update 2019. Adv Exp Med Biol [Internet]. 2020 [cited 2024 Mar 11];1268:123–39. Available from: https://pubmed.ncbi.nlm.nih.gov/32918216/
4. Swope VB, Abdel-Malek ZA. MC1R: front and center in the bright side of dark eumelanin and DNA repair. Int J Mol Sci [Internet]. 2018 Sep 8 [cited 2024 Mar 11];19(9). Available from: https://www.ncbi.nlm.nih.gov/pmc/articles/PMC6163888/
5. Skin cancer in skin of color - PubMed [Internet]. [cited 2024 Mar 11]. Available from: https://pubmed.ncbi.nlm.nih.gov/19691228/
6. Labani S, Asthana S, Rathore K, Sardana K. Incidence of melanoma and nonmelanoma skin cancers in Indian and the global regions. J Cancer Res Ther [Internet]. 2021 Jul 1 [cited 2024 Mar 11];17(4):906–11. Available from: https://pubmed.ncbi.nlm.nih.gov/34528540/
7. Hofer S, Stonig M, Wally V, Hartmann A, Fuchs D, Hermann M, et al. Contradictory effects of chemical filters in UV/ROS-stressed human keratinocyte and fibroblast cells. ALTEX [Internet]. 2019 [cited 2024 Mar 11];36(2):231–44. Available from: https://pubmed.ncbi.nlm.nih.gov/30488083/
8. Karimkhani C, Green AC, Nijsten T, Weinstock MA, Dellavalle RP, Naghavi M, et al. The global burden of melanoma: results from the Global Burden of Disease Study 2015. Br J Dermatol [Internet]. 2017 Jul 1 [cited 2024 Mar 11];177(1):134. Available from: https://www.ncbi.nlm.nih.gov/pmc/articles/PMC5575560/
9. Schneider SL, Lim HW. A review of inorganic UV filters zinc oxide and titanium dioxide. Photodermatol Photoimmunol Photomed [Internet]. 2019 Nov 1 [cited 2024 Mar 11];35(6):442–6. Available from: https://pubmed.ncbi.nlm.nih.gov/30444533/
10. Lal ST, Banipal RPS, Bhatti DJ, Yadav HP. Changing trends of skin cancer: a tertiary care hospital study in Malwa Region of Punjab. J Clin Diagn Res [Internet]. 2016 Jun 1 [cited 2024 Mar 11];10(6):PC12–5. Available from: https://pubmed.ncbi.nlm.nih.gov/27504344/
11. Ho SGY, Chan HHL. The Asian dermatologic patient. Am J Clin Dermatol 2009 10:3 [Internet]. 2012 Aug 23 [cited 2024 Mar 11];10(3):153–68. Available from: https://link.springer.com/article/10.2165/00128071-200910030-00002

12. Pega F, Momen NC, Streicher KN, Leon-Roux M, Neupane S, Schubauer-Berigan MK, et al. Global, regional and national burdens of non-melanoma skin cancer attributable to occupational exposure to solar ultraviolet radiation for 183 countries, 2000–2019: a systematic analysis from the WHO/ILO Joint Estimates of the Work-related Burden of Disease and Injury. Environ Int [Internet]. 2023 Nov 1 [cited 2024 Mar 11];181. Available from: https://pubmed.ncbi.nlm.nih.gov/37945424/
13. Brunsgaard EK, Jensen J, Grossman D. Melanoma in skin of color: part II. Racial disparities, role of UV, and interventions for earlier detection. J Am Acad Dermatol [Internet]. 2023 Sep 1 [cited 2024 Mar 11];89(3):459–68. Available from: https://pubmed.ncbi.nlm.nih.gov/35533770/
14. Menke HE. Pigment disorders and pigment manipulations. The melanin millennium: skin color as 21st century international discourse [Internet]. 2013 Aug 1 [cited 2024 Mar 2];183–205. Available from: https://link.springer.com/chapter/10.1007/978-94-007-4608-4_12
15. Yamaguchi Y, Beer JZ, Hearing VJ. Melanin mediated apoptosis of epidermal cells damaged by ultraviolet radiation: factors influencing the incidence of skin cancer. Arch Dermatol Res [Internet]. 2008 Apr [cited 2024 Mar 2];300 Suppl 1(SUPPL. 1). Available from: https://pubmed.ncbi.nlm.nih.gov/17985102/
16. Fajuyigbe D, Lwin SM, Diffey BL, Baker R, Tobin DJ, Sarkany RPE, et al. Melanin distribution in human epidermis affords localized protection against DNA photodamage and concurs with skin cancer incidence difference in extreme phototypes. FASEB J [Internet]. 2018 Jul 1 [cited 2024 Mar 5];32(7):3700–3706. Available from: https://pubmed.ncbi.nlm.nih.gov/29394104/
17. Tow R, Hanoun S, Andresen B, Shahid A, Wang J, Kelly KM, et al. Recent advances in clinical research for skin cancer chemoprevention. Cancers (Basel) [Internet]. 2023 Aug 1 [cited 2024 Mar 11];15(15). Available from: https://pubmed.ncbi.nlm.nih.gov/37568635/
18. Ravindran S, Pai B S, Shetty VM. Risk of cutaneous carcinogenesis with phototherapy in Indian subpopulation: a 10-year analysis and a review of literature. Dermatol Ther [Internet]. 2022 Jul 1 [cited 2024 Mar 11];35(7). Available from: https://pubmed.ncbi.nlm.nih.gov/35462452/
19. Kolitz E, Lopes FCPS, Arffa M, Pineider J, Bogucka R, Adamson AS. UV exposure and the risk of keratinocyte carcinoma in skin of color: a systematic review. JAMA Dermatol [Internet]. 2022 May 1 [cited 2024 Mar 11];158(5):542. Available from: https://www.ncbi.nlm.nih.gov/pmc/articles/PMC8943625/
20. Sevdem GA, Ozlem KS, Nazan Y, Nahide O. Does the risk of basal cell carcinoma increase in patients with psoriasis under treatment? Photodermatol Photoimmunol Photomed [Internet]. 2024 Mar 1 [cited 2024 Mar 11];40(2). Available from: https://pubmed.ncbi.nlm.nih.gov/38404169/
21. Lin TL, Wu CY, Chang YT, Juan CK, Chen CC, Yu SH, et al. Risk of skin cancer in psoriasis patients receiving long-term narrowband ultraviolet phototherapy: results from a Taiwanese population-based cohort study. Photodermatol Photoimmunol Photomed [Internet]. 2019 May 1 [cited 2024 Mar 11];35(3):164–71. Available from: https://pubmed.ncbi.nlm.nih.gov/30536640/
22. Mimouni I, Shulman J, Unes AA, Pavlovsky L, Pavlotsky F. Frequency of skin cancer among psoriasis, vitiligo, and mycosis fungoides patients treated with narrowband ultraviolet B phototherapy. Photodermatol Photoimmunol Photomed [Internet]. 2024 Jan 1 [cited 2024 Mar 11];40(1). Available from: https://pubmed.ncbi.nlm.nih.gov/38059681/
23. Lopes FCPS, Sleiman MG, Sebastian K, Bogucka R, Jacobs EA, Adamson AS. UV exposure and the risk of cutaneous melanoma in skin of color: a systematic review. JAMA Dermatol [Internet]. 2021 Feb 1 [cited 2024 Mar 11];157(2):213–9. Available from: https://pubmed.ncbi.nlm.nih.gov/33325988/
24. Mulliken JS, Russak JE, Rigel DS. The effect of sunscreen on melanoma risk. Dermatol Clin [Internet]. 2012 Jul [cited 2024 Mar 11];30(3):369–376. Available from: https://pubmed.ncbi.nlm.nih.gov/22800545/

25. Marionnet C, de Dormael R, Marat X, Roudot A, Gizard J, Planel E, et al. Sunscreens with the new MCE filter cover the whole UV spectrum: improved UVA1 photoprotection in vitro and in a randomized controlled trial. JID Innov [Internet]. 2021 Jan 1 [cited 2024 Mar 3];2(1). Available from: https://pubmed.ncbi.nlm.nih.gov/35072138/
26. Green A, Williams G, Neale R, Hart V, Leslie D, Parsons P, et al. Daily sunscreen application and betacarotene supplementation in prevention of basal-cell and squamous-cell carcinomas of the skin: a randomised controlled trial. Lancet [Internet]. 1999 Aug 28 [cited 2024 Mar 3];354(9180):723–729. Available from: https://pubmed.ncbi.nlm.nih.gov/10475183/
27. Frost CA, Green AC, Williams GM. The prevalence and determinants of solar keratoses at a subtropical latitude (Queensland, Australia). Br J Dermatol [Internet]. 1998 [cited 2024 Mar 11];139(6):1033–9. Available from: https://pubmed.ncbi.nlm.nih.gov/9990367/
28. Dennis LK. Cumulative sun exposure and melanoma in a population-based case–control study: does sun sensitivity matter? Cancers (Basel) [Internet]. 2022 Feb 1 [cited 2024 Mar 11];14(4). Available from: https://www.ncbi.nlm.nih.gov/pmc/articles/PMC8870683/
29. Panda S. Nonmelanoma skin cancer in India: current scenario. Indian J Dermatol [Internet]. 2010 Oct [cited 2024 Mar 11];55(4):373. Available from: https://www.ncbi.nlm.nih.gov/pmc/articles/PMC3051301/
30. Carvalho LADC, Aguiar FC, Smalley KSM, Possik PA. Acral melanoma: new insights into the immune and genomic landscape. Neoplasia [Internet]. 2023 Dec 1 [cited 2024 Mar 11];46:100947–1476. Available from: https://www.ncbi.nlm.nih.gov/pmc/articles/PMC10637990/
31. Gosman LM, Țăpoi DA, Costache M. Cutaneous melanoma: a review of multifactorial pathogenesis, immunohistochemistry, and emerging biomarkers for early detection and management. Int J Mol Sci. 2023 [Internet]. 2023 Nov 1 [cited 2024 Mar 11];24(21):15881. Available from: https://www.mdpi.com/1422-0067/24/21/15881/htm
32. Young AR, Boles J, Herzog B, Osterwalder U, Baschong W. A sunscreen's labeled sun protection factor may overestimate protection at temperate latitudes: a human in vivo study. J Invest Dermatol [Internet]. 2010 [cited 2024 Mar 11];130(10):2457–2462. Available from: https://pubmed.ncbi.nlm.nih.gov/20535128/
33. Diffey B. New sunscreens and the precautionary principle. JAMA Dermatol [Internet]. 2016 May 1 [cited 2024 Mar 11];152(5):511–2. Available from: https://pubmed.ncbi.nlm.nih.gov/26885870/
34. Van Der Pols JC, Williams GM, Pandeya N, Logan V, Green AC. Prolonged prevention of squamous cell carcinoma of the skin by regular sunscreen use. Cancer Epidemiol Biomarkers Prev [Internet]. 2006 Dec [cited 2024 Mar 11];15(12):2546–8. Available from: https://pubmed.ncbi.nlm.nih.gov/17132769/
35. Green AC, Williams GM, Logan V, Strutton GM. Reduced melanoma after regular sunscreen use: randomized trial follow-up. J Clin Oncol [Internet]. 2011 Jan 20 [cited 2024 Mar 11];29(3):257–63. Available from: https://pubmed.ncbi.nlm.nih.gov/21135266/
36. Thompson SC, Jolley D, Marks R. Reduction of solar keratoses by regular sunscreen use. N Engl J Med [Internet]. 1993 Oct 14 [cited 2024 Mar 11];329(16):1147–51. Available from: https://pubmed.ncbi.nlm.nih.gov/8377777/
37. International Agency for Research on Cancer. Sunscreens. Handbooks of cancer prevention, vol. 5. Lyon: International Agency for Research on Cancer; 2001. Google Search [Internet]. [cited 2024 Mar 11]. Available from: https://www.google.com/search?q=%E2%80%9CInternational+Agency+for+Research+on+Cancer.%2C%E2%80%9D+Sunscreens.+Handbooks+of+cancer+prevention%2Cvol.+5.+Lyon+%28France%29%3A+International+Agency+for+Research+on+Cancer%3B+2001..+&sca_esv=d1b5aeb9d701f53b&ei=7cLuZbmpKfaQnesP0-yD6AY&ved=0ahUKEwj50_yu5-uEAxV2SGcHHVP2AG0Q4dUDCBE&uact=5&oq=%E2%80%9CInternational+Agency+for+Research+on+Cancer.%2C%E2%80%9D+Sunscreens.+Handbooks+of+cancer+prevention%2Cvol.+5.+Lyon+%28France%29%3A+International+Agency+for+Research+on+Cancer%3B+2001..+&gs_lp=Egxnd3Mtd2l6LXNlc-nAiqgHigJxJbnRlcm5hdGlvbmFsIEFnZW5jeSBmb3IgUmVzZWFyY2ggb24gQ2FuY2VyLi

zigJ0gU3Vuc2NyZWVucy4gSGFuZGJvb2tzIG9mIGNhbmNlciBwcmV2ZW50aW9uLHZ-
vbC4gNS4gTHlvbiAoRnJhbmNlKTogSW50ZXJuYXRpb25hbCBBZ2VuY3kgZm9yIFJl-
c2VhcmNoIG9uIENhbmNlcjsgMjAwMS4uIDIUEAAYgAQY4wQY6QQY6gIYtALYAQEy
FBAAGIAEGOMEGOkEGOoCGLQC2AEBMhQQABiABBjjBBjpBBjq
Ahi0AtgBATIWEC4YAxiPARjlAhjqAhi0AhiMA9gBAjIWEAAYAxiPARjlAhjqAhi0AhiM
A9gBAjIWEAAYAxiPARjlAhjqAhi0AhiMA9gBAjIWEAAYAxiPARjlAhjq
Ahi0AhiMA9gBAjIWEC4YAxiPARj
lAhjqAhi0AhiMA9gBAjIWEAAYAxiPARjlAhjqAhi0AhiMA9gBAjIWEAAYAxiPARjlAh
jqAhi0AhiMA9gBAkilClAAWJkHcAF4AZABA-
JgBAKABAKoBALgBA8gBAPgBAfgBApgCAaA
CGqgCCpgDGroGBAgBGAe6BgQIAhgKkgcBMaAHAA&sclient=gws-wiz-serp

38. Rueegg CS, Stenehjem JS, Egger M, Ghiasvand R, Cho E, Lund E, et al. Challenges in assessing the sunscreen-melanoma association. Int J Cancer [Internet]. 2019 Jun 1 [cited 2024 Mar 11];144(11):2651–68. Available from: https://pubmed.ncbi.nlm.nih.gov/30447006/
39. Ma Y, Yoo J. History of sunscreen: an updated view. J Cosmet Dermatol [Internet]. 2021 Apr 1 [cited 2024 Mar 15];20(4):1044–9. Available from: https://pubmed.ncbi.nlm.nih.gov/33583116/
40. Weinstock MA. Do sunscreens increase or decrease melanoma risk: an epidemiologic evaluation. J Investig Dermatol Symp Proc [Internet]. 1999 [cited 2024 Mar 13];4(1):97–100. Available from: https://pubmed.ncbi.nlm.nih.gov/10537017/
41. Moyal DD, Fourtanier AM. Broad-spectrum sunscreens provide better protection from solar ultraviolet-simulated radiation and natural sunlight-induced immunosuppression in human beings. J Am Acad Dermatol [Internet]. 2008 May [cited 2024 Mar 11];58(5 Suppl 2). Available from: https://pubmed.ncbi.nlm.nih.gov/18410801/
42. Fourtanier A, Moyal D, Seite S. UVA filters in sun-protection products: regulatory and biological aspects. Photochem Photobiol Sci [Internet]. 2012 [cited 2024 Mar 11];11(1):81–9. Available from: https://pubmed.ncbi.nlm.nih.gov/21904741/
43. Cole C, Appa Y, Ou-Yang H. A broad spectrum high-SPF photostable sunscreen with a high UVA-PF can protect against cellular damage at high UV exposure doses. Photodermatol Photoimmunol Photomed [Internet]. 2014 [cited 2024 Mar 11];30(4):212–219. Available from: https://pubmed.ncbi.nlm.nih.gov/24806442/
44. Ekstein SF, Hylwa S. Sunscreens: a review of UV filters and their allergic potential. https://home.liebertpub.com/derm [Internet]. 2023 May 17 [cited 2024 Apr 4];34(3):176–90. Available from: https://www.liebertpub.com/doi/10.1097/DER.0000000000000963
45. Sayre RM, Dowdy JC, Gerwig AJ, Shields WJ, Lloyd R V. Unexpected photolysis of the sunscreen octinoxate in the presence of the sunscreen avobenzone. Photochem Photobiol [Internet]. 2005 [cited 2024 Mar 11];81(2):452. Available from: https://pubmed.ncbi.nlm.nih.gov/15560736/
46. Ginzburg AL, Blackburn RS, Santillan C, Truong L, Tanguay RL, Hutchison JE. Zinc oxide-induced changes to sunscreen ingredient efficacy and toxicity under UV irradiation. Photochem Photobiol Sci [Internet]. 2021 Oct 1 [cited 2024 Apr 6];20(10):1273. Available from: https://pubmed.ncbi.nlm.nih.gov/34647278/
47. Gholap AD, Sayyad SF, Hatvate NT, Dhumal V V., Pardeshi SR, Chavda VP, et al. Drug delivery strategies for avobenzone: a case study of photostabilization. Pharmaceutics 2023 [Internet]. 2023 Mar 21 [cited 2024 Mar 11];15(3):1008. Available from: https://www.mdpi.com/1999-4923/15/3/1008/htm
48. Marshall SW, Poole C, Waller AE. Sunscreen use and malignant melanoma risk: the jury is still out. Am J Public Health [Internet]. 2003 Jan [cited 2024 Mar 11];93(1):11-b-12. Available from: https://pubmed.ncbi.nlm.nih.gov/12511370/
49. Green A, Battistutta D, Hart V, Leslie D, Marks G, Williams G, et al. The Nambour Skin Cancer and Actinic Eye Disease Prevention Trial: design and baseline characteristics of participants. Control Clin Trials [Internet]. 1994 [cited 2024 Mar 11];15(6):512–522. Available from: https://pubmed.ncbi.nlm.nih.gov/7851112/

50. Williams JD, Maitra P, Atillasoy E, Wu MM, Farberg AS, Rigel DS. SPF 100+ sunscreen is more protective against sunburn than SPF 50+ in actual use: results of a randomized, double-blind, split-face, natural sunlight exposure clinical trial. J Am Acad Dermatol [Internet]. 2018 May 1 [cited 2024 Mar 11];78(5):902–910.e2. Available from: https://pubmed.ncbi.nlm.nih.gov/29291958/
51. Serpone N. Sunscreens and their usefulness: have we made any progress in the last two decades? Photochem Photobiol Sci 2021 20:2 [Internet]. 2021 Feb 18 [cited 2024 Mar 3];20(2):189–244. Available from: https://link.springer.com/article/10.1007/s43630-021-00013-1
52. Autier P, Doré J -F, Schifflers E, Cesarini J -P, Bollaerts A, Koelmel KF, et al. Melanoma and use of sunscreens: an EORTC case-control study in Germany, Belgium and France. The EORTC Melanoma Cooperative Group. Int J Cancer [Internet]. 1995 [cited 2024 Mar 11];61(6):749–55. Available from: https://pubmed.ncbi.nlm.nih.gov/7790106/
53. Alli S, LeBeau J, Hasbani A, Lagacé F, Litvinov I V., Peláez S. Understanding the perceived relationship between sun exposure and melanoma in Atlantic Canada: a consensual qualitative study highlighting a "sunscreen paradox." Cancers 2023, Vol 15, Page 4726 [Internet]. 2023 Sep 26 [cited 2024 Mar 11];15(19):4726. Available from: https://www.mdpi.com/2072-6694/15/19/4726/htm
54. Sánchez G, Nova J, Rodriguez-Hernandez AE, Medina RD, Solorzano-Restrepo C, Gonzalez J, et al. Sun protection for preventing basal cell and squamous cell skin cancers. Cochrane Database Syst Rev [Internet]. 2016 Jul 25 [cited 2024 Mar 13];7(7). Available from: https://pubmed.ncbi.nlm.nih.gov/27455163/
55. Diffey BL. The impact of topical photoprotectants intended for daily use on lifetime ultraviolet exposure. J Cosmet Dermatol [Internet]. 2011 Sep [cited 2024 Mar 13];10(3):245–250. Available from: https://pubmed.ncbi.nlm.nih.gov/21896139/
56. Diffey B. Sunscreens and melanoma: the future looks bright. Br J Dermatol [Internet]. 2005 Aug [cited 2024 Mar 13];153(2):378–81. Available from: https://pubmed.ncbi.nlm.nih.gov/16086753/
57. Huncharek M, Kupelnick B. Use of topical sunscreens and the risk of malignant melanoma: a meta-analysis of 9067 patients from 11 case–control studies. Am J Public Health [Internet]. 2002 [cited 2024 Mar 13];92(7):1173. Available from: https://www.ncbi.nlm.nih.gov/pmc/articles/PMC1447210/
58. Berry EG, Bezecny J, Acton M, Sulmonetti TP, Anderson DM, Beckham HW, et al. Slip versus slop: a head-to-head comparison of UV-protective clothing to sunscreen. Cancers (Basel) [Internet]. 2022 Feb 1 [cited 2024 Mar 3];14(3):542. Available from: https://www.mdpi.com/2072-6694/14/3/542/htm
59. Hao OY, Jiang LI, Meyer K, Wang SQ, Farberg AS, Rigel DS. Sun protection by beach umbrella vs sunscreen with a high sun protection factor: a randomized clinical trial. JAMA Dermatol [Internet]. 2017 Mar 1 [cited 2024 Mar 27];153(3):304–8. Available from: https://pubmed.ncbi.nlm.nih.gov/28114650/
60. Koch S, Pettigrew S, Strickland M, Slevin T, Minto C. Sunscreen increasingly overshadows alternative sun-protection strategies. J Cancer Educ [Internet]. 2017 Sep 1 [cited 2024 Mar 13];32(3):528–31. Available from: https://pubmed.ncbi.nlm.nih.gov/26792784/
61. Neale R, Williams G, Green A. Application patterns among participants randomized to daily sunscreen use in a skin cancer prevention trial. Arch Dermatol [Internet]. 2002 Oct 1 [cited 2024 Mar 29];138(10):1319–25. Available from: https://pubmed.ncbi.nlm.nih.gov/12374537/
62. Federal Register:: sunscreen drug products for over-the-counter human use [Internet]. [cited 2024 Mar 20]. Available from: https://www.federalregister.gov/documents/2019/02/26/2019-03019/sunscreen-drug-products-for-over-the-counter-human-use
63. Darlington S, Williams G, Neale R, Frost C, Green A. A randomized controlled trial to assess sunscreen application and beta carotene supplementation in the prevention of solar keratoses. Arch Dermatol [Internet]. 2003 Apr 1 [cited 2024 Mar 13];139(4):451–5. Available from: https://pubmed.ncbi.nlm.nih.gov/12707092/

64. Roewert-Huber J, Stockfleth E, Kerl H. Pathology and pathobiology of actinic (solar) keratosis—an update. Br J Dermatol [Internet]. 2007 Dec [cited 2024 Mar 13];157 Suppl 2(SUPPL. 2):18–20. Available from: https://pubmed.ncbi.nlm.nih.gov/18067626/
65. Pandeya N, Purdie DM, Green A, Williams G. Repeated occurrence of basal cell carcinoma of the skin and multifailure survival analysis: follow-up data from the Nambour Skin Cancer Prevention Trial. Am J Epidemiol [Internet]. 2005 Apr 15 [cited 2024 Mar 13];161(8):748–54. Available from: https://doi.org/10.1093/aje/kwi098
66. Van Der Pols JC, Williams GM, Neale RE, Clavarino A, Green AC. Long-term increase in sunscreen use in an Australian community after a skin cancer prevention trial. Prev Med (Baltim) [Internet]. 2006 Mar [cited 2024 Mar 13];42(3):171–6. Available from: https://pubmed.ncbi.nlm.nih.gov/16325898/
67. Jayaratne N, Russell A, van der Pols JC. Sun protection and vitamin D status in an Australian subtropical community. Prev Med (Baltim) [Internet]. 2012 Aug [cited 2024 Mar 13];55(2):146–50. Available from: https://pubmed.ncbi.nlm.nih.gov/22634425/
68. Lawrence KP, Sarkany RPE, Acker S, Herzog B, Young AR. A new visible light absorbing organic filter offers superior protection against pigmentation by wavelengths at the UVR-visible boundary region. J Photochem Photobiol B. 2022;227:112372.

Chapter 5
Effects of Sun Exposure in Skin of Colour

Abbreviations

HEVL	High-energy visible light
IUCD	Intrauterine contraceptive device
MASI	Melasma Area and Severity Index
MC1R	Melanocortin 1 receptor
MELASQoL	Melasma Quality of Life Index
MMP	Matrix metalloproteinases
MSH	Melanocyte-stimulating hormone
NIR	Near-infrared light
OCP	Oral contraceptive pills
OPN-3	Opsin-3
PIH	Postinflammatory hyperpigmentation
PMLE	Polymorphous light eruption
PP-PMLE	Pinpoint papular variant of PMLE
PUVA	Psoralen and ultraviolet A therapy
SOC	Skin of colour
TRP	Tyrosinase-related protein
TSH	Thyroid-stimulating hormone
UV	Ultraviolet
UVR	Ultraviolet radiation
VL	Visible Light

Key Objectives

- The differential response in SOC to sunlight underlies the high concentration of melanin in such skin types.
- Pigmentary conditions such as melasma and PIH are very common in SOC populations, with implications for solar light across all of its spectra.
- Broad-spectrum sunscreens with coverage reaching deep into the VL and IR spectrum are recommended for SOC.

R. Rajan, *Sunscreens for Skin of Color*,
https://doi.org/10.1007/978-981-97-3195-4_5

- Understanding the need for balanced protection across all subcomponents of the solar spectrum is a prerequisite to choosing the correct sunscreen for SOC individuals.

5.1 Photoageing in SOC

Solar radiation is the main cause of premature skin ageing, second only to genetic predisposition [1, 2]. People who live in areas of high ultraviolet (UV) index and do not practice sun protection behaviour are perceived as appearing older than peers who do [3]. Skin of colour is innately protected from photoaging, due to the presence of melanin with its ability to absorb sunlight across a wide spectrum, ranging from the gamma spectrum, through UV and visible light to the infrared zone [4]. However, in skin of colour, pigmentary changes are noted to be a major aspect of photoaging, with UVA inducing significantly more pigmentation than UVB [5]. Suberythemal doses of UVA can cumulatively cause tissue damage, premature skin ageing and wrinkling, and also immunosuppression [6].

Skin of colour typically includes Fitzpatrick phototypes IV–VI. In general, the notion of skin of colour covers anyone who is not considered a non-Hispanic White. This includes anyone who identifies as Asian, Hispanic, African/Black, Native American, Pacific Islander, but considering the intermixing of races since world transport came into vogue may include other smaller groups as well [7].

UV-induced photoageing is likely the result of direct photochemical modifications or posttranslational changes in skin proteins, culminating in denaturation of skin collagen and elastin [8]. Though initially thought to be related to a similar UV range as erythema, typically UVB, recent studies have noted a larger contribution from the UVA, VL, and IR parts of the solar spectrum towards photoageing. Visible light (VL) and UVA are known to individually and synergistically promote skin pigmentation [9]. Other than UVA and VL, the near-infrared spectrum has also been noted to generate free radicals, at a higher level in darker skin [7]. The impact of free radicals generated by near-infrared light (NIR) is thought to induce photoaging by causing direct mitochondrial damage.

The main impact of solar radiation on skin is mediated through the generation of free radicals, which damage or destroy vital cellular elements such as DNA, RNA, proteins, and lipids. The solar spectrum between wavelengths 290 and 700 nm is capable of generating these free radicals, with UVA being a prominent contributor [8]. Much of the generated free radicals are quenched by melanin. Eumelanin is the dominant melanin in higher skin types and has considerable free-radical scavenging abilities. While the amount of melanin and number of melanosomes are higher in SOC, the distribution and fate of melanosomes vary across ethnicities. The number of melanocytes remains the same across races, for a given anatomical location [10]. The presence of melanin in skin type VI Black individuals reduces transmission into the dermis, by 75% and 70%, respectively, for UVB and UVA, compared to White individuals [11].

While it is clear that higher phototypes are inherently better protected, the level of such protection afforded by constitutive pigmentation varies depending on the endpoint. Compared to a light skinned individual, dark skin offers 10–15 fold more protection in terms of developing erythema, but the protection factor increases to 500–1000 fold for developing skin cancer. For Hispanics, the protection factor ranges from 2.5 times for erythema to twice that for protection against cancer. Ethnicity, and therefore melanin quantity and distribution, seems to influence differentially, symptoms related to sun exposure like erythema here or outcomes such as skin cancer [12].

In a study comparing ethnic populations in the same city and therefore at the same UV index and geographical conditions, wrinkles were found to develop least in African Americans and Asians, compared to Hispanics, who in turn have lesser photoageing-related wrinkles compared to Caucasians [7]. Melanin mitigates the effect of matrix metalloproteinases (MMPs) in causing photo-induced dermal collagen breakdown and eventual solar elastosis [11]. With the overall significant attenuation of oxidative damage in SOC due to melanin, the onset of photoageing appears at a later date in SOC. Wrinkles have been noted to appear at least 10–20 years later in Asian skin compared to Caucasian skin [13].

Evaluating female faces across five ethnicities, Chinese, Japanese, French, Indian, and South African, researchers found that skin gloss, wrinkles, and sagging were the main attributes that relate to a perception of ageing. For skin health, the criteria were skin gloss, skin tone, and wrinkling. Perception of attractiveness was related to the presence of wrinkles and sagging. Nearly all of these features are affected by the solar spectrum. An uneven skin tone is one of the most common terms that patients use to express the changes that occur as a result of photoageing in SOC, especially in Asia. In a comparison between Chinese, French, Japanese, Indian, and South African women, lack of a uniform and homogenous skin tone, or the presence of significant contrast in skin pigmentation in different parts of the face, was noted predominantly in the latter two groups [14]. As homogenous facial skin colour is perceived as attractive, patchiness of skin pigmentation or a lack of uniformity of skin tone can create a perception of ageing by up to 20 years [2]. In faces standardized for shape and features, an even skin colouration led to higher attractiveness ratings, compared to less homogenous images. Further, participants tended to gaze longer at faces with more homogenous skin tone, with increased overall dwell times [15]. Across these five ethnic groups, sagging and wrinkling of skin were identified as signs of ageing, surprisingly, in agreement. However, facial sagging and volume of facial sagging were perceived to be the highest in Indian women, followed by South African women. Skin colouration was perceived as a sign of skin health, even compared to aspects of skin surface topography [14]. Loss of skin elasticity with sagging is noted to be more pronounced in photoaging, compared to chrono-ageing [16].

While for the most part melanin plays the role of a photoprotector, it can also be of concern in SOC, which responds to most cellular injury with an increase in pigmentation. Specifically, the role of visual light in the pathogenesis of photoaggravated pigmentary disorders in SOC has been well established in recent years. In dark-skinned individuals, intermittent and chronic sun exposure have been associated with tanning as well as pigmentation responses, which are not seen in light-skinned individuals. A higher UV exposure resulting in pigmentation conditions has been noted in Indian and South African women, despite higher protection against UV radiation (UVR) afforded by the increased skin pigmentation [17]. One would even go on to say that the darker skin phototypes age with pigmentation, as compared to the lighter skin types where photoaging is characterized by more of textural than pigmentary effects [18]. Though the number of melanocytes decreases with age, focal areas of localized hyperpigmentation occur as a component of photoaging in SOC [17]. Thus, the seeming advantage of SOC over the other group, as regards photoaging, seems to be quickly lost when it comes to disorders of pigmentation, with Asians noted to develop more hyperpigmentation and actinic lentigines, compared to Caucasians [13].

Pigmentation is an important component of photoaging, characterized by cellular senescence as per recent research. Photopigmentation is considered largely driven by UVA. The increase in skin melanin and therefore of pigmentation, brought about by UV rays, is usually uniform and homogenous. However, in skin of colour, there is a tendency to irregular and uneven increase in pigmentation, leading to the appearance of hyperpigmented lesions on sun exposure [5, 19]. Of late, the role of visible light and NIR is being aggressively explored, with particular relevance to photopigmentation disorders in SOC. Antioxidants in sunscreens are considered an effective way to reduce infrared (IR) induced photoaging, while future research may bring out filters with a specific ability to protect against the IR component of the solar spectrum [13].

Loss of skin surface reflectance or reduced skin gloss, with increased surface dehydration is one of the components of photoaging. Skin gloss refers to the contrast between the skin surface reflection and the darkness of the subsurface reflection, i.e., skin tone, and is perceived as a sign of skin health and youth. This parameter of attractiveness is easily perceived by humans, and loss of skin gloss is considered a sign of ageing [14].

Recently, the concepts of atrophic and hypertrophic photoaging have come to be recognized, though with lesser data for SOC [20–23]. Atrophic photoaging is found to be associated with erythema and telangiectasia and a higher tendency to the development of actinic keratosis, seborrheic keratosis, and skin cancer. Hypertrophic photoaging, however, is characterized by abundant skin wrinkling, increased skin thickness, sallowness, lesser erythema, and an overall higher score on photoaging. Though hypertrophic skin ageing is considered to be more common among higher skin types compared to Fitzpatrick (FST) I and II, even within FST I, II, and III, variabilities exist between the two types of ageing, related to gender, ancestry and sun exposure [23, 24].

The dermal extracellular matrix (ECM) plays a potential role in skin cancer, and differential changes in the ECM microenvironment between the two types of photoaging could explain the increased propensity for skin cancer development in those noted to have atrophic photoaging. Hypertrophic photoaging is characterized by plenty of solar elastosis, with resultant yellowness and sallowing of skin. However, the stiff elastotic material may also be considered to provide some protection against tumour growth and expansion of nonmelanoma skin cancers (NMSCs). On the contrary, increased vascularity in atrophic ageing may contribute to tumour development. The melanocortin 1 receptor (MC1R) gene is considered to play a role in the determination of atrophic versus hypertrophic photoageing [22].

Preageing is a new concept of skin ageing, reported mainly in Asian populations, typically from the far East. Proposed by Anwar et al., preageing is defined as changes in the skin that are seen as emerging signs of skin ageing, perceived by women in the 18–35 age group [24]. The typical signs reported include dull skin, uneven skin tone, dryness, transient wrinkles, lack of skin firmness, and slower recovery from pigmentary conditions like phototanning and post-acne marks. Though these changes are not typically considered as ageing by dermatologists, they are significant concerns to the individuals, and are thought to reflect an inability of repair mechanisms to keep up with accumulation of skin damage in the form of telomere shortening and impaired protein and DNA repair [24, 25]. Earlier onset of skin ageing has also been noted in areas with high solar impact like Australia, with skin ageing changes seen in early teens [26]. Photoaging features peculiar to preaging seem to be triggered by light exposure, pollution, poor sleep, psychological stress, poor nutrition, and lack of adequate sleep, apart from genetically modulated intrinsic processes. Addressing these lifestyle habits and the adoption of a skin care routine comprising sunscreens, moisturizers, and antioxidants may delay ageing and provide clinically visible results for this indication [24].

5.2 PIH

The principal response of SOC to most injuries of the skin is postinflammatory hyperpigmentation (PIH), which can be considered a prototype for pigmentary disorders in skin of colour. PIH can occur with the most common of skin conditions, with over 58.2% of individuals experiencing PIH after acne in an Asian cohort of FST III–VI, spanning 10 countries [27]. Further, the PIH was persistent for more than a year in over half of the study participants and up to 5 years in 22.3%. The incidence of PIH postacne was even higher in a recent Middle Eastern study, PIH was present in 87.2% of the subjects, with persistence up to a year in a little over half the study population [28]. Notably, PIH worsens on sun exposure [7] and sadly, even with ambient light [13], and improves with the use of sunscreens [29]. PIH in Indonesian women was also noted to be less in older women, probably in response to lesser sun exposure with increasing age [30].

Histopathologically, PIH has been identified to be of two types: epidermal and dermal. The dermal pigment type shows a lower epidermal pigmentation and a higher pigmentation in the upper dermis along with intense perivascular lymphocytic infiltrates. In contrast, the epidermal type is seen as increased pigmentation in the epidermal basal layer [31].

PIH is also a concern following cosmetic and aesthetic procedures in SOC [32–38]. Typically, post-laser pigmentation is noticeable about 7–14 days after the procedure and can persist for up to 3 months or longer [39]. Increased melanocyte activity with resultant increased pigmentation was noted to appear starting a week after an alexandrite laser irradiation in a Korean sequential histological study, which also showed the thwarting of this pigmentary response by the application of a topical corticosteroid [40]. For ablative resurfacing with the fractional CO_2 laser, it was found that the use of a broad-spectrum sunscreen along with anti-inflammatory agent, licochalcone-A, from the first postprocedure day, resulted in a lower melanin index indicating a lesser occurrence of PIH [41]. For all procedural treatments in SOC, regular use of a broad-spectrum sunscreen is recommended as a standard of care [42]. Sunscreens are also a daily baseline skin care recommendation for preventing pigmentation resulting from increased sun sensitivity in oncology patients, with a minimum SPF of 15 and with suitable UVA-PF as appropriate for the phototype [43]. Epidermal growth factors containing topical agents have been found to be variably useful in reducing the incidence of post-laser PIH in SOC [44–48]. The mechanism of action is expected to be an inhibition of melanin production from laser-treated keratinocytes, acting through the tyrosinase and prostaglandin E2 pathways, which are upregulated by laser treatment [49].

5.3 Melasma

The other commonly prevalent pigmentary condition in SOC is melasma. From being considered as a hormonally triggered event, the position of melasma is being reconsidered of late, as a photoaging disorder in genetically predetermined individuals. Melasma is disproportionately more common in SOC, with prevalence ranging from 15% to 25% of men in India, 19% of Kashmiri paddy field workers, and up to 34% women in Brazil, all the way to 100% in Indonesian women [30, 50–52].

In revisiting the causes of melasma as applied to the modern day scenario, studies found that only 20% of melasma was related to pregnancy. Also, men with melasma form a significant proportion of cases. At some level, socioeconomic factors play an exposome role in the management of melasma and in the prevention of further pigmentation. Cost was considered a deterrent factor for the use of sunscreens, in a North African study [53]. A certain level of awareness and educational status also seems to be necessary for successful and consistent adaptation of photoprotective behaviour, including sun avoidance and sunscreen use [54]. However, the psychosocial impact of melasma is undeniably more perceived as to reflect a higher likelihood of sunscreen usage, at an odds ratio of 6.7 times higher as compared to those with PIH [55].

The entire solar spectrum, and visible light in particular, has been found to exacerbate melasma. Sun exposure is considered the most significant exposome factor for melasma, with both direct stimulation of melanocytes to produce more melanin and indirectly through paracrine stimulation from cells in the epidermis and the dermis. Melasma intensity varies in geographies with seasonal variation of solar radiation [56]. UV increases the levels of melanocyte-stimulating hormone (α-MSH), corticotropin, and lipid peroxidation end products (LOX) in lesional skin of melasma, leading to increased pigmentation. UVB further upregulates melanocyte-specific genes causing increased expression of tyrosinase, tyrosinase-related protein (TRP-1), and dopachrome tautomerase in affected sites [56].

In favour of a solar contribution to melasma, lesional skin demonstrated increased elastolysis, increased vascularity, and an increase in dermal mast cells, in addition to increased epidermal and dermal melanin. Passeron et al. outline the presence of basal membrane alterations, molecular degradation, and protein denaturation in lesions of melasma, as evidence for solar-induced photodamage. Further promelanogenic paracrine factors secreted by fibroblasts, endothelial cells, and sebocytes are postulated to influence the appearance and anatomical distribution of melasma lesions on the face [57]. Sebocytes in particular are being revisited for their ability to stimulate melanocytes through the secretion of paracrine propigmentation mediators like α-MSH. Further, sebocytes sustain the locally inflamed and photoaged milieu in melasma lesions, working together with dermal fibroblasts [58].

Due to the depth of its penetration, visible light is able to sustain the inflammatory processes in the dermis and contributes to chronic exacerbation of melasma [57]. Acting through opsin 3 receptor (OPN-3), the blue-violet short wavelength high-energy visible light (HEVL) component of visible light, stimulates melanocytes to synthesize melanin [59]. The sensitivity of skin to blue light increases with age, due to the accumulation of the age pigment, lipofuscin. Made up of proteins and undegraded lipids, lipofuscin moieties act as photosensitizers and can aggravate VL-induced skin pigmentation and photoageing [60]. Considering that lipofuscin itself is generated by UVA, its ability to become photosensitive on VL stimulation underscores the close interaction between UVA and VL in causing photodamage [61]. Therefore, the use of sunscreens in general and tinted sunscreens with VL blocking ability in addition to coverage of the UV spectrum are foundational for long-term management of melasma [62].

In a 12-week study on Indian women, Sarkar et al. demonstrated the beneficial impact of sun protection on melasma, using sunscreens as a solo agent for pigment reduction. The pigmentation severity computed using Melasma Area and Severity Index (MASI) score reduced significantly from baseline, with a corresponding increase in the perceived quality of life captured by Melasma Quality of Life Index (MELASQoL) [63]. In addition using sunscreens as the only intervention as above, the use of sunscreens along with depigmenting agents like hydroquinone has shown to be more beneficial than using hydroquinone alone [64]. Going by studies where a sunscreen routine was used as the placebo arm, melasma was found to improve by 10–20%, using the MASI [65]. Similar studies have reported a lightening effect with the use of sunscreen alone in patients with melasma [66]. Broad-spectrum sunscreens have been effective in reducing melasma during pregnancy by almost 50% [39], underscoring sun exposure as a significant factor in melasma pathogenesis. Castanedo-Cazares et al. were able to show the additive benefit of using VL blocking sunscreens in addition to UV blockade, with a 75% reduction in MASI score compared to a 60% reduction with blocking UV alone [67].

The most common depigmenting agents used for melasma cannot be continued long term, due to their side effect profile. Relapses in melasma are therefore commonly expected and frequently witnessed in clinical practice. Managing a relapse of melasma is fairly difficult. Sunscreens have been found to be effective measures for maintaining melasma in some level of remission.

Though the melasma story is being rewritten as one of photoaging [57, 68], with solar elastosis being seen in up to 93% of patients with melasma [62], the hormonal contribution to pigmentation in melasma cannot be ignored. Oestrogens together with UVB exposure have been known to aggravate pigmentation and melasma [69]. Though not all women experience a reduction in melasma on stopping oral contraceptive pills, an improvement in pigmentation severity has been recorded on switching from oral contraceptive pills (OCPs) to a hormonal Intrauterine Contraceptive Device (IUCD) carrying progesterone with resultant reduced systemic exposure to the steroid hormones [70].

To conclude, melasma can be considered a clinical expression of the interplay between sun exposure, impaired repair of oxidative damage, propigmentary hormonal stimuli, coming together in a genetically susceptible population [59]. Sunscreens, preferably with antioxidants and/or pigments, are a standard of care in managing melasma [71], which benefits from targeting the multiple players involved in the pathogenesis.

5.4 PMLE

Polymorphous light eruption (PMLE) is a fairly common condition [72], known to occur in 10–20% of the general population in India, with a peak incidence between 20 and 30 years. The pruritic eruption occurs after 1 or 2 days of sun exposure and is a papulovesicular rash, occurring on sun-exposed areas [5]. Polymorphous skin eruption, also known as polymorphic skin eruption or prurigo aestivalis [73], is considered the most common photodermatoses in skin of colour, followed by chronic actinic dermatosis [74, 75]. PMLE has a female predominance, and a potential genetic predisposition, with a family history being reported in 12–16% of those with PMLE [72, 76]. This familial predisposition was not noted to be observed in Indian studies [72].

Globally, the predominant representation of darker coloured races in PMLE is well documented. In a large case series by Kerr and Lim, PMLE was noted to be significantly more common in African Americans compared to Caucasians [77, 78]. Following through on this study, Nakamura et al. documented the higher prevalence of PMLE in African Americans at 86.2% compared to 54% in Caucasians [79]. However, some authors consider it to be quite common even in lighter skin type [73, 80].

Uniquely in skin of colour, the lesion morphology is significantly variable with the appearance of hyperpigmented, normopigmented, and hypopigmented lesions with variable erythema. Pigmentary lesions were noted to occur in up to 50% of cases, based on the Indian scenario described by Karthikeyan and Aishwarya [72]. It is not uncommon for the hypo- or hyperpigmentation to persist for some time after the clearance of lesions themselves. Though described as polymorphous, in a given individual, the lesions usually tend to be monomorphic [72, 80]. Specific clinical variants include juvenile spring eruption, seen seasonally, during spring or summer, as vesicles on the ears of young boys, and PMLE sine eruption, characterized by pruritus on sun-exposed parts without the occurrence of any skin lesions [73]. Increased expression of intercellular adhesion molecule-1 (ICAM-1) has been noted to occur relative to the development of skin lesions [81]. Hardening, which reduced severity of the skin rash and reduced itching, is noted as a result of repeated sun exposure, with lesions occurring less commonly on the face and the arms and also less commonly towards the end of the summer [72]. The condition improves within 2 weeks of cessation of exposure to UV. Hardening to sun exposure takes about 4–6 weeks to result in better sun tolerance in individuals with photosensitivity [82].

A recent variant described from East Asia is the pinpoint papular variant of PMLE, also called PP-PMLE, recorded in darker skin types in Singapore and Japan, where it is known as micropapular light eruption. A similar micropapular form known to occur in Indians has been called the summertime actinic lichenoid eruption, and all these three variants may represent different morphological points in the clinical PMLE spectrum in dark-skinned individuals [80]. The scoring system to denote the severity of PMLE was developed by Hadshiew [83] and is as below, Table 5.1. Histopathological severity grading was described by Bansal et al. [84], with interface liquefactive changes, considered to be diagnostic, Table 5.2.

PMLE is considered to be a delayed-type hypersensitivity reaction to novel antigens uncovered by sun exposure. These antigens are yet to be characterized, but interestingly photohardening with exposure to narrow band UVB or psoralen and ultraviolet A therapy (PUVA) therapy has been demonstrated to reduce the sensitivity to sun exposure [85]. PMLE is generally presumed to be triggered predominantly by UVA [86], though some Indian data points to the involvement of UVB in photo patch testing studies [72, 87], though less commonly, both UVA and UVB

Table 5.1 PMLE severity scoring by Hadshiew et al. [83]

Score	Description	Interpretation
0	No PMLE	Pigmentation, Plane erythema, no papulovesicles
0.5	Doubtful PMLE	Patchy erythema and pruritus
1	Mild PLE (positive PMLE reaction)	Papulovesicles/papules≤10 or plaques ≤30% at the site of photoprovocation and pruritus
2	Moderate PMLE	Papulovesicles/papules >10 and ≤30% at the site of photoprovocation and pruritus
3	Severe PMLE	Papulovesicles/papules >30 or plaques >50% or haemorrhage or bullae at the site of photoprovocation and severe pruritus

Table 5.2 Histopathology grading of PMLE by Bansal et al. [84]

Grading	Epidermis	Basal cell degeneration	Dermis
Diagnostic	Hyperkeratosis/atrophy/spongiosis	Liquefactive-degeneration present	Dense perivascular lymphocytic infiltrate in upper and mid dermis
Possible	Atrophy/spongiosis	Not present	Sparse perivascular lymphocytic infiltrate
Probable	No changes	Not present	Minimal perivascular lymphocytic infiltrate

may be implicated [81]. UVA, particularly the UVA1 spectrum, induces photo-immunosuppression by modulating genes related to immunity with upregulation of inflammatory molecules. This altered immune response is said to play a role in the development of PMLE [88]. Underscoring the role of UVA1, persistent PMLE has been known to occur in patients receiving UVA1 phototherapy [89].

Sunscreens with a higher UVA-PF are more protective for PMLE, at an equivalent SPF, highlighting a larger role for UVA in the development of this photodermatosis [5]. An ectoin containing sunscreen was found to significantly reduce the occurrence of PMLE. In addition to ectoin claim of having the ability to reduce UVA-induced stress responses in the skin, the sunscreen also contained octocrylene, titanium dioxide, butyl methoxydibenzoylmethane, and bis-ethylhexyloxyphenol methoxyphenyl triazine [81]. The presence of 2 UVA filters, ecamsule and avobenzone, in an SPF 40 sunscreen cream was found to confer better protection against PMLE than test sunscreen formulations which contained only one UVA filter [90].

Considering an immunologically mediated phenomenon, PMLE was recently found to be associated with underlying biochemical thyroid abnormalities. Thyroid-stimulating hormone (TSH) values were found to be elevated in 93.3% of cases, significantly higher than controls at 3.3%. A commonly acting autoimmune pathway may be responsible for the generation of autoantibodies, and this early finding by Mishra et al. warrants further elucidation in larger cohorts [76].

Sunscreens for PMLE should be broad-spectrum and have adequate protection against UVA. To ensure this, a critical wavelength criterion of more than 370 nm, and a higher protection factor (PF) rating on the label, should be looked for while selecting a sunscreen. Seeking shade and other methods of physical sun protection such as clothing and the use of an umbrella should always be recommended.

Chronic actinic dermatitis, collagen vascular diseases, atopic dermatitis, actinic lichen planus, and lichen planus pigmentosus are the other common photodermatosis reported in Indians, typically of skin type IV and V, in an incidence comparable to SOC globally [75].

5.5 Sunscreens for SOC

The purpose of sunscreens in skin of colour (SOC) is uniquely distinct, compared to other skin types. SOC ethnicities are constitutively better protected against the most widely known effect of sunlight, namely photocarcinogenesis, due to the high epidermal melanin content [91]. Even photoageing occurs with different manifestations in skin of colour [92]. However, the high melanin content also predisposes this population to a range of pigmentary disorders, which can be associated with a significant burden of disease, even if the outcomes themselves are not life threatening [92, 93]. The differential outcomes of sun exposure are due to the specific ways in which skin of colour responds to the exposome of solar radiation, an exploration of which is warranted, to arrive at the exact positioning of sunscreens for SOC.

Sunscreen use in Asia closely mirrors the long standing preference for lighter skin in this part of the world. Sun avoidance and physical methods of sun protection have always been practised since ancient times by Asians, with an emphasis on fairer skin, and the sunscreens may be understood as a natural extension of the same thought process. However, the routine use of sunscreens in skin of colour has come under debate.

In a pertinent article, Taneja et al. question the benefit of regular sunscreen use in people who have no pre-existing photoaggravated skin disorder [94]. The authors rightly wonder if the increased demand for sunscreens as a means of skin lightening or complexion improvement might not have stemmed from the ever-growing obsession in this part of the world, for fair skin. The need for general physical sun protection is also debated in this article, considering the ability of highly melanized black skin to filter out close to 92.6% of UVB and 82.5% of UVA, compared to 76% of UVB and 45% of UVA in white skin. A similar sentiment is echoed in a recent article by Brian Diffey, widely considered to be a pioneer of modern sunscreen science [95]. In a recent article, Diffey makes a case for avoiding sunscreen application at times where there may be no biological advantage. Particularly, he opines there may be no need to use sunscreens at latitudes ≥45° North, during the winter month. However, for latitudes within 30°North, there is a need to use sunscreens throughout the year. By using sunscreen where there is likely to be a significant UV load and avoiding at other times, the photobiologist suggests that sunscreen use may be brought down globally by at least 25%, reducing the load on the environment. The role of clothing and shade seeking behaviour complements this rational use of sunscreen.

But what may justify the regular use of sunscreens even in skin of colour is the predisposition to develop pigmentary conditions as one of the main manifestations of photoaging [95]. It has been suggested that if skin darkening is a result of sun exposure, the regular use of sun protection products may lead to skin lightening. In other words, sunscreen products may be considered as remedial options to address sun-induced facultative skin pigmentation [19]. That there is a significant reduction in skin pigmentation in SOC on sunscreen use has been well established in different ethnic groups. Halder et al. demonstrated the overall skin lightening in 85% and reduction in pigmented macules in 81% of African American and Hispanic women with the use of sunscreen for 8 weeks [39, 96]. This study also highlighted the advantage of using higher SPF sunscreens even in SOC. Sarkat et al. demonstrated a significant reduction in MASI scores with the solo use of sunscreens in Indian patients with melasma, over a 12-week period. This study used a sunscreen with an SPF of 19, but with PA +++ rating, highlighting the importance of broad-spectrum protection in melasma [63].

With the increase in the number of people, globally and regionally, using sunscreens for photoaging benefits, sunscreen may be seen as serving an aesthetic goal over and above a health goal. Further, the rise in pigmentary conditions with rising levels of pollution [97–100], particularly in the Asian continent, may eventually bring sunscreens back into the health domain, as the cornerstone of managing pigmentary disorders in at least some individuals and preventing these disorders in others.

Sunscreen Requirements for Skin of Colour

1. Broad Spectrum: Sunscreens recommended for people with SOC should address the ability of the given product to protect against pigmentation. Since pigmentation can result from exposure to all parts of the solar spectrum, sunscreens meant for SOC should be essentially broad spectrum.
2. Provide HEVL Cover: Given the role of HEVL in causing skin pigmentation, sunscreens should specifically provide attenuation in this zone. This can be achieved through the addition of antioxidants with proven protection in the longer end of the UVA and HEVL spectrum, use of tinted sunscreens, and deployment of newer UV filters with proven benefits for this range of UV spectrum.
3. Use of antioxidants, melanin, lignin, tannin, and similar agents which reduce free radical damage can likely prevent and delay photoageing-related photopigmentation with resultant improvement in skin health.
4. Sunscreens meant for SOC should not contain photosensitizers like bergamot oil, psoralens, and other potential photosensitizers, as the risk for photocontact pigmentation is high in skin of colour. Agents such as henna and its derivative lawsone, which has been used in tanning sunscreens and tanning cosmetics are to be avoided in SOC, due to the high potential for photosensitization and pigment contact dermatitis [101].

5.6 Summary

The key differences between solar-induced responses between skin of colour and lighter skin types lie in the domain of photoageing and skin pigmentation. Melasma, a common condition in SOC, is triggered by multiple components within solar light, from UV to VL to IR, and therefore, sunscreens for this condition need to address coverage in each of these domains. Similarly, PIH is a very common condition in SOC and merits a comprehensive discussion and planning to prevent hyperpigmentation after skin treatments and laser procedures. Allergy to sunlight in the form of PMLE is triggered mainly by the UVA component, with some contribution from UVB. Overall, sunscreens are used in SOC more for conditions other than photocarcinogenesis and therefore must be formulated after understanding the role of solar or UV stimulation in the pathogenesis of these conditions. Physicians must be aware of the specific spectral coverage of modern day sunscreens to effectively include sunscreens as co-prescriptions as part of their treatment strategy.

References

1. Zastrow L, Meinke MC, Albrecht S, Patzelt A, Lademann J. From UV protection to protection in the whole spectral range of the solar radiation: new aspects of sunscreen development. Adv Exp Med Biol [Internet]. 2017 [cited 2024 Mar 3];996:311–8. Available from: https://pubmed.ncbi.nlm.nih.gov/29124711/
2. Matts PJ, Nash JF. Sunscreens—another endangered species? Int J Cosmet Sci [Internet]. 2023 Oct 1 [cited 2024 Mar 3];45 Suppl 1(S1):20–32. Available from: https://pubmed.ncbi.nlm.nih.gov/37799079/
3. Avila FR, Carter RE, McLeod CJ, Bruce CJ, Giardi D, Guliyeva G, et al. Perceived age in patients exposed to distinct UV indexes: a systematic review. Indian J Plast Surg [Internet]. 2023 May 4 [cited 2024 Mar 13];56(2):103. Available from: https://www.ncbi.nlm.nih.gov/pmc/articles/PMC10159705/
4. Hanel A, Carlberg C. Skin colour and vitamin D: an update. Exp Dermatol [Internet]. 2020 Sep 1 [cited 2024 Mar 2];29(9):864–875. Available from: https://pubmed.ncbi.nlm.nih.gov/32621306/
5. Moyal D. Need for a well-balanced sunscreen to protect human skin from both Ultraviolet A and Ultraviolet B damage. Indian J Dermatol Venereol Leprol [Internet]. 2012 Jun 1 [cited 2024 Mar 22];78(SUPPL.1):24. Available from: https://ijdvl.com/need-for-a-well-balanced-sunscreen-to-protect-human-skin-from-both-ultraviolet-a-and-ultraviolet-b-damage/
6. Parisi A V., Turnbull DJ, Kimlin MG. Influence of solar UVA on erythemal irradiances. Phys Med Biol [Internet]. 2006 Jun 21 [cited 2024 Mar 3];51(12):3241–9. Available from: https://pubmed.ncbi.nlm.nih.gov/16757874/
7. Tsai J, Chien AL. Reinforcing photoprotection for skin of color: a narrative review. Dermatol Ther (Heidelb) [Internet]. 2023 Sep 1 [cited 2024 Mar 13];13(9):1935–58. Available from: https://pubmed.ncbi.nlm.nih.gov/37495857/
8. Gasparro FP. Sunscreens, skin photobiology, and skin cancer: the need for UVA protection and evaluation of efficacy. Environ Health Perspect [Internet]. 2000 [cited 2024 Mar 13];108(Suppl 1):71. Available from: https://www.ncbi.nlm.nih.gov/pmc/articles/PMC1637776/
9. Kohli I, Chaowattanapanit S, Mohammad TF, Nicholson CL, Fatima S, Jacobsen G, et al. Synergistic effects of long-wavelength ultraviolet A1 and visible light on pigmentation and erythema. Br J Dermatol [Internet]. 2018 May 1 [cited 2024 Mar 14];178(5):1173–80. Available from: https://pubmed.ncbi.nlm.nih.gov/28877342/
10. Del Bino S, Duval C, Bernerd F. Clinical and biological characterization of skin pigmentation diversity and its consequences on UV impact. Int J Mol Sci [Internet]. 2018 Sep 8 [cited 2024 Mar 2];19(9). Available from: https://www.ncbi.nlm.nih.gov/pmc/articles/PMC6163216/

11. Kaidbey KH, Agin PP, Sayre RM, Kligman AM. Photoprotection by melanin--a comparison of black and Caucasian skin. J Am Acad Dermatol [Internet]. 1979 [cited 2024 Mar 14];1(3):249–60. Available from: https://pubmed.ncbi.nlm.nih.gov/512075/
12. Objective determination of Fitzpatrick skin type—PubMed [Internet]. [cited 2024 Mar 14]. Available from: https://pubmed.ncbi.nlm.nih.gov/20682135/
13. Passeron T, Lim HW, Goh CL, Kang HY, Ly F, Morita A, et al. Photoprotection according to skin phototype and dermatoses: practical recommendations from an expert panel. J Eur Acad Dermatol Venereol [Internet]. 2021 Jul 1 [cited 2024 Mar 14];35(7):1460–1469. Available from: https://pubmed.ncbi.nlm.nih.gov/33764577/
14. Voegeli R, Campiche R, Biassin R, Rawlings A V., Shackelford TK, Fink B. Predictors of female age, health and attractiveness perception from skin feature analysis of digital portraits in five ethnic groups. Int J Cosmet Sci [Internet]. 2023 Oct 1 [cited 2024 Mar 5];45(5):672–687. Available from: https://pubmed.ncbi.nlm.nih.gov/37338195/
15. Fink B, Matts PJ, Klingenberg H, Kuntze S, Weege B, Grammer K. Visual attention to variation in female facial skin color distribution. J Cosmet Dermatol [Internet]. 2008 Jun [cited 2024 Mar 14];7(2):155–61. Available from: https://pubmed.ncbi.nlm.nih.gov/18482022/
16. de Moura JP, de Moura Fernandes ÉP, Lustoza Rodrigues TCM, Messias Monteiro AF, de Sousa NF, dos Santos AMF, et al. Targets involved in skin aging and photoaging and their possible inhibitors: a mini-review. Curr Drug Targets [Internet]. 2023 Jul 20 [cited 2024 Mar 14];24(10):797–815. Available from: https://pubmed.ncbi.nlm.nih.gov/37469150/
17. Rawlings A V. Ethnic skin types: are there differences in skin structure and function?1. Int J Cosmet Sci [Internet]. 2006 Apr 1 [cited 2024 Mar 3];28(2):79–93. Available from: https://onlinelibrary.wiley.com/doi/full/10.1111/j.1467-2494.2006.00302.x
18. Vierkötter A, Hüls A, Yamamoto A, Stolz S, Krämer U, Matsui MS, et al. Extrinsic skin ageing in German, Chinese and Japanese women manifests differently in all three groups depending on ethnic background, age and anatomical site. J Dermatol Sci [Internet]. 2016 Sep 1 [cited 2024 Mar 14];83(3):219–25. Available from: https://pubmed.ncbi.nlm.nih.gov/27289339/
19. Moyal D. Prevention of ultraviolet-induced skin pigmentation. Photodermatol Photoimmunol Photomed [Internet]. 2004 Oct [cited 2024 Mar 4];20(5):243–7. Available from: https://pubmed.ncbi.nlm.nih.gov/15379874/
20. Langton AK, Ayer J, Griffiths TW, Rashdan E, Naidoo K, Caley MP, et al. Distinctive clinical and histological characteristics of atrophic and hypertrophic facial photoageing. J Eur Acad Dermatol Venereol [Internet]. 2021 Mar 1 [cited 2024 Mar 14];35(3):762–8. Available from: https://pubmed.ncbi.nlm.nih.gov/33275818/
21. Sachs DL, Varani J, Chubb H, Fligiel SEG, Cui Y, Calderone K, et al. Atrophic and hypertrophic photoaging: clinical, histologic, and molecular features of 2 distinct phenotypes of photoaged skin. J Am Acad Dermatol [Internet]. 2019 Aug 1 [cited 2024 Mar 14];81(2):480–8. Available from: https://pubmed.ncbi.nlm.nih.gov/30954583/
22. Guida S, Ciardo S, De Pace B, De Carvalho N, Farnetani F, Pezzini C, et al. Atrophic and hypertrophic skin photoaging and melanocortin-1 receptor (MC1R): the missing link. J Am Acad Dermatol [Internet]. 2021 Jan 1 [cited 2024 Mar 14];84(1):187–90. Available from: https://pubmed.ncbi.nlm.nih.gov/32335180/
23. Langton AK, Ali Z, Hann M, Ayer J, Watson REB, Griffiths CEM. Prevalence of atrophic and hypertrophic skin ageing phenotypes: a UK-based observational study. Acta Derm Venereol [Internet]. 2020 [cited 2024 Mar 14];100(19):1–3. Available from: https://pubmed.ncbi.nlm.nih.gov/33241421/
24. Anwar SS, Smith SD, Pongprutthipan M, Kim JY, Yuan C, van Steensel M. Preageing of the skin among Asian populations. JEADV Clin Pract [Internet]. 2022 Jun 1 [cited 2024 Mar 14];1(2):88–95. Available from: https://onlinelibrary.wiley.com/doi/full/10.1002/jvc2.22
25. Anwar SS, Apolinar MA, Ma L. Perception, understanding, and association between psychological stress and skin aging: quantitative surveys of Asian women aged 18–34 years, dermatologists, and psychologists in China and Japan. J Cosmet Dermatol [Internet]. 2023

Aug 1 [cited 2024 Mar 14];22(8):2297–307. Available from: https://onlinelibrary.wiley.com/doi/full/10.1111/jocd.15732

26. Green AC, Wallingford SC, McBride P. Childhood exposure to ultraviolet radiation and harmful skin effects: epidemiological evidence. Prog Biophys Mol Biol [Internet]. 2011 Dec [cited 2024 Mar 14];107(3):349. Available from: https://www.ncbi.nlm.nih.gov/pmc/articles/PMC3409870/
27. Abad-Casintahan F, Chow SKW, Goh CL, Kubba R, Hayashi N, Noppakun N, et al. Frequency and characteristics of acne-related post-inflammatory hyperpigmentation. J Dermatol [Internet]. 2016 Jul 1 [cited 2024 Mar 14];43(7):826–828. Available from: https://pubmed.ncbi.nlm.nih.gov/26813513/
28. Abanmi A, Al-Enezi M, Al Hammadi A, Galadari I, Kibbi AG, Zimmo S. Survey of acne-related post-inflammatory hyperpigmentation in the Middle East. J Dermatolog Treat [Internet]. 2019 Aug 18 [cited 2024 Mar 14];30(6):578–81. Available from: https://pubmed.ncbi.nlm.nih.gov/30426810/
29. Sarkar R, Garg VK, Jain A, Agarwal D, Wagle A, Flament F, et al. A randomized study to evaluate the efficacy and effectiveness of two sunscreen formulations on Indian skin types IV and V with pigmentation irregularities. Indian J Dermatol Venereol Leprol [Internet]. 2019 Mar 1 [cited 2024 Mar 14];85(2):160–8. Available from: https://pubmed.ncbi.nlm.nih.gov/30381582/
30. Du Y, Doraiswamy C, Mao J, Zhang Q, Liang Y, Du Z, et al. Facial skin characteristics and concerns in Indonesia: a cross-sectional observational study. Skin Res Technol [Internet]. 2022 Sep 1 [cited 2024 Mar 14];28(5):719–728. Available from: https://onlinelibrary.wiley.com/doi/full/10.1111/srt.13189
31. Park JY, Park JH, Kim SJ, Kwon JE, Kang HY, Lee ES, et al. Two histopathological patterns of postinflammatory hyperpigmentation: epidermal and dermal. J Cutan Pathol [Internet]. 2017 Feb 1 [cited 2024 Mar 14];44(2):118–24. Available from: https://pubmed.ncbi.nlm.nih.gov/27766668/
32. Laser skin resurfacing. Pre- and posttreatment guidelines—PubMed [Internet]. [cited 2024 Mar 14]. Available from: https://pubmed.ncbi.nlm.nih.gov/7496667/
33. Goldman MP. Universal classification of skin type. Simplified Facial Rejuvenation [Internet]. 2008 [cited 2024 Mar 5];47–50. Available from: https://link.springer.com/chapter/10.1007/978-3-540-71097-4_3
34. Goodman GJ. Carbon dioxide laser resurfacing: preliminary observations on short-term follow-up. A subjective study of 100 patients' attitudes and outcomes. Dermatol Surg [Internet]. 1998 [cited 2024 Mar 14];24(6):665–72. Available from: https://pubmed.ncbi.nlm.nih.gov/9648575/
35. Bernstein LJ, Kauvar ANB, Grossman MC, Geronemus RG. The short- and long-term side effects of carbon dioxide laser resurfacing. Dermatol Surg [Internet]. 1997 [cited 2024 Mar 14];23(7):519–25. Available from: https://pubmed.ncbi.nlm.nih.gov/9236869/
36. Nanni CA, Alster TS. Complications of carbon dioxide laser resurfacing. An evaluation of 500 patients. Dermatol Surg [Internet]. 1998 [cited 2024 Mar 14];24(3):315–20. Available from: https://pubmed.ncbi.nlm.nih.gov/9537005/
37. Laser skin resurfacing treatment outcome of facial scars and wrinkles in Asians with skin type III/IV with the Unipulse CO2 laser system—PubMed [Internet]. [cited 2024 Mar 14]. Available from: https://pubmed.ncbi.nlm.nih.gov/12008773/
38. Single-pass CO2 laser skin resurfacing of light and dark skin: extended experience with 52 patients—PubMed [Internet]. [cited 2024 Mar 14]. Available from: https://pubmed.ncbi.nlm.nih.gov/12745598/
39. Fatima S, Braunberger T, Mohammad T, Kohli I, Hamzavi I. The role of sunscreen in melasma and postinflammatory hyperpigmentation. Indian J Dermatol [Internet]. 2020 Jan 1 [cited 2024 Mar 14];65(1):5. Available from: https://www.ncbi.nlm.nih.gov/pmc/articles/PMC6986132/

40. Song HS, Park JY, Kim SJ, Kang HY. In vivo time-sequential histological study focused on melanocytes: suggestion of golden time for intervention to prevent post-laser pigmentary changes. J Eur Acad Dermatol Venereol [Internet]. 2016 Feb 1 [cited 2024 Mar 14];30(2):306–10. Available from: https://pubmed.ncbi.nlm.nih.gov/25731745/
41. Wanitphakdeedecha R, Phuardchantuk R, Manuskiatti W. The use of sunscreen starting on the first day after ablative fractional skin resurfacing. J Eur Acad Dermatol Venereol [Internet]. 2014 Nov 1 [cited 2024 Mar 29];28(11):1522–8. Available from: https://pubmed.ncbi.nlm.nih.gov/24320057/
42. Amici JM, Cogrel O, Jourdan M, Raimbault C, Canchy L, Kerob D, et al. Expert recommendations on supportive skin care for non-surgical and surgical procedures. J Eur Acad Dermatol Venereol [Internet]. 2023 Mar 1 [cited 2024 Mar 14];37 Suppl 3(S3):16–33. Available from: https://pubmed.ncbi.nlm.nih.gov/36635618/
43. Bensadoun RJ, Humbert P, Krutman J, Luger T, Triller R, Rougier A, et al. Daily baseline skin care in the prevention, treatment, and supportive care of skin toxicity in oncology patients: recommendations from a multinational expert panel. Cancer Manag Res [Internet]. 2013 Dec 9 [cited 2024 Mar 14];5(1):401–8. Available from: https://pubmed.ncbi.nlm.nih.gov/24353440/
44. Ying J, Zhang Y, Qiu Y, Xiang W. The role of epidermal growth factor-containing topical products on recovery and post-inflammatory hyperpigmentation prevention after laser surgeries: a systematic review and meta-analysis. J Cosmet Dermatol [Internet]. 2024 Feb 1 [cited 2024 Mar 14];23(2):382–90. Available from: https://pubmed.ncbi.nlm.nih.gov/37853844/
45. Kim HO, Kim HR, Kim JC, Kang SY, Jung MJ, Chang SE, et al. A randomized controlled trial on the effectiveness of epidermal growth factor-containing ointment on the treatment of solar lentigines as adjuvant therapy. Medicina (Kaunas) [Internet]. 2021 Feb 1 [cited 2024 Mar 14];57(2):1–11. Available from: https://pubmed.ncbi.nlm.nih.gov/33668564/
46. Wattanakrai P, Sindhusen S, Ploydaeng M. Effectiveness of an epidermal growth factor-containing cream on postinflammatory hyperpigmentation after 1064-nm Q-switched neodymium-doped yttrium aluminum garnet laser treatment of acquired bilateral nevus of Ota-like macules (Hori's nevus) in Asians: a split-face, double-blinded, randomized controlled study. J Cosmet Dermatol [Internet]. 2022 May 1 [cited 2024 Mar 14];21(5):2031–7. Available from: https://pubmed.ncbi.nlm.nih.gov/35066982/
47. Disphanurat W, Kaewkes A, Suthiwartnarueput W. Comparison between topical recombinant human epidermal growth factor and Aloe vera gel in combination with ablative fractional carbon dioxide laser as treatment for striae alba: a randomized double-blind trial. Lasers Surg Med [Internet]. 2020 Feb 1 [cited 2024 Mar 14];52(2):166–75. Available from: https://onlinelibrary.wiley.com/doi/full/10.1002/lsm.23052
48. Techapichetvanich T, Wanitphakdeedecha R, Iamphonrat T, Phothong W, Eimpunth S, Jane Hidajat I, et al. The effects of recombinant human epidermal growth factor containing ointment on wound healing and post inflammatory hyperpigmentation prevention after fractional ablative skin resurfacing: a split-face randomized controlled study. J Cosmet Dermatol [Internet]. 2018 Oct 1 [cited 2024 Mar 14];17(5):756–761. Available from: https://pubmed.ncbi.nlm.nih.gov/29956440/
49. Yun WJ, Bang SH, Min KH, Kim SW, Lee MW, Chang SE. Epidermal growth factor and epidermal growth factor signaling attenuate laser-induced melanogenesis. Dermatol Surg [Internet]. 2013 Dec [cited 2024 Mar 14];39(12):1903–11. Available from: https://pubmed.ncbi.nlm.nih.gov/24131350/
50. Sarkar R, Jagadeesan S, Basavapura Madegowda S, Verma S, Hassan I, Bhat Y, et al. Clinical and epidemiologic features of melasma: a multicentric cross-sectional study from India. Int J Dermatol [Internet]. 2019 Nov 1 [cited 2024 Mar 14];58(11):1305–10. Available from: https://pubmed.ncbi.nlm.nih.gov/31187480/
51. Ishiy PS, e Silva LR, Penha MÁ, Handel AC, Miot HA. Skin diseases reported by workers from UNESP campus at Rubião Jr, Botucatu-SP (Brazil). An Bras Dermatol [Internet]. 2014

[cited 2024 Mar 14];89(3):529. Available from: https://www.ncbi.nlm.nih.gov/pmc/articles/PMC4056724/

52. Bashir S, Hassan I, Wani RT, Zeerak S, Shah F. Pattern of skin diseases and occupational dermatoses among paddy field workers in Kashmir Valley: a cross-sectional study from North India. Indian J Community Med [Internet]. 2021 Oct 1 [cited 2024 Mar 14];46(4):610–613. Available from: https://pubmed.ncbi.nlm.nih.gov/35068719/
53. Seetan K, Shatanawi M, Ali A, Khamees A, Alsheikh A, Alawneh A, et al. Disease characteristics, determinants, and perception of use of sunscreen and sun-protective behaviors among patients of color with melasma: a cross-sectional study. Photodermatol Photoimmunol Photomed [Internet]. 2022 Sep 1 [cited 2024 Mar 14];38(5):495–500. Available from: https://pubmed.ncbi.nlm.nih.gov/35108414/
54. Nazli EC, Avcı C, Akarsu S. The effect of patient characteristics on illness perception and sun protection behaviors in melasma. J Cosmet Dermatol [Internet]. 2022 Dec 1 [cited 2024 Mar 14];21(12):7107–15. Available from: https://pubmed.ncbi.nlm.nih.gov/36136352/
55. Maymone MBC, Neamah HH, Wirya SA, Patzelt NM, Zancanaro PQ, Vashi NA. Sun-protective behaviors in patients with cutaneous hyperpigmentation: A cross-sectional study. Journal of American Dermatology [Internet]. 2017 [cited 2024 Mar 14];76:841–846.e2. Available from: https://doi.org/10.1016/j.jaad.2016.12.018
56. Liu W, Chen Q, Xia Y. New Mechanistic Insights of Melasma. Clin Cosmet Investig Dermatol [Internet]. 2023 [cited 2024 Mar 14];16:429–42. Available from: https://pubmed.ncbi.nlm.nih.gov/36817641/
57. Passeron T, Picardo M. Melasma, a photoaging disorder. Pigment Cell Melanoma Res [Internet]. 2018 Jul 1 [cited 2024 Mar 14];31(4):461–465. Available from: https://pubmed.ncbi.nlm.nih.gov/29285880/
58. Flori E, Mastrofrancesco A, Mosca S, Ottaviani M, Briganti S, Cardinali G, et al. Sebocytes contribute to melasma onset. iScience [Internet]. 2022 Mar 18 [cited 2024 Mar 14];25(3). Available from: https://pubmed.ncbi.nlm.nih.gov/35252805/
59. Espósito ACC, Cassiano DP, da Silva CN, Lima PB, Dias JAF, Hassun K, et al. Update on Melasma-Part I: Pathogenesis. Dermatol Ther (Heidelb) [Internet]. 2022 Sep 1 [cited 2024 Mar 4];12(9):1967–88. Available from: https://pubmed.ncbi.nlm.nih.gov/35904706/
60. Le Digabel J, Filiol J, Lauze C, Redoulès D, Josse G. In vivo method for evaluating sunscreen protection against high-energy visible light. J Eur Acad Dermatol Venereol [Internet]. 2023 Oct 1 [cited 2024 Mar 14];37 Suppl 6(S6):6–11. Available from: https://pubmed.ncbi.nlm.nih.gov/37671998/
61. Tonolli PN, Chiarelli-Neto O, Santacruz-Perez C, Junqueira HC, Watanabe IS, Ravagnani FG, et al. Lipofuscin Generated by UVA Turns Keratinocytes Photosensitive to Visible Light. J Invest Dermatol [Internet]. 2017 Nov 1 [cited 2024 Mar 14];137(11):2447–50. Available from: https://pubmed.ncbi.nlm.nih.gov/28711386/
62. Piętowska Z, Nowicka D, Szepietowski JC. Understanding melasma-how can pharmacology and cosmetology procedures and prevention help to achieve optimal treatment results? A narrative review. Int J Environ Res Public Health [Internet]. 2022 Oct 1 [cited 2024 Mar 2];19(19). Available from: https://pubmed.ncbi.nlm.nih.gov/36231404/
63. Sarkar R, Ghunawat S, Narang I, Verma S, Garg VK, Dua R. Role of broad-spectrum sunscreen alone in the improvement of melasma area severity index (MASI) and Melasma Quality of Life Index in melasma. J Cosmet Dermatol [Internet]. 2019 Aug 1 [cited 2024 Mar 29];18(4):1066–1073. Available from: https://pubmed.ncbi.nlm.nih.gov/31033184/
64. Pennitz A, Kinberger M, Avila Valle G, Passeron T, Nast A, Werner RN. Self-applied topical interventions for melasma: a systematic review and meta-analysis of data from randomized, investigator-blinded clinical trials. Br J Dermatol [Internet]. 2022 Sep 1 [cited 2024 Mar 14];187(3):309–317. Available from: https://pubmed.ncbi.nlm.nih.gov/35290681/
65. Cassiano DP, Espósito ACC, da Silva CN, Lima PB, Dias JAF, Hassun K, et al. Update on melasma-part II: treatment. Dermatol Ther (Heidelb) [Internet]. 2022 Sep 1 [cited 2024 Mar 14];12(9):1989–2012. Available from: https://pubmed.ncbi.nlm.nih.gov/35906506/

66. Topical isotretinoin for melasma in Thai patients: a vehicle-controlled clinical trial—PubMed [Internet]. [cited 2024 Mar 14]. Available from: https://pubmed.ncbi.nlm.nih.gov/10561942/
67. Castanedo-Cazares JP, Hernandez-Blanco D, Carlos-Ortega B, Fuentes-Ahumada C, Torres-Álvarez B. Near-visible light and UV photoprotection in the treatment of melasma: a double-blind randomized trial. Photodermatol Photoimmunol Photomed [Internet]. 2014 Feb [cited 2024 Mar 14];30(1):35–42. Available from: https://pubmed.ncbi.nlm.nih.gov/24313385/
68. Kwon SH, Na JI, Choi JY, Park KC. Melasma: Updates and perspectives. Exp Dermatol [Internet]. 2019 Jun 1 [cited 2024 Mar 14];28(6):704–8. Available from: https://pubmed.ncbi.nlm.nih.gov/30422338/
69. Kim JC, Park TJ, Kang HY. Skin-Aging Pigmentation: Who Is the Real Enemy? Cells [Internet]. 2022 Aug 1 [cited 2024 Mar 14];11(16). Available from: https://pubmed.ncbi.nlm.nih.gov/36010618/
70. Locci-Molina N, Wang A, Kroumpouzos G. Melasma Improving spontaneously upon switching from a combined oral contraceptive to a hormone-releasing intrauterine device: a report of four cases. Acta Derm Venereol [Internet]. 2015 [cited 2024 Mar 14];95(5):624–5. Available from: https://pubmed.ncbi.nlm.nih.gov/25394784/
71. González-Molina V, Martí-Pineda A, González N. Topical treatments for melasma and their mechanism of action. J Clin Aesthet Dermatol [Internet]. 2022 May 1 [cited 2024 Mar 14];15(5):19. Available from: https://www.ncbi.nlm.nih.gov/pmc/articles/PMC9122278/
72. Karthikeyan K, Aishwarya M. Polymorphous light eruption– an Indian scenario. Indian Dermatol Online J [Internet]. 2021 Mar 1 [cited 2024 Mar 14];12(2):211. Available from: https://www.ncbi.nlm.nih.gov/pmc/articles/PMC8088173/
73. Oakley AM, Ramsey ML. Polymorphic light eruption. European Handbook of dermatological treatments, Third Edition [Internet]. 2023 Aug 8 [cited 2024 Mar 14];757–61. Available from: https://www.ncbi.nlm.nih.gov/books/NBK430886/
74. Sharma VK, Sahni K, Wadhwani AR. Photodermatoses in pigmented skin. Photochem Photobiol Sci [Internet]. 2013 [cited 2024 Mar 14];12(1):65–77. Available from: https://pubmed.ncbi.nlm.nih.gov/23123922/
75. Wadhwani AR, Sharma VK, Ramam M, Khaitan BK. A clinical study of the spectrum of photodermatoses in dark-skinned populations. Clin Exp Dermatol [Internet]. 2013 Dec [cited 2024 Mar 14];38(8):823–9. Available from: https://pubmed.ncbi.nlm.nih.gov/23758593/
76. Mishra R, Talanikar H, Raheja A, Deora MS, Yadav S, Poulose D. Biochemical correlation of thyroid dysfunction among patients presenting with polymorphic light eruption. Cureus [Internet]. 2022 Mar 8 [cited 2024 Mar 14];14(3). Available from: https://pubmed.ncbi.nlm.nih.gov/35411278/
77. Lew R, Jacob J. Polymorphous light eruption: a common skin disease uncommonly recognized in the Hispanic population. Oxf Med Case Reports [Internet]. 2014 [cited 2024 Mar 14];2014(8):145. Available from: https://www.ncbi.nlm.nih.gov/pmc/articles/PMC4369994/
78. Kerr HA, Lim HW. Photodermatoses in African Americans: a retrospective analysis of 135 patients over a 7-year period. J Am Acad Dermatol [Internet]. 2007 Oct [cited 2024 Mar 14];57(4):638–43. Available from: https://pubmed.ncbi.nlm.nih.gov/17630044/
79. Nakamura M, Henderson M, Jacobsen G, Lim HW. Comparison of photodermatoses in African-Americans and Caucasians: a follow-up study. Photodermatol Photoimmunol Photomed [Internet]. 2014 Oct 1 [cited 2024 Mar 14];30(5):231–6. Available from: https://pubmed.ncbi.nlm.nih.gov/24118606/
80. Chen YA, Lee JYY. Clinicopathologic study of solar dermatitis, a pinpoint papular variant of polymorphous light eruption in Taiwan, and review of the literature. J Formos Med Assoc [Internet]. 2013 Mar [cited 2024 Mar 14];112(3):125–30. Available from: https://pubmed.ncbi.nlm.nih.gov/23473524/
81. Duteil L, Queille-Roussel C, Aladren S, Bustos X, Trullas C, Granger C, et al. Prevention of polymorphic light eruption afforded by a very high broad-spectrum protection sunscreen containing ectoin. Dermatol Ther (Heidelb) [Internet]. 2022 Jul 1 [cited 2024 Mar 14];12(7):1603–13. Available from: https://pubmed.ncbi.nlm.nih.gov/35716331/

82. Wong LC, Jamil A, Md Nor N. The effect of pre-phototest sun exposure on minimal erythema dose and minimal melanogenic dose among skin phototypes III, IV and V. Photodermatol Photoimmunol Photomed [Internet]. 2018 Nov 1 [cited 2024 Mar 3];34(6):400–4. Available from: https://pubmed.ncbi.nlm.nih.gov/29953669/
83. Hadshiew IM, Treder-Condrad C, Bülow R V., Klette E, Mann T, Stäb F, et al. Polymorphous light eruption (PLE) and a new potent antioxidant and UVA-protective formulation as prophylaxis. Photodermatol Photoimmunol Photomed [Internet]. 2004 Aug [cited 2024 Mar 14];20(4):200–4. Available from: https://pubmed.ncbi.nlm.nih.gov/15238098/
84. Bansal I, Kerr H, Janiga JJ, Qureshi HS, Chaffins M, Lim HW, et al. Pinpoint papular variant of polymorphous light eruption: clinical and pathological correlation. J Eur Acad Dermatol Venereol [Internet]. 2006 Apr [cited 2024 Mar 14];20(4):406–10. Available from: https://pubmed.ncbi.nlm.nih.gov/16643137/
85. Guarrera M. Polymorphous Light Eruption. Adv Exp Med Biol [Internet]. 2017 [cited 2024 Mar 14];996:61–70. Available from: https://pubmed.ncbi.nlm.nih.gov/29124691/
86. Maier T, Korting HC. Sunscreens—which and what for? Skin Pharmacol Physiol [Internet]. 2005 Nov [cited 2024 Mar 3];18(6):253–62. Available from: https://pubmed.ncbi.nlm.nih.gov/16113595/
87. Indian Journal of Dermatology [Internet]. [cited 2024 Mar 15]. Available from: https://journals.lww.com/ijd/pages/default.aspx
88. Marionnet C, de Dormael R, Marat X, Roudot A, Gizard J, Planel E, et al. Sunscreens with the new MCE filter cover the whole UV spectrum: improved UVA1 photoprotection in vitro and in a randomized controlled trial. JID Innov [Internet]. 2021 Jan 1 [cited 2024 Mar 3];2(1). Available from: https://pubmed.ncbi.nlm.nih.gov/35072138/
89. Aljasser MI, Lui H, Ball NJ, Kalia S. Persistent polymorphous light eruption after ultraviolet A1 phototherapy. Photodermatol Photoimmunol Photomed [Internet]. 2013 Feb [cited 2024 Mar 14];29(1):52–4. Available from: https://pubmed.ncbi.nlm.nih.gov/23281698/
90. A new ecamsule-containing SPF 40 sunscreen cream for the prevention of polymorphous light eruption: a double-blind, randomized, controlled study in maximized outdoor conditions—PubMed [Internet]. [cited 2024 Mar 14]. Available from: https://pubmed.ncbi.nlm.nih.gov/19326695/
91. Ho SGY, Chan HHL. The Asian dermatologic patient: review of common pigmentary disorders and cutaneous diseases. Am J Clin Dermatol [Internet]. 2009 [cited 2024 Mar 14];10(3):153–68. Available from: https://pubmed.ncbi.nlm.nih.gov/19354330/
92. Krutmann J, Piquero-Casals J, Morgado-Carrasco D, Granger C, Trullàs C, Passeron T, et al. Photoprotection for people with skin of colour: needs and strategies. Br J Dermatol [Internet]. 2023 Feb 1 [cited 2024 Mar 14];188(2):168–75. Available from: https://pubmed.ncbi.nlm.nih.gov/36763874/
93. Ho SGY, Chan HHL. The Asian dermatologic patient. Am J Clin Dermatol 2009 10:3 [Internet]. 2012 Aug 23 [cited 2024 Mar 11];10(3):153–68. Available from: https://link.springer.com/article/10.2165/00128071-200910030-00002
94. Taneja A, Mittal A, Beniwal R. Do we really need sunscreens? Indian J Dermatol Venereol Leprol [Internet]. 2017 Jan 1 [cited 2024 Mar 14];83(1):7. Available from: https://ijdvl.com/do-we-really-need-sunscreens/
95. Agbai ON, Buster K, Sanchez M, Hernandez C, Kundu R V., Chiu M, et al. Skin cancer and photoprotection in people of color: a review and recommendations for physicians and the public. J Am Acad Dermatol [Internet]. 2014 [cited 2024 Mar 14];70(4):748–62. Available from: https://pubmed.ncbi.nlm.nih.gov/24485530/
96. Evaluation and effectiveness of a photoprotection composition (sunscreen) on subjects of skin of color. J Am Acad Dermatol [Internet]. 2015 May 1 [cited 2024 Mar 14];72(5):AB215. Available from: http://www.jaad.org/article/S0190962215009901/fulltext
97. Grether-Beck S, Felsner I, Brenden H, Marini A, Jaenicke T, Aue N, et al. Air pollution-induced tanning of human skin. Br J Dermatol [Internet]. 2021 Nov 1 [cited 2024 Mar 14];185(5):1026–34. Available from: https://pubmed.ncbi.nlm.nih.gov/33991337/

98. Pollution as a risk factor for the development of melasma and other skin disorders of facial hyperpigmentation—is there a case to be made?—PubMed [Internet]. [cited 2024 Mar 15]. Available from: https://pubmed.ncbi.nlm.nih.gov/25844605/
99. Nkengne A, Robic J, Lua BL. The effect of air pollution on the skin colour and tone of Chinese women: A multicentre cohort study. Skin Res Technol [Internet]. 2021 May 1 [cited 2024 Mar 15];27(3):428–34. Available from: https://pubmed.ncbi.nlm.nih.gov/33111363/
100. Puri P, Nandar SK, Kathuria S, Ramesh V. Effects of air pollution on the skin: a review. Indian J Dermatol Venereol Leprol [Internet]. 2017 Jul 1 [cited 2024 Mar 15];83(4):415–423. Available from: https://pubmed.ncbi.nlm.nih.gov/28195077/
101. Kim MS, Chung BY, Chang SE, Oh SH, Ryu HJ, Kim DH, et al. Pigmented contact dermatitis and hair dyes: A retrospective case-control multicentre study in Korea. J Eur Acad Dermatol Venereol [Internet]. 2023 Dec 1 [cited 2024 Mar 15];37(12):2543–9. Available from: https://pubmed.ncbi.nlm.nih.gov/37528459/

Chapter 6
An Introduction to Sunscreens

Abbreviations

BEF	Biologically effective protective factor
BEMT	bis-ethylhexyloxyphenol methoxyphenyl triazine
DHHB	Diethylamino hydroxybenzoyl hexyl benzoate
EHT	ethylhexyl triazone
EORTC	European Organization for Research and Treatment of Cancer
EU	European union
GRASE	Generally recognized as safe and effective.
HEVL	High energy visible light
IMC	Isoamyl methoxycinnamate
IR	Infrared
MBBT	methylene bis-benzotriazolyl tetramethylbutylphenol
MUsT	Maximum usage trial
SOC	Skin of colour
SPF	Sun protection factor
USFDA	United States Food and Drug Administration
VOC	Volatile organic compounds

Key Objectives

- The spectral coverage differs between sunscreen filters, and a complementary use of these agents is requisite for broad spectrum coverage with spectral homeostasis.
- Regional and national guidelines provide an overarching framework for regulating sunscreens.
- Nonfiltering agents in sunscreen formulations can impact the SPF levels significantly. This is important to explore, keeping in mind the importance of formulation type and spreadability in influencing sunscreen testing methodologies and again in cutaneous absorption of sunscreens.

R. Rajan, *Sunscreens for Skin of Color*,
https://doi.org/10.1007/978-981-97-3195-4_6

- Sunscreen sprays, while popular, may be associated with risk of inhalation of UV filters.
- Other sunscreen formats such as sticks and wipes may not be comparable to traditional sunscreen types, since quantification of protection varies.

Sunscreens are simply defined as personal care products sold to consumers for protection against solar radiation. Erstwhile considered necessary only for protection from the ultraviolet (UV) spectrum, and primarily for skin cancer, sunscreens are currently used to protect against the entire biophysically relevant spectrum of sunlight, for outcomes such as prevention of pigmentation and photoageing.

Sunscreens can be classified as organic and inorganic based on the presence or absence of a carbon molecule in the chemical structure. There are only two inorganic sunscreens as of now, and since they both are minerals, titanium and zinc, inorganic sunscreens have also come to be called as mineral sunscreens [1]. When both chemical and physical filters are present in a sunscreen, such products are called hybrid sunscreens. Sunscreens can also be sorted into different groups based on the spectral coverage they provide. The search for an ideal sunscreen remains as relevant today, as a century ago, thanks to the huge consumer interest in this personal care product.

The ideal sunscreen should be able to cover the entire spectrum of solar radiation, across which significant negative photobiological effects are anticipated for the human skin. The UV protection spectrum of sunscreen filters are shown in Fig. 6.1. Typically, this would indicate protection not only across UVA and UVB, but also address the need for visible light and infrared protection. The ideal sunscreen should also be able to dissipate the absorbed photons in the form of excited state energy, safely and quickly, ideally within femtoseconds or picoseconds at best. This is crucial to avoid cellular damage in the form of molecular fragmentation and to avoid generation of triplet oxygen free radicals. While thus protecting the skin, the ideal filter should be stable and not create pro-oxidant changes itself. It is important that the sunscreen is not absorbed in any relevant quantity into the viable epidermis, and then into the bloodstream. Furthermore, in case of any such absorption, the sunscreen filter should not have the potential to impact human health negatively. It is also highly desirable for sunscreen to have pleasant aesthetic attributes, without appearing obvious on the skin. The sunscreen should provide durable protection to avoid the need for reapplication, which is both seen as inconvenient by the user and as inconsistent by the health care provider. A once daily application would be desirable. Sunscreens with activities like antioxidants would provide users an added advantage depending on the intended outcome of the active—from antiaging to pigmentation relief [2, 3]. While such an ideal sunscreen does not exist, advances in sunscreen science have come very close to achieving this. The approved list of sunscreens in the USA and the EU are given in Tables 6.1 and 6.2.

GRASE certification implies that a particular drug or product is safe and effective. Three criteria are involved. Firstly, the product must be backed by evidence-based medicine, for claims of safety and efficacy. Secondly, such evidence must be published in relevant medical literature for scrutiny by peers. Thirdly, there must be

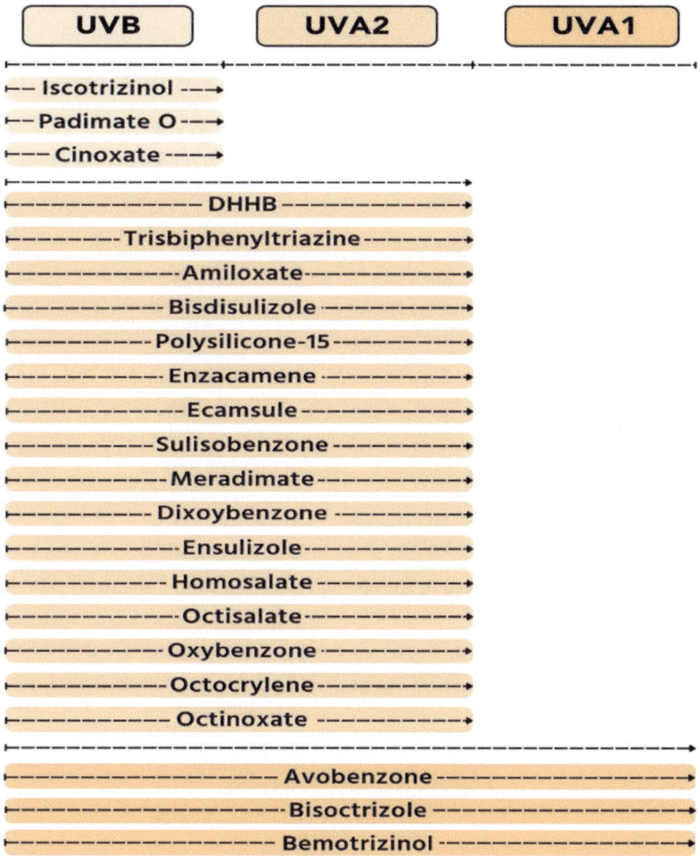

Fig. 6.1 Protection spectrum of sunscreen filters

acceptance among suitably qualified experts that the said product is safe and effective, based on the available literature [4, 5]. FDA approved non-GRASE sunscreens are considered for OTC use as 'Marketed Unapproved Drugs', with the understanding that they not have been subject to the same rigorous evaluation, as is needed for GRASE I [6].

For the sake of broader coverage, and in cognisance of the biological activity of sunscreens in the high energy visible light (HEVL) spectrum, newer filters which provide protection in the UVA1, HEVL spectrum have recently been added to the sunscreen list, at least in the European union (EU) [7, 8]. Extensive data is now available to establish the role of UVA in photocarcinogenesis, photoageing, and photopigmentation, alone or in combination with high energy visible radiation (HEVR). HEVR denotes the spectral range between 380 and 450 nm and has been shown to cause increased skin pigmentation, free radical damage, oxidative stress

Table 6.1 GRASE status of UV filters approved in the USA [5, 6]

GRASE certification		
Category I	Approved as GRASE	Zinc oxide Titanium dioxide
Category II	Non-GRASE	PABA Trolamine salicylate
Category III	Non-GRASE	Avobenzone Cinnoxate Dioxybenzone Ensulizole Homosalate Meradimate Octinoxate Octisalate Octocrylene Oxybenzone Padimate O Sulizobenzone

GRASE generally recognized as safe and effective

Table 6.2 List of UV Filters approved in Europe and the USA from Pantelic et al. [11]

Sunscreen filters approved in Europe	Sunscreen filters approved in both Europe Union and the USA
4-Methylbenzylidene camphor Benzylidene camphor sulfonic acid Diethylhexyl butamido triazone Bemotrizinol Disodium phenyl dibenzimidazole tetrasulfonate Bisoctrizole Camphor benzalkonium methosulfate Diethylamino hydroxybenzoyl hexyl benzoate Polysilicone-15 Drometrizole trisiloxane Ethylhexyl triazone Isoamyl p-methoxycinnamate Ethoxylated ethyl 4-aminobenzoate Benzophenone-5 Tris-biphenyl triazine (nano) Phenylene bis-diphenyl triazine Methoxy propyl amino cyclohexenylidene ethoxyethylcyanoacetate	Oxybenzone Octisalate Homosalate Avobenzone OD PABA Titanium dioxide Zinc oxide Octinoxate Octocrylene Ensulizole Ecamsule

with damage to cellular DNA and also immune suppression, acting similar to the UV spectrum [9, 10].

Currently, there are 17 UV filters approved in the USA. In the European Union, the number of approved UV filters is 29, of which 18 are approved only in the EU [8, 11].

A larger particle size and therefore a reduced chance of systemic absorption and a reduced incidence of cutaneous toxicity have been considered by the EU for approval of sunscreens. Accordingly, filters that satisfy these criteria in the UVB spectrum include ethylhexyl triazone (EHT), isoamyl methoxycinnamate (IMC), and 4 methyl benzylidene camphor (4 MBC). Photostable and stabilizing UV filters like octocrylene and bemotrizinol which have a larger particle size to deter systemic absorption are recommended to be added to innately photounstable sunscreens like avobenzone [9]. Newer filters are also expected to be skin friendly, and more relevantly be able to deliver protection measured across some relevant biological effective protection factors (BEPFs). For the UVA spectrum, Mexoryl SX, and for broad spectrum coverage, drometrizole trisiloxane, bemotrizinol, and bisoctrizole are considered as satisfying these requirements [9].

Today, sunscreen ingredients are also widely present in makeup products, toothpastes, food products, and in personal care products such as body washes and shampoos as well. In the latter, their addition is for the purpose of preventing photooxidation of the product itself, and not for any skin protection. Similarly, sunscreen filters are also present in other industrial products such as paints and textiles, resulting in significant interaction of these agents with humans and our ecosystem.

6.1 *Sunscreens*: A Historical Perspective

If the earliest evidence of sun worship by humans can be dated back to 6000 BC, sun protection methods do not seem to have lagged behind by much. Around 4000 BC, Egyptians were recorded to have used plant extracts for sun protection, very much like the present day, and for reasons suspected to very similar to those in modern times—to protect the skin from tanning in the sun [12, 13]. Darker skin was, and in some parts of the world still is, associated with lower social rank, and using sun protection agents was considered a way to avoid the social labelling. It is of interest that these agents, rice, jasmine, and lupine extracts, used by Egyptians are considered to have UV protective, and/or skin lightening properties and are still in use in the modern cosmetic formulations of today [13, 14].

Zinc oxide as a sun protection agent has been described in the ancient Indian medical text, the Charaka Samhita, around 500 BC, the first physical sunscreen. Physical sun protection agents have also been depicted in ancient texts, showing the intention towards sun avoidance and/or protection. Umbrellas were found to have been used in ancient China, India, Egypt, and Mesopotamia [12, 15].

The UV spectrum in sunlight was first described by Johann Wilhelm Ritter, in 1801, just a few years after the description of a photosensitivity dermatosis, eczema solare by Robert Willan, the father of modern dermatology [16]. The ability of UV rays to damage the skin was established by the end of the same century, though the role of sunlight in skin burn was established in 1820 by Everard Hume. In 1878, tannins which are now being reexplored as sun protection factor (SPF) boosters were considered as sun protection agents, but given up as they failed to deliver on the cosmetic appeal, an issue which plagues sunscreens till date. The first chemical sunscreen was created by Friedrich Hammer in 1891, based on Widmark's earlier experiments on the ability of quinine sulphate to protect against sunburn [15]. Shortly thereafter, Paul Unna further explored solar radiation induced skin cancer and developed sunscreens containing aesculin obtained from chestnut extracts. While the UV protection properties of aesculin remain relevant till dates, Unna's sunscreens, failed on the cosmetic appeal. But to be fair, peer approval did happen for aesculin by Leopold Freund, who was the first to discover that shorter wavelengths around 325 nm were mainly responsible for the erythema [15].

The first animal study to prove a link between skin cancer and sun exposure by G M Findlay was published in the 1920s, also the same period when 'sunbathing' was popularized as a concept of high fashion by Coco Chanel. Following through on the tanning trend, Eugene Schueller in 1935, developed Amber Solaire, a tanning oil with photoprotective properties—marketed for 'tanning without burning'. The 1940s saw a rapid increase in the number of commercial sunscreens, some of which were conceived on the battlefields of the World Wars. Given the medical and sociocultural importance that was being rapidly acquired by sunscreens, regulations followed suit with the SPF rating system developed in the early 1960s. The importance of the UVA spectrum in causing damage was established thereafter, but UVA specific filters and rating systems came into vogue in the 1990s. Further research continues to fine-tune the process of sunscreen development, with the introduction of antioxidants and agents that target the visible light part of the solar spectrum, to protect against skin pigmentation and photoageing, in addition to the always recognized need for protection from photocarcinogenesis [13].

Newer sunscreen formulations are available more commonly in the European Union, containing unique filters, developed, and approved for proprietary use by cosmetic companies like L'Oreal and Pierre Fabre Laboratories [17]. However, in the USA, a much lesser number of UV filters are available for use in sunscreens. Chemical UV filters considered as new generation, compared to older generation UV filters like octinoxate and octocrylene, such as diethylamino hydroxybenzoyl hexyl benzoate (DHHB), methylene bis-benzotriazolyl tetramethylbutylphenol (MBBT), ethylhexyl triazone (EHT), and bis-ethylhexyloxyphenol methoxyphenyl triazine (BEMT), are in wide use in the EU, but yet to gain approval in the USA [18]. Of these, bemotrizinol is currently awaiting FDA approval, the first filter to be put through the new maximum usage trial (MUsT) protocol for ensuring sunscreen safety [19]. The MUsT protocol is a new safeguard instituted by the recognition of, and concern around, systemic absorption of sunscreens. Absorption of sunscreens into the human body and subsequently attaining plasma levels well beyond set thresholds was demonstrated by Matta et al., in 2019–2020 [20, 21]. The research findings came to be widely publicized, and along with the reported detection of benzene in sunscreens, worked to create a global wave of awareness led by social media, but also increased consumer paranoia about sunscreen use. This has also fuelled the popularity of mineral sunscreens, as seen by the trends on social media, where recommendations for sunscreens are not always led by experts or dermatologists [22].

The potential for sunscreens to create endocrine disruption in humans has been a matter of debate with increasing research in the domain [23]. Though the timeline for such impact is debated, the potential still remains significant due to the presence of UV filtering chemicals in multiple everyday use products, other than sunscreens, with a resultant increase in cumulative exposure. With their detection in maternal urine samples and breast milk, the outcomes of foetal exposure to chemical filters which have a potential endocrine disrupting ability are currently under significant debate [24–27].

The rapid increase in sunscreen awareness and the extensive use of sunscreens by populations that are not known to be predisposed to skin cancer, but for the purpose of protection against photoageing and pigmentation, has led to a huge global burden of sunscreens on the planet [28]. More than 15,000 tons of sunscreen is expected to be let out into the Mediterranean Sea, a popular tourist zone every year as a conservative estimate [18, 29]. Sunscreens have been linked to coral bleaching, disruption of marine life and have been detected in the carcasses of larger, vertebrate marine animals such as dolphins [18, 30, 31]. The potential for this large impact on the environment has prompted significant research and some key legislative action. Working to protect its coral resources, Hawaii introduced legislation to ban certain organic sunscreen ingredients citing threat to marine life in 2018 [32–34]. Researchers are now working to improve sunscreen formulation using frameworks that focus on safe-by-design and sustainable-by-design principles, which evaluate the impact of a sunscreen product across its entire life cycle [35]. Key metrics that assess environmental sustainability such as Global Warming Potential and Cumulative Energy Demand are assessed against toxicity metrics such as human and freshwater toxicity potentials to arrive at balanced formulations that are both safe and effective [36, 37]. Multitarget machine learning algorithms are now evolving to assess product optical properties and transparency that impact SPF and performance efficacy, and the potential for toxicity arising out of photocatalytic action—in an attempt to create safe-by-design sunscreens for the future [38]. Green synthesis of raw materials, high natural content of sunscreens with high biodegradability, and lesser product utilization by producing durable sunscreens which do not require reapplication are all ways in which to make sunscreen use sustainable for both people and the planet [39].

With sunscreens, history seems to have come full circle, pivoting from protecting with sunscreens, to protecting from sunscreens.

6.2 Anatomy of a Sunscreen

A topical sunscreen is defined as a cosmetic preparation that is applied on the skin to protect against ultraviolet radiation by absorbing, scattering, or reflecting the incident rays [1, 40]. Adding to this, sunscreens today are also expected to protect against the entire spectrum of solar radiation, including visible light and infrared rays, which have now been shown to penetrate deeper into the skin, with resultant damage in the epidermis and the dermis. The main functions of a sunscreen are centred around four domains, temporally understood. They range from protecting the skin from the short-term effects of sun exposure such as sunburns to immediate term changes such as pigment darkening to midterm outcomes such as dyspigmentation and further on, to long-term changes, namely photoageing and photocarcinogenesis [41, 42]. Therefore, today's consumers are interested in using sunscreen to protect not just against sunburn, but against the complete spectrum of solar induced skin damage [42]. Furthermore, sunscreens as cosmetic agents must also have additional attributes such as aesthetic appeal and elegant skin feel, and of course, not have any irritant or allergic properties.

In contrast to other cosmetic and personal care products, the formulation of a sunscreen begins with a goal of achieving the desired level of sun protection, usually in terms of the SPF number [10, 43]. This depends on the intended purpose of the sunscreen as 'primary' meant for recreational or beach usage, and 'secondary' sunscreen, when intended for daily use, or as moisturizers, foundations, or lip care cosmetics [9, 44, 45]. So, the first step is to identify the sunscreen active ingredients to be deployed in the formulation. The United States Food and Drug Administration (USFDA) defines a sunscreen active ingredient as an agent that absorbs at least 85% of UV radiation in wavelengths between 290 and 320 nm, though the limit was later extended to 400 nm [45]. Subsequently, the UV filters, mostly in combination and ideally, each at the lowest concentration that would be sufficient to achieve the targeted SPF, are selected. Combining different filters with absorption maxima either in the UVA or UVB spectrum allows the coverage of complete UV region [45]. The determination of the quantity of a sun filter within a formulation is a crucial step. Sunscreens are built to provide efficient sun protection, with their performance efficacy evaluated by specific extinction in the spectral range from 290 to 400 nm. Denoted as <E11>, this parameter measures the extinction of a 1% dispersion of the UV filter along a 1-cm optical path. In simple terms, the <E11> indicates the amount of sun filter that would be required to achieve sufficient sun protection comparable to another filter, per unit quantity. Sunscreen ingredients with a lower efficacy would need to be used at a higher concentration compared to those that are more efficient, even at lower concentrations [46].

The process of formulation from hereon is standard, balancing the SPF to be achieved against factors like feel, aesthetic aspects, and/or economy and may be enhanced by certain hero ingredients for a better product story to suit commercial expectations. Apart from the active ingredients as above, sunscreen formulations also contain ionic, non-ionic, or amphoteric emulsifiers to stabilize the aqueous and lipid phases, producing a complex but homogeneous colloidal system. The formula may also contain other supportive and structural ingredients such as gums, preservatives, photostabilizers, chelators, and agents that improve aesthetics like fragrances and skin feel enhancers [47]. These additional agents have significant impact on the structure, stability, sensorial feel, and performance of sunscreens, interacting with each other in complex ways [47].

As of now, sunscreens are available in a wide range of physical formulations as creams, lotions, oils, sticks, sprays, gels, powders, pastes, mousses [45]. Sunscreen creams, pastes, and lotions are typically water in oil emulsions (W/O), ranging in viscosity between 50,000 and 500,000 centipoises. However, lighter sunscreen formulations which are oil in water emulsions (O/W), or more advanced formulations in W/O/W or O/W/O in stable systems, enable the wide range of texture and skin feel of sunscreen products, available in the market today. Gel sunscreens are mostly aqueous preparations containing solubilizers which ensure the transparency of the product. However, with their large proportion of water, these gel sunscreens tend to get washed away easily by water and sweat, and are not therefore, durable. Furthermore, these tend to be low SPF products, because of the poor solubility of UV filters in water, with a resultant inability to load more lipids into the formula. Hydroalcoholic gels contain water along with alcohol, typically ethanol, which is able to accommodate higher levels of UV filters, and therefore are able to provide a higher SPF than water based gels. Due to the presence of the alcohol, these sunscreens provide a cooling, refreshing skin feel but can also cause stinging of the eyes and potential irritant reactions [48]. Furthermore, alcohol-based sunscreens seem to increase cutaneous absorption of sunscreens [45]. Other formulation types such as microemulsions, though elegant, may be irritant to the skin and anhydrous sunscreens, though capable of being very durable and water resistant, may cause occlusion and acne in susceptible individuals and in humid environments. While sunscreen powders are popular for their cosmetic appeal, they are classified as GRASE III by the US FDA, other novel consumer interest formulations such as sunscreen wipes, towelettes, body washes, and shampoos are processed as new drugs by the FDA, and not inherently based on the filters therein as over the counter products [6, 49]. Aerosol sunscreens are very popular among users, due to their ease of use. A variety of technologies are used to deliver a sunscreen as an aerosol, an airborne suspension of fine particles or droplets. In aerosol sunscreens where a canister is used, the sunscreen is mixed with a liquified propellant gas, which generates an aerosol containing both the sunscreen product and the propellant, on activating a valve on the canister. In a pump spray system, the force to aerosolize the product is generated using mechanical force. A newer application called the bag on valve technology uses the propellant outside a bag within which the sunscreen is held, so that the propellant still provides the force to emit the sunscreen as an aerosol, but there is no direct contact of the sunscreen with the propellant, itself [5]. Despite the attractiveness of aerosol or spray sunscreens in terms of convenience of use, several sunscreen filters are associated with inhalational toxicity, titanium dioxide being a typical example. Furthermore, spray sunscreens are associated with uneven skin coverage and potential wastage, apart from eye irritation. Aerosol sunscreens also contribute to volatile organic compounds (VOC) emissions into the atmosphere, related to either the propellant, sunscreen filters like ethylhexyl salicylate and homosalate or to the solvent [50, 51]. Spray sunscreens are classified under Category I under the GRASE classification used by the US FDA, alongside sunscreen oils, lotions, creams, gels, butters, pastes, ointments, and sticks [5]. Newer formats like sunscreen sticks are very popular, due to their portability and ease of usage. However, they are high in wax and petrolatum and can feel very occlusive on the skin. They are of three types—transparent, containing mostly chemical filters, matte with mostly mineral sunscreen ingredients, and semi-transparent, which carries both chemical and mineral sunscreening agents [48]. More advanced formulation innovations include the hydrogel format incorporating unique ecofriendly and biocompatible ingredients like yeast, gelatin, hyaluronic acid, tannic acid, and poly L glutamic acid. These hydrogels are three-dimensional polymeric water loving network meshes which provide very good sensorial benefits like softness, superior skin feel, and flexibility along with robust solar protection [52–54]. Oleogels are tunable complexes of vegetable oils with organic filters and are anticipated to enhance ecofriendliness of sunscreen filters [55].

For mineral sunscreens, another important parameter is the zeta potential which reflects formulation stability. Mineral sunscreens are intrinsically active in formulation and do not tolerate several excipients, demand strict formulation conditions like pH ranges, need chelation agents, and are also best formulated as water in oil emulsions. On the other hand, chemical sunscreens are more tolerant and can be formulated either as water in oil or as oil in water emulsions. Measured by electrophoresis, the zeta potential indicates the adequacy of repulsive forces between the different phases within the sunscreen, enough to avoid flocculation or otherwise phase separation within the formulation [56].

The solvent of sunscreen significantly impacts its performance. With lower polarity, the UVA protection of sunscreens decreases, while SPF itself seems to be less affected. Iterating polarity of sunscreen formulations among other parameters is an effective way to enhance sunscreen performance without adding more filters or more of filters [57].

The sunscreen formulation process must also address potential concerns of systemic absorption, since sunscreens are leave on products that are also expected to frequently be reapplied, producing a constant presence on the skin, to ensure protection. For example, encapsulated versions and nonpermeable formats of UV filters are now available to use in formulations to limit skin penetration and systemic uptake [58, 59].

Newer advances in nanotechnology are being effectively employed in sunscreen formulations with multiple advantages. Polymeric nanoparticles are useful for handling volatile particles in formulation, while nanoemulsions reduce the chances of flocculation and improve formulation characteristics. Nanocrystals are suited for hydrophobic ingredients, while mesoporous silica particles are unique for their biodegradability among nanomaterials [60]. Solid-lipid nanoparticles find applications in incorporating plant ingredients, such as spinach extracts in sunscreens, triggering the exploration of a newer innovative class, the herbal nanocosmeceuticals [61, 62]. Nanostructured lipid carriers, nanosomes, and niosomes are newer tools available for cosmetic formulations, though they are also more expensive [60].

Sunspheres are novel materials of approximately 325 nm and made of copolymers of styrene or acrylate. These structures have water within the sphere which moves out to be replaced by air, on application on the skin, which increases the layers that the sunlight is scattered before it reaches the skin. While the sunspheres themselves do not have UV protection abilities, they can accommodate both organic and inorganic UV filters [60].

The wide range of sunscreen types and the increasing focus on skin feel, texture, and consumer acceptability underline the popularity of sunscreens as one of the most commonly used personal care products. Ultimately, the best sunscreen is the one that the user is happily compliant to use, in terms of both product application and skin feel.

There are important differences that need to be addressed when formulating a sunscreen for skin of colour (SOC). The use of promelanogenic agents in sunscreens is one of these.

As a mainly Western concept of photoprotection against skin cancer, sunscreens were developed to protect against skin damage, while increasing the melanin content in the skin for ongoing photoprotection. This is why photosensitizing agents like bergamot oil and lemon oil made their way into sunscreens. This approach, while satisfying a presumed Western consumer need for a 'safer tan', is unacceptable in SOC for obvious reasons. With a very low risk of skin cancer, the predominant use of sunscreens in Asian populations with higher skin types, such as in India, is for preventing photoageing and protecting against pigmentation. So, sunscreens which contain promelanogenic agents are counterproductive to user intention in SOC. Agents like bergamot oil have been well established to be phototoxic, with bergapten, the active component of bergamot oil capable of producing sunburn cells in the skin, when stimulated by UVA exposure with significant DNA damage [63–65]. Also, the active photo tumorigenic moiety in bergamot oil was identified to be 5 methoxy psoralen [66]. Notably, sunscreens with agents like psoralens which were intended to promote photopigmentation for skin protection were found to increase the risk for melanoma according to the European Organization for Research and Treatment of Cancer (EORTC) study group [67]. Adding to the confusion, the phototoxicity of bergamot oil was shown to vary across different sources of supply, suggesting difficulties in standardization [68].

Another important difference is in the spectrum of coverage offered by sunscreens. For SOC, coverage across UVA, HEVL, and infrared (IR) are as important as coverage across UVB. Therefore, indices such as the critical wavelength which shows how far the sunscreen's protection reaches into the UVA spectrum and the ratio of the UVA to UVB may be more important than the SPF factor. For skin of colour, the ability of a sunscreen to protect against pigmentation is a key indicator of performance. The pigmentation protection factor (PPF) of a sunscreen is used to denote this. The UVA protection factor (UVA-PF) value should be at least 1/3rd the value of the SPF, for the sunscreen to be considered as providing adequate protection in the pigmentation producing UVA zone. Sunscreens whose UVA-PF values approach SPF values are being introduced into the market, as specifically beneficial for preventing photoageing related pigmentation, but it is also important to note that sufficient coverage must be achieved with regard to SPF values to ensure protection against UVB generated potential photocarcinogenic effects in the skin. Furthermore, skin pigmentation can also be induced by UVB, typically as delayed tanning—but since the penetration of UVB is only until the epidermis, the site of pigmentation tends to be relatively superficial. Usually, this pigmentation tends to be reduced with normal epidermal turnover in about a month's time [69].

Today, the user predominantly understands sunscreens in terms of the number on the label. Regardless of difficulties or inconsistencies in test methodologies, these numbers have come to be very important to the sunscreen industry for all stakeholders—regulatory bodies, physicians, manufacturers, formulators, and of course, consumers. These numbers have driven the advancement of sunscreen science, and these numbers have also been blamed for a paradoxical increase in melanoma occurrence [10]. The next chapter deals with an understanding of sunscreen metrics and label advisories based on currently available guidelines.

6.3 Chapter Summary

This chapter provides an introduction to sunscreens, highlighting the spectrum they cover, regional and international guidelines and formulation basics which affect sunscreen performance and output. Combining filters that protect across different parts of the spectrum or using newer filters that protect in a broad based way are all options aimed at achieving full spectrum cover. Over years, sunscreens have evolved from crude preparations with limited coverage, mostly in the UVB zone, to elegant and aesthetically pleasing personal care products in various formats such as creams, lotions, sprays, gels, powders, wipes, and sunscreen sticks. Given the practical difficulties in sunscreen testing and the lack of repeatability of results, the newer formats of sunscreens do not have adequate data to test their efficacy. However, since the strong emergence of sunscreens as a popularly used skin care product, further research and refinements are on the anvil towards developing sunscreens with high safety and efficacy, which are also able to inspire high levels of compliance among users.

References

1. Serpone N. Sunscreens and their usefulness: have we made any progress in the last two decades? Photochem Photobiol Sci 2021 20:2 [Internet]. 2021 Feb 18 [cited 2024 Mar 3];20(2):189–244. Available from: https://link.springer.com/article/10.1007/s43630-021-00013-1
2. Holt EL, Rodrigues N d. N, Cebrián J, Stavros VG. Determining the photostability of avobenzone in sunscreen formulation models using ultrafast spectroscopy. Phys Chem Chem Phys [Internet]. 2021 Nov 14 [cited 2024 Mar 15];23(42):24439–48. Available from: https://pubmed.ncbi.nlm.nih.gov/34694312/
3. (PDF) Cutaneous photoprotection: a review of the current status and evolving strategies [Internet]. [cited 2024 Mar 3]. Available from: https://www.researchgate.net/publication/340352263_Cutaneous_Photoprotection_A_Review_of_the_Current_Status_and_Evolving_Strategies
4. Fivenson D, Sabzevari N, Qiblawi S, Blitz J, Norton BB, Norton SA. Sunscreens: UV filters to protect us: part 2-increasing awareness of UV filters and their potential toxicities to us and our environment. Int J Womens Dermatol [Internet]. 2021 Jan 1 [cited 2024 Mar 15];7(1):45. Available from: https://www.ncbi.nlm.nih.gov/pmc/articles/PMC7838327/
5. Federal Register:: Sunscreen drug products for over-the-counter human use [Internet]. [cited 2024 Mar 20]. Available from: https://www.federalregister.gov/documents/2019/02/26/2019-03019/sunscreen-drug-products-for-over-the-counter-human-use

6. Federal Register:: Amending over-the-counter monograph m020: sunscreen drug products for over-the-counter human use; over the counter monograph proposed order; availability [Internet]. [cited 2024 Mar 20]. Available from: https://www.federalregister.gov/documents/2021/09/27/2021-20780/amending-over-the-counter-monograph-m020-sunscreen-drug-products-for-over-the-counter-human-use-over
7. Sabzevari N, Qiblawi S, Norton SA, Fivenson D. Sunscreens: UV filters to protect us: part 1: changing regulations and choices for optimal sun protection. Int J Womens Dermatol. 2021;7(1):28–44.
8. Egambaram OP, Kesavan Pillai S, Ray SS. Materials science challenges in skin UV protection: a review. Photochem Photobiol [Internet]. 2020 Jul 1 [cited 2024 Mar 3];96(4):779–97. Available from: https://pubmed.ncbi.nlm.nih.gov/31886889/
9. Aguilera J, Gracia-Cazaña T, Gilaberte Y. New developments in sunscreens. Photochem Photobiol Sci [Internet]. 2023 Oct 1 [cited 2024 Mar 3];22(10):2473–82. Available from: https://pubmed.ncbi.nlm.nih.gov/37543534/
10. Young AR, Boles J, Herzog B, Osterwalder U, Baschong W. A sunscreen's labeled sun protection factor may overestimate protection at temperate latitudes: a human in vivo study. J Invest Dermatol [Internet]. 2010 [cited 2024 Mar 11];130(10):2457–62. Available from: https://pubmed.ncbi.nlm.nih.gov/20535128/
11. Pantelic MN, Wong N, Kwa M, Lim HW. Ultraviolet filters in the United States and European Union: a review of safety and implications for the future of US sunscreens. J Am Acad Dermatol [Internet]. 2023 Mar 1 [cited 2024 Mar 3];88(3):632–46. Available from: https://pubmed.ncbi.nlm.nih.gov/36442611/
12. Ma Y, Yoo J. History of sunscreen: an updated view. J Cosmet Dermatol [Internet]. 2021 Apr 1 [cited 2024 Mar 15];20(4):1044–9. Available from: https://pubmed.ncbi.nlm.nih.gov/33583116/
13. Drissi M, Carr E, Housewright C. Sunscreen: a brief walk through history. Proc (Bayl Univ Med Cent) [Internet]. 2022 [cited 2024 Mar 15];35(1):121. Available from: https://www.ncbi.nlm.nih.gov/pmc/articles/PMC8682817/
14. Dupont E, Gomez J, Bilodeau D. Beyond UV radiation: a skin under challenge. Int J Cosmet Sci [Internet]. 2013 Jun [cited 2024 Mar 15];35(3):224–32. Available from: https://pubmed.ncbi.nlm.nih.gov/23406155/
15. Urbach F. The historical aspects of sunscreens. J Photochem Photobiol B [Internet]. 2001 Nov 15 [cited 2024 Mar 15];64(2–3):99–104. Available from: https://pubmed.ncbi.nlm.nih.gov/11744395/
16. [Johann Wilhelm Ritter (1776–1810) and the discovery of ultraviolet irradiation 185 years ago]—PubMed [Internet]. [cited 2024 Mar 15]. Available from: https://pubmed.ncbi.nlm.nih.gov/3301744/
17. Bacqueville D, Jacques-Jamin C, Lapalud P, Douki T, Roullet N, Sereno J, et al. Formulation of a new broad-spectrum UVB + UVA and blue light SPF50+ sunscreen containing Phenylene Bis-Diphenyltriazine (TriAsorB), an innovative sun filter with unique optical properties. J Eur Acad Dermatol Venereol [Internet]. 2022 Jun 1 [cited 2024 Mar 15];36 Suppl 6(S6):29–37. Available from: https://pubmed.ncbi.nlm.nih.gov/35738811/
18. Varrella S, Danovaro R, Corinaldesi C. Assessing the eco-compatibility of new generation sunscreen products through a combined microscopic-molecular approach. Environ Pollut. 2022;314:120212.
19. D'Ruiz CD, Plautz JR, Schuetz R, Sanabria C, Hammonds J, Erato C, et al. Preliminary clinical pharmacokinetic evaluation of bemotrizinol—a new sunscreen active ingredient being considered for inclusion under FDA's over-the-counter (OTC) sunscreen monograph. Regul Toxicol Pharmacol [Internet]. 2023 Mar 1 [cited 2024 Mar 15];139. Available from: https://pubmed.ncbi.nlm.nih.gov/36738872/
20. Matta MK, Florian J, Zusterzeel R, Pilli NR, Patel V, Volpe DA, et al. Effect of sunscreen application on plasma concentration of sunscreen active ingredients: a randomized clinical

trial. JAMA [Internet]. 2020 Jan 21 [cited 2024 Mar 27];323(3):256–67. Available from: https://jamanetwork.com/journals/jama/fullarticle/2759002

21. Matta MK, Zusterzeel R, Pilli NR, Patel V, Volpe DA, Florian J, et al. Effect of sunscreen application under maximal use conditions on plasma concentration of sunscreen active ingredients: a randomized clinical trial. JAMA—Journal of the American Medical Association [Internet]. 2019 Jun 4 [cited 2024 Apr 2];321(21):2082–91. Available from: https://www.cosmeticsandtoiletries.com/formulas-products/sun-care/article/21835866/feel-and-function-attuning-attributes-in-mineral-sunscreens
22. Shareef S, Shoemaker WB, Abdelnour A, Albazi E, Ashack K. Assessing public interest in sunscreen safety during pregnancy and lactation. Int J Womens Dermatol [Internet]. 2022 Jun 1 [cited 2024 Mar 15];8(2). Available from: https://pubmed.ncbi.nlm.nih.gov/35619671/
23. Mustieles V, Balogh RK, Axelstad M, Montazeri P, Márquez S, Vrijheid M, et al. Benzophenone-3: comprehensive review of the toxicological and human evidence with meta-analysis of human biomonitoring studies. Environ Int [Internet]. 2023 Mar 1 [cited 2024 Mar 15];173. Available from: https://pubmed.ncbi.nlm.nih.gov/36805158/
24. Wang SQ, Burnett ME, Lim HW. Safety of oxybenzone: putting numbers into perspective. Arch Dermatol [Internet] 2011 Jul 1 [cited 2024 Mar 15];147(7):865–6. Available from: https://jamanetwork.com/journals/jamadermatology/fullarticle/1105240
25. Onyango DO, Selman BG, Rose JL, Ellison CA, Nash JF. Comparison between endocrine activity assessed using ToxCast/Tox21 database and human plasma concentration of sunscreen active ingredients/UV filters. Toxicol Sci [Internet]. 2023 Oct 30 [cited 2024 Mar 15];196(1):25–37. Available from: https://doi.org/10.1093/toxsci/kfad082
26. Krause M, Frederiksen H, Sundberg K, Jørgensen FS, Jensen LN, Nørgaard P, et al. Presence of benzophenones commonly used as UV filters and absorbers in paired maternal and fetal samples. Environ Int [Internet]. 2018 Jan 1 [cited 2024 Mar 15];110:51–60. Available from: https://pubmed.ncbi.nlm.nih.gov/29100749/
27. Krause M, Klit A, Blomberg Jensen M, Søeborg T, Frederiksen H, Schlumpf M, et al. Sunscreens: are they beneficial for health? An overview of endocrine disrupting properties of UV-filters. Int J Androl [Internet]. 2012 Jun [cited 2024 Mar 15];35(3):424–36. Available from: https://pubmed.ncbi.nlm.nih.gov/22612478/
28. Syder NC, Elbuluk N. Rising interest in sunscreen for skin of color: an analysis of Google trends. J Drugs Dermatol [Internet]. 2023 Jul 1 [cited 2024 Mar 15];22(7):712–3. Available from: https://pubmed.ncbi.nlm.nih.gov/37410040/
29. Casas-Beltran DA, Hernández-Pedraza M, Alvarado-Flores J. Estimation of the Discharge of Sunscreens in Aquatic Environments of the Mexican Caribbean. Environments [Internet]. 2020 Feb 20 [cited 2024 Mar 28];7(2):15. Available from: https://www.mdpi.com/2076-3298/7/2/15/htm
30. Gago-Ferrero P, Alonso MB, Bertozzi CP, Marigo J, Barbosa L, Cremer M, et al. First determination of UV filters in marine mammals. Octocrylene levels in Franciscana dolphins. Environ Sci Technol [Internet]. 2013 Jun 4 [cited 2024 Apr 2];47(11):5619–25. Available from: https://pubmed.ncbi.nlm.nih.gov/23627728/
31. Yuan S, Huang J, Jiang X, Huang Y, Zhu X, Cai Z. Environmental fate and toxicity of sunscreen-derived inorganic ultraviolet filters in aquatic environments: a review. Nanomaterials (Basel) [Internet]. 2022 Feb 1 [cited 2024 Mar 15];12(4). Available from: https://pubmed.ncbi.nlm.nih.gov/35215026/
32. Ouchene L, Litvinov I V., Netchiporouk E. Hawaii and other jurisdictions ban oxybenzone or octinoxate sunscreens based on the confirmed adverse environmental effects of sunscreen ingredients on aquatic environments. J Cutan Med Surg [Internet]. 2019 Nov 1 [cited 2024 Mar 16];23(6):648–9. Available from: https://pubmed.ncbi.nlm.nih.gov/31729915/
33. Raffa RB, Pergolizzi J V., Taylor R, Kitzen JM. Sunscreen bans: coral reefs and skin cancer. J Clin Pharm Ther [Internet]. 2019 Feb 1 [cited 2024 Mar 16];44(1):134–9. Available from: https://pubmed.ncbi.nlm.nih.gov/30484882/

34. Peyrot C, Mention MM, Brunissen F, Allais F. Sinapic acid esters: octinoxate substitutes combining suitable UV protection and antioxidant activity. Antioxidants [Internet]. 2020 Aug 24 [cited 2024 Mar 16];9(9):782. Available from: https://www.mdpi.com/2076-3921/9/9/782/htm
35. Battistin M, Pascalicchio P, Tabaro B, Hasa D, Bonetto A, Manfredini S, et al. A safe-by-design approach to "reef safe" sunscreens based on ZnO and organic UV filters. Antioxidants (Basel) [Internet]. 2022 Nov 1 [cited 2024 Mar 28];11(11). Available from: https://pubmed.ncbi.nlm.nih.gov/36358585/
36. Tsalidis GA, Soeteman-Hernández LG, Noorlander CW, Saedy S, Ruud van Ommen J, Vijver MG, et al. Safe-and-sustainable-by-design framework based on a prospective life cycle assessment: lessons learned from a nano-titanium dioxide case study. Int J Environ Res Public Health [Internet]. 2022 Apr 1 [cited 2024 Mar 16];19(7). Available from: https://www.ncbi.nlm.nih.gov/pmc/articles/PMC8998679/
37. Salieri B, Righi S, Pasteris A, Olsen SI. Freshwater ecotoxicity characterisation factor for metal oxide nanoparticles: a case study on titanium dioxide nanoparticle. Sci Total Environ [Internet]. 2015 Feb 1 [cited 2024 Mar 16];505:494–502. Available from: https://pubmed.ncbi.nlm.nih.gov/25461051/
38. Li S, Barnard AS. Safety-by-design using forward and inverse multi-target machine learning. Chemosphere [Internet] 2022 Sep 1 [cited 2024 Mar 16];303(Pt 1). Available from: https://pubmed.ncbi.nlm.nih.gov/35618055/
39. Singh T, Sharma S, Singh R, Pal DB, Ahmad I, Alam MM, et al. Sustainable approaches towards green synthesis of TiO2 nanomaterials and their applications in photocatalysis-mediated sensing to monitor environmental pollution. Luminescence [Internet]. 2023 Jul 1 [cited 2024 Mar 16];38(7):999–1010. Available from: https://pubmed.ncbi.nlm.nih.gov/35997211/
40. Addor FAS anna, Barcaui CB, Gomes EE, Lupi O, Marçon CR, Miot HA. Sunscreen lotions in the dermatological prescription: review of concepts and controversies. An Bras Dermatol [Internet]. 2022 Mar 1 [cited 2024 Apr 2];97(2):204–22. Available from: https://pubmed.ncbi.nlm.nih.gov/35039207/
41. Shetty N, Schalka S, Lim HW, Mohammad TF. The effects of UV filters on health and the environment. Photochem Photobiol Sci [Internet]. 2023 Oct 1 [cited 2024 Mar 3];22(10):2463–71. Available from: https://pubmed.ncbi.nlm.nih.gov/37344707/
42. Guan LL, Lim HW, Mohammad TF. sunscreens and photoaging: a review of current literature. Am J Clin Dermatol [Internet]. 2021 Nov 1 [cited 2024 Mar 16];22(6):819–28. Available from: https://pubmed.ncbi.nlm.nih.gov/34387824/
43. Nash JF, Tanner PR. Relevance of UV filter/sunscreen product photostability to human safety. Photodermatol Photoimmunol Photomed [Internet]. 2014 [cited 2024 Mar 16];30(2–3):88–95. Available from: https://pubmed.ncbi.nlm.nih.gov/24433498/
44. Matts PJ, Nash JF. Sunscreens—another endangered species? Int J Cosmet Sci [Internet]. 2023 Oct 1 [cited 2024 Mar 3];45 Suppl 1(S1):20–32. Available from: https://pubmed.ncbi.nlm.nih.gov/37799079/
45. Benson HAE. Assessment and clinical implications of absorption of sunscreens across skin. Am J Clin Dermatol [Internet]. 2000 [cited 2024 Mar 16];1(4):217–24. Available from: https://pubmed.ncbi.nlm.nih.gov/11702366/
46. Pawlowski S, Herzog B, Sohn M, Petersen-Thiery M, Acker S. EcoSun Pass: a tool to evaluate the ecofriendliness of UV filters used in sunscreen products. Int J Cosmet Sci [Internet]. 2021 Apr 1 [cited 2024 Mar 16];43(2):201–10. Available from: https://pubmed.ncbi.nlm.nih.gov/33289148/
47. Mansour OT, Venero DA. Insights into the structure of sunscreen lotions: a small-angle neutron scattering study. RSC Adv [Internet]. 2021 Apr 9 [cited 2024 Mar 16];11(24):14306–13. Available from: https://pubmed.ncbi.nlm.nih.gov/35423975/
48. Ngoc LTN, Tran V Van, Moon JY, Chae M, Park D, Lee YC. Recent trends of sunscreen cosmetic: an update review. Cosmetics [Internet]. 2019 Nov 1 [cited 2024 Mar 16];6(4):64. Available from: https://www.mdpi.com/2079-9284/6/4/64/htm

49. Wang J, Ganley CJ. Safety threshold considerations for sunscreen systemic exposure: a simulation study. Clin Pharmacol Ther [Internet]. 2019 Jan 1 [cited 2024 Mar 16];105(1):161–7. Available from: https://pubmed.ncbi.nlm.nih.gov/30094825/
50. Nicole W. skin protection dilemma: testing detects benzene in some sun care products. Environ Health Perspect [Internet]. 2022 May 1 [cited 2024 Apr 2];130(5). Available from: https://www.ncbi.nlm.nih.gov/pmc/articles/PMC9113541/
51. Yeoman AM, Shaw M, Ward M, Ives L, Andrews SJ, Lewis AC. Gas phase emissions of volatile organic compounds arising from the application of sunscreens. Int J Environ Res Public Health [Internet]. 2023 Jun 1 [cited 2024 Mar 16];20(11):5944. Available from: https://www.mdpi.com/1660-4601/20/11/5944/htm
52. Lu Y, Liu M, Cao Y, Yin J, Zhou H, Yu W, et al. Hydrogel sunscreen based on yeast /gelatin demonstrates excellent UV-shielding and skin protection performance. Colloids Surf B Biointerfaces [Internet]. 2021 Sep 1 [cited 2024 Mar 16];205. Available from: https://pubmed.ncbi.nlm.nih.gov/34091373/
53. Gwak MA, Hong BM, Park WH. Hyaluronic acid/tannic acid hydrogel sunscreen with excellent anti-UV, antioxidant, and cooling effects. Int J Biol Macromol [Internet]. 2021 Nov 30 [cited 2024 Mar 16];191:918–24. Available from: https://pubmed.ncbi.nlm.nih.gov/34597695/
54. Wang R, Wang X, Zhan Y, Xu Z, Xu Z, Feng X, et al. A dual network hydrogel sunscreen based on poly-γ-glutamic acid/tannic acid demonstrates excellent anti-UV, self-recovery, and skin-integration capacities. ACS Appl Mater Interfaces [Internet]. 2019 Oct 16 [cited 2024 Mar 16];11(41):37502–12. Available from: https://pubs.acs.org/doi/abs/10.1021/acsami.9b14538
55. Slabu AI, Miu L, Ghibu E, Stavarache CE, Stan R, Teodorescu F. Bioconjugation of vegetable oils with UV absorbers: new approach in skin photoprotection. Molecules [Internet]. 2023 Nov 1 [cited 2024 Mar 16];28(22):7550. Available from: https://www.mdpi.com/1420-3049/28/22/7550/htm
56. Seixas VC, Serra OA. Stability of sunscreens containing CePO4: proposal for a new inorganic UV filter. Molecules [Internet]. 2014 [cited 2024 Mar 16];19(7):9907–25. Available from: https://pubmed.ncbi.nlm.nih.gov/25010465/
57. Sohn M, Amorós-Galicia L, Krus S, Martin K, Herzog B. Effect of emollients on UV filter absorbance and sunscreen efficiency. J Photochem Photobiol B [Internet]. 2020 Apr 1 [cited 2024 Mar 16];205. Available from: https://pubmed.ncbi.nlm.nih.gov/32065958/
58. Touitou E, Godin B. Skin nonpenetrating sunscreens for cosmetic and pharmaceutical formulations. Clin Dermatol [Internet]. 2008 Jul [cited 2024 Mar 16];26(4):375–9. Available from: https://pubmed.ncbi.nlm.nih.gov/18691518/
59. Cozzi AC, Perugini P, Gourion-Arsiquaud S. Comparative behavior between sunscreens based on free or encapsulated UV filters in term of skin penetration, retention and photo-stability. Eur J Pharm Sci [Internet]. 2018 Aug 30 [cited 2024 Mar 16];121:309–18. Available from: https://pubmed.ncbi.nlm.nih.gov/29874551/
60. Chavda VP, Acharya D, Hala V, Daware S, Vora LK. Sunscreens: a comprehensive review with the application of nanotechnology. J Drug Deliv Sci Technol. 2023;86:104720.
61. Taniyadukkam V, Jose J, Maliyakkal N, Beeran AA, Almoyad MAA, Aleya L, et al. Development and evaluation of sunscreen cream containing solid lipid nanoparticles of Spinacia oleraceae. Environ Sci Pollut Res Int [Internet]. 2023 Apr 1 [cited 2024 Mar 16]; 30(18):51782–91. Available from: https://pubmed.ncbi.nlm.nih.gov/36820973/
62. Vaishampayan P, Rane MM. Herbal nanocosmecuticals: a review on cosmeceutical innovation. J Cosmet Dermatol [Internet]. 2022 Nov 1 [cited 2024 Mar 16];21(11):5464–83. Available from: https://pubmed.ncbi.nlm.nih.gov/35833365/
63. Yasui H, Hirone T. Action spectrum for bergamot-oil phototoxicity measured by sunburn cell counting. J Dermatol [Internet]. 1994 [cited 2024 Mar 16];21(5):319–22. Available from: https://pubmed.ncbi.nlm.nih.gov/8051317/
64. Moysan A, Morlière P, Averbeck D, Dubertret L. Evaluation of phototoxic and photogenotoxic risk associated with the use of photosensitizers in suntan preparations: application to

tanning preparations containing bergamot oil. Skin Pharmacol [Internet]. 1993 [cited 2024 Mar 16];6(4):282–91. Available from: https://pubmed.ncbi.nlm.nih.gov/8198814/

65. Binder S, Hanáková A, Tománková K, Pížová K, Bajgar R, Manišová B, et al. adverse phototoxic effect of essential plant oils on NIH 3T3 cell line after UV light exposure. Cent Eur J Public Health [Internet]. 2016 [cited 2024 Mar 16];24(3):234–40. Available from: https://pubmed.ncbi.nlm.nih.gov/27755863/
66. Young AR, Walker SL, Kinley JS, Plastow SR, Averbeck D, Morlière P, et al. Phototumorigenesis studies of 5-methoxypsoralen in bergamot oil: evaluation and modification of risk of human use in an albino mouse skin model. J Photochem Photobiol B [Internet]. 1990 [cited 2024 Mar 16];7(2–4):231–50. Available from: https://pubmed.ncbi.nlm.nih.gov/2128326/
67. Autier P, Doré J -F, Schifflers E, Cesarini J -P, Bollaerts A, Koelmel KF, et al. Melanoma and use of sunscreens: an Eortc case-control study in Germany, Belgium and France. The EORTC Melanoma Cooperative Group. Int J Cancer [Internet]. 1995 [cited 2024 Mar 11];61(6):749–55. Available from: https://pubmed.ncbi.nlm.nih.gov/7790106/
68. Kejlová K, Jírová D, Bendová H, Kandárová H, Weidenhoffer Z, Kolářová H, et al. Phototoxicity of bergamot oil assessed by in vitro techniques in combination with human patch tests. Toxicol In Vitro [Internet]. 2007 [cited 2024 Mar 16];21(7):1298–303. Available from: https://pubmed.ncbi.nlm.nih.gov/17669618/
69. Moyal D. Need for a well-balanced sunscreen to protect human skin from both Ultraviolet A and Ultraviolet B damage. Indian J Dermatol Venereol Leprol [Internet]. 2012 Jun 1 [cited 2024 Mar 22];78(SUPPL.1):24. Available from: https://ijdvl.com/need-for-a-well-balanced-sunscreen-to-protect-human-skin-from-both-ultraviolet-a-and-ultraviolet-b-damage/

Chapter 7
Sunscreen Metrics and Labelling Guidelines

Abbreviations

ASEAN	Association of Southeast Asian Nations
BEPF	Biological effective protection factors
BIS	Bureau of Indian Standards.
CIE	Commission Internationale de l'Eclairage
COLIPA	The European Cosmetic and Perfumery Association
EEE	The erythemal effective dose
EU	European Union
GPF	Genotoxic protection factor
HDRS	Hybrid diffuse reflectance spectroscopy
HEVL	High-energy visible light
ICNIRP	International Commission on Non-Ionizing Radiation Protection
IPF	Immune protection factor
ISO	International Organization for Standardization
ISO/CIE	International Organization for Standardization/International Commission on Illumination
ITA	Individual typology angle
JCIA	Japanese Cosmetic Industry Association
MED	Minimal erythema dose
MISD	Minimal immune suppression dose
MPPD	Minimal persistent pigment dose
MPPDD	Minimal persistent pigment darkening dose
NHP	Natural Health Products
NIPH	National Institute of Public Health
OTC	Over the counter
PMMA	Polymethyl methacrylate
PPD	Persistent pigment darkening
PPF	Pigmentation protection factor
RPF	Radical protection factor
SED	Standard erythema dose

R. Rajan, *Sunscreens for Skin of Color*,
https://doi.org/10.1007/978-981-97-3195-4_7

SOC	Skin of colour
SPF	Sun protection factor
SPT	Skin phototype
SSR	Solar-simulated radiation
UK	United Kingdom
UNEP	United Nations Environment Programme
US FDA	United States Food and Drug Administration
US	United States
UV	Ultraviolet
UVA-PF	Ultraviolet A-protection factor
UVI	UV index
WHO	World Health Organization
WMO	World Meteorological Organization

Key Objectives

- Sunscreens are performance-based skin care products, where a certain level of protection is required, tied to a certain volume of application. Therefore, measurement or quantification of the protection provided is central to ensuring optimal photoprotection outcomes.
- SPF and UVA-PF are the main metrics to evaluate the UV protection capacity of a sunscreen. Standards are available for in vivo and in vitro testing for both parameters. However, since significant inconsistencies exist in test results, standardization and validation is an ongoing, international collaborative effort.
- Monochromatic testing for specific solar subdomains such as VL and IR is now coming into prominence, as are methods like HDRS which offer the scope for non-invasive testing across all skin colours.
- Biological effective protective factors (BEPF) are more relevant measures to evaluate the effectiveness of sunscreens in domains such as UV-induced immunosuppression and DNA damage, which may be more sensitive to capture the entirety of solar-induced skin damage beyond an erythema end point.

There are two widely used standards for representing the photoprotection of a sunscreen. These are the sun protection factor (SPF) measurement for assessing UVB, and the ultraviolet A-protection factor (UVA-PF) to measure ultraviolet A (UVA) radiation [1].

SPF as a performance metric followed the introduction of minimal erythema dose (MED) as a useful indicator of sun protection on forearm skin, in 1934 by Ellinger. The first commercial sunscreen had just hit the US (United States) market a few years earlier. In 1956, the metric was formally introduced by Schulze in Germany, as a ratio of MED between sunscreen-protected and unprotected skin [2]. The method was improved upon further by Greiter and in 1978, the Food and Drug Administration (FDA) adopted the SPF metric. Originally, SPF measurement involved using natural sunlight at high altitudes. Eventually, artificial light sources were recommended to be used in the methodology, by both the FDA and in Europe

[3]. As mentioned, SPF testing employs skin redness or erythema as a visual end point to assess sunscreen efficacy. The assessment is performed using solar-simulated radiation (SSR) that mostly mimics the sun at a high elevation in low latitudes, with a higher proportion of UVB relative to UVA, as compared to actual solar radiation received at the equator. Therefore, this system, in effect, measures UVB protection primarily [4]. Over the last few decades, SPF measurement has come to be the most understood measure of sunscreen protection, from a consumer point of view.

SPF is calculated as the least amount of UVB energy required to produce minimal erythema on sunscreen-protected skin, compared to skin not protected by sunscreen [5, 6].

Formula

$$\text{SPF} = \text{MED of protected skin} / \text{MED of unprotected skin}$$

An SPF value of 15 would mean that it would take 15 times longer for the sunscreen-protected skin to develop erythema after UV exposure, as compared to sunscreen unprotected skin. Also, this sunscreen with SPF 15 would be able to filter out 93% of incident UV. SPF 30 and SPF 50 sunscreens are able to filter out 96% and 98% of UVB, respectively [1, 7].

The main evaluation metric used in SPF testing, the minimal erythema dose (MED) is the lowest UV energy required to produce just perceptible redness in previously unexposed human skin. It varies between skin types, from 150 to 600 J/cm^2 for skin types I–IV [8]. Researchers have also noted higher MED requirements in skin of colour (SOC), up to 885 J/cm^2 for skin phototype (SPT) IV in Columbia, for UVB [9]. The shortcomings of the MED are that it is not a standard metric, but a variable measure dependant on multiple factors, such as skin type, individual sensitivity to UV light, optical and radiometric fidelity of the light source, field size, dose increment, skin pigmentation, skin thickness, and anatomical site. In addition, observer related factors such as the time of reading of the erythema, definition of the end point, and the ambient illumination at the time of reading the result also influence the outcome. To overcome the lack of consistency produced by these variables, the concept of standard erythema dose (SED) was proposed [8].

SED is defined by International Organization for Standardization/International Commission on Illumination (ISO/CIE) standard as an erythemal exposure of 100 J/cm^2, assuming constant irradiance during this period [10]. It is possible to easily express the MED in relation to the SED. For example, the MED for skin types I–IV ranges from 150 to 600 J/cm^2, which is about 1.5–6 SED. So now, the SED simply denotes the UV radiation received—objectively, without the need for determination using a biological, and therefore, variable, and subjective end point. From here, it is also possible to characterize the duration required for this standard dose to be delivered, either from natural or artificial sources. It is estimated that a person in Northern Europe gets an exposure of 1 SED during the weekends in summer [4]. The minimum time required for exposure of 1 SED for UVA was found to be half that of winter, for summer. The SED in Iceland, where the global UV index is low compared to other Nordic countries, can go up to 32 in summer, while being 20 in June and the average Icelander may expect to get a sunburn after 4–6 SED [11]. Thus, it may be possible to compare exposures more easily using SED than MED. However, due to the wide extent of its use in sunscreen testing, MED is still the recommendation as per the latest guidelines, though both these parameters may be used to denote the dose of UVR [12, 13].

The United States Food and Drug Administration (US FDA) has been revising the maximum labelled SPF for sunscreens, from 30 in its 1999 monograph, to 50 in 2011, and now to 60+ in 2019 [13, 14]. Further, in 2019, the US FDA also approved the marketing of sunscreens with SPF claims of up to 80, to allow the development of products with more UVA coverage and to allow for lab test variations in sunscreens labelled as SPF 60+. However, the earlier labelling guidelines under the Code of Federal Regulations which have been stayed indefinitely continue to include sunscreens with SPF as low as 2 [15]. However, sunscreens with SPF below 15 are expected to carry a warning on the label stating that the product is only known to protect against sunburn but may not offer reliable protection against skin cancer or skin ageing [13, 16].

The current SPF classification as per different country guidelines is as below [17]. UV filters are regulated as OTC drugs in the US, cosmetics in Europe, quasi-drugs in Japan, and therapeutic drugs in Australia, for SPF > 15. In Canada, sunscreens with inorganic filters are considered as natural health products (NHPs), while the chemical sunscreens are considered as over the counter (OTC) drugs. In India, sunscreens are classed under cosmetics, and Bureau of Indian Standards (BIS) regulatory guidelines for testing broadly adopt the International Organization for Standardization (ISO) guidelines with some minor iterations [18–21]. According to the FDA, the value on the sunscreen label would be mentioned as a precise numerical value for those sunscreens with an SPF range of 2–14. For SPF above 15, the number on the label should be in increments of 5, for the range between 15 and 29, and corresponding to the lowest value in a range, as 15, 20, and 25. For SPF above 30, the values should be mentioned in the label in increments of 10, as 40, 50, and 60+, shown in Table 7.1.

According to the guidelines followed in the European Union, the minimum SPF for a sunscreen is 6 [22]. The EU recommendation requires that the UVA protection value, UVA-PF should be at least 1/3rd that of the SPF value, and that the critical wavelength exceeds 370 nm, Table 7.2.

The rating system followed by the Association of Southeast Asian Nations (ASEAN) is similar to that followed in the European Union (EU) and requires a minimum SPF of 6, Table 7.3. The ASEAN guidelines apply to 10 Southeast Asian nations, namely Indonesia, Malaysia, Philippines, Singapore, Thailand, Brunei Darussalam, Vietnam, Lao People's Democratic Republic (Lao PDR), Myanmar, and Cambodia [23].

The Australian Sunscreen Standard provides the labelling guidelines for Australia and New Zealand based on SPF, broad-spectrum coverage, and water resistance

Table 7.1 Sunscreen labels recommended by FDA guidelines [15, 16]

Labelled category	**SPF value**
Low	2–14.9
Medium	15–29.9
High	30–59.9
Very high	>60

However, the FDA Final Rule and Proposed Rules, issued in 2021, carry a simplified label guideline as below, retaining the FDA recommendation suggested in 2019 [13].

Range of determined SPF values	**Associated labelled SPF value**
60–80*	60+
50–59	50
40–49	40
30–39	30
25–29	25
20–24	20
15–19	15
2–14	Determined SPF value

*The OTC Monograph also recognizes sunscreens with SPF > 80.

Table 7.2 Sunscreen labelling recommendation of The Commission of the European Communities [22]

Labelled category	Labelled SPF	Measured SPF
Low protection	6	6–9.9
	10	10–14.9
Medium protection	15	15–19.9
	20	20–24.9
	25	25–29.9
High protection	30	30–49.9
	50	50–59.9
Very high protection	50+	≥60

Table 7.3 ASEAN sunscreen labelling guideline [23]

Label	SPF level
Low	≤6 < 15
Medium	≤15 < 30
High	≤30 < 50
Very high	≥50

SPF 50+ label may also be used to denote sunscreens with SPF above 50

claims. The rating starts at a minimum SPF value of 4 and increases in increments of 2 up to SPF 10, in increments of 5 between SPF 15 and 29, and in increments of 10 thereafter, in a similar fashion as the FDA rating, Table 7.4. Sunscreens with an SPF less than 4, or secondary sunscreens in cosmetic products such as lip balms or tinted bases and foundations with an SPF of 4 or more, and moisturizing skin care

Table 7.4 Australia and New Zealand Sunscreen Standard [24]

Description/level of protection	SPF claim on label	SPF
NA	NA	0–4
Low protection	4, 6, 8, 10	4–14
Medium or moderate protection	15, 20, 25	15–29
High protection	30, 40, 50	30–59
Very high protection	50+	60 or higher

Table 7.5 Boots star rating of UVA/UVB ratio from Polonini et al. [104]

Requirements		Initial mean UVA:UVB ratio			
		0.0–0.59	0.6–0.79	0.8–0.89	0.9 and over
Postexposure mean UVA:UVB ratio	0.0–0.56	No rating	No rating	No rating	No rating
	0.57–0.75	No rating	***	***	***
	0.76–0.85	No rating	***	****	****
	0.86 and over	No rating	***	****	*****

products, sunbathing skin care products with an SPF between 4 and 15, but without water resistance claims, in specified pack sizes are exempt from listing as therapeutic sunscreens, a mandatory requirement for sale in Australia [24].

The SPF system is widely in place across many countries; however, the story is relatively recent for UVA. This is because, though UVA was identified by Albert Kligman as causing structural damage to the skin, when he coined the term 'photoaging' in the late 1960s, sunscreens with UVA protection did only debut in the early 1980s. More recently, the role of UVA in photocarcinogenesis has been well recognized in the light-skinned population [13, 25, 26]. The idea of measuring sunscreens for UVA protection was first conceived in the early 1990s. At present, three systems are in place to assess UVA protection.

The Boots star rating, a proprietary method which is mostly used in the United Kingdom (UK), was introduced in 1992 and subsequently revised in 2008 and 2011, Table 7.5. It is an in vitro method, involving the application of sunscreen at a density of 1.3 mg/cm^2 on abraded polymethyl methacrylate (PMMA) plates, which are then irradiated with a fixed dose of UV from a xenon arc solar simulator at 17.5 J/cm^2, implying an equivalence to 1 h of standard sunlight. The ratio of the mean absorbance values in the UVA and the UVB ranges is compared, before and after irradiation and then used to arrive at the star rating [27–29]. For a complete interpretation of the sun protection efficacy, one needs to know the SPF in addition to the star rating.

Currently, the most common method of measuring UVA protection is the UVA-PF. This metric compares the ability of a sunscreen to prevent permanent pigment darkening, compared to sunscreen unprotected skin. The JCIA (Japanese Cosmetic Industry Association) rating for expressing the UVA protection has been widely used as the PA factor, shown in Table 7.6. Currently, there are 4 categories, compared to 3 earlier. The UVA-PF values are arrived at using the ISO 24442 in vivo method, discussed further below [20, 29].

Table 7.6 Japan Cosmetic Industry Association rating for UVA-PF [29]

UVA-PF values	PA rating
2 to less than 4	+
4 to less than 8	++
8 to less than 16	+++
16 or more	++++

Thus far, the UVA -PF is not required to be mentioned as an absolute number on sunscreen labels. However, for SOC, UVA protection is at least as important as UVB protection, and therefore, the UVA-PF value should receive an equal importance as the SPF. The UVA_PF value of a sunscreen gives a clear idea of the protection provided by the product in the UVA domain, independent of SPF [30]. Therefore, it should ideally be stated as an absolute value on the label.

It is interesting to note that sunscreens with an SPF up to 99 are allowed in certain countries, like Brazil [31].

7.1 SPF Testing

Sunscreen testing for SPF and UVA-PF is performed both in vivo and in vitro. The in vitro methods are influenced by the substrate, manner of application of the product and the spreading technique, environmental conditions, and UV irradiation dose and source [32]. Variations in film thickness and/or integrity, especially for zinc oxide based formulations, and due to temperature differences causing potential interference from infrared rays, create inconsistencies in measuring the exact level of protection provided by the sunscreen [33, 34]. The determination of SPF using in vivo techniques has challenges of its own. In vivo testing is prone to significant interlaboratory variations. Further, the source of light, natural versus artificial, creates significant differences in the outcome, owing to the spectral composition and the differences in the erythemal effective energy from the various subcomponent wavelength zones. Standardization of UV doses is difficult, due to the difference in response elicited by the same dose, but from different sources. For example, UVR at a dose of 1 J/cm^2 may elicit no response in a light-skinned individual, when the source is a UVA fluorescent lamp, compared to a sunburn like response with violaceous erythema, when the emitting source is a mercury arc lamp. This may result in significant differences in the reported SPF, for example. The SPF of a sunscreen product may vary depending on the amount of UVB in the light source used for testing. The erythemal effective dose (EEE) of UVA from SSR is 1/3rd that of the EEE from sun exposure. However, it is well known that even suberythemal doses of UVA can cumulatively induce cutaneous erythema, introducing a variability factor in SPF testing [4]. Finally in vivo testing involves significant human exposure to UV, a well-recognized carcinogen [35].

The latest standards for measuring in vivo SPF are the ISO 24444:2019 and the FDA 2019 [17, 19]. For in vivo UVA-PF, the most recently updated standard is ISO

24442:2022, and for in vitro UVA-PF, the recommended standard is ISO 24443:2021. ISO committee draft, ISO/CD 23678 is a protocol currently in development as an in vitro standard for SPF, and ISO/CD 23698 is being developed to standardize sunscreen testing using hybrid diffuse reflectance spectroscopy (HDRS) [3, 30].

These methods listed above represent the most current efforts in international collaboration and harmonization of standards, to present a clearer picture of sunscreen efficacy to the end user. Multiple iterations have been carried out over the years, in an attempt to remove or reduce discrepancies and accommodate the latest clinical information across different skin types as it becomes available. Considerable interlaboratory variations occur when testing for SPF using the in vivo tests, probably a pointer to the fact that while the testing parameters for ISO 24444 have been standardized, the validation standpoint needs further exploration [30].

The in vivo SPF testing can be performed in individuals with FST I, II, or III, or those have an ITA value above 28. The Indian BIS standards observe an ITA range of 28–41, stating that this range is more relevant to the skin colour of the Indian population [21].

In contrast, for UVA-PF testing as per the ISO 24442:2022, the most recent updates recommend abolishment of Fitzpatrick skin typing, and its replacement with individual typology angle, with the range expanded to include ITA up to 18 (range being 18–43) [36], whereas for in vivo SPF testing, the recommended ITA cut off is 28 [3], as above. Newer updates from the ISO may likely harmonize the ITA range for SPF testing as well.

The general format for the SPF in vivo test is as below. The volunteers who meet the inclusion criteria are selected, it is recommended that subjects who are new to testing be interviewed by a health care professional before the test. The test and the standard sunscreen products are applied over the test site, the back, at a density of 2 mg/cm^2 and allowed to dry for 15–30 min, depending on the standard used. The standards provide clear recommendations for the exact method of spreading the sunscreen over the test area. The test area is then subjected to predetermined dosages of UV, predicted based on ITA, with incremental increases as per protocol, in either a sitting or a prone position. The end point of MED is read after 16–24 h from the time of exposure of the last test site, by an experienced evaluator, in standardized ambient light conditions. Minor variations exist between the standards, but overall, the assessment is done after giving careful attention to a number of factors related to subject, method, and evaluation. For example, in subjects with hair on the back, it is acceptable to clip the hair, but to not shave the hair. This is because the latter process may remove some portion of the stratum corneum, which may interfere with the erythema response and therefore, the test results [3, 17]. The erythema response is graded as shown in Table 7.7 [21, 37].

Table 7.7 Grading of erythema for SPF testing from Donglikar et al. [21, 40]

Grading	Description
0	No response
0.5	Equivocal response
1	Unambiguous erythema
1.5	Well-defined erythema with sharp borders
2	Bright erythema

In vivo SPF testing may be inaccurate in the case of sunscreens which have an anti-inflammatory effect. Couteau et al. identified that some sun filters have significant anti-inflammatory effects with oedema inhibition percentage, ranging from 92% for iscotrizinol, to 90% for benzophenone-5 (BP-5) and titanium dioxide (TiO2), to 70% for diethylamino hydroxybenzoyl hexyl benzoate (DHHB) and bis-ethylhexyloxyphenol methoxyphenyl triazine (BEMT). Due allowance must be given for the suppression of the inflammatory end point, resulting from the inherent anti-inflammatory capacity of the sunscreen [38].

In vitro SPF testing awaits the development of a new standard, ISO/CD 23675; however, protocols are available for in vitro SPF testing using UV spectrometers.

UV spectrometry measures two aspects of sunscreen protection—absorbance and transmittance. Absorbance refers to the ability of the UV filter to absorb light and is proportionate to the amount of filtering molecules present in a sunscreen formulation. This criterion was found to linearly correlate with SPF results, demonstrating that the SPF label on a product gives a valuable idea of the level of blockage of UVB rays [39, 40]. Another parameter, transmittance measures the amount of light that passes through the sunscreen to reach the skin and can give an idea about what proportion of UVR reaches the skin. The higher the light absorbed in passing through the skin, less of it reaches the skin surface. At UV max, the higher the SPF, the lower the quantum of UVR that reaches the skin [39]. The method for determining SPF using the absorption principle of the UV spectrophotometer involves serial dilution with ethanol and then comparing spectral absorption in the range between 290 and 450 nm, with ethanol as the blank. However, results may be inconsistent depending on the formulation type and its interaction with ethanol [37]. The SPF determination using the transmittance principle, specifically with the Labsphere UV 2000S ultraviolet transmittance analyser, involves the measurement of the ratio of the illumination passed through a sample to the illumination impinging on the sample. The provided PMMA plate is loaded with sunscreen at a density of 2 µl/cm^2 and spread using standard recommendations, and then the plate is irradiated with a xenon flash lamp, to evaluate the transmittance through the plate. Pre-irradiation of the sample in this method helps evaluate the photostability of sunscreens containing UVA absorbers [37]. While this closely reflects the European Cosmetic and Perfumery Association (COLIPA) standard, the National Institute of Public Health (NIPH) method uses a sheet of Mikelanta covering paper with 2 mg/cm^2 of product, and Výzkumný ústav organických syntéz (VUOS) [41] protocol uses surgical tape affixed to a quartz layer and loaded with 1.2 mg/cm^2 to calculate SPF using transmittance principles [1]. These in vitro methods and the new standards in development may help develop universal guidelines for SPF testing, applicable to all skin types, including SOC, as higher skin types are currently excluded from in vivo testing for UVB [17].

7.2 UVA -PF Testing

In vivo testing for UVA-PF is similar to the method for in vivo SPF testing. The light source used here delivers only UVA, and the end point of persistent pigment darkening (PPD) is evaluated at 2 h after irradiation and graded as below. The UVA-PF is the ratio of the sunscreen-protected minimal persistent pigment darkening dose (MPPDD) to the unprotected MPPDD that produces a ≥ 1 grade of pigmentation [37], shown in Table 7.8.

Since the publication of the ISO standard for in vivo testing for UVA-PF [19], several countries like Japan and Australia have updated their national guidelines to follow the ISO standard, the latest being 24442:2022. While the earlier methods like CEN 2006 and FDA 2007 laid the groundwork for optimal testing, harmonization of the standards is the way towards internationally more uniform sunscreen testing. The updated guidelines recommend the inclusion of volunteers in the ITA range 18–43, with the test end point used is persistent pigment darkening.

The minimal persistent pigment darkening dose (MPPDD) has been redefined in the recent update as the lowest UVA dose that is able to produce the first perceptible, unambiguous, persistent pigment darkening response involving more than 50% of the UV exposure subsite, observed between 2 and 24 h after the end of the UVA exposure. Where earlier systems used the IPD (immediate pigment darkening), the CEN 2006 and FDA 2007, and further revisions up to the ISO 24442:2022, use PPD as the determinant for arriving at the UVA-PF. IPD measures the ability of UVA exposure to oxidize preformed melanosomes, reflected as a change in the colour of the skin to greyish brown [5, 20, 32, 42]. However, since this effect is maximally observed only within the first few minutes after sun exposure, its practical applicability and lack of reproducibility made it a less preferred option to PPD, which also allows for evaluation of sunscreen stability. As per the FDA 2007 testing guidelines for in vivo UVA-PF, the readings for minimum pigment darkening (MPD) are taken after 3–24 h of irradiation, and after 2–4 h from the last irradiation for CEN 2006, where the pigment darkening is deemed to be most stable [32].

Though the in vivo methods have been recommended for their precision, repeatability, and increased relevance due to their being applied on human subjects, there are pitfalls. The most important one is the lack of representation of skin of colour in the selection criteria of study subjects. The lowest that the sunscreen in vivo testing allows is ITA 18, which effectively excludes the brown and dark skin types, and about half the people in the tan group of the ITA scale [43] in Fig. 7.1.

Table 7.8 Grading of PPD for UVA-PF testing from Donglikar et al. [21, 40]

Grading	Description
0	No response
0.5	Equivocal response
1	Unambiguous dark grey or brown pigmentation
1.5	Well-defined dark grey or brown pigmentation with sharp borders
2	Deep pigmentation

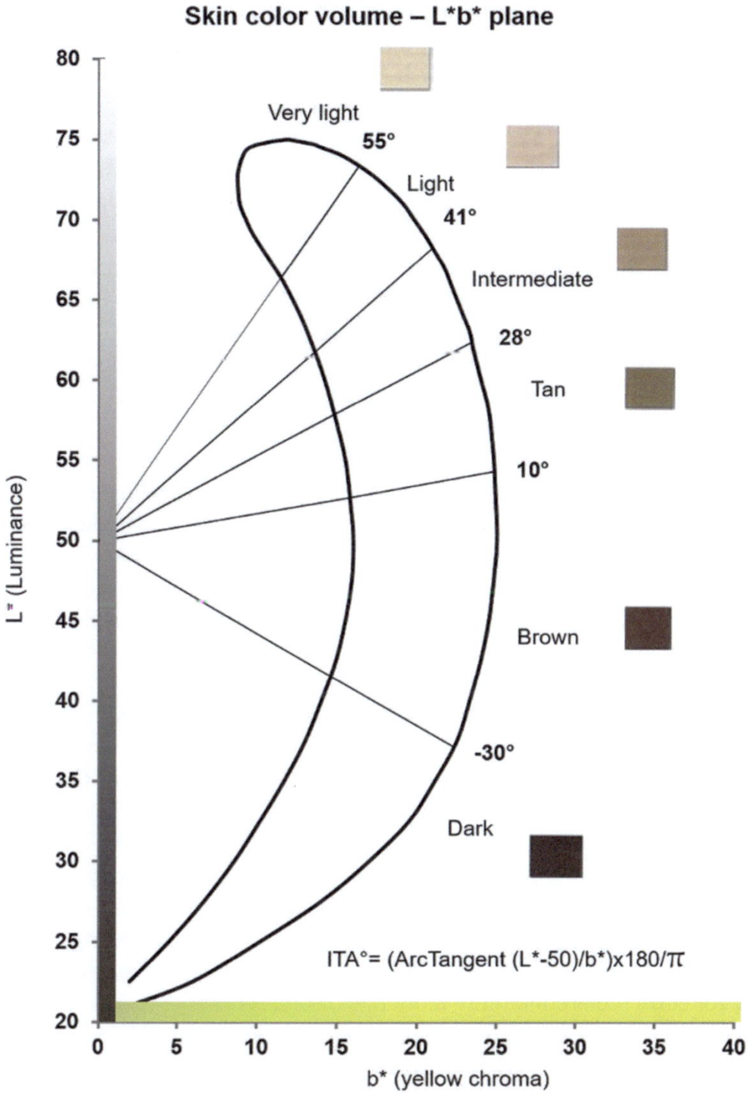

Fig. 7.1 Skin colour volume allows for objective quantification and classification of skin colour into six groups: very light, light, intermediate, tan, brown, and dark [44, 45]. The skin colour volume aligns the colorimetric 1976 CIE L*a*b* parameters with the ITA value. The L* (luminance) value of the skin colour is represented on the vertical axis and the b* (yellow-blue) component is on the horizontal axis. The ITA of the corresponding skin colour can be obtained from the L* and b* values according to the formula. The colour swatches are representative average skin colours for each colour group that match the L'Oréal Skin Color Chart [46]. CIE Commission Internationale de l'Eclairage, ITA individual typology angle. (Obtained with permission from Ly et al. [101])

Unlike the erythema response end point in UVB testing, which is accomplished in a shorter period of time, UVA-PF testing has a pigmentation end point, which may take up to an hour for development of the end point. This involves a significant exposure of the test subjects to UVR, even up to 750 J/cm^2 of UVA, especially when testing for products with high efficacy of protection [3]. Since UVA is now established as capable of photocarcinogenesis, in vivo testing may not be feasible in the long run given the duration of exposure [30]. Including only lighter skin types involves exposing subjects who are predisposed to photocarcinogenesis, for test durations of up to 30 min, but potentially longer, and simultaneously, leaves out higher phototypes, aka SOC, who look for robust UVA protection from the point of view of photopigmentation, a disadvantage on both counts.

For these reasons, the in vitro measurements, particularly the latest ISO 24443, seem attractive. The in vitro measurement of UVA-PF using ISO 24443 has been found to be consistently comparable to persistent pigment darkening, the criterion used in the in vivo tests as well. So, ISO 24443 may well be considered an efficient surrogate measure of UVA-PF. Three other in vitro methods are available, of which the FDA 2011 and the ISO 24443 both use a standardized two-phase application method. A 2 mg/cm^2 of product loading was used by the CEN 2006 and FDA 2007 methods, while the updated ISO 24443 uses 1.3 mg/cm^2. The FDA 2011 method recommends the use of 0.75 mg/cm^2 of sunscreen [32]. Considering consumer behaviour studies that note that people generally apply sunscreens at the usage rate of 0.5–1.5 mg/cm^2 [6, 47–49], the lower volumes may be more realistic and practical.

Given the larger role of UVA in developing and promoting conditions of concern to skin of colour, such as pigmentation and photoageing, further work in quantifying the UVA protection ability in these populations is warranted. One hindrance seems to be the lack of a reliable and sufficient generation of UVA light by solar simulators compared to natural sunlight. The cost of the xenon arc lamp instituted as the light source for ISO 24443:2021 is also considered high, and researchers have proposed modifications that may allow the use of cheaper light-emitting diode (LED) light sources with good UVA fidelity, as options for increasing the access to the UVA-PF in vitro testing [6, 33]. In vivo testing for UVA-PF is considered more accurate for sunscreens containing inorganic particles or those that are likely to have issues related to film formulation. In such cases, the in vitro UVA-PF is likely to show a lower value than in vivo measurement [50].

Moyal calculated that the minimum required UVA-PF for sun protection in India would be 12–17 in winter to a maximum of 29–30 in summer, based on season-based meteorological dose of UVA per day, along with other factors such as anatomical skin area exposed to UVR, duration of such exposure, skin type, and behavioural constructs such as a realistic sunscreen usage level [51].

SPF testing using the in vitro method involves the use of roughened PMMA plates on to which the sunscreen is 'plated' at an application density of 1.3 mg/cm^2 for UVA testing. The transmission of UV radiation through this film is then measured. The roughening of the PMMA plate is done by sandblasting, which creates significant plate-to-plate variation. Uniformity here is crucial, as the roughness of the PMMA plates plays a role in the final SPF output. Ferrero et al. identified the availability of two substrates, one with a surface roughness of 2 microns, and the other with a roughness of 6 microns, which have been used in different publications. The plate with the lower roughness accommodated an application density of 0.75–1 mg/cm^2, while the similar value for the high roughness plate was 1.2–1.4 mg/cm^2, closer to the intended value of 1.3 mg/cm^2. Correlation with in vivo testing was obtained using the 6 micron roughness plate, at application densities of 1.2 mg/cm^2 validating the recommended value as above. Injection moulding is a newer solution to this problem of varied roughness noted with sandblasting to roughen the PMMA plates. Testing in vitro protection using these plates was also found to correlate well with in vivo measurements [17, 52].

As seen above, no test method is considered perfect when it comes to sunscreen testing, and the need to find better substitutes for in vivo testing is well understood by researchers, world over. Newer alternatives have already begun to evolve, with technologies like HDRS, newer in vitro SPF testing protocol the ISO/CD 23675, in silico calculation of transmittance, UV photography, and machine learning models to predict the protection capabilities of a sunscreen based on the ingredients, presence of pigment, type of formulation, and product type [30, 53]. Much earlier, Diffey et al. had proposed that a filter such as zinc oxide, avobenzone, or titanium dioxide may be considered a required but not adequate way to cover the UVA spectrum based on the understanding of critical wavelength [54]. In silico models were able to predict the differential levels of sun protection capacity of sunscreens with the same UV filters but in different physical formulations [55]. Such calculations and modelling have been shown to be useful for formulation design, prediction of vitamin D synthesis even when using sunscreens, for sustainable-by-design and safe-by-design concepts, and for performance metrics such as water resistance and sun protection efficacy cross biological end points [56].

HDRS is the latest and most advanced technology, which is anticipated to reduce human exposure risk to UV during sunscreen testing. HDRS uses a combination of in vivo measurements using diffuse reflectance spectroscopy and in vitro measurement of transmission through a film of sunscreen applied on a roughened polymethyl methacrylate (PMMA) plate. The HDRS method shows good correlation with current ISO standard 24444. The advantage of the HDRS method is the lack of dependence on erythema as an end point. This new hybrid technology aims to reduce the variability of outcomes that are noted with current sunscreen testing methods, thereby increasing the reproducibility, and also reduces the radiation risk for subjects in in vivo assessments, since MED measurements are not applicable for this method. Further, UVA-PF values can also be calculated simultaneously and show good correlation to ISO 24443 standards. Further, lack of interobserver variations in defining and reading MED, and applicability for all sunscreen types, including high SPF formulations, indicate that the future of sunscreen testing may have arrived with HDRS [57].

As the next step towards developing an ISO-HDRS standard, a total of 25 sunscreen emulsions and sprays were evaluated using HDRS equipment from multiple manufacturers, at different laboratories. Concurrence of results was obtained within a narrow range for both SPF and UVA-PF values, from all participating labs, and was not affected by operator related or equipment manufacture related factors, confirming the reliability and objectivity of the HDRS technology [58].

7.3 Broad-Spectrum Protection with Sunscreens

Sun protection in both UVA and UVB domains is considered a requisite for all sunscreens that are made available to the public today. All countries have updated their guidelines to reflect this requirement, through easily understood parameters.

As per the European Commission standards of 2006, the numerical value of the UVA-PF must be at least 1/3rd that of the numerical value of the SPF for the sunscreen to be considered broad spectrum as per European Union (EU) standards [1, 59]. The more recent FDA proposal recommends a ratio of 0.7 or greater, for UVA1: UV, in addition to satisfying a critical wavelength requirement of >370 nm, to ensure adequate sun protection in the UVA1 spectrum, relative to the entire UV spectrum [13, 16, 59]. The Boots star rating recommends a more complete UVA–UVB coverage with at least 0.9:1 ratio of UVA-PF:SPF values. This ratio is considered the toughest of sunscreen metrics [20, 48, 54]. Comprehensive sunscreen testing devices such as the Labsphere 2000S display this metric as part of the results.

An even protection across both UVA and UVB spectra is considered the ideal standard—elegantly expressed as 'spectral homeostasis' or 'spectral uniformity'. This is achieved only with a higher protection in the UVA range, with the UVA-PF value approaching the SPF value numerically or by a higher critical wavelength. A sunscreen even with a lower SPF 15, a UVA-PF value of 15, and a critical wavelength around 389 nm is considered to provide a level of sun protection, as provided by a tightly woven, dark clothing, due to achievement of spectral homeostasis [30].

To understand broad-spectrum protection, the concept of critical wavelength must be understood, first.

7.4 Critical Wavelength

In the USA, broad-spectrum sun protection across both the UVB and the UVA spectra is indicated by a metric called critical wavelength, Fig. 7.2.

Critical wavelength represents the wavelength below which 90% of the absorbance of a sunscreen falls, indicating how far into the UVA spectrum, the protection of the said product extends [25, 30]. This is an in vitro parameter and needs to be performed in addition to the in vivo tests employed for sunscreen testing. The US FDA simply requires the critical wavelength to be above 370 nm, creating a pass/fail binary criterion for labelling a sunscreen as broad spectrum. This is supported by studies by Diffey et al. on commercial sunscreens that demonstrated correlation between UVA protection and achieving a critical wavelength above 370 nm [13, 54]. However, it is possible that products with similar SPF and critical wavelength pass criterion can have very different levels of protection in the UVA spectrum, when measured by a biological end point such as the PPD in calculating UVA-PF [30, 54].

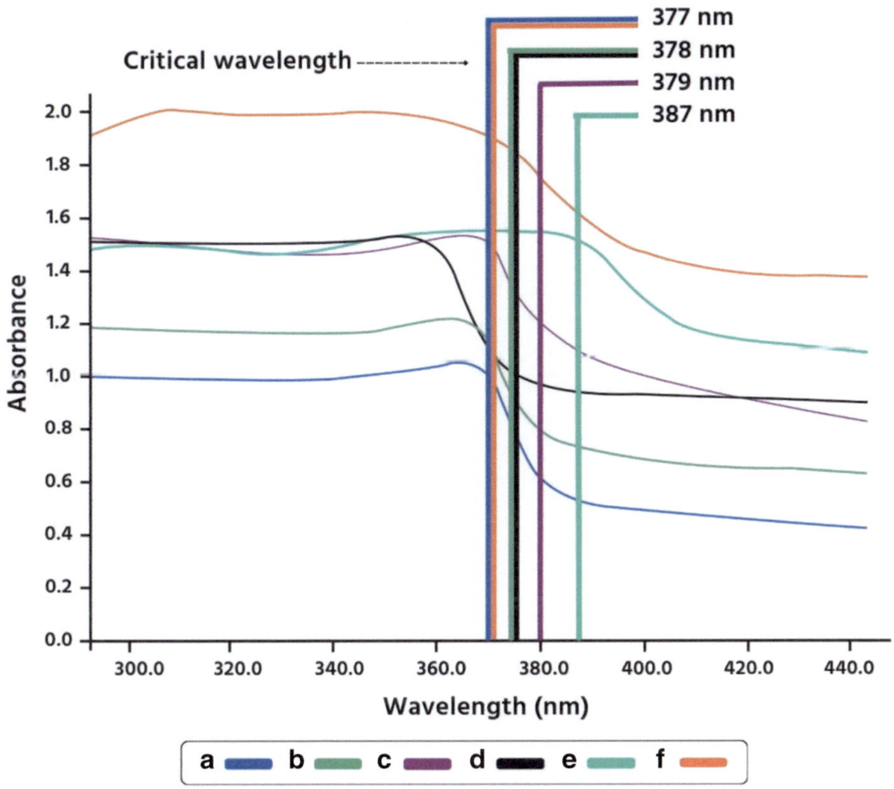

Fig. 7.2 Critical wavelengths of different sunscreen formulations, containing (A) non-nano zinc oxide as the only UV filter (377 nm), (B) non-nano zinc oxide with silymarin antioxidant (378 nm), (C) non-nano zinc oxide with antioxidant Pycnogenol (379 nm), (D) bemotrizinol with vegetable melanin (378 nm), (E) bisoctrizole, titanium dioxide, and iron oxide, tinted sunscreen (387 nm), and (F) non-nano zinc oxide coated with silica (377 nm). The protection of the sunscreen further into the UVA spectrum can be extended by adding both pigmented antioxidants and iron oxide tints. Addition of antioxidants also increases absorbance by a factor of 1.5 times. Absorbance also increased with silica-coated non-nano zinc, though the critical wavelength remains the same as that of uncoated non-nano zinc. The UV spectrophotometer measures critical wavelength up to 389 nm. (Images with permission from Dr Renita Lourdhurajan)

While support for this metric arises from it being non-invasive, critics point to the lack of a biological end point in this criterion. However, since the complete photobiological impact of UVA in the skin is yet to be thoroughly elucidated, this critical wavelength may be a simple number on the sunscreen label, easily understood by the customer. Gasparro proposes replacing the term 'critical wavelength' to a more neutral and less judgmental 'Long Wave Index', expressed with a rating method, as in Table 7.9 [60]. The Long Wave Index (LWI) is proposed to be used for finished sunscreen formulations and not for individual UV filters [60]. This is important since multiple nonfiltering ingredients play a role in determining the final sun protection ability of a sunscreen product [1].

Table 7.9 Long wave index rating recommended by Gasparro F. P. [60]

Wavelength range (nm)	LWI rating
<320	0
321–340	1
341–360	2
361–380	3
381–400	4
>400	5

To conclude, at this point spectral uniformity or spectral homeostasis seems to be the main requirement from a good sunscreen, for which the UVA-PF must be commensurate with SPF to ensure broad-spectrum coverage [28, 30, 61]. Proposals for newer methods of testing, including in silico methods to determine output, in terms of protection, as a function of input, in terms of ingredients, are exciting as they would support sunscreen development, right from the formulation stage to be of improved efficiency [30]. Despite the significant progress made in this field of sun protection testing, in addition to the admitted difficulty in obtaining repeatable results, the quantification of protection against visible and infrared spectrum remains to be tackled.

7.5 VL-PF

Recent research acknowledges the visible light spectrum as an important photobiologically active part of the solar spectrum, with impacts on photoaging, pigmentation, and erythema [18, 62, 63]. The need for sunscreens to be able to specifically protect in this spectrum is also well established, as is the need to develop metrics to measure the efficacy of such protection.

VL-PF is designated as the metric to arrive at the visible light protecting efficiency of a sunscreen, which is calculated in a manner similar to that of SPF, both in vivo and in vitro, but using a light source that irradiates in the visible light wavelengths [64].

The in vitro tests mostly use a PMMA plate loaded with sunscreens at densities between 0.75 and 2 mg/cm^2, but most commonly 1.3 mg/cm^2 [64]. Using UV spectrophotometers to analyse the reduction in transmittance, Schalka et al. suggested the classification of sunscreens based on visible light protection factor and also an in vitro pigmentation protection factor (PPF) for denoting the benefit provided by the sunscreen in blocking UVA+ blue light (BL), in a manner similar to SPF and UVA-PF and proposed classifying sunscreens based on their ability to protect against VL as in Table 7.10 [65].

Based on available information on VL-PF testing, Lim et al. suggested a harmonization of test methods, in 2021 [64]. The proposed range of ITA for visible light testing is 10 to −40, to include a representative melanocompetent population that can demonstrate detectable pigmentary changes. Light sources

Table 7.10 Proposed classification of sunscreens by range of protection against visible light

Protection against VL	Stars	PF-VIS	Transmittance reduction (%TR)
Very high	★★★★	>5.0	>60%
High	★★★☆	4.1–5.0	
Medium	★★☆☆	3.1–4.0	
Weak	★☆☆☆	2.1–3.0	
Absent	☆☆☆☆	<2.0	<60%

From Schalka, S. et al. Clinical, Cosmetic and Investigational Dermatology 2019 12 605-616' Originally published by, adapted and used with permission from Dove Medical Press Ltd [62]

that mimic solar radiation as closely as possible, but without a significant IR component are recommended to obtain results with good fidelity. Two protocols exist, one involving a single exposure and the other, repeated exposure over 4 days [63, 66]. The harmonized guidelines recommend a single exposure protocol to reduce drop outs and limit the number of variables to ensure better standardization [64].

Using pigmentation as the end point, in vivo VL-PF is calculated as the ratio of change in ITA between exposed and nonexposed skin, at day 7 after a single exposure of 480 J/cm^2 using a VL light source with 94–98% spectral output between 400 and 700 nm, administered 30 min following the test product application, typically on anatomical test sites such as the lower back or buttocks in at least 10 individuals with ITA ranging between 10 and −40 [62]. In vitro tests to measure the absorption or transmission spectrum of formulations containing visible light filters, typically but not exclusively iron oxides, using the visible light source, and using artificial skin substrates have been described. To avoid interference with immediate pigment darkening, restricting the visible light bandwidth to 400–600 nm is suggested [18, 67]. In 2022, Duteil et al. demonstrated that in vitro testing correlated well with a 4-day in vivo test protocol for VL-PF and highlighted the beneficial effects of tinted sunscreen in blocking HEVL. Specifically, the most critical spectrum to block seems to be in the 400–469 nm region, which corresponds to the absorption spectrum of Opsin-3, whose role has been recently well established in promoting VL-induced pigmentation. The authors also proposed that VL-PF be represented as a percentage denoted by pVL-PF, and calculated as (1-(1/VL-PF)) × 100, for ease of understanding for dermatologists and consumers who seek sunscreens offering specific protection from VL-induced pigmentation [68]. Further iterations and standardizations are expected before the VL-PF can be seen on product labels, depicted in a meaningful way.

Use of multispectral imaging to demonstrate sunscreen protection in the visible light spectrum, using light reflectance maps, was described by Le Digabel et al. In principle, the methodology is similar to the HDRS but has the advantage of visualizing sunscreen spread. While this technology may help consumer awareness around sunscreens that predominantly absorb and not reflect light, the research applications of this technology and similar approaches like ultraviolet camera photography are unclear at present [69].

7.6 Water Resistance

Substantivity of a sunscreen is defined as its ability to resist being washed off the skin on exposure to water or be removed from the skin by sweating during exercise, while photosubstantivity is the ability of the sunscreen to provide the intended sun protection, without undergoing photodegradation [60]. Sunscreen protection and performance are both affected by sweating and exposure to water [3]. Water resistance testing on sunscreens is compliant to the FDA 2021 and the ISO 16217:2020 standards, the latter having been adopted by countries such as Australia and New Zealand. In Europe, the COLIPA 2005 method is used. The US FDA allows the labelling of water resistance on sunscreens as Water Resistant (40 min) and Water Resistant (80 min), translating into water-resistant claims and very-water resistant claims used earlier. An in vivo testing method is recommended, similar to the standards followed in other countries. The water resistance protocol involves the testing of sunscreen applied on volunteers performing moderate activity in water in a hot tub, indoor fresh water pool or whirlpool, at 23–32 °C, in 2 sessions of 20 min separated by a 15-min period for claiming water resistance for 40 min, and 4 such sessions for 80 min, without towelling [3, 16]. Label claims for water resistance are made on the SPF tested after water exposure in the US and Australia. For Europe, a water resistance claim can be made if the SPF drops by less than 50% after water exposure compared to the original SPF [3]. The Australia and New Zealand adaptation of the ISO guidelines requires immersion for 4 h, compared to the shorter periods of 40 and 80 min, used in other countries [19].

In vitro water resistance testing measures have been proposed by multiple researchers, but as of now, none has been officially approved for standard use. Different substrates have been used, such as pig skin and explants, but PMMA is the most popular. Pissavini et al. conducted immersion experiments using an agitated water bath to simulate COLIPA conditions of in vivo testing; however, suitable correlations could not be established with the latter method. Similar immersion methods by other workers found that the PMMA plate method was inherently an issue for in vitro testing, due to the variable affinity of the sunscreen to the plate, and the lack of uniform film formation. An in silico method using ethanol was suggested by Sohn et al. which was found to be superior to the plate method [19, 70].

Water resistance is equated to sweat resistance for practical use [16]. Apart from the testing methodologies, sunscreen water resistance performance is also influenced by formulation. Sunscreen formulas that were either anhydrous or emulsions of water in oil were found not to get rinsed off exposures mimicking sea water bathing, for up to 40 min. Saxe et al. tested the tendency of sunscreens to get rinsed off during recreational bathing in the sea, by simulating the conditions with synthetic sea water and sunscreens applied on porcine skin. A total of 22 sunscreens containing 6 UV filters, zinc oxide, titanium dioxide, avobenzone, homosalate, octisalate, and octocrylene were tested. At least 90% of the product was found to stay on the porcine skin at the end of 40 min, in 19 out of 22 sunscreens. Oil in water emulsion type of formulations was found to rinse off relatively easily, compared to waterless formulations or water in oil formulations, where lipids form the continuous phase [71]. Anhydrous or hydrophobic sunscreen formulations themselves may act as barrier-protecting agents and protect the skin from extended periods of water exposure [72].

7.7 Biological Effective Protection Factors (BEPF)

SPF and UVA-PF are standard measures of sun protection efficacy of sunscreens. Typically, the component of erythema is expressed as SPF, thus far implied as a measure of protection against photocarcinogenesis. Though the most widely known metric, SPF and therefore, erythema is no way a complete measure for changes that occur in the skin, predating photocarcinogenesis. This is because even sub-MED doses have been shown to hasten photoageing, modulate immune responses, and DNA damage [1, 6]. Further, there are still gaps in understanding the complete bio-physiological activity of UVA. Outcome points which capture the biological processes in photoexposed skin over a larger scope are more relevant for efficient protection.

BEPFs represent defined metrics which take into account factors other than SPF and UVA-PF, from a holistic protection perspective. They are calculated for predetermined UV-mediated skin responses, based on transmission measurements, typically defined by the Diffey method, but modified by other workers. Simply stated, BEPFs express the number of times a person with a photoprotective agent can be exposed to sunlight, compared to a control [73–75].

It is well established that UVR induces cutaneous immunosuppression in addition to causing DNA damage. This immunosuppression then allows the DNA damaged cells to escape immune surveillance and eventually progress into cutaneous malignancies [76–78]. The immune protection factor (IPF) uses the principle of cutaneous hypersensitivity to arrive at the ability of a sunscreen to inhibit UVR-induced immunosuppression. Contact hypersensitivity is assessed by applying haptens to UV-irradiated skin and then looking for an erythema response. For delayed hypersensitivity, a subcutaneous antigen challenge is done, to assess UV-induced suppression of an elicitation phase response. The ability of a sunscreen to prevent blunting of the induction or elicitation arm of these hypersensitivity responses is assessed to arrive at the IPF. Damian et al. first attempted to characterize the IPF of a sunscreen by defining the minimal immune suppression dose (MISD) as the amount of UV that reduces the mean nickel cutaneous hypersensitivity response by 20%. Sunscreen IPF was then calculated as a ratio of MISD on sunscreen-protected skin to MISD on unprotected skin [77, 79, 80]. It was recently shown that sunscreens are only able to reduce immune suppression by only 50% of their SPF value [60, 76]. The action spectrum of UV-induced immunosuppression has two peaks, one in the UVB zone at around 300 nm, and a much larger peak in the UVA zone between 364 and 385 nm. This is evidence that UVA contributes to the bulk of UV-induced immunosuppression and underlines the need for broad-spectrum UV protection [81–83]. Though there is a dire need for discussion around UV-induced immunosuppression in view of its contribution to photocarcinogenesis, a reliable and easy to understand metric is yet to be finalized [77, 84].

Another attempt has been to quantify the ability of the sunscreen to suppress signature p53 mutations induced by UVB exposure on skin, the mutation protection factor. P53 protection factor rates the ability of a sunscreen to protect against solar-induced production of p53 activation, while genotoxic protection factor (GPF) looks at the number of sunburn cells between sunscreen-protected and unprotected skin, after sun exposure. The DNA protection factor is evaluated using monoclonal antibodies to detect thymine dimers and 6–4 photoproducts in addition to image analysis to indicate DNA damage in cells [85]. Young et al. demonstrated that this metric correlated meaningfully with SPF, indicating that erythema may be a relevant and easy to identify marker for DNA damage with a potential for skin cancer [86, 87]. Another widely known BEPF to assess the role of UV-induced immunosuppression is the trans to cis isomerization of urocanic acid on photoexposed skin. Cis urocanic acid accumulates in the stratum corneum after multiple exposures to UV, with a reduction in levels occurring only by protection by the use of broad-spectrum sunscreens with UVA and UVB coverage [88, 89]. Maturation of these indices may help address the impact of UV on the skin, over and beyond sunburn into the domain of impending photocarcinogenesis [6, 79, 90].

Radical protection factor (RPF) of a sunscreen is a newer concept and aims to evaluate the ability of a sunscreen to prevent free radical generation in the skin on UVR exposure. The RPF of a sunscreen is a ratio of the time required for the generation of free radicals on unprotected skin versus sunscreen-protected skin [91]. Short acting reactive oxygen species and more long-lived lipid peroxidation photoproducts (LOX) can be generated at UV doses that may not always correlate with the SPF label. Hence, a clear characterization of sun protection through RPF values, stated independently or in relation to the SPF, may be more useful to the consumer and the clinicians while advocating sun protection behaviour for prevention of cancer and of pigmentation in SOC [92].

Simply put, BEFPs reflect selected meaningful biological downstream effects of sun exposure across any part of the solar spectrum and the ability of a sunscreening agent to protect against the same. These may include ingredient-related factors like an ability to reduce lipid peroxidation, photoageing, and elastosis for the UVA spectrum and photocarcinogenesis, singlet oxygen generation, DNA damage in addition to immunosuppression as above, for the UVB spectrum [75]. Newer BEPFs continue to be explored as potential non-invasive biomarkers of sunscreen efficacy in preventing photocarcinogenesis [92, 93]. Further elucidation of BEPFs specific to skin pigmentation would be a welcome step for photoprotection in SOC.

7.8 Environmental Indices Affecting Solar Impact on the Skin

7.8.1 UV Index

To keep the messaging simple and to indicate a way for people to understand the level of sun protection needed related to geographical location and climate conditions, the World Health Organization (WHO) developed the concept of a UV index through the INTERSUN Project, in collaboration with international agencies such as World Meteorological Organization (WMO), United Nations Environment Programme (UNEP), and the International Commission on Non-Ionizing Radiation Protection (ICNIRP) in 1995. The UV index (UVI) represents the biologically effective ambient solar UVR at different geographical points on the earth's surface [94, 95].

The Global Solar UV Index (UVI) is a unitless metric, ranging from 0 to 20. Values of 11 and above are represented as a single category, extreme. Each unit on the index reflects a terrestrial UV radiation of 25 mW/m^2, assuming a Diffey-weighted UV irradiance of 250 mW/m^2 for midday summer sun. The exact energy is slightly variable, subject to ozone levels and a few environmental parameters that affect the terrestrial UV radiation levels [92]. Peak levels of UV radiation occur when the sun is highest in the sky, around midday. For temperate climates, this is most appreciated during the summer months, while a seasonal change is not as evident in the tropics. Further, the UV index in the tropics is mostly in the extreme category, indicating the need for sun protection for vulnerable populations, year round. Comparing the 4 metros of India, except for Delhi, UV indices were above 11 for Mumbai, Kolkata, and Chennai, going up to 13 in the summer months [96]. The UV index is also higher closer to the equator. Clouds may attenuate UV by 50–90%; however, clouds may also increase overall UVR through the scattering principle. Albedo refers to the fraction of radiation that is reflected off a surface. Snow reflects 30–80% of incident UVR, sand and sea foam reflect 15 and 25%, respectively. Water by itself has a lower albedo at 5%. Further, UVR also increases by 10–12% for every 1000 m increase in altitude [94, 97].

With subsequent revisions since its inception, the UVI has evolved to be a harmonized public education tool which can be used easily and effectively to communicate sun protection advice [98]. A few countries have embraced the metric for issuing regional sunscreen guidelines. New Zealand and Australia, in the Sunscreen Summit in 2019, recommended the use of sunscreens on all exposed parts when the UV index exceeded 3 on the scale. For outdoor exposure, additional sun protection measures are to be used alongside sunscreen. The UV index has been shown to correlate with measurement of skin erythema, similar to the SPF values. However, research has shown that suberythmogenic levels of UVR also contribute to cutaneous carcinogenesis, and the impact of these may therefore not be adequately addressed by the UVI. Despite being meant for global use, the adaptation of the UV Index still remains to be fully executed, Figs. 7.3 and 7.4 [99, 100].

EXPOSURE CATEGORY	UVI RANGE
LOW	< 2
MODERATE	3 TO 5
HIGH	6 TO 7
VERY HIGH	8 TO 10
EXTREME	11+

Fig. 7.3 UV radiation exposure categories (Obtained with permission from WHO Global solar UV index: a practical guide [102])

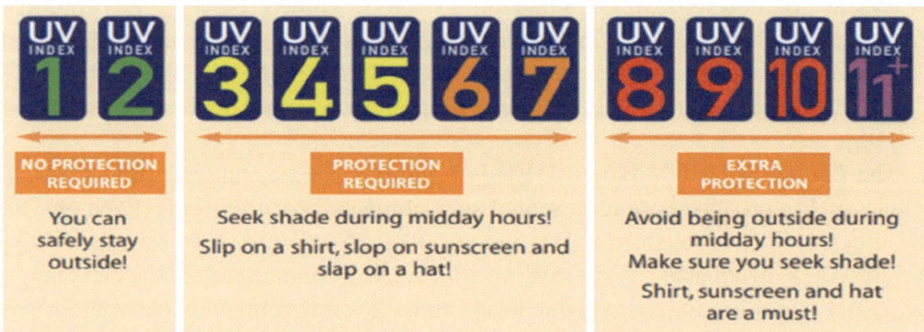
UV INDEX 1
UV INDEX 2
UV INDEX 3
UV INDEX 4
UV INDEX 5
UV INDEX 6
UV INDEX 7
UV INDEX 8
UV INDEX 9
UV INDEX 10
UV INDEX 11+
NO PROTECTION REQUIRED
You can safely stay outside!
PROTECTION REQUIRED
Seek shade during midday hours!
Slip on a shirt, slop on sunscreen and slap on a hat!
EXTRA PROTECTION
Avoid being outside during midday hours!
Make sure you seek shade!
Shirt, sunscreen and hat are a must!

Fig. 7.4 UV Index (UVI) guidance according to the WHO (From Lehmann et al. et al. [103], an open access article distributed under the terms and conditions of the Creative Commons Attribution (CC BY) license (http://creativecommons.org/licenses/by/4.0/) [103])

The quantification of performance by elaborate metrics as above is unique to sunscreens among all personal care products. Over time, current in vivo testing methods which involve some level of human exposure may be replaced by in vitro testing which provides the scope for assessing monochromatic protection factors, which is the quantification of protection across specific domains such as the HEVL and IR [30]. Further efforts towards the harmonization of metrics across countries, and the development of non-invasive testing methodologies such as HDRS, underscore the public health importance of sunscreens.

7.9 Chapter Summary

This chapter traces the evolution of sunscreen testing from SPF factor to the more recent biological effective protection factors (BEPF). Likewise, the progression of refinement of standards used for testing and the testing methodologies to the latest work in progress, sunscreen testing by non-invasive HDRS techniques, are outlined. Regional and national guidelines for sunscreen labelling and testing, water resistance testing protocols, and specific protocols in development such as for visible light, are discussed, allowing the clinician adequate scope to recommend the right level of sun protection across different skin types and use cases. Inclusion of the ITA for subject selection for in vivo sunscreen testing is a welcome step; however, higher skin types are not represented. Ironing out of inconsistencies in sunscreen testing, harmonization of standards, and focused testing for monochromatic protection factors for domains such as VL and IR of interest to SOC are all anticipated in the immediate future.

References

1. González S, Aguilera J, Berman B, Calzavara-Pinton P, Gilaberte Y, Goh CL, et al. Expert recommendations on the evaluation of sunscreen efficacy and the beneficial role of non-filtering ingredients. Front Med (Lausanne). 2022;9:790207.
2. Li L, Chong L, Huang T, Ma Y, Li Y, Ding H. Natural products and extracts from plants as natural UV filters for sunscreens: a review. Animal Model Exp Med [Internet]. 2023 Jun 1 [cited 2024 Mar 3];6(3):183–95. Available from: http://www.ncbi.nlm.nih.gov/pubmed/36536536
3. Bielfeldt S. Performance metrics of sunscreen formulations: in vitro and in vivo techniques. Curr Probl Dermatol [Internet]. 2021 Oct 1 [cited 2024 Mar 20];55:124–32. Available from: https://pubmed.ncbi.nlm.nih.gov/34698029/
4. Young AR, Boles J, Herzog B, Osterwalder U, Baschong W. A sunscreen's labeled sun protection factor may overestimate protection at temperate latitudes: a human in vivo study. J Invest Dermatol [Internet]. 2010 [cited 2024 Mar 11];130(10):2457–62. Available from: https://pubmed.ncbi.nlm.nih.gov/20535128/
5. Gilaberte Y, González S. Update on photoprotection. Actas Dermosifiliogr (Engl Ed). 2010;101(8):659–72.
6. Maier T, Korting HC. Sunscreens—which and what for? Skin Pharmacol Physiol [Internet]. 2005 Nov [cited 2024 Mar 3];18(6):253–62. Available from: https://pubmed.ncbi.nlm.nih.gov/16113595/
7. Ngoc LTN, Bui VKH, Moon JY, Lee YC. In-vitro cytotoxicity and oxidative stress induced by cerium aminoclay and cerium oxide nanoparticles in human skin keratinocyte cells. J Nanosci Nanotechnol [Internet]. 2019 Apr 26 [cited 2024 Mar 20];19(10):6369–75. Available from: https://pubmed.ncbi.nlm.nih.gov/31026963/
8. Diffey BL, Jansen CT, Urbach F, Wulf HC, Morison WL. The standard erythema dose: a new photobiological concept. Photodermatol Photoimmunol Photomed [Internet]. 1997 [cited 2024 Mar 4];13(1–2):64–6. Available from: https://pubmed.ncbi.nlm.nih.gov/9361131/
9. Valbuena Mesa MC, Nova Villanueva JA, Sánchez Vanegas G. Minimal erythema dose: correlation with Fitzpatrick skin type and concordance between methods of erythema assessment in a patient sample in colombia. Actas Dermosifiliogr [Internet]. 2020 Jun [cited 2024 Mar 4];111(5):390–7. Available from: https://pubmed.ncbi.nlm.nih.gov/32408973/
10. Parisi A V., Turnbull DJ, Kimlin MG. Influence of solar UVA on erythemal irradiances. Phys Med Biol [Internet]. 2006 Jun 21 [cited 2024 Mar 3];51(12):3241–9. Available from: https://pubmed.ncbi.nlm.nih.gov/16757874/
11. Sigurgeirsson B, Wulf HC. [Erythemogenic UV rays]. Laeknabladid [Internet]. 2011 [cited 2024 Mar 20];97(7–8):417–20. Available from: https://pubmed.ncbi.nlm.nih.gov/21849709/
12. Morton SK, Harrison SL. Slip, slop, slap, slide, seek and sport: a systematic scoping review of sun protection in sport in Australasia. Curr Oncol [Internet]. 2022 Jan 1 [cited 2024 Mar 20];30(1):401–15. Available from: https://pubmed.ncbi.nlm.nih.gov/36661682/
13. Federal Register:: Sunscreen drug products for over-the-counter human use [Internet]. [cited 2024 Mar 20]. Available from: https://www.federalregister.gov/documents/2019/02/26/2019-03019/sunscreen-drug-products-for-over-the-counter-human-use

14. Labeling and effectiveness testing; sunscreen drug products for over-the-counter human use. [cited 2024 Mar 20]; Available from: http://www.fda.gov/Drugs/
15. CFR—Code of Federal Regulations Title 21.
16. Federal Register:: Amending over-the-counter monograph m020: sunscreen drug products for over-the-counter human use; over the counter monograph proposed order; availability [Internet]. [cited 2024 Mar 20]. Available from: https://www.federalregister.gov/documents/2021/09/27/2021-20780/amending-over-the-counter-monograph-m020-sunscreen-drug-products-for-over-the-counter-human-use-over
17. Hedayat K, Ahmad Nasrollahi S, Firooz A. Quick and brief review: comparison between different in vivo SPF determination methods. J Cosmet Dermatol [Internet]. 2019 Dec 1 [cited 2024 Mar 20];18(6):1617–23. Available from: https://pubmed.ncbi.nlm.nih.gov/30969008/
18. Geisler AN, Austin E, Nguyen J, Hamzavi I, Jagdeo J, Lim HW. Visible light. Part II: photoprotection against visible and ultraviolet light. J Am Acad Dermatol [Internet]. 2021 May 1 [cited 2024 Mar 20];84(5):1233–44. Available from: https://pubmed.ncbi.nlm.nih.gov/33640513/
19. Zou W, Ramanathan R, Urban S, Sinclair C, King K, Tinker R, et al. Sunscreen testing: a critical perspective and future roadmap. TrAC—Trends in Analytical Chemistry [Internet]. 2022 Dec 1 [cited 2024 Mar 20];157:1–19. Available from: https://researchrepository.rmit.edu.au/esploro/outputs/9922155909201341
20. Latha MS, Martis J, Shobha V, Shinde RS, Bangera S, Krishnankutty B, et al. Sunscreening agents: a review. J Clin Aesthet Dermatol [Internet]. 2013 Jan [cited 2024 Mar 20];6(1):16. Available from: https://www.ncbi.nlm.nih.gov/pmc/articles/PMC3543289/
21. Bureau of Indian Standards.
22. Commission Recommendation of 22 September 2006 on the efficacy of sunscreen products and the claims made relating thereto (notified under document number C(2006) 4089) (Text with EEA relevance)—Google Search [Internet]. [cited 2024 Mar 20]. Available from: https://www.google.com/search?q=COMMISSION+RECOMMENDATION+of+22+September+2006+on+the+efficacy+of+sunscreen+products+and+the+claims+made+relating+thereto+(notified+under+document+number+C(2006)+4089)+(Text+with+EEA+relevance)&oq=COMMISSION+RECOMMENDATION+of+22+September+2006+on+the+efficacy+of+sunscreen+products+and+the+claims+made+relating+thereto+(notified+under+document+number+C(2006)+4089)+(Text+with+EEA+relevance)&gs_lcrp=EgZjaHJvbWUyBggAEEUYOdIBCTU5MzNqMGoxNagCALACAA&sourceid=chrome&ie=UTF-8
23. ASEAN 2015 SPF labeling guidelines—Google Search [Internet]. [cited 2024 Mar 21]. Available from: https://www.google.com/search?q=ASEAN+2015+SPF+labeling+guidelines&sca_esv=c27c31a5ed104b1d&ei=RbT7ZYqID7agnesP8K4Q&ved=0ahUKEwjKvtabv4SFAxU2UGcHHXAXBAAQ4dUDCBA&oq=ASEAN+2015+SPF+labeling+guidelines&gs_lp=Egxnd3Mtd2l6LXNlcnAiIkFTRUFOIDIwMTUgU1BGIGxhYmVsaW5nIGd1aWRlbGluZXMyCBAAGIAEGKIEMggQABiABBiiBEi1FlCsCFisCHABeACQAQCYAeI-BoAHiAaoBAzItMbgBDMgBAPgBAfgBApgCAqAC-wGoAgrCAhYQABgDGI8BGOUCGOoCGLQCGIwD2AEBwgIWEC4YAxiPARjlAhjqAhi0AhiMA9gBAZgDFboGBAgBGAqSBwUxLjAuMaAH6wE&sclient=gws-wiz-serp
24. Australian regulatory guidelines for sunscreens ARGS. 2023.
25. Berry EG, Bezecny J, Acton M, Sulmonetti TP, Anderson DM, Beckham HW, et al. Slip versus slop: a head-to-head comparison of UV-protective clothing to sunscreen. Cancers (Basel) [Internet]. 2022 Feb 1 [cited 2024 Mar 3];14(3):542. Available from: https://www.mdpi.com/2072-6694/14/3/542/htm
26. Ma Y, Yoo J. History of sunscreen: an updated view. J Cosmet Dermatol [Internet]. 2021 Apr 1 [cited 2024 Mar 15];20(4):1044–9. Available from: https://pubmed.ncbi.nlm.nih.gov/33583116/
27. Do sunscreens have a role in preventing skin cancer? Drug Ther Bull [Internet]. 2011 Jun [cited 2024 Mar 21];49(6):69–72. Available from: https://pubmed.ncbi.nlm.nih.gov/21632608/

28. Wang SQ, Stanfield JW, Osterwalder U. In vitro assessments of UVA protection by popular sunscreens available in the United States. J Am Acad Dermatol [Internet]. 2008 Dec [cited 2024 Mar 21];59(6):934–42. Available from: https://pubmed.ncbi.nlm.nih.gov/18835064/
29. https://cdnmedia.eurofins.com/apac/media/601375/boots-star.pdf.—Google Search [Internet]. [cited 2024 Mar 21]. Available from: https://www.google.com/search?q=https%3A%2F%2Fcdnmedia.eurofins.com%2Fapac%2Fmedia%2F601375%2Fboots-star.pdf.&sca_esv=652ec1b02583bbe2&ei=acX7ZeDGGfqPseMPzYmcqAg&ved=0ahUKEwign4_Iz4SFAxX6R2wGHc0EB4UQ4dUDCBA&uact=5&oq=https%3A%2F%2Fcdnmedia.eurofins.com%2Fapac%2Fmedia%2F601375%2Fboots-star.pdf.&gs_lp=Egxnd3Mtd2l6LXNlcnAiP2h0dHBzOi8vY2RubWVkaWEuZXVyb2ZpbnMuY29tL2FwYWMvbWVkaWEvNjAxMzc1L2Jvb3RzLXN0YXIucGRmLkgAUABYAHAAeACQAQCYAQCgAQCqAQC4AQPIAQD4AQGYAgCgAgCYAwCSBwCgBwA&sclient=gws-wiz-serp
30. Surber C, Osterwalder U. Challenges in sun protection. Curr Probl Dermatol (Switzerland). 2021;55:1–43.
31. Addor FAS anna, Barcaui CB, Gomes EE, Lupi O, Marçon CR, Miot HA. Sunscreen lotions in the dermatological prescription: review of concepts and controversies. An Bras Dermatol [Internet]. 2022 Mar 1 [cited 2024 Apr 2];97(2):204–22. Available from: https://pubmed.ncbi.nlm.nih.gov/35039207/
32. Hedayat K, Nasrollahi SA, Firooz A, Rastegar H, Dadgarnejad M. Comparison of UVA protection factor measurement protocols. Clin Cosmet Investig Dermatol [Internet]. 2020 [cited 2024 Mar 3];13:351. Available from: https://www.ncbi.nlm.nih.gov/pmc/articles/PMC7244352/
33. Minaberry YS, Svarc FE. Sun protection, progress, myths, and inconsistencies (a proposal for the democratization of ISO 24443). Photochem Photobiol [Internet]. 2024 Jan 1 [cited 2024 Mar 21];100(1):244–53. Available from: https://pubmed.ncbi.nlm.nih.gov/37344925/
34. McCormick PG, Tsuzuki T. In vitro testing of zinc oxide sunscreens. Int J Cosmet Sci [Internet]. 2012 Aug [cited 2024 Mar 21];34(4):291–7. Available from: https://pubmed.ncbi.nlm.nih.gov/22591031/
35. Osterwalder U, Surber C. [Characterization of sun protection performance: Quo vadis?]. Hautarzt [Internet]. 2022 Apr 1 [cited 2024 Mar 21];73(4):276–82. Available from: https://pubmed.ncbi.nlm.nih.gov/35333933/
36. Cosmetics-Sun protection test methods-In vivo determination of sunscreen UVA protection. 2022 [cited 2024 Mar 21]; Available from: www.iso.org
37. Donglikar M, Deore S, Deore S, Deore S. Sunscreens: a review. Pharm J. 2016;8(3):171–9.
38. Couteau C, Chauvet C, Paparis E, Coiffard L. UV filters, ingredients with a recognized anti-inflammatory effect. PLoS One [Internet]. 2012 Dec 20 [cited 2024 Mar 21];7(12). Available from: https://pubmed.ncbi.nlm.nih.gov/23284607/
39. Chou J. Rapid comparison of UVB absorption effectiveness of various sunscreens by UV-Vis spectroscopy. 2017.
40. Egambaram OP, Kesavan Pillai S, Ray SS. Materials science challenges in skin UV protection: a review. Photochem Photobiol [Internet]. 2020 Jul 1 [cited 2024 Mar 3];96(4):779–97. Available from: https://pubmed.ncbi.nlm.nih.gov/31886889/
41. Pelizzo M, Zattra E, Nicolosi P, Peserico A, Garoli D, Alaibac M. In vitro evaluation of sunscreens: an update for the clinicians. ISRN Dermatol. 2012;2012:1–4.
42. Campiche R, Curpen SJ, Lutchmanen-Kolanthan V, Gougeon S, Cherel M, Laurent G, et al. Pigmentation effects of blue light irradiation on skin and how to protect against them. Int J Cosmet Sci [Internet]. 2020 Aug 1 [cited 2024 Mar 4];42(4):399–406. Available from: https://onlinelibrary.wiley.com/doi/full/10.1111/ics.12637

43. Amano K, Xiao K, Wuerger S, Meyer G. A colorimetric comparison of sunless with natural skin tan. PLoS One. 2020;15(12 December):e0233816.
44. Chardon A, Cretois I, Hourseau C. Skin colour typology and suntanning pathways. Int J Cosmet Sci. 1991;13(4):191–208. https://doi.org/10.1111/j.1467-2494.1991.tb00561.x. PMID: 19291061.
45. Del Bino S, Ito S, Sok J, Nakanishi Y, Bastien P, Wakamatsu K, Bernerd F. Chemical analysis of constitutive pigmentation of human epidermis reveals constant eumelanin to pheomelanin ratio. Pigment Cell Melanoma Res. 2015;28(6):707–17. https://doi.org/10.1111/pcmr.12410. Epub 2015 Sep 22. PMID: 26285058.
46. de Rigal J, Abella ML, Giron F, Caisey L, Lefebvre MA. Development and validation of a new Skin Color Chart. Skin Res Technol. 2007;13(1):101–9. https://doi.org/10.1111/j.1600-0846.2007.00223.x. PMID: 17250540.
47. Couteau C, Diarra H, Coiffard L. Effect of the product type, of the amount of applied sunscreen product and the level of protection in the UVB range on the level of protection achieved in the UVA range. Int J Pharm [Internet]. 2016 Mar 16 [cited 2024 Mar 22];500(1–2):210–6. Available from: https://pubmed.ncbi.nlm.nih.gov/26806467/
48. Osterwalder U, Sohn M, Herzog B. Global state of sunscreens. Photodermatol Photoimmunol Photomed [Internet]. 2014 [cited 2024 Mar 22];30(2–3):62–80. Available from: https://pubmed.ncbi.nlm.nih.gov/24734281/
49. Green A, Williams G, Neale R, Hart V, Leslie D, Parsons P, et al. Daily sunscreen application and betacarotene supplementation in prevention of basal-cell and squamous-cell carcinomas of the skin: a randomised controlled trial. Lancet [Internet]. 1999 Aug 28 [cited 2024 Mar 3];354(9180):723–9. Available from: https://pubmed.ncbi.nlm.nih.gov/10475183/
50. Poh Agin P. Measuring ultraviolet A protection in sunscreen products. J Am Acad Dermatol [Internet]. 2017 Sep 1 [cited 2024 Mar 22];77(3):e81. Available from: http://www.jaad.org/article/S0190962217317255/fulltext
51. Moyal D. Need for a well-balanced sunscreen to protect human skin from both Ultraviolet A and Ultraviolet B damage. Indian J Dermatol Venereol Leprol [Internet]. 2012 Jun 1 [cited 2024 Mar 22];78(SUPPL.1):24. Available from: https://ijdvl.com/need-for-a-well-balanced-sunscreen-to-protect-human-skin-from-both-ultraviolet-a-and-ultraviolet-b-damage/
52. Ferrero L, Pissavini M, Doucet O. How a calculated model of sunscreen film geometry can explain in vitro and in vivo SPF variation. Photochem Photobiol Sci [Internet]. 2010 [cited 2024 Mar 22];9(4):540–51. Available from: https://pubmed.ncbi.nlm.nih.gov/20354649/
53. Shim J, Lim JM, Park SG. Machine learning for the prediction of sunscreen sun protection factor and protection grade of UVA. Exp Dermatol [Internet]. 2019 Jul 1 [cited 2024 Mar 22];28(7):872–4. Available from: https://onlinelibrary.wiley.com/doi/full/10.1111/exd.13958
54. Coyne EQ, Lichtman MK, Simons J, Sarkar AK, Rünger TM. In vitro assessment of the broad-spectrum ultraviolet protection of clothing. J Am Acad Dermatol [Internet]. 2018 Aug 1 [cited 2024 Mar 27];79(2):373–5. Available from: https://pubmed.ncbi.nlm.nih.gov/29317283/
55. Sohn M, Herzog B, Osterwalder U, Imanidis G. Calculation of the sun protection factor of sunscreens with different vehicles using measured film thickness distribution—comparison with the SPF in vitro. J Photochem Photobiol B [Internet]. 2016 Jun 1 [cited 2024 Mar 22];159:74–81. Available from: https://pubmed.ncbi.nlm.nih.gov/27045276/
56. Herzog B, Sohn M. The formula for best sunscreen performance: Beer-Lambert's Law under the microscope. Curr Probl Dermatol [Internet]. 2021 Oct 1 [cited 2024 Mar 22];55:133–43. Available from: https://pubmed.ncbi.nlm.nih.gov/34698036/
57. Rohr M, Ernst N, Schrader A. Hybrid diffuse reflectance spectroscopy: non-erythemal in vivo testing of sun protection factor. Skin Pharmacol Physiol [Internet]. 2018 Jun 1 [cited 2024 Mar 22];31(4):220–8. Available from: https://pubmed.ncbi.nlm.nih.gov/29791917/
58. Ruvolo E, Rohr M, Oliveira S, Nogueira L, Carvalho J, Cole C. Multi-laboratory study of hybrid diffuse reflectance spectroscopy to assess sunscreen SPF and UVA-PFs. Photodermatol

Photoimmunol Photomed [Internet]. 2021 Nov 1 [cited 2024 Mar 22];37(6):511–20. Available from: https://pubmed.ncbi.nlm.nih.gov/34060681/
59. Aguilera J, Gracia-Cazaña T, Gilaberte Y. New developments in sunscreens. Photochem Photobiol Sci [Internet]. 2023 Oct 1 [cited 2024 Mar 3];22(10):2473–82. Available from: https://pubmed.ncbi.nlm.nih.gov/37543534/
60. Gasparro FP. Sunscreens, skin photobiology, and skin cancer: the need for UVA protection and evaluation of efficacy. Environ Health Perspect [Internet]. 2000 [cited 2024 Mar 13];108(Suppl 1):71. Available from: https://www.ncbi.nlm.nih.gov/pmc/articles/PMC1637776/
61. Dudley DK, Laughlin SA, Osterwalder U. Spectral homeostasis—The fundamental requirement for an ideal sunscreen. Curr Probl Dermatol [Internet]. 2021 Oct 1 [cited 2024 Mar 23];55:72–92. Available from: https://pubmed.ncbi.nlm.nih.gov/34698022/
62. Ezekwe N, Maghfour J, Kohli I. Visible Light and the Skin. Photochem Photobiol [Internet]. 2022 Nov 1 [cited 2024 Mar 3];98(6):1264–9. Available from: https://onlinelibrary.wiley.com/doi/full/10.1111/php.13634
63. Kohli I, Nahhas AF, Braunberger TL, Chaowattanapanit S, Mohammad TF, Nicholson CL, et al. Spectral characteristics of visible light-induced pigmentation and visible light protection factor. Photodermatol Photoimmunol Photomed [Internet]. 2019 Nov 1 [cited 2024 Mar 3];35(6):393–9. Available from: https://pubmed.ncbi.nlm.nih.gov/31152612/
64. Lim HW, Kohli I, Granger C, Trullàs C, Piquero-Casals J, Narda M, et al. Photoprotection of the skin from visible light–induced pigmentation: current testing methods and proposed harmonization. J Invest Dermatol [Internet]. 2021 Nov 1 [cited 2024 Mar 23];141(11):2569–76. Available from: https://pubmed.ncbi.nlm.nih.gov/34112516/
65. Schalka S, Corrêa M de P, Sawada LY, Canale CC, de Andrade TN. A novel method for evaluating sun visible light protection factor and pigmentation protection factor of sunscreens. Clin Cosmet Investig Dermatol [Internet]. 2019 [cited 2024 Mar 23];12:605–16. Available from: https://pubmed.ncbi.nlm.nih.gov/31695466/
66. Duteil L, Esdaile J, Maubert Y, Cathelineau AC, Bouloc A, Queille-Roussel C, et al. A method to assess the protective efficacy of sunscreens against visible light-induced pigmentation. Photodermatol Photoimmunol Photomed [Internet]. 2017 Sep 1 [cited 2024 Mar 25];33(5):260–6. Available from: https://pubmed.ncbi.nlm.nih.gov/28602025/
67. Ruvolo E, Fair M, Hutson A, Liebel F. Photoprotection against visible light-induced pigmentation. Int J Cosmet Sci [Internet]. 2018 Dec 1 [cited 2024 Mar 25];40(6):589–95. Available from: https://pubmed.ncbi.nlm.nih.gov/30428143/
68. Duteil L, Cadars B, Queille-Roussel C, Giraud I, Drulhon F, Graizeau C, et al. A new in vitro method to predict in vivo photoprotection of skin hyperpigmentation induced by visible light. J Eur Acad Dermatol Venereol [Internet]. 2022 Jun 1 [cited 2024 Mar 25];36(6):922–6. Available from: https://pubmed.ncbi.nlm.nih.gov/35224781/
69. Le Digabel J, Filiol J, Lauze C, Redoulès D, Josse G. In vivo method for evaluating sunscreen protection against high-energy visible light. J Eur Acad Dermatol Venereol [Internet]. 2023 Oct 1 [cited 2024 Mar 14];37 Suppl 6(S6):6–11. Available from: https://pubmed.ncbi.nlm.nih.gov/37671998/
70. Pissavini M, Alard V, Heinrich U, Jenni K, Perier V, Tournier V, et al. In vitro assessment of water resistance of sun care products: a reproducible and optimized in vitro test method. Int J Cosmet Sci [Internet]. 2007 Dec [cited 2024 Mar 25];29(6):451–60. Available from: https://www.researchgate.net/publication/5361860_In_vitro_assessment_of_water_resistance_of_sun_care_products_A_reproducible_and_optimized_in_vitro_test_method
71. Saxe JK, Mullins L, Jones R, Lewis A, Sun F, Reynertson KA. Influence of sunscreen formulation on the transfer of mineral and organic ultraviolet filters from skin to seawater in simulated ocean bathing tests. Int J Cosmet Sci [Internet]. 2023 Oct 1 [cited 2024 Mar 25];45(S1):84–92. Available from: https://onlinelibrary.wiley.com/doi/full/10.1111/ics.12901

72. Shyr T, Ou-Yang H. Sunscreen formulations may serve as additional water barrier on skin surface: a clinical assessment. Int J Cosmet Sci [Internet]. 2016 Apr 1 [cited 2024 Mar 25];38(2):164–9. Available from: https://pubmed.ncbi.nlm.nih.gov/26309044/
73. Solano F. Photoprotection and skin pigmentation: melanin-related molecules and some other new agents obtained from natural sources. Molecules [Internet]. 2020 [cited 2024 Mar 2];25(7). Available from: https://pubmed.ncbi.nlm.nih.gov/32230973/
74. Bernerd F, Marionnet C, Duval C. Solar ultraviolet radiation induces biological alterations in human skin in vitro: relevance of a well-balanced UVA/UVB protection. Indian J Dermatol Venereol Leprol [Internet]. 2012 Jan 1 [cited 2024 Mar 25];78(SUPPL.1):15–23. Available from: https://www.researchgate.net/publication/227706545_Solar_ultraviolet_radiation_induces_biological_alterations_in_human_skin_in_vitro_Relevance_of_a_well-balanced_UVAUVB_protection
75. de la Coba F, Aguilera J, Korbee N, de Gálvez MV, Herrera-Ceballos E, Álvarez-Gómez F, et al. UVA and UVB photoprotective capabilities of topical formulations containing mycosporine-like amino acids (MAAs) through different biological effective protection factors (BEPFs). Mar Drugs [Internet]. 2019 Jan 14 [cited 2024 Mar 25];17(1). Available from: https://pubmed.ncbi.nlm.nih.gov/30646557/
76. Kelly DA, Seed PT, Young AR, Walker SL. A commercial sunscreen's protection against ultraviolet radiation-induced immunosuppression is more than 50% lower than protection against sunburn in humans. J Invest Dermatol [Internet]. 2003 [cited 2024 Mar 25];120(1):1–7. Available from: https://pubmed.ncbi.nlm.nih.gov/12535199/
77. Fourtanier A, Moyal D, Maccario J, Compan D, Wolf P, Quehenberger F, et al. Measurement of sunscreen immune protection factors in humans: a consensus paper. J Invest Dermatol. 2005;125(3):403–9.
78. Cooper KD, Baron ED, Matsui MS. Implications of UV-induced inflammation and immunomodulation. Cutis [Internet]. 2003 Sep 1 [cited 2024 Mar 25];72(3 Suppl):11–6. Available from: https://pubmed.ncbi.nlm.nih.gov/14533825/
79. Al-Jamal MS, Griffith JL, Lim HW. Photoprotection in ethnic skin. Dermatol Sin. 2014;32(4):217–24.
80. Measurement of in vivo sunscreen immune protection factors in humans—PubMed [Internet]. [cited 2024 Mar 25]. Available from: https://pubmed.ncbi.nlm.nih.gov/10628302/
81. Damian DL, Matthews YJ, Phan TA, Halliday GM. An action spectrum for ultraviolet radiation-induced immunosuppression in humans. Br J Dermatol [Internet]. 2011 Mar [cited 2024 Mar 25];164(3):657–9. Available from: https://pubmed.ncbi.nlm.nih.gov/21375518/
82. Moyal DD, Fourtanier AM. Broad-spectrum sunscreens provide better protection from solar ultraviolet-simulated radiation and natural sunlight-induced immunosuppression in human beings. J Am Acad Dermatol [Internet]. 2008 May [cited 2024 Mar 11];58(5 Suppl 2). Available from: https://pubmed.ncbi.nlm.nih.gov/18410801/
83. Damian DL, Halliday GM, Barnetson RSC. Broad-spectrum sunscreens provide greater protection against ultraviolet-radiation-induced suppression of contact hypersensitivity to a recall antigen in humans. J Invest Dermatol [Internet]. 1997 [cited 2024 Mar 26];109(2):146–51. Available from: https://pubmed.ncbi.nlm.nih.gov/9242499/
84. Methods used to evaluate the immune protection factor of a sunscreen: advantages and disadvantages of different in vivo techniques—PubMed [Internet]. [cited 2024 Mar 25]. Available from: https://pubmed.ncbi.nlm.nih.gov/15603218/
85. Schuch AP, Lago JC, Yagura T, Menck CFM. DNA dosimetry assessment for sunscreen genotoxic photoprotection. PLoS One [Internet]. 2012 Jun 29 [cited 2024 Mar 3];7(6). Available from: https://pubmed.ncbi.nlm.nih.gov/22768281/
86. Young AR, Sheehan JM, Chadwick CA, Potten CS. Protection by ultraviolet A and B sunscreens against in situ dipyrimidine photolesions in human epidermis is comparable to protection against sunburn. J Invest Dermatol [Internet]. 2000 [cited 2024 Mar 25];115(1):37–41. Available from: https://pubmed.ncbi.nlm.nih.gov/10886505/

87. Young AR, Greenaway J, Harrison GI, Lawrence KP, Sarkany R, Douki T, et al. Sub-optimal application of a high SPF sunscreen prevents epidermal DNA damage in vivo. Acta Derm Venereol [Internet]. 2018 [cited 2024 Mar 25];98(9):880–7. Available from: https://pubmed.ncbi.nlm.nih.gov/29944164/
88. Van Der Molen RG, Out-Luiting C, Driller H, Claas FHJ, Koerten HK, Mommaas AM. Broad-spectrum sunscreens offer protection against urocanic acid photoisomerization by artificial ultraviolet radiation in human skin. J Invest Dermatol [Internet]. 2000 [cited 2024 Mar 25];115(3):421–6. Available from: https://pubmed.ncbi.nlm.nih.gov/10951278/
89. Krien PM, Moyal D. Sunscreens with broad-spectrum absorption decrease the trans to cis photoisomerization of urocanic acid in the human stratum corneum after multiple UV light exposures. Photochem Photobiol [Internet]. 1994 [cited 2024 Mar 25];60(3):280–7. Available from: https://pubmed.ncbi.nlm.nih.gov/7972382/
90. Young AR. The adverse consequences of not using sunscreens. Int J Cosmet Sci [Internet]. 2023 Oct 1 [cited 2024 Mar 11];45 Suppl 1(S1):11–9. Available from: https://pubmed.ncbi.nlm.nih.gov/37799076/
91. Herrling T, Jung K, Fuchs J. Measurements of UV-generated free radicals/reactive oxygen species (ROS) in skin. Spectrochim Acta A Mol Biomol Spectrosc [Internet]. 2006 Mar 13 [cited 2024 Mar 3];63(4):840–5. Available from: https://pubmed.ncbi.nlm.nih.gov/16543118/
92. Zastrow L, Meinke MC, Albrecht S, Patzelt A, Lademann J. From UV protection to protection in the whole spectral range of the solar radiation: new aspects of sunscreen development. Adv Exp Med Biol [Internet]. 2017 [cited 2024 Mar 3];996:311–8. Available from: https://pubmed.ncbi.nlm.nih.gov/29124711/
93. Keurentjes AJ, Jakasa I, John SM, Ulrich C, Bekkenk MW, Rustemeyer T, et al. Tape stripping the stratum corneum for biomarkers of ultraviolet radiation exposure at sub-erythemal dosages: a study in human volunteers. Biomarkers [Internet]. 2020 [cited 2024 Mar 25];25(6):490–7. Available from: https://pubmed.ncbi.nlm.nih.gov/32657162/
94. Global Solar UV Index—a practical guide [Internet]. [cited 2024 Mar 25]. Available from: https://www.who.int/publications/i/item/9241590076
95. Ultraviolet index—Wikipedia [Internet]. [cited 2024 Mar 26]. Available from: https://en.wikipedia.org/wiki/Ultraviolet_index
96. Bera B, Bhattacharjee S, Shit PK, Sengupta N, Saha S. Variation and correlation between ultraviolet index and tropospheric ozone during COVID-19 lockdown over megacities of India. Stochastic Environmental Research and Risk Assessment [Internet]. 2022 Feb 1 [cited 2024 Mar 26];36(2):409. Available from: https://www.ncbi.nlm.nih.gov/pmc/articles/PMC8164408/
97. Matts PJ, Nash JF. Sunscreens—another endangered species? Int J Cosmet Sci [Internet]. 2023 Oct 1 [cited 2024 Mar 3];45 Suppl 1(S1):20–32. Available from: https://pubmed.ncbi.nlm.nih.gov/37799079/
98. Gies P, Van Deventer E, Green AC, Sinclair C, Tinker R. Review of the Global Solar UV Index 2015 workshop report. Health Phys [Internet]. 2018 Jan 1 [cited 2024 Mar 26];114(1):84. Available from: https://www.ncbi.nlm.nih.gov/pmc/articles/PMC5728586/
99. Italia N, Rehfuess EA. Is the Global Solar UV Index an effective instrument for promoting sun protection? A systematic review. Health Educ Res [Internet]. 2012 Apr [cited 2024 Mar 26];27(2):200–13. Available from: https://www.ncbi.nlm.nih.gov/books/NBK109305/
100. Whiteman DC, Neale RE, Aitken J, Gordon L, Green AC, Janda M, et al. When to apply sunscreen: a consensus statement for Australia and New Zealand. Aust N Z J Public Health [Internet]. 2019 Apr 1 [cited 2024 Mar 26];43(2):171–5. Available from: https://pubmed.ncbi.nlm.nih.gov/30681231/
101. Ly BCK, Dyer EB, Feig JL, Chien AL, Del Bino S. Research techniques made simple: cutaneous colorimetry: a reliable technique for objective skin color measurement. J Invest Dermatol [Internet]. 2020 Jan 1 [cited 2024 Mar 2];140(1):3–12.e1. Available from: https://www.researchgate.net/publication/338303610_Research_Techniques_Made_Simple_Cutaneous_Colorimetry_A_Reliable_Technique_for_Objective_Skin_Color_Measurement

102. Global Solar UV Index: a practical guide." World Health Organization—Google Search [Internet]. [cited 2024 Apr 8]. Available from: https://www.google.com/search?q=Global+Solar+UV+Index%3A+A+Practical+Guide.%2C%E2%80%9D+World+Health+Organization&oq=GLOBAL+SOLAR+UV+INDEX&gs_lcrp=EgZjaHJvbWUqBggCEEUYO-zIHCAAQABiABDIGCAEQRRhAMgYIAhBFGDsyBggDEEUYOzINCAQQABiGAxiABBiKBTINCAUQABiGAxiABBiKBTINCAYQABiGAxiABBiKBTINCAcQABiGAxiA-BBiKBdIBCDIzODBqMGo3qAIIsAIB&sourceid=chrome&ie=UTF-8

103. Lehmann M, Pfahlberg AB, Sandmann H, Uter W, Gefeller O. public health messages associated with low UV index values need reconsideration. Int J Environ Res Public Health [Internet]. 2019 Jun 1 [cited 2024 Apr 8];16(12). Available from: https://www.ncbi.nlm.nih.gov/pmc/articles/PMC6617134/

104. Polonini HC, Lopes RS, Beatriz A, Gomes RS, Silva AO, De Lima R V., et al. Synthesis and evaluation of octocrylene-inspired compounds for UV-filter activity. Quim Nova [Internet]. 2014 [cited 2024 Apr 8];37(6):1004–9. Available from: https://www.researchgate.net/publication/272908525_Synthesis_and_evaluation_of_octocrylene-inspired_compounds_for_UV-filter_activity

Chapter 8
Topical Sunscreening Agents

Abbreviations

AL-PDA	Polydopamine grafted lignin
ASEAN	Association of Southeast Asian Nations
BDBP	Bis-(diethylaminohydroxybenzoyl benzoyl)
BEMT	Bis-ethylhexyloxyphenol methoxyphenyl triazine
BEPF	Biological effective protection factors
BMDM	Butylmethoxy dibenzoylmethane
BMI	Body mass index
BP-3	Benzophenone-3
BP-4	Benzophenone-4
BP-8	Benzophenone-8
CDC	Centres for Disease Control and Prevention
CHF	Contact hypersensitivity factor
CNS	Central nervous system
COLIPA	European Cosmetic and Perfumery Association
CPD	Cyclobutane pyrimidine dimers
DBT	Diethylhexyl butamido triazone
DHHB	Diethylamino hydroxybenzoyl hexyl benzoate
DHICA	5,6-dihydroxyindole-2-carboxylic acid
DPDT	Disodium phenyl dibenzimidazole tetrasulfonate
DRT	Drometrizole trisiloxane
ECM	Extracellular matrix
EGCG	epigallocatechin-3-gallate
EHS	Ethylhexyl Salicylate
EHT	Ethylhexyl triazone
EU	European union
FDA	Food and Drug Administration
GI	Gastrointestinal
GRAS	Generally recognized as safe
GRASE	Generally Recognized As Safe and Effective.

R. Rajan, *Sunscreens for Skin of Color*,
https://doi.org/10.1007/978-981-97-3195-4_8

HEVL	High energy visible light
HIF	Human immunoprotection factor
HS	Homosalate
IARC	International Agency for Research on Cancer
INCI	International Nomenclature Cosmetic Ingredient
ISO	International Organization for Standardization
IVPT	In vitro permeation test
MAA	Mycosporine-like amino acids
MBBT	Methylene bis-benzotriazolyl tetramethylbutylphenol
MCE	Methoxypropylamino Cyclohexenylidene Ethoxyethylcyanoacetate
MMP	Matrix metalloproteinases
MUsT	Maximum usage trial
NDA	New drug application
NIR	Near-infrared light
NSAID	Non-steroidal anti-inflammatory drugs
OCR	Octocrylene
OD- PABA	Octyl dimethyl PABA
OMC	Octyl methoxycinnamate
OTC	Over the counter
PABA	Para-amino benzoic acid
PBSA	Phenylbenzimidazole sulfonic acid
PCOS	Polycystic ovary syndrome
PEG 25 PABA	Polyethylene glycol 25 p-aminobenzoic acid
PMLE	Polymorphous light eruption
PMMA	Polymethyl methacrylate
PPAR	Peroxisome proliferator-activated receptors
ROS	Reactive oxygen species
RPF	Radical protection factor
SCCS	Scientific Committee on Consumer Safety
SLE	Systemic lupus erythematosus
SLN	Solid lipid nanoparticles
SPF	Sun protection factor
TBT	Tris biphenyl triazine
TDSA	Terephthalylidene dicamphor sulfonic acid
TDSA	Terephthalylidene dicamphor sulfonic acid
TEA salicylate	Triethanolamine salicylate
TiO2	Titanium dioxide
US FDA	United States Food and Drug Administration
USA	United States of America
USAN	United States Adopted Names
UV	Ultraviolet
UVA	Ultraviolet-A
UVB	Ultraviolet-B
UVR	Ultraviolet radiation

VOC	Volatile organic compounds
VS	Visible light
ZnO	Zinc oxide
2 -EMC	2-ethoxy ethyl 4-methoxycinnamate
4 MBC	4-Methylbenzylidene camphor
6–4PP	Pyrimidine-pyrimidone 4,6 photoproducts
8OHdG	8-hydroxy-2-deoxyguanosine

Key Objectives

- UV filters in topical sunscreens have undergone rapid advancements in the last few years, from development of new filters to strict regulation of older ones.
- The specific spectrum of each filter, regional regulations, safety and performance attributes, impact on human and environmental health have been succinctly listed in a biodata format to provide the reader a quick understanding of the sunscreen filter.
- Information on sensitization potential, interaction with other filters in a finished formulation, and the endocrine disruption properties of each filter helps the clinician to provide informed choices when counselling a patient on the use of sunscreen.

According to the Sunscreen Innovation Act in the United States of America (USA), a 'sunscreen active ingredient' refers to an active ingredient that is intended for application to the skin of humans for purposes of absorbing, reflecting, or scattering ultraviolet radiation (UVR). In Europe, an ultraviolet (UV) filter is defined as a substance intended to protect the skin against UV radiation by absorbing, reflecting, or scattering the incident UVR [1]. UV filters are broadly classified as chemical, or organic, which work by absorbing UV energy, and as mineral or inorganic or particulate filters which protect by reflecting or scattering incident UV. More recently, the classification has evolved to now be organic, organic particulate, polymers, and inorganic particulate filters [2].

In referring to sunscreens, United States Adopted Names (USAN) have been used throughout this book, for the sake of brevity and clarity. USAN is a nonproprietary name for an entity, provided by the USAN Council ensuring safety, consistency, and logic in nomenclature of drugs. Compared to using International Nomenclature Cosmetic Ingredient (INCI) names, USAN names have the advantage of being relatively simple, and therefore as easy to use among experts as among the public. They are also more specific compared to the trade names. In the individual sections, the trade names and the INCI have been used where needed, for relevance and context [3, 4].

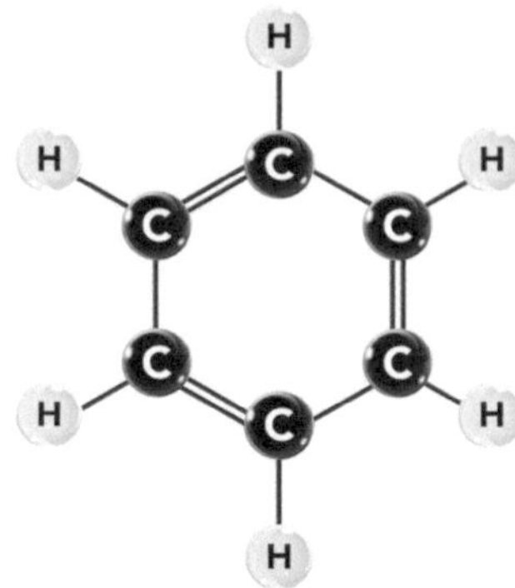

Fig. 8.1 Structure of benzene(C6H6) ring

Benzene Detection in Personal Care Products, Fig. 8.1

In 2021, Valisure LLC registered a Citizen's Petition with the United States Food and Drug Administration (US FDA) about the presence of benzene in some of the commercially available sunscreens, exceeding the conditional FDA restriction of 2 ppm [5]. This prompted the FDA to issue a formal alert to manufacturing companies on the risk of benzene contamination and the need for stringent testing. This was also followed by a number of product recalls—not just of sunscreens, but also of hand sanitizers, deodorants, hand, and foot care products between April 2021 and April 2022 [6].

Benzene is a known human carcinogen and may be present in products as a contaminant, as it is not meant to be added intentionally. Exposure to benzene occurs mainly via two routes—inhalation and skin contact. Environmental exposures occur from sources of indoor air pollution such as glues, paints, furniture coatings, detergents, cigarette smoke, fireplaces, furnaces and from vehicles parked in indoor garages [7]. Potential sources of benzene contamination in a finished product are aerosol propellants used in spray type products, fragrances, and/or in formulation stabilising agents [6, 8]. Processes such as packaging, storage, heating, irradiation, and sources such as water may all contribute to the presence of benzene in personal care products [7].

Pal et al. evaluated 50 commercial sunscreens available in the USA and found the presence of three volatile organic compounds (VOCs), benzene, toluene, and styrene in 80, 92, and 58%, respectively, of the samples tested. Notably, extrapolating from the level of detection, 44% of children's sunscreens and 38% of sunscreens meant for adults, yielded a lifetime cancer risk, exceeding the acceptable benchmark level of 1.0×10^{-6}, or 1 ppm (part per million) [9]. The research group compared the exposure to these three VOCs in hand sanitizers and observed the presence of benzene, toluene, and styrene in 31, 25, and 32% of 200 samples. The lifetime cancer risk from exposure was noted to exceed benchmark levels, similar to the observations in sunscreens [10]. Propellants in aerosol sunscreens are also likely to contribute to higher emissions of volatile organic compounds (VOC) such as benzene, toluene, ethylbenzene, o-xylene, and p-xylene. Ethanol obtained from fossil fuels is considered a source of VOCs in these sunscreen aerosols as are certain sunscreen filters like homosalate and ethyl hexyl salicylate, and volatile silicones used to enhance skin feel in sunscreens [8]. Yeoman et al. quantified that a toddler might inhale up to 10 mg of ethanol from one facial application of sunscreens, while adults may be exposed to 26–30 mg of ethanol with each application of sunscreen on the face. The group characterized the VOCs emitted from cream and lotion sunscreen products to contain contaminants at a concentration of 0.0119% for toluene, 0.0006% for benzene, and 0.0018% for ethylbenzene per total product weight and noted that this was higher than VOCs emitted from facial moisturizers. This could be due to the fact that the usage volume of sunscreens is higher than that for face moisturizers [8].

The most recent evaluation by Valisure highlighted the detection of benzene in chemical sunscreen sprays in excess of the 2 ppm threshold, more commonly as compared to the lotion formulations. Aerosol propellants used in sprays may be considered a possible point of contamination; however, this was not the case for mineral sunscreen sprays. After sun care products were also found to contain benzene at levels over the above threshold. This evaluation included crowdsourced samples as well, to the tune of 400 samples, highlighting the high public interest in the matter [6, 11].

8.1 Physical Sunscreens

The last few years have seen a sudden increase in the popularity of mineral filters [12, 13]. This almost viral awareness, triggered by the sunscreen ban in Hawaii, and amplified by the detection of benzene in certain sunscreens, and studies reporting the finding of sunscreen ingredients in the human bloodstream above permissible levels of safety, created a perception of safety around inorganic sunscreen filters [5, 14]. Also, the megatrend for natural products further catapulted the popularity of these mineral or 'physical' sunscreens as safer and more natural than 'chemical' sunscreens [15, 16]. The two approved inorganic filters in use today are zinc oxide and titanium dioxide.

Though traditionally considered to protect from sun on the principle of reflection, recent studies suggest that even inorganic filters use energy absorption as an important mechanism for photoprotection. Within the long UVA spectrum and the visible light (VL) zone, both the inorganic filters work by reflecting light up to 60%, acting as micromirrors, and can be said to be nonabsorbing. However, when the entire breadth of the UV spectrum is considered, the reflection component falls to only 4–5%. The rest of the means of photoprotection is attributable to the semiconductor band gap driven absorbance of energy. With lowered size of filters through micronization, the reflectance mechanism is reduced furthermore [17, 18].

Zinc oxide and titanium dioxide are the only UV filters that are Food and Drug Administration (FDA) approved as Generally Recognized As Safe and Effective (GRASE) I. Once considered inelegant for the white cast or the Kabuki mask appearance on using these filters, the production and consumption of sunscreens based on these filters has increased dramatically in recent years, due to reasons cited above. When used as such, the size of the particle ranges from 200 to 400 nm for zinc oxide and from 150 to 300 nm for titanium dioxide. At this size, the visual perception of reflected light makes these sunscreens appear as white or grey, which is not preferred by users [13, 19]. Both the mineral filters are available as nanoparticles as well, where the particle size is 100 nanometers or less, and in this form, are considered more acceptable cosmetically [16, 19]. At this nanosize, the visibility of the particles on the skin is lesser, making the sunscreen more cosmetically acceptable. But, with nanominerals, absorption is a large component of the photoprotection mechanism, such that the inorganic filters behave similar to chemical UV filters.

Zinc and titanium nanoparticles exist in three physical forms—primary particles, aggregates, and agglomerates. The smallest of the three, primary particles are around 5–20 nm in size. In formulation as a suspension, these particles aggregate to form 30 to 150 nm sized particles, in which form they are present in sunscreens. Larger agglomerates are formed when the aggregates bind together in clumps of sizes 1 micron or larger. Prolonged homogenization and stabilization during the manufacturing process ensures that these clumps are broken down to aggregates in the final formulation [19–21]. The aggregation may also be impacted by other formulation factors such as pH, zeta potential, and ionic strength, and the sufficient addition of chelators, Fig. 8.2.

Inorganic mineral filters are not known to be absorbed into the skin in any significant amount [22]. This lack of interaction with any of the components of the living epidermis—Langerhans cells, keratinocytes, and melanocytes—accounts for the extremely low, practically nonexistent possibility of allergic contact dermatitis with mineral filters. This advantage of inertness may be lost in the case of nanosized particles, with potential penetration of metal ions into the hair follicle openings, and eventual rendezvous with epidermal cells, however, the practical implication of this scenario is not clear as of now [22, 23]. Zinc oxide provides broad-spectrum coverage, while titanium is more effective in the UVB spectrum, and has a higher <E11> compared to zinc. Both the minerals have protective effects against visible light, but only in the non-nano, pigmentary grade and not in the nano-form [24]. Mineral sunscreens are effective right after application, but a settling time of about 15 min may allow the product to form a better film on the skin's surface [16].

The section below details the two mineral sunscreens, and a brief description of a potential new addition to the inorganic filter range, cerium oxide.

8.1.1 Zinc Oxide

Zinc oxide is widely available as a UV filter world over and is one of the only two inorganic filters currently approved for use in sunscreens, the other being titanium Table 8.1, Fig. 8.3. It is a photostable filter with a broad-spectrum coverage, across

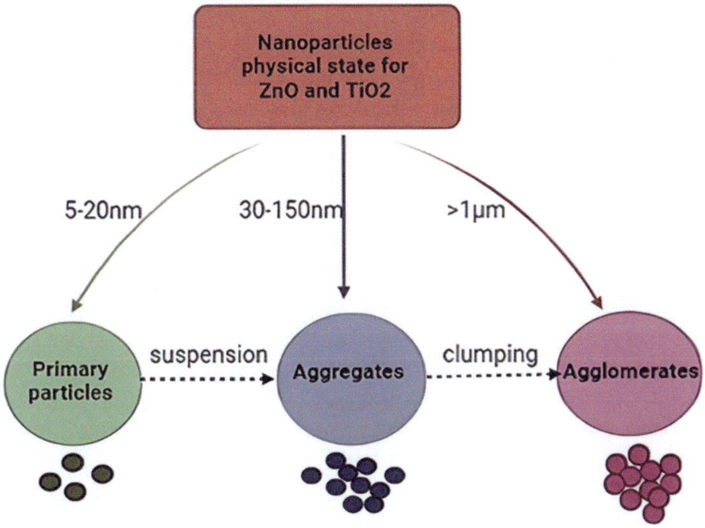

Fig. 8.2 Zinc and titanium nanoparticles may occur in different forms, as primary particles, aggregates and agglomerates and are classified according to their size and physical properties. Obtained from Mascarenhas-Melo et al., Inorganic nanoparticles in dermopharmaceutical and cosmetic products: Properties, formulation development, toxicity, and regulatory issues. (Image obtained from open access article distributed under the terms of the Creative Commons CC-BY licence https://creativecommons.org/licenses/by/4.0/ [19])

Table 8.1 Profile snapshot of zinc oxide UV filter

Zinc Oxide (ZnO), Fig. 8.3	
Approval status	Approved in the USA as GRASE I, European union (EU), Japan, Australia, Association of Southeast Asian Nations (ASEAN) [25]
Mechanism of photoprotection	Reflect, absorb, and deflect UV photons [26, 27].
Maximum concentration in a sunscreen	Up to 25% in the USA and EU, no upper limit in Australia and Japan [28] [29] [30].
Spectrum	UVB, UVA2, UVA1 HEVL (non-nano, pigment grade) [24, 25]
Systemic absorption	Zinc oxide is not known to penetrate into the viable epidermis [31].
Safety in pregnancy	Considered safe [30]
Ecological concerns	Potential aquatic toxicity, nanozinc has been known to be associated with coral bleaching [12, 13]
Endocrine disruptor potential	Not known to possess endocrine disruption potential [32]
Sensitization potential	Not known to sensitize skin [26]
Photostability	Photostable [33]
Areas of concern	Aquatic toxicity of nanoparticles, skin dryness, white cast

Fig. 8.3 Chemical structure of zinc oxide

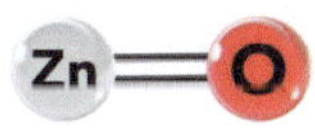

both the UVA and the UVB regions of solar radiation [13, 26]. Its position as the second most abundant trace mineral in the human body, added to the widespread and safe long-term use of topical zinc for several dermatological conditions [16, 34], the safety of oral zinc supplements, give zinc oxide its easy familiarity—both to the physician and to the sunscreen user. The US FDA notes this long history of usage of zinc mineral in multiple skin care and dermatology products in its approval of zinc as GRASE certified. In its natural state, zinc occurs in one of two forms—wurtzite and zincblende. Wurtzite is the form that is used in sunscreens and has an optical refractive index of 2.3–2.0 in the visible light zone (or from 375 to 900 nm), and therefore gives a lesser white cast compared to titanium dioxide in formulations [26].

The inorganic filter is available in nano and non-nano sizes either as an uncoated powder or with specialized coatings to reduce the reactivity of the mineral. The coated zinc oxide may either be a powder or an emulsion, the latter allowing ready incorporation of the filter into the formulation. Zinc oxide is permitted in sunscreens at a concentration of up to 25% in the USA and the EU and can be used in higher levels without a defined upper limit in Japan and Australia [26, 29]. The need for a higher concentration may be due to the lower <E11> of zinc, despite its broad-spectrum action [35]. Despite such higher concentrations in sunscreens, zinc does not get absorbed systemically due to its lack of solubility in aqueous media and in biological fluids at a neutral pH. At both nano and non-nano sizes, zinc is not expected to penetrate deeper than the nonviable layers of the human epidermis and is thought to simply stay on the skin's surface extending into the superficial skin furrows and along the hair follicle. Any deeper penetration of the filter into the dermis results in its dissociation into zinc and oxygen atoms [26]. Furthermore, skin naturally contains zinc at a concentration of 60 μg/g in the epidermis and at 40 μg/g in the upper dermis [34]. Inbuilt mechanisms to maintain homeostasis, the lack of any significant absorption into the viable layers of the skin, broader spectrum of coverage compared to titanium, and being one of the just two FDA GRASE I approved sunscreen filters have made zinc oxide a popular filter. Zinc is not known to cause any photoallergic or photoirritant reactions on human skin [26].

Topical zinc oxide in sunscreen formulations may offer potential benefit as an anti-acne sunscreen. This is due to the antibacterial, antifungal, and anti-inflammatory properties of zinc, with an ability to reduce the population of *Cutibacterium acnes* by inhibiting microbial lipases. Furthermore, zinc regulates sebum by exerting an antiandrogenic effect [36, 37]. While this may prove advantageous to those with oily, acne prone skin types, inherently, zinc oxide does not offer significant moisturizing benefits in a sunscreen [19]. Additional moisturization may be necessary.

In the non-nano particle sizes, between 200 and 400 nm, zinc oxide can leave a distinct, unappealing white cast. With micronization of the filter to achieve a smaller size, typically a particle size of <100 nm, the aesthetics of this filter improves remarkably. With the decrease in size, comes an increase in the total surface area, which leads to a potential increase in the reactivity of zinc in the environment. Also at lower particle sizes, the mechanism of photoprotection moves from being predominantly reflective and scattering to absorption, much like a chemical filter. Coating with silica and similar inert materials reduces photocatalysis on UV exposure and mitigates free radical generation [12]. As both nano and non-nano versions of zinc oxide are not expected to penetrate into the viable epidermis either form may be considered safe for human use. Zinc does not experience a reduction in UVA coverage with micronization to a smaller size, a change which is noted with the other mineral filter, titanium [13, 26, 36]. In particular, zinc has very good UV attenuation properties in the UVA spectrum, capable of providing protection in the band >360 nm. When combined with titanium dioxide (TiO_2) to overcome the disadvantages of nanonization, zinc oxide (ZnO) was shown to completely protect against the induction of DNA damage as indicated by cyclobutane pyrimidine dimers (CPD) and p53 markers [16].

UVR is able to produce dissociation of zinc oxide generating Zn2+ ions, which are then capable of inducing reactive oxygen species with some level of cytotoxicity to the human epidermal keratinocytes, demonstrated in cellular studies. However, the magnitude of such change is expected to be small and to be quenched by the skin's antioxidants [13, 26].

Animal studies show that the use of zinc metal oxide sunscreens is safe in pregnancy [13]. Considering lack of significant absorption, and the historical safety, zinc sunscreens may be considered safe and effective for preventing pregnancy-induced pigmentary conditions in SOC, typically melasma [30].

While physiologically safe for human use, zinc nanoparticles have been studied to cause some level of environmental impact, especially in its nanoform. Zinc oxide was shown to cause more significant coral bleaching as compared to titanium. Overall, though, the reactivity of titanium nanoparticles was found to be ten times that of zinc nanoparticles in an experiment to assess the photoreactive generation of free radicals from either filter, using methylene blue in water [13]. Zinc nanoparticles, along with nanotitanium particles contribute to over 90% of all engineered nanomaterials in personal care products. In 2014, the sunscreen use in the USA was estimated to be 90,000 metric tons per year, which included engineered nanomaterials at 2300–2700 metric tons per year. If anything, mineral sunscreen use has only increased over the last decade, implying that more nano-materials are being released into the environment [38].

Recently, the effect of combining zinc oxide with avobenzone, as representative of chemical filters, showed that the combination was not synergistic both for nano and microsized zinc particles [39]. Except in a few instances, zinc does not appear to benefit from combining with most other filters, though such addition extends broad-spectrum coverage [21, 40].

Zinc sunscreens have some inherent handicaps when undergoing in vitro tests for sun protection factor (SPF). This is because of the nonuniformity of the sunscreen film on the polymethyl methacrylate (PMMA) plates, especially at higher concentrations of the mineral filter. Consequently, in vitro SPF testing produces lower values compared to in vivo testing. To some extent, this may be managed with the higher density of 1.3 mg/cm^2 in the International Organization for Standardization (ISO) standards compared to the 0.75 mg/cm^2 in the earlier

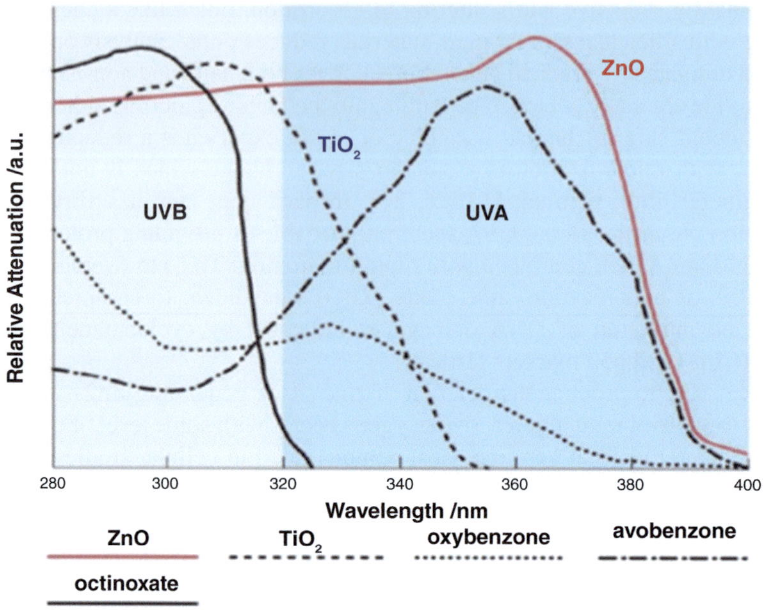

Fig. 8.4 Image illustrating the relative attenuation spectra of the UVB/UVA radiation by oxybenzone, octinoxate, avobenzone (Parsol 1789), zinc oxide, and (anatase) titanium dioxide reproduced from a social media forum [43]

European Cosmetic and Perfumery Association (COLIPA) methods. Both these methods, though, have not been validated for higher concentrations of mineral sunscreens [41, 42], Fig. 8.4 [43].

8.1.2 Titanium Dioxide

Titanium dioxide has been used as a sunscreen since 1952, Table 8.2, Fig. 8.5 and is available as one of three forms, rutile, brookite, and anatase [19, 26, 27], with the absorption spectrum as shown below, Fig. 8.6 [26].

The particle size of titanium ranges from 200 to 400 nm, but with micronization, nanoparticles are generated which reduce the size to <100 nm [13, 26, 47]. Titanium is a naturally occurring mineral, which is known to be thermally stable, corrosion resistant, and is insoluble in water. Of the three forms of titanium dioxide, namely rutile, brookite, and anatase, rutile is the most stable, with a higher refractive index of 4.0, and is most suited for photoprotective functions due to its characteristic white pigment. The anatase form follows closely with a refractive index of 3.6 [19]. Though more reactive, coated anatase forms are also used commercially in sunscreens, where they have a potential to generate free radical species [48]. Titanium dioxide absorbs up to 70% of incident light and is said to provide substantial UV shielding [13, 26]. Compared to zinc oxide, titanium dioxide has a higher refractive

Table 8.2 Profile snapshot of titanium dioxide UV filter

Titanium dioxide (TiO_2), Fig. 8.5	
Approval status	Approved in the USA as GRASE I, and in the EU, Japan, Australia, ASEAN [25]
Mechanism of photoprotection	Reflect, absorb, and deflect UV photons [26, 27]
Maximum concentration in a sunscreen	Up to 25% in the USA, EU and Australia, no upper limit in Japan [28–30, 44]
Spectrum	UVB, UVA2 [26, 33] Weak HEVL (non-nano, pigment grade) [24, 25]
Systemic absorption	Penetration into the upper dermis, no significant systemic absorption [26, 31, 45]
Safety in pregnancy	Considered to be safe [30], new concerns related to genotoxicity [46]
Ecological concerns	Potential aquatic toxicity with titanium nanoparticles [12, 13]
Endocrine disruptor potential	Not known to possess endocrine disruption potential [32]
Sensitization potential	Not known to sensitize skin [26, 28, 47]
Photostability	Photostable [30, 33]
Areas of concern	Potential genotoxicity [46], aquatic toxicity, white cast

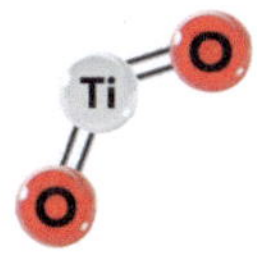

Fig. 8.5 Chemical structure of titanium dioxide

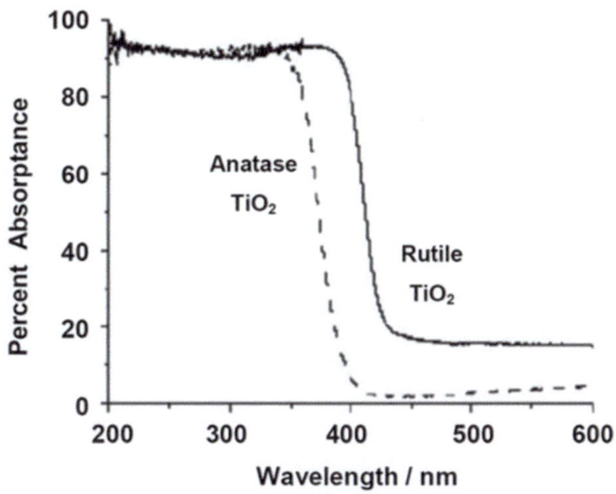

Fig. 8.6 Percent absorptance spectra of anatase TiO2 versus rutile TiO2. (Obtained with permission from Serpone [26])

index, and therefore, a higher tendency to produce a white cast when used in cosmetics.

Titanium dioxide nanoparticles are not expected to penetrate the skin significantly. The formulation type plays a role in determining the level of penetration, with the powder forms of nano titanium, showing no skin penetration, even with a smaller particle size of 38 nm, similar to the rod shaped rutile form at 20 nm. However, oil in water emulsions and water in oil emulsions which are found as agglomerates in formulation may show some level of penetration in the upper layers of the skin, at a minimal level. Clumping of titanium dioxide nanoparticles into aggregates in formulation may affect sunscreen performance compared to that provided by intact spherical rutile titanium particles in suspension [19].

Due to its inert and biocompatible behaviour, titanium has been utilized in a number of biomedical applications and is extensively used in the food and personal care industry. However, its behaviour in sunscreens is significantly different. On irradiation, titanium dioxide in general and nanoforms in particular are capable of reactive hydroxyl radicals with DNA damage, both in vitro and in cell models. The anatase forms are noted to be significantly more reactive with UVR compared to the rutile form [48]. Titanium dioxide was notified as a Group 2B carcinogen (possibly carcinogenic to humans) by the International Agency for Research on Cancer (IARC) Union in February 2020, most likely related to the inhalational toxicity of the mineral [49]. Based on this, the European Commission in its Regulation 2020/217 proceeded to classify and label titanium dioxide, when used in a powder form containing 1% or more of particles at sizes at or below 10 μm as suspected of being carcinogenic to humans, through the inhalation route [50]. However, the Court of Justice of the European Union, annulled the above classification of titanium stating that the methodology adopted, and the data used to label titanium dioxide as carcinogenic by inhalation in certain powders did not satisfy the required criteria [51].

An Austrian group working to establish the level of titanium dioxide contamination from suspended particulate matter, in the old Danube Lake in Vienna, found it difficult to differentiate naturally occurring titanium mineral from those attributable to sunscreens. However, the overall levels of titanium in the recreational lake increased during the summer months, indicating an influx of tourists into the area, and therefore sunscreens into the lake. Titanium dioxide nanoparticles are known to possess significant aquatic toxicity and given the volume of sunscreen usage across the world and the rising popularity of mineral sunscreens, this can be a considerable ecological problem [52, 53].

Titanium dioxide particles seem to require some level of coating to prevent reactivity. Specifically, nanoparticles of titanium as seen in the more cosmetically acceptable formulations require coating with inert material to reduce the generation of free radicals [23, 27, 54]. Passivization of titanium dioxide nanoparticles can be achieved with hydrated silica, aluminium oxide, or aluminium hydroxide. Such coating with aluminium oxide increases formulation stability, increases the dispersion of titanium dioxide, reduces direct contact of titanium dioxide with the skin, and potentially decreases photocatalytic activity, free radical generation, and oxidative stress [19, 27]. Further coating by aluminium nanoparticles also increases the soft focus or blur effect, increasing the cosmetic appeal of the finished product. It is important to note that aluminium in sunscreens has been reported to cause allergic contact dermatitis in children with preexisting allergy to aluminium, but the potential for allergies with aluminium nanoparticles to coat inorganic sunscreen filters, is unclear [55].

Titanium dioxide nanoparticles are allowed in sunscreens with the following proviso, as per the EU Commission regulations. The titanium nanomaterials are not to be used in applications that have any risk of inhalational exposure to the end user. The nanomaterials must have a purity not less than 99%, must be of the rutile form or if anatase is present, the latter to constitute not more than 5%, with a mean particle size based on number size distribution not less than 30 nm, with crystalline structure and physical appearance as clusters of needle, spherical, or lanceolate shaped particles. The aspect has been specified to be from 1 to 4.5, and volume specific surface area not more than $460 m^2/cm^3$. The nanoparticles must be coated with one of the following materials silica, hydrated silica, alumina, aluminium hydroxide, aluminium stearate, stearic acid, trimethoxycaprylylsilane, glycerin, dimethicone, hydrogen dimethicone, simethicone, resulting in a reduction of photocatalytic activity by 90% compared to the corresponding noncoated or nondoped reference. Finally, the nanoparticles must be photostable in the final formulation [56].

Titanium has been found to be more reactive than zinc, in the nanoform, however, the overall magnitude of the impact of titanium nanoparticles in the environment from sunscreens remains unclear. This is also due to the widespread usage of titanium in the food industry, notably in candies and chewing gum and in other personal care products such as toothpastes and make up. It is estimated that children in the USA aged 10 years or less are exposed to 1–2 mg of titanium dioxide/kg body weight/day. Several authors recommend the quantification of titanium exposure from nonsunscreen sources to arrive at the actual size of titanium nanoparticle toxicity [13, 26, 36]. Despite their huge popularity, sunscreen sprays containing titanium dioxide are not recommended, however, controversy exists as to the toxicity potential of the inhalational exposure to titanium dioxide [29].

In formulation, titanium behaves similar to zinc, enhancing the photodegradation of chemical filters such as avobenzone, and to a much lesser, though significant extent, octocrylene and octinoxate [26]. Since titanium dioxide is also present in a number of cosmetic products other than sunscreen, it is important to remember this photocatalytic potential of titanium when used alongside other chemical filters. About 5000 tonnes of titanium dioxide are said to be produced every year, with a titanium dioxide sunscreen market volume of 1500 tonnes per year. These numbers underscore the potential magnitude for environmental impact considering that titanium nanoparticles along with zinc, contribute to 94% of environmentally relevant engineered nanomaterials [38, 57].

Recently, titanium nanoparticles have been evaluated to have potential genotoxicity to humans, dependent on crystal size, type, and shape [46]. Safe-and-sustainable-by-design concepts, which integrate aspects of safety, sustainability, and functionality throughout a product's life cycle, along with in silico methods to predict and understand the real-time behaviour of finished formulations can help engineer safer sunscreens based on this versatile and easily available mineral [58]. Biomineralization concepts to develop titanium hydroxyapatite nanoparticles with low photoactivity, high UV reflectance, good biocompatibility, ecosafe, synergistic with organic filters and less prone to cutaneous penetration, are being explored currently [59].

Understanding White Cast in Sunscreens [26]

The scattering effect of mineral sunscreens of light from its incident point on the skin is perceived by the observer's eye as white. The dreaded white cast or Kabuki mask like appearance is the result of this photo scattering phenomenon of incident white light. Though zinc and titanium tend to have attenuations in their filtering capacity near the 400 nm mark, their opacity makes them still valuable options for protection against UV light. The white cast from these inorganic sunscreens, though considered to be a deterrent for sunscreen use from the consumer point of view, is testimony to the scattering of incident light on the skin. Zinc oxide has a lesser tendency to create a white cast, compared to titanium dioxide, with the latter scattering white light four times as much as zinc oxide [29, 60, 61].

Which Mineral?

Which Mineral: Zinc Oxide Versus Titanium Dioxide, Fig. 8.7 [49]

Mineral sunscreens have become very popular with consumers preferring physical sunscreens, due to perceived lack of 'harmful or harsh chemicals', and the need for more 'natural' options. With only two physical sunscreens currently available, choice is highly limited. Still, consumers and formulators may prefer one over the other based on some of the aspects below.

Spectral Performance:

Couteau et al. noted that TiO2 was a more effective filter than ZnO, by a factor of three times at maximal dosage levels with a higher <E11> compared to zinc [62]. In other research, compared to microfine titanium, microfine zinc at similar concentrations provided better protection against solar radiation at all wavelengths, but particularly in the band between 340 and 380 nm. For skin of colour, protection in the UVA spectrum is necessary, which is achieved with zinc oxide, while titanium is primarily an attenuator in the UVB spectrum [60, 63].

Compared at similar concentrations, zinc oxide provides a more stable UVA coverage with higher UVA-PF values even for the same SPF, than titanium. This suggests that TiO_2 should not be considered a substitute for ZnO where broad-spectrum coverage is desired [64]. The main strength of zinc oxide in sunscreens is its high performance in terms of achieving adequate UVA-PF. For the same SPF, sunscreens with higher UVA- PF were found to be more efficient at preventing dermal damage. An SPF to UVA-PF ratio of ≤ 3 denotes a higher level of protection against UVA- and UVA-induced pigmentation [65].

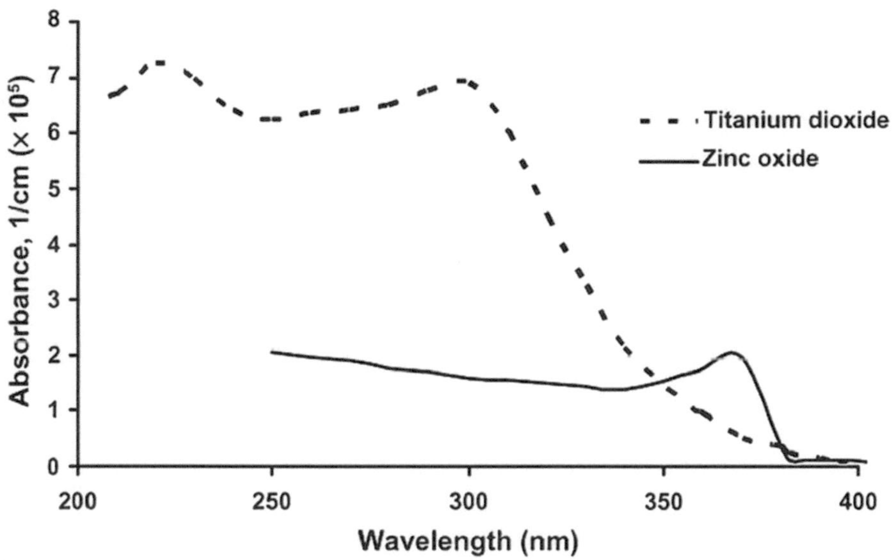

Fig. 8.7 Absorbance of bulk titanium dioxide and zinc oxide at room temperature. Despite the high absorbance in the UVB spectrum for titanium dioxide, zinc oxide has a better protection in the UVA spectrum of relevance to SOC. (Obtained from Nanotechnology, Science and Applications 2011 4 95–112 Originally published by and used with permission from Dove Medical Press Ltd. [49])

Safety:

Zinc nanoparticles are not expected to penetrate the viable epidermis to any significant level. Titanium nanoparticles may not be absorbed to any significant extent, however, certain formulation types may show minimal penetration into the top layers of the skin [19, 45]. Nanoparticles of both mineral filters are expected to have inhalational toxicity, titanium dioxide more than zinc oxide. Both the mineral filters are considered as nonallergenic, and therefore recommended as suitable for use by individuals with autoimmune skin disease [28, 66].

Aesthetics:

Titanium has more likelihood for white cast compared to zinc oxide due to the higher scattering ability [60]. The refractive index for zinc oxide is 1.9–2.0 compared to 2.5–4 for titanium. A lower refractive index allows for a more transparent product [67]. Zinc sunscreens, on the other hand, do not provide adequate moisturizing feel [19].

Ecoreactivity:

Titanium nanoparticles were found to be more reactive than zinc nanoparticles, however, the latter have been documented to cause more coral bleaching. Specific coatings to increase particle inertness are required for eco-tolerance of both the inorganic filters [13].

Overall, the impact of both the mineral sunscreens on the ecosystem seems to be more benign than that of chemical sunscreens. However, this could also be biased by the wider use of chemical sunscreens which are inherently more aesthetically pleasing. But also, it must be admitted that there is some difficulty in quantifying zinc and titanium minerals in ecosystems, which occur naturally in the environment, versus those introduced into an ecosystem through sunscreens and may under represent the impact of mineral filters on the environment [52].

8.1.3 Iron Oxides

Though not classified as a sunscreen filter per se, iron oxides are discussed here, due to their relevance as important photoprotective agents in SOC. Their utility in protecting against visible light-induced photomelanosis has attracted a lot of attention. Cole et al. noted that less than 2% of commercially available sunscreens contained iron oxide tints, in the Philadelphia region, in 2023 [68]. However, the tinted sunscreen trend is catching up, due to larger consumer awareness and better formulation options.

For SOC, protection in the UVA-VL zone is of high importance, due to the demonstrated ability of this spectrum to produce and/or worsen cutaneous hyperpigmentation. Currently available tinted sunscreens mostly contain iron oxides with titanium dioxide, though iron oxides are also available in an uncomplexed form, to add to the formulation [69]. Iron oxides are mostly available in three colours, red, yellow and black, listed as by their colour index as CI 77491, CI77492 and CI 77499, respectively, Fig. 8.8 [70]. The colour depends on the level of oxidation. The hue or the tint is dependent on the ratio of the iron oxides in the formulation. Only synthetic iron oxides are preferred in cosmetic products as per the US FDA, as natural iron oxides may contain heavy metal contaminants [69]. Natural iron oxides are permitted in cosmetics in the European Union, provided the products have been assayed to not exceed the limits stipulated for heavy metals such as lead, arsenic, mercury, cadmium, nickel, copper, barium, chromium, and zinc.

Iron oxides act similar to metal oxides in protecting against solar light—by absorption, reflection, and scattering [71]. Tinted sunscreens containing iron oxides are able to protect better in the VL-UVA1 spectrum, compared to non-tinted sunscreens. Addition of iron oxides increases the critical wavelength of sunscreens, indicating protection in the UVA-HEVL zone. Specifically, sunscreens containing iron oxides with titanium dioxide provided better protection compared to zinc oxides with iron oxide, even with a higher concentration of tint in the latter formulations [71]. This could be due to the higher refractive index of titanium dioxide,

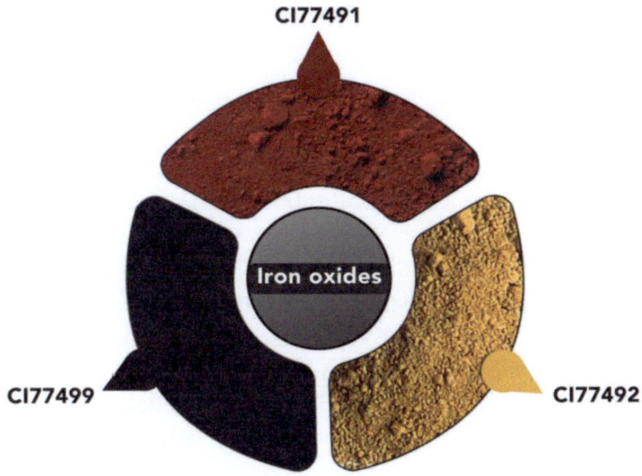

Fig. 8.8 Red, yellow, and black iron oxides

3.6–4, compared to zinc oxide, 2.0–2.3, providing a whitening effect to boost the tint [49].

Tinted sunscreens have now come to be recommended as a standard of care for all skin types, according to the recently published International Consensus on Antiaging Dermocosmetics and Skin Care for Clinical Practice. However, the cosmetic acceptability of such tinted sunscreens remains to be seen, as the availability of colour matched products for SOC has been low until now. Cole et al. found that only 1.7% of facial sunscreen products included iron oxides, and shade matching was not available in 99.5% of all sunscreen products tested, except for those meant for use on the lips [68].

Iron oxides are considered nontoxic and nonirritant and well tolerated even by those with sensitive skin. They may also have some antioxidant potential with free radical quenching abilities. However, iron oxide nanoparticles were observed to penetrate into the viable epidermis up to the stratum granulosum and also reach the deeper portions of the hair follicles, entering through hair follicle orifices [72]. The link between facial sunscreens, including those with tints and frontal fibrosing alopecia attributable to the interaction of UV protecting agents, including metal oxides, with hair follicles, needs further exploration [73].

Natural antioxidants such as silymarin, polypodium leucotomos extracts, pycnogenol, and astaxanthin also provide a subtle tint which can improve sunscreen acceptability in skin of colour; however, these agents may not offer the coverage provided by iron oxides, often complexed to titanium dioxide with its whitening, masking effect. The masking of skin pigmentation and dyschromias in addition to providing ongoing protection, as in the case of 'foundation' sunscreens, CC (complexion corrector) creams, and BB (beauty balm or blemish balm) products, is of importance both functionally and aesthetically to SOC [73].

8.1.4 Newer Inorganic Filters

Compared to the slow, but steady increase in organic filters currently available, newer options for inorganic filters are scarce.

In consideration are a few contenders, the most notable of them being cerium compounds. The others in consideration include hydroxyapatite and hydrotalcite [74].

Inorganic filters have the advantage of being photostable and providing broad-spectrum coverage with negligible systemic absorption. However, inorganic oxides are also opaque and to the consumer, a white cast has low cosmetic appeal, even if the performance of the sunscreen itself is efficient [75]. The whiteness of the zinc and titanium sunscreens is due to the high refractive index. Also, inorganic filters, typically titanium dioxide also have photoreactive behaviour with a potential for oxidative damage in skin cells.

Cerium is a new, rare earth element proposed as a novel inorganic filter for use in suncare and cosmetic formulations. Cerium oxide has a low refractive index and appears nearly transparent on skin, without the white cast typical of inorganic sunscreens. In addition, cerium oxide is said to have a lower photocatalytic activity compared to titanium and zinc oxides [75]. Cerium nanoparticles act by scattering UV rays [76].

Cerium oxide particles are also known to have a catalytic tendency to oxidize organic materials, and hence their application for use in sunscreens has been mostly in the research stage thus far. This led to the development of cerium phosphate nanoparticles with lesser photocatalytic properties and improved antioxidant function providing anti-inflammatory and antiageing benefits. Cerium oxide has a wide optical absorption spectrum ranging from 320 to 600 nm, while absorption bands have been identified around 208 nm and around 274 nm [77]. The significant ability of the cerium phosphate nanoparticles to protect in the visible spectrum, as shown in the image below, is attributed to the phosphate moiety which contributes protection in the near-infrared light (NIR) range [78].

In experiments comparing titanium dioxide with cerium dioxide, the former was found to have significant photocatalytic effects with pro-oxidant, mutagenic outcomes with evidence of cellular damage. In contrast, cerium dioxide was not only found to have none of the above effects, but also to have a protective antioxidant behaviour, by quenching oxidation and reducing DNA damage, leading to amelioration of mutagenesis. Cerium particles also increased the speed of DNA repair, and increased the viability of UV irradiated cells, and was also seen to protect cellular damage caused by titanium dioxide. This raises the possibility of cerium being used as an antiaging, anticancer sun filter, but also opens up the possibility of being a free radical quencher and antioxidant when combined with UV filters with a known ability to protect against sunlight [79].

While addition of zinc or titanium oxides to organic filters has been known to result in potential loss of stability [36], addition of cerium phosphate was shown to nearly double the shelf life of sunscreen formulations containing avobenzone, octinoxate, and octocrylene. In the same experiment, a slight decrease in shelf life was seen on the addition of zinc oxide to octinoxate, no change was noted for zinc oxide added to octocrylene, and when added to avobenzone, the shelf life was found to increase significantly. For titanium dioxide shelf life was found to reduce in addition to octinoxate and avobenzone, each, with no significant change for octocrylene [75].

Cerium particles are spherical with a size between 15 and 25 nm, thus a larger surface area may be responsible for the higher catalytic activity [76]. Cerium compounds are being developed with larger particle sizes up to 50 nm. A larger sized cerium compound, the cerium aminoclay is also being considered for its potential benefit in sunscreens [80].

Cerium compounds have been used in multiple other biomedical applications. Notably, cerium nanoparticles are used in regenerative applications to treat hydroxychloroquine-induced retinal toxicity to reduce oxidative stress to the rods and cones and also to improve high light-induced macular degeneration [81]. Considering that nanoceria operate in these applications on the principle of preventing oxidative damage, it would be interesting to observe what these particles have to offer in sunscreens.

Further studies with relevant human data are awaited, before cerium phosphate can be approved to be formulated in a cosmetically elegant mineral filter with broad-spectrum coverage.

8.2 Chemical Sunscreens

According to the EU Cosmetics Regulation [Regulation (EC) No 1223/2009], UV filters are defined as substances which are exclusively or mainly intended to protect the skin against certain UV radiations by absorbing, reflecting, or scattering mechanisms. Traditionally, mineral filters are understood to reflect or scatter sunlight and the chemical filters to absorb light. Of late, these lines are blurring, and as detailed in the section on nanominerals in sunscreens, smaller particles in mineral sunscreens act predominantly by absorption, even up to 95%. On the contrary, newer particulate chemical filters are now able to scatter light in addition to the absorption mechanism. However, the level of scattering is expected to be smaller, as with the mineral sunscreens [25, 26, 36, 82].

Chemical sunscreens are used widely and represent one of the largest and most growing segments within the sun care domain. Though each of the chemical filters are unique in their potency and spectrum of coverage, a comparison by Couteau et al. using in vitro testing, ranks chemical filters from least effective to most effective as below,

3-Benzylidene camphor (1.66) < oxybenzone (3.01) < octylsalicylate (3.12) < PABA (3.36) < polysilicone 15 (3.64) < methylene bis-benzotriazolyl tetramethylbutylphenol (3.68) < PEG25 PABA (3.81) < benzophenone-4 (3.85) < 4-methylbenzylidene camphor (4.22) < homosalate (4.33) < octyltriazone (7.80) < phenylbenzimidazole sulfonic acid (8.31) < octyldimethyl PABA (8.71) < octocrylene (10.41) < octylmethoxycinnamate (10.42) < diethylhexylbutamidotriazone (12.58) < isoamylparamethoxycinnamate (15.14) < anisotriazine (20.0). Figure 8.9 [83]. In the upcoming segment, we shall explore the different filters in some detail. Figures 8.10 and 8.11 [47, 84, 85].

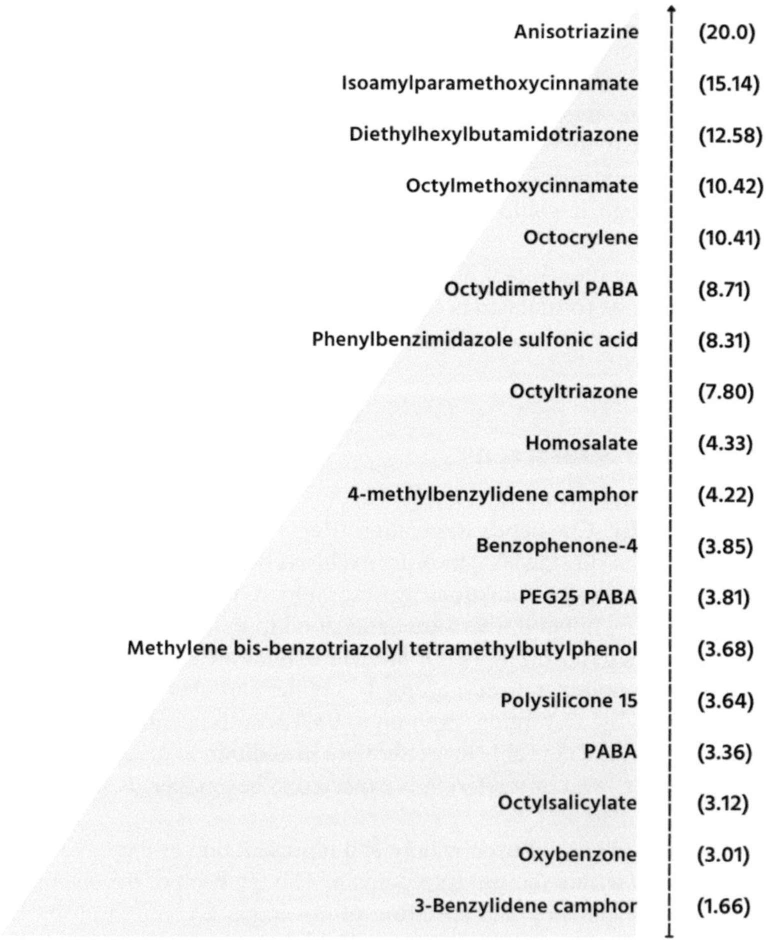

Fig. 8.9 Filtering efficacy of chemical UV filters based on data from Couteau et al. [83]

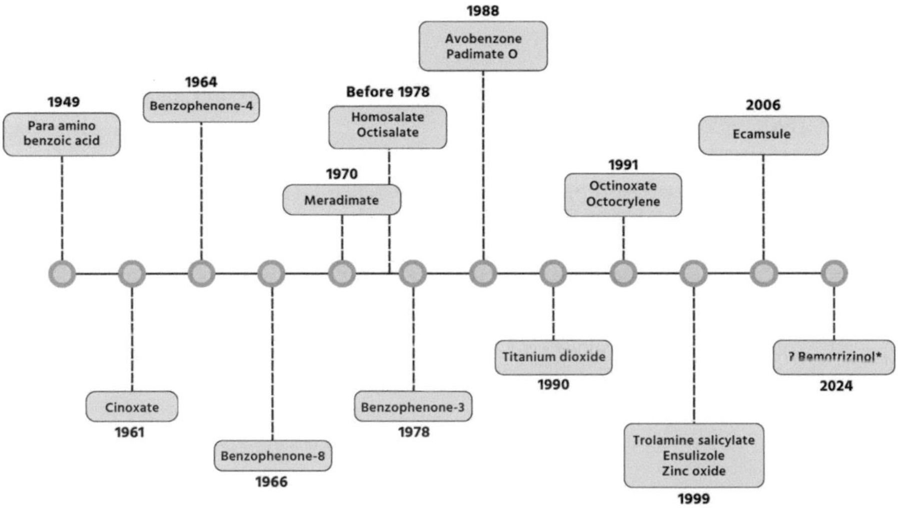

Fig. 8.10 Time line—US FDA Approved UV filters. *in consideration for approval [84, 85]

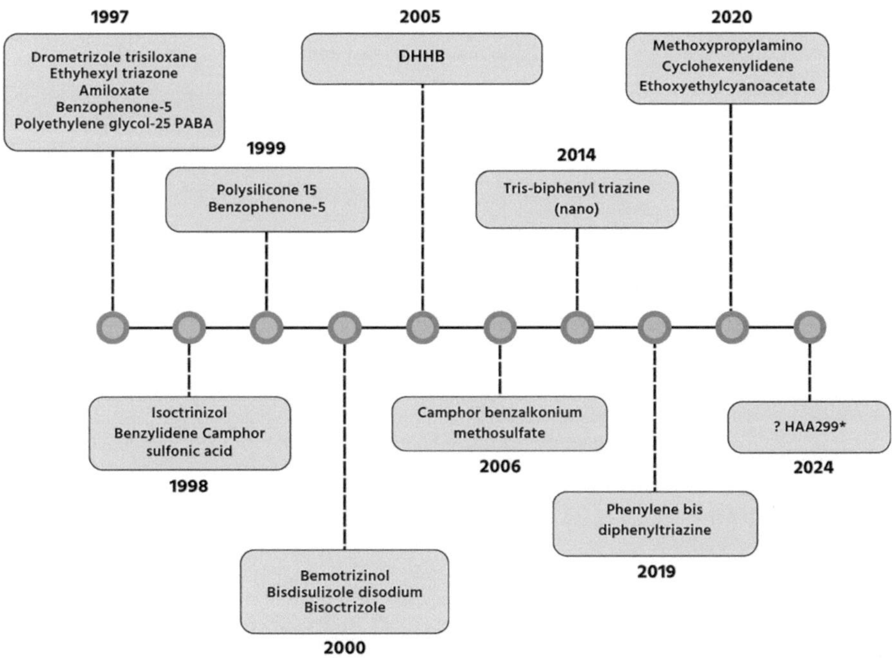

Fig. 8.11 Timeline—EU approved UV filters [48]. *in consideration for approval [84] [85]

8.2.1 PABA

PABA was one of the earliest sunscreen filters to be commercially available to consumers Table 8.3, Fig. 8.12. Launched in the 1920s, the popularity of PABA was enhanced by the fact that it was water resistant. Over the next few decades, however, the nitrosamine degradation products of PABA were identified as potentially carcinogenic, with potential for cellular toxicity. Additionally, PABA was known to cause allergic contact dermatitis and photosensitization, with skin reactions seen in up to 8% of users [26, 30]. Systemic absorption was also a concern, and PABA use was also related to autoimmune conditions like systemic lupus erythematosus (SLE). Coupled with a tendency to stain clothing, these multiple problems made PABA fall out of favour [30, 61], especially with the advent of multiple newer filters with better coverage, lesser tendency for skin irritation, improved safety profile and most relevant to the consumer, improved aesthetic user experience [28, 36].

Table 8.3 Profile snapshot of PABA UV filter

PABA (Para-amino benzoic acid, Amino benzoic acid) Fig. 8.12	
Approval status	Non-GRASE, Category II, not commonly used in the USA Not approved in the EU [30, 86, 87]
Mechanism of photoprotection	Absorbs UV to release thermal energy [30]
Maximum concentration in a sunscreen	15% [30]
Spectrum	UVB
Systemic absorption	Risk of systemic absorption present, detected in urine
Safety in pregnancy	No current data
Ecological concerns	No current data
Endocrine disruptor potential	No current data
Sensitization potential	High, up to 8% [26]
Photostability	Stable, however, photodegradation has been documented [88]
Areas of concern	Potential carcinogen, predisposition to photoallergic and allergic contact dermatitis, potential link to autoimmune disorders [26, 30]

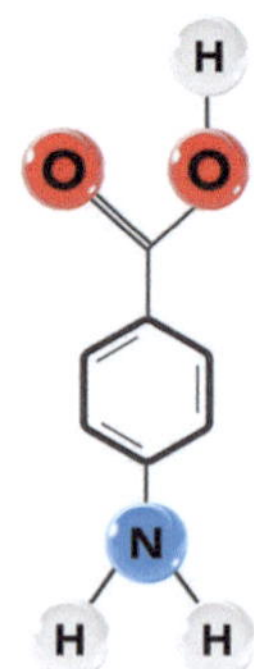

Fig. 8.12 Chemical structure of para-amino benzoic acid, amino benzoic acid

PABA still features in the FDA sunscreen list in the most recent monograph with a maximum permissible level of 15% in sunscreen products. It is, however, listed as GRASE II, along with trolamine sulphate and is not expected to be commercially marketed in the USA. PABA is not allowed as a sunscreen filter in the EU [30, 45]. PEG-25 PABA or polyethylene glycol PABA is approved in sunscreens in the EU at concentrations up to 10% [89].

8.2.2 Trolamine Salicylate

Trolamine salicylate protects against light in the spectrum between 250 and 355 nm, providing coverage across UVB and UVA2 Table 8.4, Fig. 8.13. It is allowed to be used in sunscreens up to a maximum concentration of 12%, though products with this compound are not currently available [45, 86].

Trolamine salicylate is also marketed as an analgesic, the salicylate moiety in this filter functioning as an NSAID. Its performance in this capacity infers that there is some level of percutaneous penetration, which is not desirable for its function as a sunscreen, in which role it would be preferred that the product stay on the skin without uptake beyond the nonviable epidermis. Analgesic products containing this filter carry label instructions for the product to be applied only to the affected areas, not more than 3–4 times a day, and not beyond 7 days of usage. However, as a sunscreen this product would expect to be labelled as being required to be used every 2 h, going by the current guidelines.

In view of these ambiguities, and due to the availability of more effective and efficient sunscreen filters, the use of trolamine salicylate in sunscreens is rare [26, 45].

Table 8.4 Profile snapshot of Trolamine salicylate

Trolamine salicylate (TEA salicylate, triethanolamine salicylate), Fig. 8.13	
Approval Status	Non-GRASE, Category II, not used in the USA since 2019 [30, 47, 86]
Mechanism of photoprotection	Absorbs UV
Maximum concentration in a sunscreen	12% in the USA, Canada, and Australia, 2.5% in the EU [30, 47, 86]
Spectrum	UVB
Safety in pregnancy	Risk of salicylism [30]
Systemic absorption	Percutaneous absorption possible, systemic absorption suggests toxicity (GI distress, bleeding, ototoxicity, and hypersensitivity) from use over large body surface area [30]
Areas of concern	Ambiguity in use since the product is also marketed as an analgesic, recommended for limited use

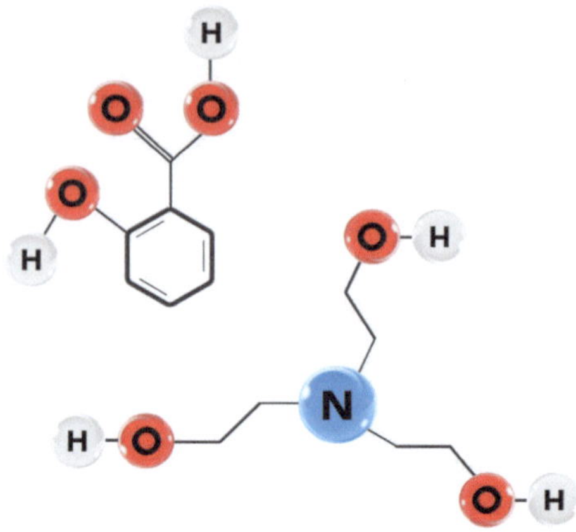

Fig. 8.13 Chemical structure of trolamine salicylate

8.2.3 *Ecamsule*

Ecamsule was approved in the USA through an FDA NDA process, exclusively for La Roche Posay products, in 2016 Table 8.5, Fig. 8.14. It is not formally listed in the FDA OTC Monograph, nor allotted a GRASE category [90]. However, there are no MuST (maximal usage trial) studies for ecamsule as yet, which is considered requisite for the United States Food and Drug Administration (US FDA) approval of chemical filters [86].

Ecamsule was developed by L'Oreal Laboratories, as a filter for the UVA range in the early 1990s. With an absorption max at 345 nm, ecamsule was expected to be a welcome addition to the UVA spectrum, after avobenzone. Early animal studies showed a successful amelioration of UVA-induced dermal changes such as decrease in total collagen, decreased hydroxylation of collagen, increased ratio of type III collagen to type I, and fibronectin synthesis [93]. In a subsequent study, ecamsule was shown to delay the development of UVR-induced murine skin tumours by 6 weeks, with a tumour protection factor of 2.4 [94]. Later, in vitro studies demonstrated that ecamsule was able to protect against UV-induced cell damage, using several parameters such as comet assays to evaluate DNA damage and DNA repair, p53 expression, structural alterations in plasmid DNA, and induction of pigmentation in human melanocyte cultured cells [95]. Ecamsule at 5% was able to protect against sub erythemal UVA-induced photoageing, denoted by alteration in elastin and collagen on histopathology [96]. Additionally, ecamsule 5% was also shown to inhibit UVA-induced disappearance of dermal fibroblasts [97]. In combination with octocrylene and avobenzone, ecamsule was found to mitigate UVA-induced cutaneous changes signalling photoageing, in human volunteers [98] and to have a dose-dependent effect on reducing UVR skin pigmentation, alone and in combination with drometrizole trisiloxane [99].

Ecamsule is specifically found to be useful in individuals with photosensitivity disorders like systemic lupus erythematosus (SLE) [66] or those with photoallergic

Table 8.5 Profile snapshot Ecamsule

Ecamsule (Terephthalylidene dicamphor sulfonic acid, TDSA, Mexoryl SX), Fig. 8.14	
Approval status	Approved in the USA through a New Drug Application (NDA) process for use in sunscreens manufactured by La Roche Posay, no GRASE status [30]. Approved in the EU, Japan, Australia [47]
Mechanism of photoprotection	Absorbs UV [30]
Maximum concentration in a sunscreen	3% in the USA, up to 10% in EU, Japan, and Australia [30]
Spectrum	UVB (partial), UVA2, UVA1(partial) [25]
Systemic/percutaneous absorption	Systemic absorption was reported by Matta et al. [14, 90].
Safety in pregnancy	Not recommended [30]
Ecological concerns	None identified based on ECHA reporting [91]
Endocrine disruptor potential	No conclusive data
Sensitization potential	Less likely to have allergenic potential [92]
Photostability	Photostable [63]
Areas of concern	Systemic absorption has been demonstrated, however, systemic toxicity is unclear [30]

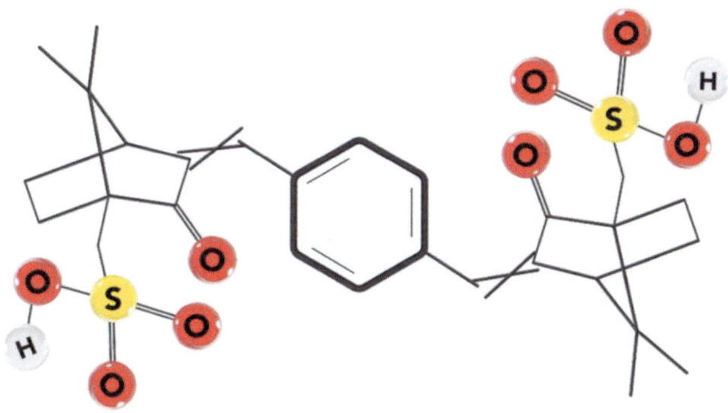

Fig. 8.14 Chemical structure of ecamusule

reactions to other UV filters (Schmidt T), due to its low potential for contact dermatitis. Foutanier et al. reviewed the clinical applications of ecamsule and concluded that addition of this filter provided a dose-dependent protection against UV-induced pigmentation [100].

Dermal penetration and systemic uptake were not considered significant for ecamsule, with less than 0.1% expected to be absorbed systemically [101]. However, more recently, Matta et al. demonstrated that plasma levels of 0.5 ng/ml were exceeded using maximal use case tests [90]. Ecamsule is approved at a maximum of 3% in the USA, while several efficacy studies as detailed above have used this filter at 5%. Furthermore, where this filter is used maximally in Europe, concentrations of up to 10% are permitted [63]. While this may mean that a lesser amount of filter is used, sunscreen products are always evaluated for efficacy in the final formulation, and this difference in usage levels may not mean much in practical usage. In support, a recent study showed that an SPF 40 sunscreen containing ecamsule at 3%, along with 10% octocrylene, 2% avobenzone and titanium dioxide 5% was found to protect against PMLE flares as compared to filters with avobenzone alone or ecamsule alone [102]. Ecamsule is a good filter for sunscreens formulated to be water resistant and to be photostable [63, 94].

8.2.4 *Avobenzone*

Avobenzone is the most widely used UVA blocker, as it was introduced around the time when the role of UVA in photodamage was becoming increasingly clear Table 8.6, Fig. 8.15 [66, 107, 108]. Sunscreens with avobenzone were reported to provide adequate UVA protection [109]. The only UV filter currently available in the USA and included in the OTC Monograph, for coverage of the UVA spectrum other than zinc oxide, avobenzone is well known for its photounstable behaviour. On sun exposure, avobenzone undergoes an irreversible degradation of its keto isomer resulting in phenacyl and benzoyl photoadducts [110]. After 1 h of UV exposure, photodegradation reactions can result in a loss of 50–90% of avobenzone in formulation with resultant lack of efficacy and failure to protect against ongoing sun exposure [33].

Table 8.6 Profile snapshot of avobenzone

Avobenzone (Butylmethoxy dibenzoylmethane/BMDM/Parsol 1789), Fig. 8.15	
Approval status	NONGRASE, Category III in the USA. Approved in the EU, Australia, and Japan [45]
Mechanism of photoprotection	Absorbs UV [30]
Maximum concentration in a sunscreen	3% in the USA, 5% in the EU and Australia, 10% in Japan [25, 28]
Spectrum	UVA1, UVA2 [25]
Systemic absorption	Has been documented in several studies [14, 90], though avobenzone is considered to have low skin permeation potential [103]
Safety in pregnancy	Not recommended [30]
Ecological concerns	Potential impact on coral [104]
Endocrine disruptor potential	Potential influence on thyroid hormones, significance of impact on humans in not known [105]
Sensitization potential	Has irritation, allergenic, photoallergic, and phototoxic potential [47, 106]
Photostability	Unstable [26]
Areas of concern	Systemic absorption, photoinstability

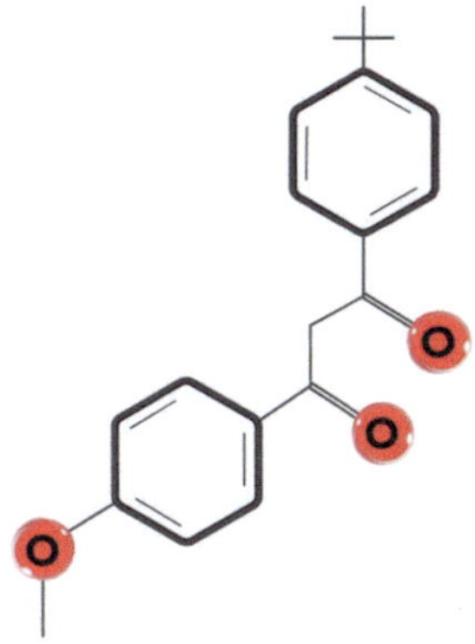

Fig. 8.15 Chemical structure of avobenzone

Avobenzone is known to have significant allergenic potential, more commonly resulting in photoallergic contact dermatitis (PACD) than allergic contact dermatitis (ACD). One of the breakdown products of avobenzone after exposure to UVR, aryl glyoxal have been considered responsible for the photocontact allergies due to the dibenzoylmethane class of sun filters, and avobenzone in particular. As a very common ingredient in sunscreens due to the UVA spectral coverage, the incidence of a higher number of allergies from avobenzone is probably attributable to its widespread use [66, 107].

Due to the inherent lack of photostability of avobenzone, careful attention must be paid to synergy of ingredients in formulations. Combinations of two photounstable classes of sunscreens such as cinnamates, eg octinoxate and dibenzoylmethanes, such as avobenzone, are discouraged [26, 45]. This combination has been studied to generate cinnamate dimers and cyclobutyl ketone photoadducts with potential oxidative damage to the skin [111]. Similarly, combinations of zinc oxide and avobenzone worsened the photostability of the sunscreen [39]. On the contrary and just as certain ingredients worsen photoinstability, certain other active and inactive sunscreen constituents may help stabilize avobenzone. Apart from filters like octocrylene and bemotrizinol, these include emollients such as tridecyl salicylate, butyloctyl salicylate, and polyester 8 [29]. Addition of antioxidants like vitamin C, vitamin E, ubiquinone, and resveratrol have also been used to increase the photostability of avobenzone, along with exploration of physical modifications like encapsulation [26, 108, 112]. Despite its lack of photostability, avobenzone is a strong protector against UVA, performing better than titanium dioxide [26].

Recently, avobenzone was identified to be a potential metabolic disrupting obesogen, acting along, and independently of peroxisome proliferator-activated receptors (PPAR) pathways [113]. Considering that avobenzone was known to persist in human plasma at higher than threshold levels for up to 3 weeks after the initial exposure, its ability to increase PPARγ transcription as an obesogen merits further watch [114].

8.2.5 Octinoxate

Octinoxate is considered to be the most commonly used UVB filter Table 8.7, Fig. 8.16 [26, 28]. It is allowed in sunscreens up to 20% in Japan, and at a lesser concentration of 10% in EU and Australia, and at 7.5% in the USA [28]. In sunscreens, octinoxate is most commonly found in combination with avobenzone, a potentially photounstable pair, whose sun protection benefits may be offset by the toxicity of photoadducts created on UV radiation [26]. Typically, the lack of meaningful sun protection, plus an added oxidation effect may actually promote carcinogenesis, which may explain the increase in skin cancers, even with increasing

Table 8.7 Profile snapshot of octinoxate

Octinoxate (Ethyl hexyl methoxycinnamate, octyl methoxycinnamate, OMC), Fig. 8.16	
Approval status	NONGRASE, Category III in the USA. Approved in the EU, Australia, and Japan [45]
Mechanism of photoprotection	UV absorption [30]
Maximum concentration in a sunscreen	7.5% in the USA, 10% in the EU and Australia, 20% in Japan [28]
Spectrum	UVB, UVA2(weak) [30, 47]
Systemic absorption	Significant, noted in several studies [14, 115], detected in human breast milk and other biological fluids [116]
Safety in pregnancy	Not recommended [30]
Ecological concerns	Aquatic toxicity, bioaccumulation, and biomagnification [106, 117]
Endocrine disruptor potential	Present [32]
Sensitization potential	Present [38]
Photostability	Photounstable [111]
Areas of concern	Endocrine disruption, systemic absorption, ecotoxicity, photounstable behaviour

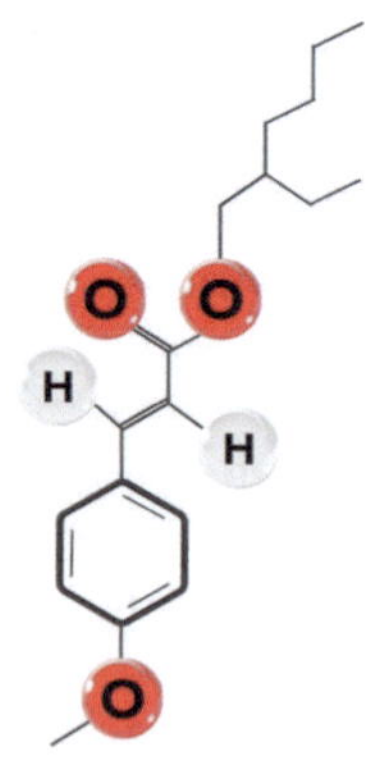

Fig. 8.16 Chemical structure of octinoxate

sunscreen use [111]. For better photostability, a higher concentration of the filter in highly polar lipid solvents is recommended, but the impact of these steps on absorption is a concern [118].

Despite concerns over its potential for endocrine disruption, octinoxate continues to be used extensively, since it is not just used in sunscreen products, but also in other personal care products to reduce product photooxidation and to increase shelf life. Overall, octinoxate is expected to be present in over 90% of personal care products, which provides multiple touch points for the consumer to be exposed to this filter, so as to call it an emerging contaminant [119, 120].

Octinoxate, cinnoxate, and octocrylene are the cinnamates commonly used in sunscreens, and as a cinnamate, octinoxate exhibits cross reactivity to both cinnamic acid and cinnamaldehyde. Positive patch test reactions to octinoxate have been reported from multiple countries, though at a much less frequency than oxybenzone, octocrylene, and avobenzone [66, 107, 121–123].

Octinoxate was found to have an oestrogenic, antithyroid, and antiprogestogenic profile, and this is of relevance to susceptible populations [124]. Krause et al. reviewed the endocrine impact of currently used UV filters and found octinoxate to impact oestrogen, progesterone, androgen, and thyroid hormone receptors and possess reproductive, developmental, CNS toxicities, in several studies [32]. Animal studies have shown an impact on the hypothalamic pituitary gonadal axis. The presence of octinoxate in breast milk has raised significant concern. As the foetal exposome is being explored as significant for future health, the impact of this filter on pregnant women, and through them, to the foetus, merits attention [116]. Examining the impact of UV filter exposure and pubertal development among Chinese adolescents, Huang et al. noted that octinoxate and its metabolites were significantly negatively correlated with testicular volume and genital development, and a later onset of pubic hair and testicular volume achievement in boys, indicating a delay in pubertal development [125]. Recent data suggests that octinoxate may act as an environmental obesogen for girls [126]. While modelling studies on the impact of UV filter exposure provide some reassurance against alarm, the long-term consequences of such exposure must be evaluated [127, 128].

The aquatic toxicity of octinoxate deserves attention because it is coupled with bioaccumulation, and biomagnification at trophic levels, exposing the human who consumes sea food to a significantly larger amount of octinoxate than what entered the food chain [106]. UV filters were found to be present in diet, including animal origin foods, and proportionately in human milk, with octisalate, octinoxate, and homosalate contributing to the bulk of the exposure. The study concluded that based on absorption, distribution, metabolism elimination kinetics, UV filters have the potential to persist in the human body [129].

Octinoxate is one of the sunscreens prohibited by the environmental ban on certain UV filters by states like Hawaii in the USA, as the endocrine disruption and impact on corals is expected to be significant at the magnitude of sun filters being let out into the beaches at these heavily visited tourist locations [27].

8.2.6 Octocrylene

Octocrylene is a UV filter with predominant action in the UVB and short UVA regions Table 8.8, Fig. 8.17. In Europe and in the USA, octocrylene is allowed up to a maximum concentration of 10% [134]. The recent Scientific Committee on Consumer Safety (SCCS) guidelines rule that octocrylene is safe for a combined use of a sunscreen cream or lotion, pump spray, face cream, hand cream, and lipstick up to 10% concentration. In sunscreen propellant sprays, a concentration limit of 9% should be maintained when used together with other products such as face cream, hand cream, or lipstick containing 10% octocrylene [135].

Octocrylene has dual advantages, both as a primary UV filter and as a stabilizer of other UV filters like octinoxate, oxybenzone, and avobenzone, which have been known to undergo photodegradation [36, 136]. The stabilization abilities of octocrylene enabled a photounstable avobenzone to be used more widely, producing sunscreens with full spectrum UV coverage, and this combination is seen in many popular sunscreens.

Along with benzophenone, octocrylene tops the list of photoallergens among UV absorbers, compared to newer UV filters which are much less commonly associated with allergenic potential [137]. Octocrylene has been considered as an emerging allergen strongly associated with contact dermatitis in children and photoallergic

Table 8.8 Profile snapshot of octocrylene

Octocrylene (OCR), Fig. 8.17	
Approval status	Approved in the USA, EU, Australia, and Japan [25, 82, 130]
Mechanism of photoprotection	UV absorption [26, 27]
Maximum concentration in a sunscreen	Up to 10% in the USA, EU, Australia, and Japan, up to 9% in propellant sprays in the EU [28, 130]
Spectrum	UVB, UVA2, partial UVA1 [25]
Systemic absorption	Present, exceeded threshold values [14]
Safety in pregnancy	Not recommended [30]
Ecological concerns	Significant [131]
Endocrine disruptor potential	Early human data linking octocrylene and PCOS [132]
Sensitization potential	Photoallergic and allergic contact dermatitis [107]
Photostability	Photostable improves the photostability of other filters [28]
Areas of concern	Degradation to benzophenone in finished formulations [133]

Fig. 8.17 Chemical structure of Octocrylene

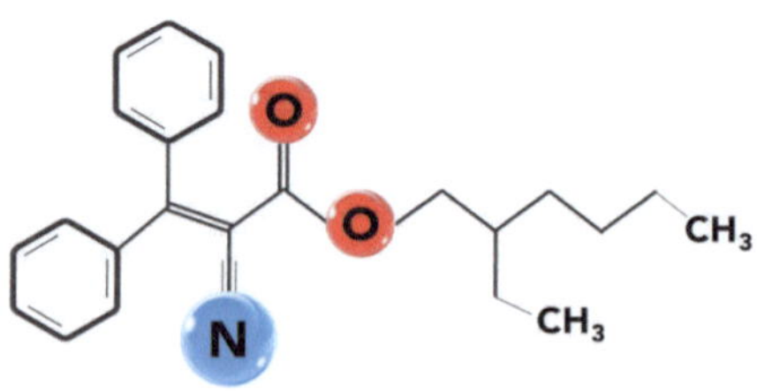

contact dermatitis (PACD) in adults. Photoallergy to octocrylene also seems to occur in relation to cross reactivity with ketoprofen, a prolific allergen, even though the structural similarity between the two molecules is limited. Octocrylene not only contains benzophenone as an impurity, but also undergoes time and temperature dependent degradation into benzophenone [133]. In individuals with photosensitization to ketotifen, photo allergic contact dermatitis to octocrylene is potentially related to its benzophenone content [138]. Individuals with allergy to any of these three components must be counselled about the need to use sunscreens without all three of these agents [139, 140].

The cutaneous penetration of octocrylene was considered to be low, with 95% of the applied product remaining on the skin's surface [134], with up to 0.4% in the epidermis. However, Matta et al. demonstrated the systemic absorption of octocrylene above permitted threshold values of 0.5 ng/ml in human volunteer studies, ranging from 2.9 to 7.8 ng/ml. Furthermore, the concentration levels in the plasma also indicated a potential accumulation of octocrylene over time. Octocrylene was also detected in breastmilk, and in urine of sunscreen users, however, animal studies did not demonstrate any significant reproductive toxicity at clinically relevant use levels, nor any teratogenicity or developmental toxicity [14, 134].

Octocrylene has also been noted to have endocrine disrupting properties. Though the majority of the data for endocrine disruption potential has been drawn from animal studies [105, 141, 142], a recent human case control study in women with PCOS merits attention. Exposure to octocrylene was found to be significantly associated with the occurrence of PCOS in women with BMI > 24, indicating a potential impact on hormonal signalling pathways due to octocrylene use [132]. Ko et al. identified octocrylene to be a potential obesogen, similar to benzophenone and avobenzone [113, 143, 144].

Although the presence of this UV filter has been documented in population relevant ecosystems [145] Toxcast in vitro screening for biological activity, found octocrylene to not have significant endocrine disruption potential [127]. However, octocrylene has been implicated as the compound with the highest concentration among 55 different legacy and emerging pollutants from Spanish marine bivalve ecosystems. Octocrylene was also detected in more than 96% of coral tissues from Hawaii, and in cod livers from Norway. The latter is a potential biomagnification concern for human beings. Typically, this UV filter has been noted to be a contaminant in most marine organisms [131]. Octocrylene has been noted to have significant bioaccumulation potential and has been detected in dolphin blubber, and early data suggests bioaccumulation in humans as well [146]. However, the magnitude and physiological significance on human health has been debated by other workers [147–149]. Octocrylene was noted to be poorly biodegradable [150].

Despite its huge popularity as a very useful and effective UV filter, the human and environmental impacts of octocrylene have recently been a source of concern. With the identification of newer filters with stabilizing benefits such as bemotrizinol, the dependance on octocrylene for its photostabilizing benefits may be reduced.

8.2.7 *Oxybenzone: Benzophenone 3*

Benzophenone or BP-3 gained popularity in the 1980s as a replacement for PABA, which, by then had fallen into disfavour due to its ability to generate nitrosamines on photodegradation Table 8.9, Fig. 8.18 [61, 108]. Given the broad spectrum of coverage, the domination of BP-3 as a sunscreen ingredient world over, was also reflected in the number of personal care products and household products with benzophenones added to protect the products themselves from photodegradation. However, recent data points to a downward trend in the popularity of BP-3 [107].

Oxybenzone is a small molecular weight, lipophilic UV filter with UVmax at 325, 287, and 243 nm, providing substantial protection throughout the UVB and UVA2 spectrum, but with some protective cover for UVA1 and even UVC [25, 153]. Upon light exposure, BP-3 very rapidly gets converted into its keto-tautomer through an electron driven internal conversion process. This is the principal mechanism through which oxybenzone protects from UV-induced free radical damage. Hofer et al. demonstrated a protective benefit of benzophenone in minimizing UV-induced free radical damage in fibroblast and keratinocyte cell culture lines, with a more pronounced effect on the former, in addition to demonstrating antioxidant properties [153].

Table 8.9 Profile snapshot of oxybenzone

Oxybenzone (Benzophenone 3, BP-3, 2 hydroxy 4 methoxy benzophenone), Fig. 8.18	
Approval status	Non-GRASE, Category III, in the USA, updated in the EU, Japan, Australia [25]
Mechanism of photoprotection	UV absorption [26]
Maximum concentration in a sunscreen	Up to 6% in the USA and in the EU, 10% in Australia, 5% in Japan [25, 30, 151] 0.5% when used for protection of products from oxidation damage [135]
Spectrum	UVB, UVA2, Partial UVA1, UVC [25, 26, 33, 151]
Systemic absorption	Significant, detected in human biological fluids [3]
Safety in pregnancy	Not recommended [30, 151, 152]
Ecological concerns	Significant [151]
Endocrine disruptor potential	Significant [151]
Sensitization potential	Significant [47, 107]
Photostability	Variable photodegradation [30, 33]
Areas of concern	Endocrine disruption, significant systemic absorption, contact dermatitis, photostability

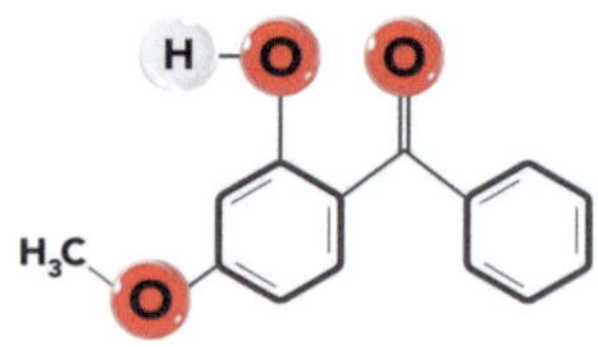

Fig. 8.18 Chemical structure of oxybenzone—benzophenone 3

In 2022, an EU Commission Regulation reduced the limit of benzophenone-3 in sunscreens, noting a potential risk to human health from the use of BP-3 in cosmetic products. Accordingly, the regulation ruled that BP-3 be allowed at a reduced concentration of 2.2%, from the earlier 6%, in body creams, propellant sprays, and pump sprays, provided that further BP-3 is not present in the same formulation for product protection. Since BP-3 is allowed up to 0.5% for the purpose of protecting the formulations, the upper limit was fixed at 1.7% for sunscreen body creams, propellant sprays, and pump sprays where BP-3 was used for product protection. The limit of 6% was retained for BP-3 as a UV filter in face cream, hand cream, and lipsticks [135].

While the photoprotective effects of BP-3 are due to its conversion to its keto-tautomer, this process also sets off the generation of toxic photoproducts with potential human toxicity in the form of endocrine disruption, allergic contact dermatitis, developmental, reproductive, and neurotoxicity [151]. Benzophenones were named Allergen of The Year 2014 [154], having accounted for up to 70% of all sunscreen allergies [151]. Among all active sunscreen ingredients currently in use, oxybenzone is considered to have the highest potential for allergic contact dermatitis and photoallergic contact dermatitis [107]. It is important to reiterate that oxybenzone and related benzophenones are present not only in sunscreens, but also in other personal care products as a product protection ingredient to reduce photooxidation. Interestingly, photoallergic contact dermatitis implying sensitization to this class of chemicals has been noted to occur from exposure to daily use articles such as magazine covers and T shirts and therefore the potential for contact dermatitis is significantly higher, than it would if benzophenone exposure was limited only to sunscreens [107, 155, 156].

In 2008, the centres for disease control and prevention (CDC) placed the level of benzophenone exposure in the general population at an extremely high 96.8% [157]. Since then, the presence of benzophenone in various human tissues has been demonstrated in multiple tissues, confirming the high level of skin penetration and systemic absorption [157, 158]. The smaller molecular size, high lipophilicity, and presence of this filter in multiple personal care products such as lipsticks, lip balms, moisturizers, body washes, hair sprays, and to enhance fragrance perception and for prevention of photo oxidation of products themselves, and even in textiles such as pantyhose contributes to the wide presence and thence, detection of this filter in human biological fluids, and in the marine ecosystem [26, 159].

A seminal study by Matta et al. demonstrated the systemic absorption of BP-3 leading to eventual blood levels at 500 times the permissible limit of 0.5 ng and in 10X concentrations compared to other UV filters in the absorption studies [90, 151]. Benzophenone-3, has been detected in urine samples in multiple studies, almost throughout the world, with concentrations as high as 22.98 ng/ml in North America, with the lowest values from Asia at 1.25 ng/ml [152]. The exposure in adolescents was found to be higher than that in adults and children, which is a potentially vulnerable phase in terms of endocrine development [152].

The proclivity of benzophenone-3 to systemic absorption is well established in in vitro permeation test (IVPT) tests, where BP-3 showed 20X higher penetration at

(>2000 ng/cm^2) compared to avobenzone and octocrylene. This is explained by the molecular size of the filters, BP-3 having the least molecular weight among the three filters weighing in at 228.2 daltons, in addition to its lipophilicity. Both avobenzone and octocrylene are larger than BP-3 by 36% and 58.4%, respectively. The skin penetration for lotion formulation was higher than that for spray [103]. Multiple researchers have studied the ready systemic absorption of oxybenzone. BP-3 and its major metabolite, benzophenone-1, has been demonstrated in urine, amniotic fluid, cord blood, placenta, breast milk, seminal plasma, and adipose tissue, demonstrating the systemic absorption and redistribution in different tissue compartments [146, 152, 160, 161]. Systemic absorption is noted to occur at a low level steady exposure from sources such as indoor air and dust, food, and textiles, with episodic, higher level peak exposures from sunscreens and cosmetics [152, 159]. There is a significant interpersonal variability in absorption of this filter, probably related to genetically driven variations in epidermal barrier function. Specifically, filaggrin loss-of-function mutations known to occur in 10% of individuals with European ancestry have been known to favour increased cutaneous penetration, with potentially higher chances of BP-3 related adverse events in this group [152, 162].

Benzophenones are able to bind to the pregnane X receptor and possess endocrine disrupting ability [114]. In 2018, the European Commission placed BP-3 in its priority list of potential endocrine disruptors [152]. Studies on uterine weight in rodents caused widespread public concern for BP-3 [116]. However, Wang et al. considered such levels of exposure as essentially unattainable, based on the extrapolative calculation from BP-3 concentrations used in this animal study, as relates to human exposure based on sunscreen use cases [163]. Subsequently, however, dermal exposure levels capable of causing increased lipid peroxidation and decreased antioxidant activity in rats were similar to levels of dermal exposure from the use of benzophenone in personal care products [151]. Furthermore, BP-3 and its main metabolite BP-1 have been shown to be oestrogenic in concentrations similar to peak concentrations in human plasma after sunscreen use [152]. BP-1 has a longer biological half-life and demonstrates higher in vitro oestrogenic potency [164]. Human observational studies point to a possible but variable risk for disruption of female hormone regulation, uterine fibroids, and endometriosis, with potential mid to long-term impact for heavy users of sunscreens and cosmetics [165–168]. BP-3 foetal exposure has been linked to Hirschsprung's disease [169–171]. Studies on the impact of BP-3 on sperm quality in men are not conclusive [162, 172]. BP-3 detection in urine has also been linked to the occurrence of osteoarthritis [131]. Benzophenone has recently been identified to be an obesogen, BP-3 being considered a full PPARγ agonist. Other benzophenones such as BP-4 have been noted to have partial agonist behaviour [143]. An association between higher BP-3 levels and lower thyroid hormones has been noted in several human studies [173, 174]. Maternal serum levels of BP-3 were found to be associated with raised triiodothyronine (T3) and tetraiodothyronine (T4) levels, particularly for mothers carrying male foetuses, while the T4 levels were found to be lower with increasing levels of BP-3, for mothers carrying female foetuses [175]. Overall, the significant impact of benzophenone-3 and its related compounds on endocrine disruption has been well established for humans, with impacts on the androgen, oestrogen, progesterone receptors, and other nuclear receptor targets as well [176].

The ecological impact of benzophenones has raised concern with these chemicals being identified in diverse waterbodies and in multiple marine species [177]. Interestingly, oxybenzone was found to be in higher concentrations in densely populated metropolitan areas with commercial and industrial waste water runoff, than in recreational locations in a study from the US [157]. Coral bleaching due to oxybenzone exposure has been well documented, as also with detection of this filter in larger vertebrate marine mammals like bottlenose dolphins [12, 178]. This led to a ban of sunscreens containing this filter in certain geographies [179], leading to some decline in the popularity and extensive use of BP-3 in sunscreens [151].

Further data on human and environmental safety will potentially decide the fate of this filter in terms of approval for continued use in sunscreens.

8.2.8 *Octisalate*

Octisalate is a weak UVB filter, with some action in the UVA2 spectrum Table 8.10, Fig. 8.19 [25]. It is structurally similar to padimate O and has a maximum absorption wavelength of 307 nm [89]. The increasing presence of this filter in sunscreens and other personal care products such as perfumes, makeup items, aftershave products, and face creams is reflected by the increasing detection of this chemical in human subjects, over the years, as reflected by a longitudinal evaluation from Germany [149, 180].

Octisalate is insoluble in water, and has a high substantivity, and therefore is a common filter in water-resistant sunscreens [30, 33]. Octisalate has been detected in

Table 8.10 Profile snapshot of octisalate

Octisalate (Ethylhexyl Salicylate, Octyl salicylate, EHS), Fig. 8.19	
Approval status	Non-GRASE, FDA Category III in the USA, approved in the EU, Australia, Japan
Mechanism of photoprotection	UV absorption [26, 27, 47]
Maximum concentration in a sunscreen	Up to 5% in the US, EU, and Australia, 10% in Japan [28–30, 44]
Spectrum	Weak UVB, Weak UVA2 [25, 28, 107]
Systemic absorption	Systemic absorption demonstrated in human studies [14, 90]
Safety in pregnancy	Not recommended [30]
Ecological concerns	Potential aquatic toxicity [117, 131]
Endocrine disruptor potential	Possible [180]
Sensitization potential	Potential cause of allergic and photoallergic contact dermatitis [107]
Photostability	Mostly photostable but photodegradation possibilities exist [30, 89]
Areas of concern	Lack of photostability, systemic absorption, ecotoxicity

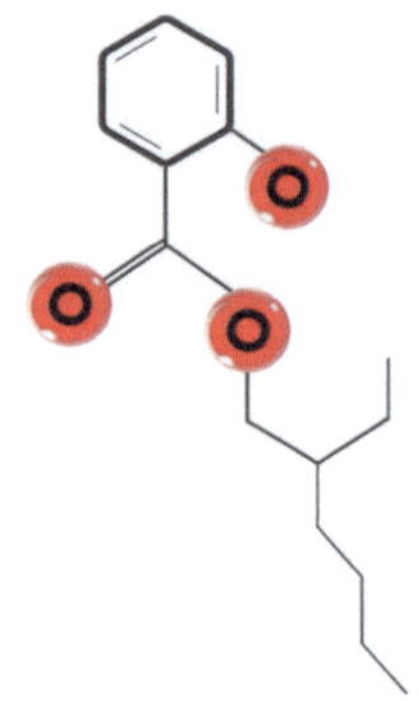

Fig. 8.19 Chemical structure of octisalate

waterways both as a result of recreational sunscreen use and from municipal and industrial wastewater drainage, though less commonly than the other organic filters such as octinoxate and octocrylene [105].

This UV filter is known to possess antiandrogenic properties, variable androgenic, oestrogenic, and antiestrogenic properties [180]. Significant systemic absorption has been demonstrated in sunscreens containing octisalate in aerosol spray, nonaerosol spray, and pump spray formats, with threshold levels being exceeded within 6 h of a single, maximal application of sunscreens containing octisalate [90]. The filter has also been detected in urine [126].

Octisalate has been reported to cause allergic and less commonly, photoallergic contact dermatitis, though some in vivo studies do not show irritation, phototoxic or photoallergic behaviour with this filter [107].

As more sunscreens are moving towards a comprehensive cover focusing on UVA, and visible light, the future importance of UVB only filters like octisalate, remains to be seen.

8.2.9 Homosalate

Homosalate, also called homomenthyl salicylate, is a lipophilic, low molecular weight UVB filter, with a maximum absorption wavelength of 306 nm Table 8.11, Fig. 8.20 [89, 181]. Homosalate is a very popular filter and is commonly used for increasing the water resistance of sunscreens, like octisalate [33]. Similar to BP-3, homosalate is allowed in concentrations up to 0.5% for UV protection of cosmetic products. However, the upper limit of 10% in sunscreens has been recently revised down to 7.34% by an EU Commission Regulation in November 2022 [85, 89] in nonspray and pump spray products meant for facial use, with a proposed further reduction to 1.4%, even which reduction may not be considered adequate for consumer safety [89, 182]. The photodegradation of homosalate is known to generate phototoxic by-products [26].

Table 8.11 Profile snapshot of homosalate

Homosalate (Homomenthyl salicylate, HS), Fig. 8.20	
Approval status	Non-GRASE, FDA Category III in the USA, approved in the EU, Australia, Japan [45]
Mechanism of photoprotection	UV absorption [26, 27, 47]
Maximum concentration in a sunscreen	15% in the USA and Australia, 10% in Japan, 7.34% in the EU [28–30, 44, 89]
Spectrum	UVB [25, 28, 107]
Systemic absorption	Systemic absorption demonstrated in human studies [14, 90]
Safety in pregnancy	Not recommended [30]
Ecological concerns	Potential aquatic toxicity [117, 131]
Endocrine disruptor potential	Exists [32, 85, 86]
Sensitization potential	Less likely than other organic filters [107]
Photostability	Mostly photostable but photodegradation possibilities exist [30, 89]
Areas of concern	Photodegradation, systemic absorption, endocrine disruption ecotoxicity

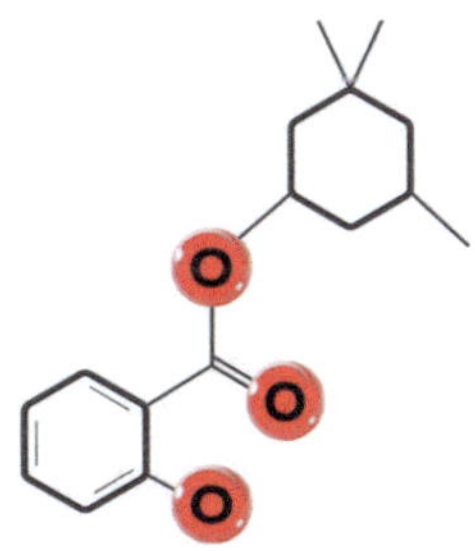

Fig. 8.20 Chemical structure of homosalate

Salicylate ingredients in sunscreens are generally considered to cause contact dermatitis. Surprisingly, homomenthyl salicylate does not have a significant level of allergic contact dermatitis, unlike other salicylates like butyl salicylate and octyl salicylate, which are known photosensitizers [107]. Also, homosalate is not a skin irritant, or a sensitiser, and is not expected to cause eye irritation [181]. However, homosalate is known to possess endocrine disrupting properties, acting on androgen, oestrogen, and progesterone receptors in humans [32]. Taking this into context for human health, a trophic magnification potential was identified for homosalate indicating food web biomagnification, a significant concern for humans, considering the identification of this filter in several aquatic organisms [108].

There has been a progressive limit restriction for the use of this filter in sunscreens, citing a lack of safety as seen above. With the advent of newer filters, the widespread use of this filter may be expected to contract over time.

8.2.10 *Padimate O*

Padimate O is a para-amino benzoic acid (PABA) ester, offering protection in the UVB range Table 8.12, Fig. 8.21. It is a lipophilic filter, with a peak absorption wavelength of 311 nm [89]. There is a concern that Padimate O may contribute to photocarcinogenesis due to its potential for increased mutagenicity on sun exposure [185]. OD-PABA is considered to be an important cause for photoallergic contact dermatitis attributed to sunscreens [107]. OD PABA exhibits potential endocrine disruptor behaviour, with Huang et al. identifying an earlier pubertal onset of breast development along with speeding up of the progression of pubic hair growth and breast development, in adolescent girls exposed to this filter [125].

Table 8.12 Profile snapshot of padimate O

Padimate O (ethylhexyl dimethyl PABA, octyl dimethyl PABA, OD- PABA), Fig. 8.21	
Approval status	Non-GRASE, FDA Category III in the USA, approved in the EU Australia, Japan [28, 30, 45]
Mechanism of photoprotection	UV absorption [89]
Maximum concentration in a sunscreen	8% in the US, EU, Australia and 10% in Japan [28, 183]
Spectrum	UVB [25]
Systemic absorption	Capable of cutaneous penetration [184], and potential organ toxicity [185]
Safety in pregnancy	Not recommended [30]
Ecological concerns	Exist, variable [27, 186]
Endocrine disruptor potential	Exists [32, 125]
Sensitization potential	Photoallergic and allergic contact dermatitis [107]
Photostability	Low photostability [89]
Areas of concern	Contact dermatitis, photounstable

Fig. 8.21 Chemical structure of padimate O

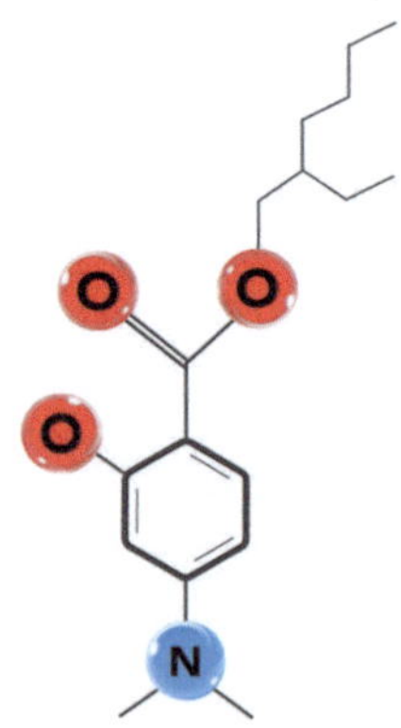

8.2.11 *Cinoxate*

This UVB filter is used less commonly in sunscreens nowadays, due to the current availability of more broad-spectrum agents. It is a cinnamic acid derivative and behaves similar to octinoxate with an absorption peak at 308 nm [89, 107]. However, compared to octinoxate, cinoxate is more water soluble and less lipophilic [89].

Cinoxate is considered to have a low allergenic potential, overall, though there are some reported cases of photoallergic contact dermatitis Table 8.13, Fig. 8.22 [107].

Table 8.13 Profile snapshot of cinoxate

Cinoxate (2-ethoxy ethyl 4-methoxycinnamate, 2 -EMC), Fig. 8.22	
Approval Status	Non-GRASE, FDA Category III in the USA, approved in Australia, Japan [28, 45]
Mechanism of photoprotection	UV absorption [30]
Maximum concentration in a sunscreen	3% in the USA and 6% in Australia (Sabzevari, January 2021), 5% in Japan [183]
Spectrum	UVB [25, 28, 107]
Systemic absorption	No current data
Safety in pregnancy	Not recommended [30]
Ecological concerns	Potential concerns [187]
Endocrine disruptor potential	No current data
Sensitization potential	Less likely than other organic filters, but occasional PACD cases have been reported [107]
Areas of concern	Not a commonly used UV filter at present

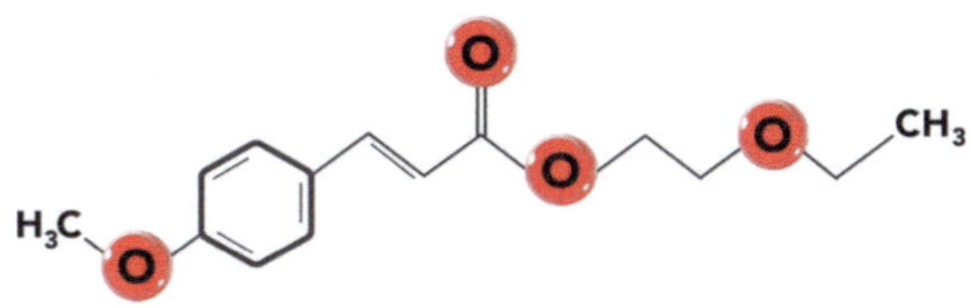

Fig. 8.22 Chemical structure of cinoxate

8.2.12 *Ensulizole*

Ensulizole absorbs UV predominantly in the UVB and UVA2 spectrum Table 8.14, Fig. 8.23, with an absorption peak at 310 nm, with an efficient absorption from 290 to 320 nm [89]. The salt of 2-phenylbenzimidazole-5-sulfonic acid, PBSA is used as a water soluble UV filter for use in aqueous sunscreen formulations, in the hydrophilic emulsion phase. Addition thus to another lipophilic filter enhances sunscreen performance while reducing input of each filter due to the synergistic increase achieved in the sun protection ability. To ensure stability of such emulsions, the final pH needs to be maintained above 7, since PBSA is poorly soluble in acidic media [188].

While ensulizole was noted to protect against the generation of CPDs on sun exposure, low level exposure stimulated the formation of oxidized guanine after UV exposure, along with generation of a variety of free radicals [89, 188]. The photoprotection ability of this filter is influenced by latitude, weather, and seasonal factors, which can promote variable photodegradation. This makes PBSA a relatively unreliable UV filter [89]. Incorporating the PBSA molecule into hydrophilic cyclodextrin derivatives increases the photostability and the steric stability of PBSA even in acidic sunscreen formulations, which are closer to the skin's pH [89, 188]. Melanova et al. described a novel way to stabilize PBSA in zinc aluminium intercalate fillers incorporated into polyurethane-acrylate lacquer with good photoprotection outcomes [189].

Table 8.14 Profile snapshot of ensulizole

Ensulizole (Phenylbenzimidazole sulfonic acid, PBSA), Fig. 8.23	
Approval status	Non-GRASE, Category III in the USA, approved in the EU, Japan, Australia [25, 30, 86]
Mechanism of photoprotection	UV absorption [26, 27]
Maximum concentration in a sunscreen	Up to 4% in the USA and Australia, 8% in the EU, and 3% in Japan [28–30, 44]
Spectrum	Partial UVA II, UVB [25]
Systemic absorption	No current data
Safety in pregnancy	Not recommended [30]
Ecological concerns	Has been detected in larger vertebrate aquatic animals [27].
Endocrine disruptor potential	No current data
Sensitization potential	Lower than other filters, but exists [107]
Photostability	Photodegradation potential, photooxidation, photostability dependent on climatic conditions [89]
Areas of concern	Photounstable, generation of free radicals on UV exposure

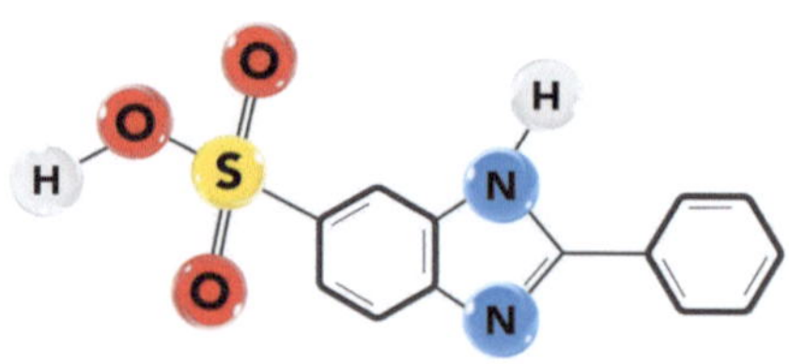

Fig. 8.23 Chemical structure of ensulizole

This filter is not known to have significant potential for allergenicity, however, some reports of photoallergic contact dermatitis do exist [107] A potential environmental impact exists, with this filter being detected in loggerhead turtles, similar to homosalate, octisalate, and BP-3 [27]. The ability of this filter to generate free radicals on sun exposure must be considered in the course of its photodegradation processes in aquatic environments [190].

8.2.13 Drometrizole Trisiloxane

Drometrizole is a lipophilic benzotriazole, with a broad-spectrum absorption across UVB and UVA Table 8.15, Fig. 8.24, with absorption maxima at 243, 298, 340 nm [192]. This filter is in wide use as a UV absorber and stabilizer in plastic, rubber, dye, detergent, adhesive, and agricultural industries among others [192]. It is used

Table 8.15 Profile snapshot of drometrizole trisiloxane

Drometrizole trisiloxane (DRT, Mexoryl XL, Silatriazole), Fig. 8.24	
Approval status	Not included in the OTC Monograph in the USA, approved in the EU, Canada, Japan, and Australia [87, 89]
Mechanism of photoprotection	UV absorption [27, 47]
Maximum concentration in a sunscreen	Up to 15% in the EU, and in Canada, 10% in Australia, 7% in Japan [89, 183, 191, 192]
Spectrum	Partial UVA1, UVA2, UVB [25, 28, 107]
Systemic absorption	Possible [192]
Safety in pregnancy	Not recommended [30]
Ecological concerns	Early concerns have been raised, significance unknown [193]
Endocrine disruptor potential	Not implicated [194]
Sensitization potential	Rare [195, 196]
Photostability	Photostable [33]
Areas of concern	Incomplete coverage, early ecological concerns

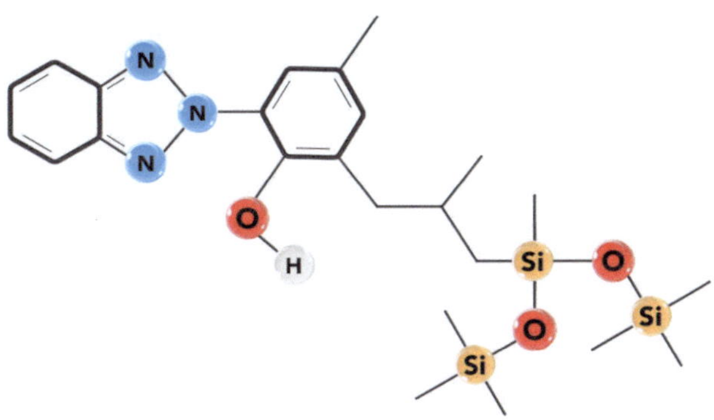

Fig. 8.24 Chemical structure of drometrizole trisiloxane

in non-colouring hair care products and nail care products as well at relatively low concentrations around 0.07%, but also up to 1% in such use cases. In sunscreens a higher concentration is allowed, up to 15% in the EU and Canada and 10% in Australia. In Japan, a concentration of up to 15% is allowed, but Korea recently revised the concentration down to 1% from 7% [183, 191]. It is not included in the Sunscreen OTC Monograph of the US FDA but is available in the USA through a Personal Care Products Council route [30]. Drometrizole is marketed as Mexoryl XL, exclusively for use in sunscreen brands owned by L'Oreal.

Moyal et al. observed that the combination of a lipophilic drometrizole and a hydrophilic ecamsule were synergistic and specifically useful to create sunscreens with complete spectral homeostasis or complete protection in the UVA and UVB domains [99]. In combination with other filters, drometrizole was found to help reduce the occurrence of UV-induced lesions in patients with SLE [197]. Mostly, the addition of drometrizole seems to be intended for enhancing UVA cover in sunscreens, while its solo use is evidently not possible due its limited spectral activity [196]. Drometrizole is considered to be photostable, however, has been known to undergo degradation on pH related stresses [89].

Being a relatively newer filter, restricted to a few brands, there is not a lot of data available on the endocrine impact and ecotoxicity of this filter. Rehfeld et al. observed drometrizole among the 'negative hits' sunscreen filters, those that were not known to have an impact on calcium signalling on human sperms, a process that underlies fertilization [194]. Allergic contact dermatitis has been rarely reported with the use of this filter, which more recently, has been linked to frontal fibrosing alopecia [195, 196]. Hughes et al. noted the lack of adequate patch testing kits to identify allergies related to the newer filters [196].

8.2.14 Dioxybenzone

BP-8 is an approved UV filter included in the FDA OTC Monograph Table 8.16, Fig. 8.25, though as non-GRASE, however, the use in commercial sunscreens is uncommon currently [47, 107]. Benzophenone-8 is one of the main metabolites of BP-3 and is considered potentially more toxic than the parent molecule [198]. However, BP-8 has been less commonly detected in human biological fluids and in the ecosystem, thus far, compared to BP-3. Placental presence of, and therefore foetal exposure to, BP-8 has been noted. Among the benzophenones found in human semen samples, the hierarchy of concern is for BP-3 first, followed by BP-1, and then BP-8 in terms of concentration [199].

Due to its low use in sunscreens, allergies to this filter are less commonly reported. However, allergic contact dermatitis has been rarely reported. Cross reactivity between benzophenones is not common [107].

Table 8.16 Profile snapshot of dioxybenzone

Dioxybenzone (Benzophenone-8, BP-8), Fig. 8.25	
Approval status	Non-GRASE, Category III in the USA, approved in Australia, and Japan [30, 45]
Mechanism of photoprotection	UV absorption
Maximum concentration in a sunscreen	3% in the USA and Australia [30]
Spectrum	Partial UVA1, UVA2, UVB [25]
Systemic absorption	No current data
Safety in pregnancy	Not recommended [30]
Ecological concerns	Significant, similar to BP-3 [198]
Endocrine disruptor potential	Potential exists, considered to be similar to benzophenone 3 [199]
Sensitization potential	Rare [107]
Photostability	Biodegradation potential exists [33]
Areas of concern	Systemic absorption

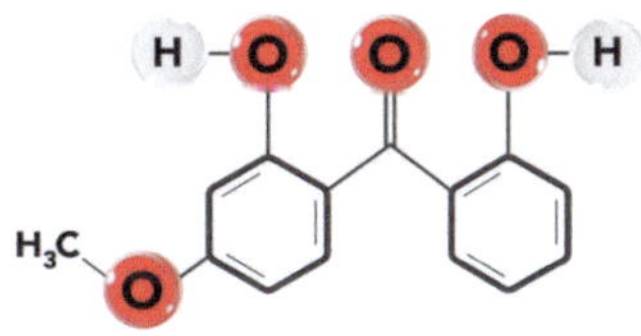

Fig. 8.25 Chemical structure of dioxybenzone

8.2.15 *Meradimate*

Menthyl anthranilate, or meradimate, is a lipophilic liquid, and hence is easily incorporated into formulations Table 8.17, Fig. 8.26. Therefore, meradimate is commonly used in lip balms, lipsticks, and moisturizers, primarily as a UVB filter. Its protection in the UVA spectrum is limited to 336 nm [89]. Meradimate is listed in the OTC Monograph and is approved in Australia and Canada, though it is used very uncommonly in Europe [47]. Rehfeld et al. reported the ability of meradimate among other UV filters to affect human sperm function behaving in a progesterone like manner [194]. Meradimate has been known to generate singlet oxygen species on photostimulation, hindering the efficient relaxation of electrons from their excited state [202]. This oxidant behaviour was found to be countered by the addition of antioxidants like tocopherol and similar vitamin E analogues [203]. While meradimate is not as photounstable as the other UVA filter avobenzone, it does require some level of stabilization itself. Both octocrylene and octinoxate were found to increase the photostability of meradimate, through triplet state quenching. The antagonistic interaction of octinoxate with avobenzone was not observed when combining meradimate with octinoxate [201]. Photoallergic contact dermatitis to meradimate has rarely been reported [107, 204].

Table 8.17 Profile snapshot of meradimate

Meradimate (Menthyl anthranilate), Fig. 8.26	
Approval status	Non-GRASE, Category III in the USA. Approved in Australia [30, 45]
Mechanism of photoprotection	UV absorption [30]
Maximum concentration	5% in the USA and Australia [28]
Spectrum	Partial UVA1, UVA2, weak UVB [24, 25, 30, 47]
Systemic absorption	No current data
Safety in pregnancy	Not recommended [30]
Ecological concerns	Unclear [200]
Endocrine disruptor potential	Progesterone mimicking behaviour reported [194]
Sensitization potential	Present [107]
Photostability	Photounstable [201]
Areas of concern	Endocrine disruption, free radical generation

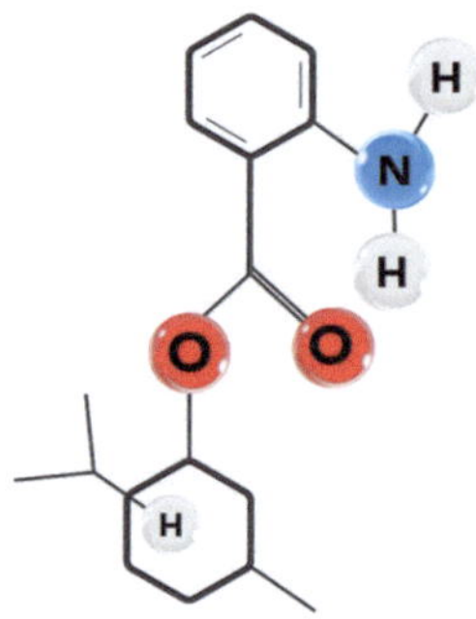

Fig. 8.26 Chemical structure of meradimate

8.2.16 *Methoxypropylamino Cyclohexenylidene Ethoxyethylcyanoacetate*

MCE-UVA1 filter is a new filter developed by L'Oreal Research and Innovation and approved for use in sunscreens up to a 3% concentration by the SCCS in 2019–20 Table 8.18, Fig. 8.27 [205–207]. This filter was developed to address the gap in UVA1 photoprotection and has been observed to protect against UV-induced pigmentation, photoageing, and immunosuppression [36, 208]. It belongs to a class of chemicals called cyclic merocyanine, which are characterized by a high absorption coefficient and provide significant photoprotection even at low concentrations as low as 1% [89, 209]. A lower concentration of the filter in the sunscreen translates to lesser systemic exposure, lesser absorption, and potentially, lesser impact on the ecosystem, though data to support these expectations are not available at this point in time. MCE is photo and thermostable [36]. This filter has not been formally approved by the US FDA yet.

Table 8.18 Profile snapshot of Methoxypropylamino Cyclohexenylidene Ethoxyethylcyanoacetate

Methoxypropylamino Cyclohexenylidene Ethoxyethylcyanoacetate, Mexoryl 400, MCE, Fig. 8.27	
Approval status	Approved in the EU in 2020 [47]
Mechanism of photoprotection	UV absorption [25]
Maximum concentration in a sunscreen	3% in the EU [56]
Spectrum	UVA1 [205]
Photostability	Stable [205]
Areas of concern	No clear data at present on systemic absorption, endocrine disruption, allergenic potential

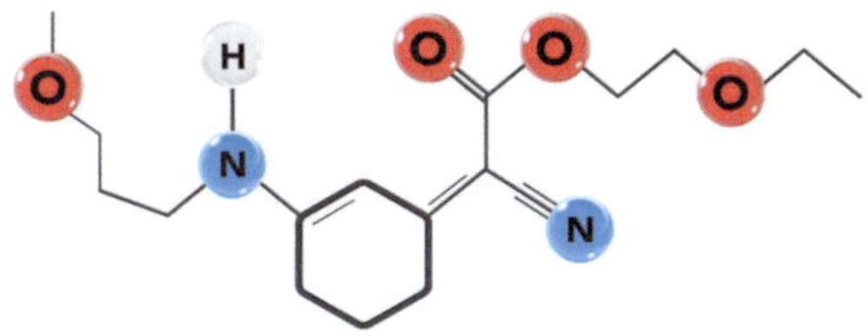

Fig. 8.27 Chemical structure of methoxypropylamino cycloxenylidene ethoxyethylcyanoactete

The SCCS cautions that as a secondary amine, MCE is susceptible to nitrosation and the formation of nitrosamines. Therefore, formulations with MCE should specifically be tailored to anticipate and prevent the generation of nitrosamines, which should be regulated to less than 50 ppb and should not include nitrosating substances. Also, this UV filter is not considered for formulations that have a risk of inhalation, such as sunscreen sprays [87, 206].

MCE has a peak absorption at 385 nm in the UVA1 spectrum with a critical wavelength of 389 nm and a potential coverage up to 400 nm [205]. Positioned as an antiageing sunscreen, Mexoryl 400 was found to have dermal protective properties acting through the inhibition of generation of matrix metalloproteinases and interleukins, 6 and 8. Overall this leads to lesser collagen breakdown by the UVA1 spectrum which is well able to penetrate up to the deep dermis [36, 205]. MCE has been tested to provide better photoprotection against ageing and pigmentation in skin types, II, III and IV, in a split face, split forearm study over 8 weeks [207].

More clarity on the long-term safety of this chemical filter is expected in the years to come.

8.2.17 *Sulizobenzone*

Compared to BP-3, sulizobenzone is less commonly used globally, and currently not in much use in Europe despite approval [47]. Sulisobenzone or BP-4 is the sulfonic acid derivative of BP-3 and is listed on the FDA OTC Monograph as non-GRASE, Category III Table 8.19, Fig. 8.28 [45]. It has two absorption peaks at

Table 8.19 Profile snapshot of sulizobenzone

Sulizobenzone (Benzophenone-4, BP-4, Escalol), Fig. 8.28	
Approval status	Non-GRASE, FDA Category III in the USA, approved in the EU, Australia, Japan [28]
Mechanism of photoprotection	UV absorption [25, 28, 107]
Maximum concentration in a sunscreen	Up to 10% in the USA, Japan, and Australia, 5% in the EU [28–30, 44]
Spectrum	Partial UVA1, UVB, UVA2 [25, 28, 107]
Systemic absorption	Detected in placental tissue with potential exposure to foetus [210]
Safety in pregnancy	Not recommended [30]
Ecological concerns	Present [211, 212]
Endocrine disruptor potential	Reported [199, 213]
Sensitization potential	Present [107, 214]
Photostability	Photostable [30]
Areas of concern	Impact on serum lipid biomarkers in humans [213]

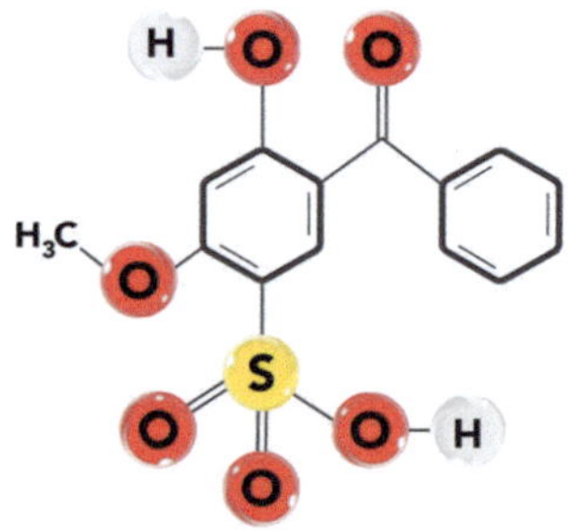

Fig. 8.28 Chemical structure of sulizobenzone

286 nm and 440 nm, giving it a fairly broad-spectrum coverage, similar to BP-3 [89]. The negative impact profile is also similar to that of BP-3.

Chen et al. identified BP-4 as a prominent player among other benzophenones in its ability to influence the level of selected target lipids suggesting endocrine disruptor potential. These lipids include docosahexaenoic acid, 18:0 phosphocholine, 18:0 phosphoethanolamine, D18:1–18:0 sphingomyelin and 18:1–18:1 diglycerol, present abundantly in the brain, and are considered as sensitive to endocrine disruption. In this study, BP-4 exposure, noted to be higher in women compared to men, was shown to influence the level of these functional lipids [213]. BP-4 has been detected in human placenta [210].

BP-4 is implicated in contact dermatitis along with BP-3, with a 8-year prevalence of patch test positivity at 2.1%. Compared to BP-3, patch test positivity was three times higher with BP-4, in contrast to earlier data where BP-4 was noted to display less allergenic potential compared to BP-3 [107]. Subjects with positive patch tests were more likely to have a history of hay fever, atopic dermatitis, and facial involvement in contact dermatitis. Co reactivity between the two benzophenones was found to be low [214].

8.2.18 *Enzacamene*

Enzacamene is predominantly a UVB filter, used at a concentration of 4% in sunscreens. It has an absorption max at 300 nm, and it is considered to be very photostable Table 8.20, Fig. 8.29 [88]. Recently, the use of this filter has been declining, and its related sunscreening compound 3- benzylidene camphor, 3 BC, has been banned in Europe [89]. Endocrine disruption potential on thyroid and oestrogen receptor targets have been documented, and there is a consideration to reduce the maximum permissible concentration in sunscreens [30]. Allergic and photoallergic contact dermatitis have been reported in the past, with cross reactivity to dexketoprofen and combined sensitivity with other sunscreen filters [219–222]. 4 MBC is considered a top priority environmental pollutant along with BP-3, with significant impact on marine life [215]. The related compound, benzylidene camphor sulfonic acid is a UVB filter allowed up to 6% in the EU, Australia and Japan. Camphor benzalkonium methosulfate or Mexoryl SO and polyacrylamidomethyl benzylidene camphor or Mexoryl SW are also approved in the EU, but less commonly used [89].

Table 8.20 Profile snapshot of enzacamene

Enzacamene (4-Methylbenzylidene camphor, 4 MBC), Fig. 8.29	
Approval status	Approved in the EU and Australia [28]
Mechanism of photoprotection	UV absorption
Maximum concentration in a sunscreen	4% in the EU, potential dose reduction likely, 4% in Australia
Spectrum	UVB and UVA2
Systemic absorption	Possible
Safety in pregnancy	Not recommended [30]
Ecological concerns	Environmental impact reported [215, 216]
Endocrine disruptor potential	Exists [89, 217]
Sensitization potential	Low, but possible [218]
Photostability	Stable
Areas of concern	Endocrine disruption, Ecotoxicity

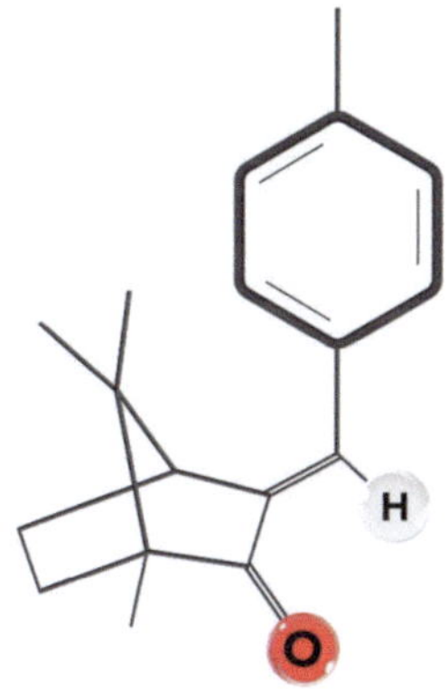

Fig. 8.29 Chemical structure of enzacamene

8.2.19 Bisdisulizole Disodium

Bisdisulizole sodium is a water soluble filter used for UVA protection in sunscreens and as a photostabilizer in cosmetics. It has a peak absorbance of 335 nm [30, 89], but also has coverage in the UVB spectrum Table 8.21, Fig. 8.30 [224]. It is commonly used in combinations with other filters due to the specific spectrum of protection. The potential for cutaneous penetration and systemic absorption is considered to be low due to its large particle size and lack of lipophilicity [89, 226]. Even though systemic absorption is low at 1%, this filter has been detected in human urine in experimental studies, where it was shown that the filter was eliminated from the body quickly [224, 225]. It is considered to be of low ecotoxic concern due to low potential for bioaccumulation [187]. An immediate reaction to this filter has been reported, potentially as a type I hypersensitivity reaction [227].

Table 8.21 Profile snapshot of bisdisulizole disodium

Bisdisulizole disodium, disodium phenyl dibenzimidazole tetrasulfonate, DPDT, Fig. 8.30	
Approval status	Approved in the EU and Australia [28]
Mechanism of photoprotection	UV absorption [25, 30]
Maximum concentration in a sunscreen	10% in the EU and Australia [25, 223]
Spectrum	Partial UVA1, UVA2, partial UVB [25, 30, 224]
Systemic absorption	Exists, but considered to be low, due to the large particle size [89, 225]
Safety in pregnancy	Not recommended [30]
Ecological concerns	Low concern [187]
Endocrine disruptor potential	No significant data at present
Sensitization potential	Low, but exists
Photostability	Stable [30]

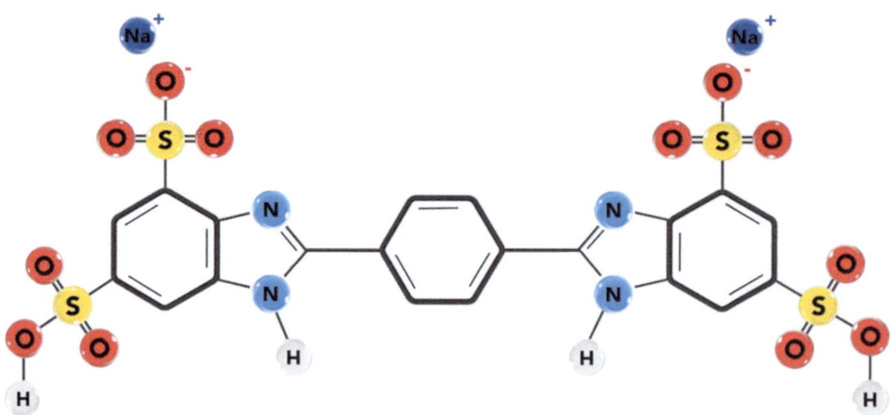

Fig. 8.30 Chemical structure of bisdisulizole disodium

8.2.20 Amiloxate

Amiloxate is a UVB filter belonging to the cinnamate family and has a maximum absorption wavelength of 308 nm Table 8.22, Fig. 8.31 [89]. Amiloxate was recently detected in children's urine, suggesting systemic absorption of this filter [126]. However, Haque et al. found that a sunscreen containing amiloxate, DHHB, and BEMT were found to not penetrate beyond 1.7 μm in the stratum corneum in a porcine model [230]. Amiloxate has been implicated along with other UV filters in the occurrence of irritant dermatitis, allergic and photoallergic contact dermatitis [229, 231]. Amiloxate is not expected to possess bioacumulation properties, although it is not readily biodegradable [187].

Table 8.22 Profile snapshot of amiloxate

Amiloxate (Isopentyl 4-methoxycinnamate, Isoamyl p-methoxycinnamate), Fig. 8.31	
Approval status	Approved in the EU and Australia [28]
Mechanism of photoprotection	UV absorption [30]
Maximum concentration in a sunscreen	10% in Australia, EU, MERCOSUR and ASEAN [2, 28]
Spectrum	Partial UVA2, UVB [25]
Systemic absorption	Reported [126]
Safety in pregnancy	Not recommended [30]
Ecological concerns	Potential risk, limited data [187]
Endocrine disruptor potential	Not reported as yet [228]
Sensitization potential	Reported [229]
Photostability	Relatively unstable [88]
Areas of concern	Photounstable, potential systemic absorption

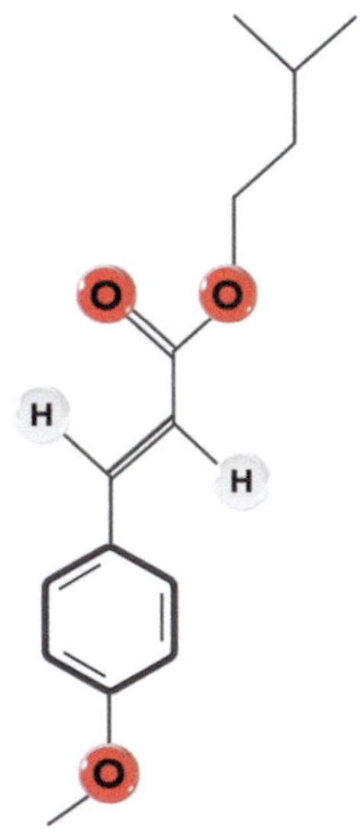

Fig. 8.31 Chemical structure of amiloxate

8.2.21 *Bemotrizinol*

Bemotrizinol is a newer broad spectrum, oil soluble sunscreen filter, expected to have lower penetration into viable skin due to its large molecular weight Table 8.23, Fig. 8.32. BEMT has better ability to integrate into the lipid phase, allowing elegant formulations in oil in water emulsions, compared to heavier water in oil emulsions, preferred to house most other UV filters [232]. Similar to octocrylene, BEMT is known to increase the photostability of sun filters, like avobenzone and octinoxate

Table 8.23 Profile snapshot of bemotrizinol

Bemotrizinol (bis-ethylhexyloxyphenol methoxyphenyl triazine, anisotriazine, BEMT Bemotrizinolum), Fig. 8.32	
Approval status	Approved in the EU, Canada, Japan, and Australia [25, 30]
Mechanism of photoprotection	UV absorption
Maximum concentration in a sunscreen	10% in EU and Australia, 6% in Canada, 3% in Japan [25, 28]
Spectrum	UVA1, UVA2, UVB [30]
Systemic absorption	Minimal skin penetration, below threshold systemic absorption [30, 232]
Safety in pregnancy	No data available [30]
Ecological concerns	Not expected to be ecotoxic, limited data [233]
Endocrine disruptor potential	No data at present
Sensitization potential	Rare [234, 235]
Photostability	Stable [89]
Areas of concern	Rare contact dermatitis

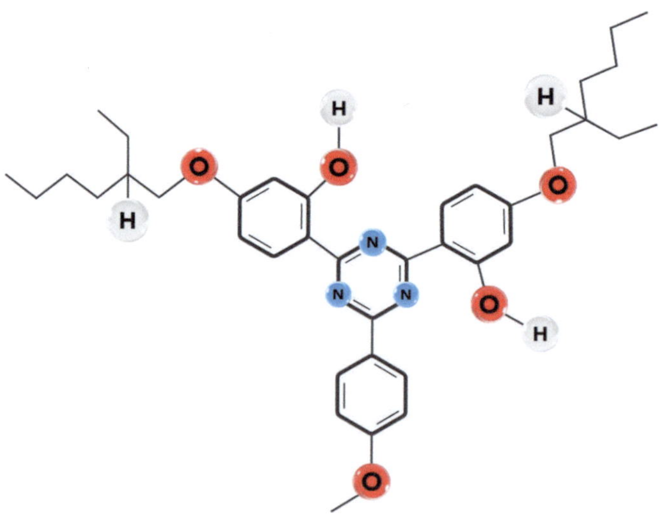

Fig. 8.32 Chemical structure of bemotrizinol

[236]. Bemotrizinol was found to increase photostability of sunscreen formulations containing retinyl palmitate along with chemical filters octocrylene, octinoxate, and benzophenone, and to a lesser extent of that containing, retinyl palmitate in combination with octocrylene, octinoxate and avobenzone. Furthermore, addition of bemotrizinol reduced the phototoxicity of the latter combination [237]. Bemotrizinol has an absorption max of 310 and 340 nm, with a critical wavelength of 373 nm.

As a filter awaiting the nod for inclusion into the OTC sunscreen monograph subject to the 2019 updated FDA GRAS guidelines, bemotrizinol was recently evaluated for systemic absorption using the in vitro skin permeation test (IVPT) and a pilot MusT pharmacokinetic evaluation, and is the first UV filter to be evaluated by the new absorption guidelines. For the maximum usage trial (MUsT), bemotrizinol was studied at a concentration of 6%, applied four times daily. While the filter was shown to penetrate the skin, based on its detection in the bloodstream, mean plasma levels were lesser than the FDA allowed threshold of 0.5 ng/ml [232]. This is in contrast to the seminal work done by Matta et al. which established the penetration and persistence of UV filters like avobenzone, oxybenzone, octocrylene, and ecamsule, in plasma levels significantly above the FDA cut off. BEMT is being considered for GRASE determination and inclusion at a concentration of 6% [232]. The molecular size of bemotrizinol and the relatively higher <E11>, twice that of bisoctrizole, allows for significant sun protection even with a lesser concentration of the filter, allowing for lesser systemic absorption and sunscreen load on the environment [226]. The skin penetration of bemotrizinol was found to be further reduced when formulated in nanostructured lipid carriers without any loss of photostability [89]. BEMT was found to not penetrate the skin to any significant extent when tested in sprayable sunscreen formulations along with other filters [238].

Due to its favourable safety profile and efficacy, along with a potential inclusion in the FDA OTC Monograph in the future, the popularity of BEMT has increased in recent years [89]. Bemotrizinol has not been known to have any teratogenic effects [228]. However, further data may be required before recommending sunscreens containing BEMT as safe in pregnancy. BEMT is considered to have a low potential for allergic reactions [89]. However, recent reports of rare contact dermatitis, in combination with other ingredients in products, have been published [234, 235]. In comparison to older generation filters, new generation filters such as BEMT, DHHB, EHT, and MBBT were found to not create significant biological effects on various organisms such as corals, crustaceans, fish, and algae [239, 240]. Sunscreen products containing only these four filters were found to be more eco-compatible compared to those that contained in addition, ethylhexyl salicylate [233]. Couteau et al. found bemotrizinol to be the most effective among currently available UV filters in the European Union based on in vitro comparison [83].

8.2.22 *Bisoctrizole*

Bisoctrizole is one of the two particulate organic filters, capable of protecting against UV both by absorption as well as scattering mechanisms, though the latter contributes to about 5% of the total effect Table 8.24, Fig. 8.33 [29]. Due to this

Table 8.24 Profile snapshot of bisoctrizole

Bisoctrizole (MBBT Methylene bis-benzotriazolyl tetramethylbutylphenol), Fig. 8.33	
Approval status	Approved in the EU, Australia, Japan, and Canada
Mechanism of photoprotection	UV absorption and scattering [30]
Maximum concentration in a sunscreen	Up to 10% of the active in the EU, Australia, Japan and 5% in Canada [28, 89]
Spectrum	UVA1, UVA2, UVB [30]
Systemic absorption	Low [89]
Safety in pregnancy	No data available [30]
Ecological concerns	Recent reports of concern, however, data is limited [233]
Endocrine disruptor potential	Potentially safe, limited data [89]
Sensitization potential	Exists [241, 242]
Photostability	Stable [88, 89]
Areas of concern	Allergic contact dermatitis, due to MBBT or other compounded moieties

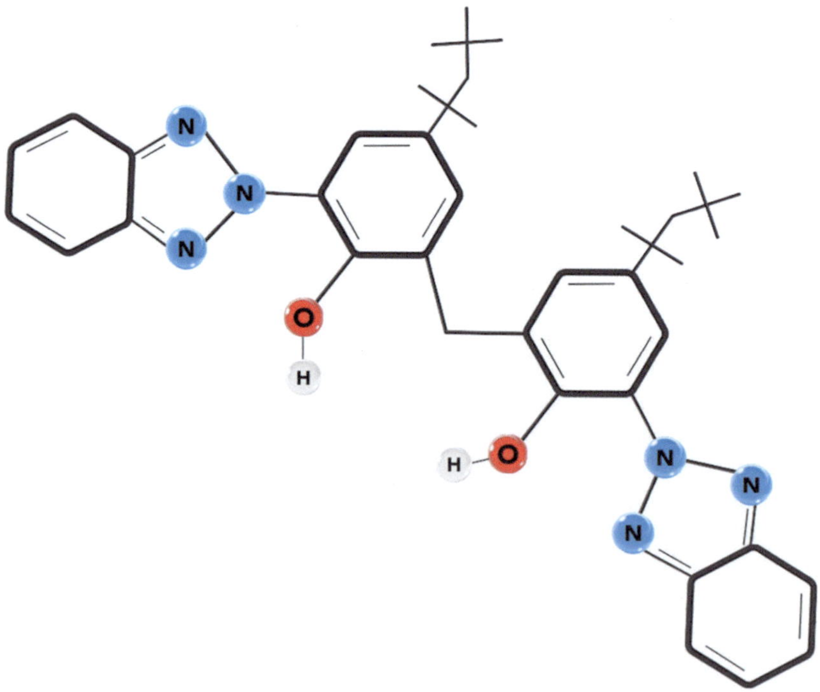

Fig. 8.33 Chemical structure of bisoctrizole

ability, bisoctrizole is able to significantly boost SPF of sunscreen formulations, beyond an additive effect [243]. Bisoctrizole is complexed with decyl glucoside, propylene glycol, xanthan gum and aqua, and marketed as Tinosorb M, as a 50% active aqueous dispersion [226]. The extinction coefficient depends on the particle size, with optimum absorption at a particle size of 80 nm [244]. Though the <E11> of MBBT at 480 (in water, 360 nm) is lesser compared to the triazone filters like BEMT and TBPT, MBBT has absorption peaks at 305 and 360 nm, yielding a critical wavelength of 380 nm for Tinosorb M [35, 226]. This provides the advantage of being able to easily yield a high level of UVA protection in sunscreens. As a large molecule, the systemic absorption of Tinosorb-M is expected to be low. Adlhart et al. demonstrated the cutaneous distribution of MBBT using tape stripping and Raman imaging and retrieved one-third of the filter from the skin's surface, another third from the superficial stratum corneum, while the deeper location of the remaining filter was attributed to the filter location in the skin's folds and furrows and along appendages [245]. Bisoctrizole was found to provide a better protection than bemotrizinol in protecting topical fluoroquinolone ointments against photodegradation [246].

The allergic contact dermatitis reported to Tinosorb-M is likely to some extent contributed by the decyl glucoside moiety [241, 242]. Bisoctrizole has also been implicated in chronic actinic dermatitis [247]. Patch testing for allergen identification is recommended to be performed with pure bisoctrizole to avoid confusion due to positive patch test reactions from cross reacting coingredients [248]. Similar to bemotrizinol, bisoctrizole is also expected to have a benevolent ecological profile [233]. However, recently bisoctrizole was found to be the main benzotriazole UV stabilizer contaminant in the Baltic sea, the impact of this is not clear at present [249]. No endocrine disruption potential has been reported thus far [89].

8.2.23 Phenylene Bis-Diphenyltriazine

Triasorb is a particulate filter similar to bisoctrizole, developed by Pierre Fabre Laboratoires, France Table 8.25, Fig. 8.34 [251]. The coverage of this filter is stated to extend from UVB through the UVA spectrum to the high energy visible light (HEVL) portion of the visible light spectrum. In the UV spectrum, the primary mode of photoprotection is as for a chemical sunscreen, namely absorption. In the HEVL range typically 400–450 nm, Triasorb acts in a hybrid way, both absorbing and reflecting sunlight, though the scattering effect is expected to be only around 5%. The filter has a critical wavelength of 388 nm [251].

This wide spectrum UV filter is insoluble in water and is neither hydrophilic nor lipophilic. In sunscreen formulations, the active ingredient is noted to be dispersed as aggregates with a particle size of >100 nm. As expected, human studies showed that dermal penetration was very limited both in normal and UV irradiated skin, probably attributable to the large molecular size of the active ingredient particular aggregates. Conceived as an alternative to older ultraviolet filters which showed a

Table 8.25 Profile snapshot of phenylene bis-diphenyltriazine

Phenylene bis-diphenyltriazine, Fig. 8.34	
Approval status	Approved in the EU, Australia, Japan, and Canada [250]
Mechanism of photoprotection	UV absorption and scattering [30]
Maximum concentration in a sunscreen	5% in the EU [25]
Spectrum	UVA1, UVA2, UVB, HEVL [251]
Systemic absorption	Anticipated to be minimal [252]
Safety in pregnancy	No data available [30]
Ecological concerns	Anticipated to be safe, minimal data availability
Endocrine disruptor potential	Anticipated to be safe, minimal data availability
Sensitization potential	No data available
Photostability	Stable [251]
Areas of concern	New filter, limited data availability

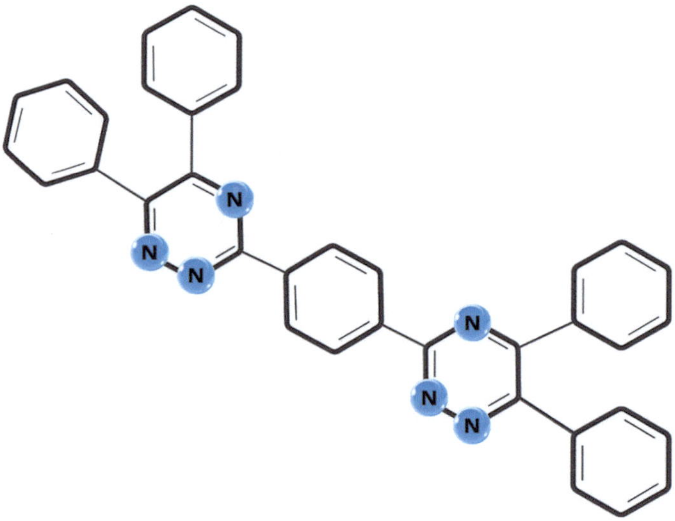

Fig. 8.34 Chemical structure of phenylene bis-diphenyltriazine

potential for binding to endocrine disruptors, Triasorb is considered to not have genotoxic, mutagenic, or endocrine disruptor potential, based on assessments thus far. Triasorb has also been evaluated on biological effective protection factors (BEPF), specifically its ability to protect against the generation of CPDs, 6–4PP (pyrimidine-pyrimidone 4,6 photoproducts) and their Dewar valence isomers (Dew) by up to 50% when used alone in formulations and by up to 90% when used along with bemotrizinol [251]. Triasorb was also found to protect the skin from blue light-induced oxidative damage. Levels of 8-hydroxy-2-deoxyguanosine (8OHdG) were found to be the same in skin protected from irradiation by the topical application of Triasorb as was nonirradiated skin. Published assessments of formulations containing this filter were not shown to be irritant to the eyes or the skin nor to be associated with skin sensitivity. Most importantly Triasorb demonstrated high photostability.

A patented SPF 50+ formulation, containing Triasorb along with bemotrizinol, DHHB, and ethylhexyl triazone, reduced the formation of 95% of measured DNA photoproducts, in protected versus sun exposed skin. A similar reduction was also noted in the occurrence of markers of DNA damage attributable to HEVL/blue light exposure. Near-infrared related lipid peroxidation was also shown to be reduced by this sunscreen formulation, though the filter itself was not demonstrated to have any significant protective benefit in the IR spectrum, while still performing better here, than bemotrizinol [252]. Clinical assessment of sunscreen formulations containing Triasorb were found to attenuate visible light-induced immediate pigmentation, with a higher performance noted for the formulation with added pigment [253]. Using multispectral imaging techniques in vivo, sunscreens containing this filter were found to have a good protection profile for HEVL [254]. Inhalation toxicity is not clearly ruled out, hence as per SCCS this ingredient is not recommended for spray formulations where there is a potential for inhalation. Scientific Committee on Consumer Safety, Opinion on the safety of cosmetic ingredients Phenylene Bis-Diphenyltriazine [250].

Though a relatively newer sunscreen with very limited data, the activity spectrum of this sunscreen is very attractive.

8.2.24 Diethylamino Hydroxybenzoyl Hexyl Benzoate (DHHB)

Diethylamino hydroxybenzoyl hexyl benzoate is a UVA filter which adds broad-spectrum coverage to sunscreen formulations Table 8.26, Fig. 8.35 [29]. It has a peak absorption wavelength of 354 nm and is highly photostable with good

Table 8.26 Profile snapshot of diethylamino hydroxybenzoyl hexyl benzoate

Diethylamino hydroxybenzoyl hexyl benzoate (DHHB), Fig. 8.35	
Approval status	Approved in the EU and Australia [25]
Mechanism of photoprotection	UV absorption [25]
Maximum concentration in a sunscreen	10% in the EU and Australia [25]
Spectrum	Partial UVA1, UVA2 [47]
Systemic absorption	Potentially low [230, 255]
Safety in pregnancy	Unknown [30]
Ecological concerns	Potentially low [233] Free radical generation on exposure to seawater
Endocrine disruptor potential	No data at present
Sensitization potential	Rare reports [256]
Photostability	Stable [89, 257]
Areas of concern	Free radical generation from swim sunscreens containing DHHB

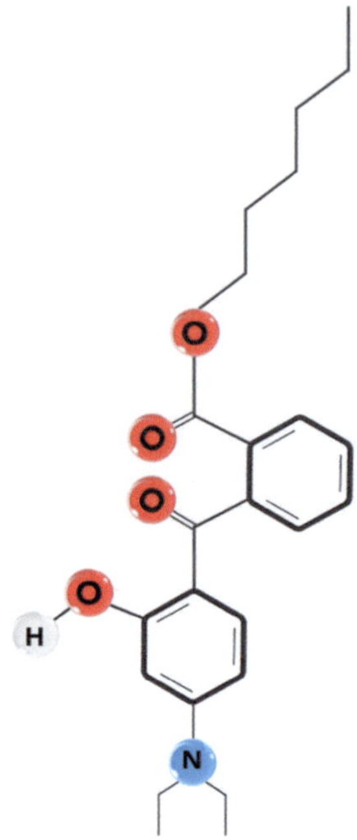

Fig. 8.35 Chemical structure of diethylamino hydroxybenzoyl hexyl benzoate (DHHB)

durability, showing only a 15% photodegradation at 6 h of extended irradiation [89, 257]. However, it tends to rapidly degrade in water and to promote the generation of transformation by-products with oxidative potential on sun exposure and exposure to chlorine in swimming pools. Therefore, DHHB is not a good candidate for swim sunscreens. The potential for such free radical generation by DHHB on exposure to water is higher for sea water than for tap water [258]. Improvement of this handicap has been possible with surfactant stabilization using surfactants like sodium dodecyl sulphate which enhanced the water solubility and reduced particle aggregation and photoexcitation. This is similar to the use of decyl glucoside surfactant stabilization of bisoctrizole [259]. Encapsulation of DHHB using silica mesoporous particles was found to increase the photostability, reduce free radical generation, and retention of the filter in the stratum corneum preventing deeper penetration into the skin [260]. DHHB was found to be more eco-friendly compared to the earlier generation UV filters like octinoxate [233]. This filter has been implicated in a case of sensitization resulting in frontal fibrosing alopecia and acquired dermal macular hyperpigmentation [256].

8.2.25 *Ethylhexyl Triazone*

EHT is a UVB filter with a peak absorption at 314 nm similar to OD PABA but has a higher absorbance capacity with an <E11> of 420 Table 8.27, Fig. 8.36 [35]. It is an oil soluble filter, used widely in sunscreens, however, its incorporation into water

Table 8.27 Profile snapshot of Ethylhexyl triazone

Ethylhexyl Triazone (EHT, Octyl Triazone, OT), Fig. 8.36	
Approval status	Approved in the EU, Australia, Japan [25]
Mechanism of photoprotection	UV absorption
Maximum concentration in a sunscreen	5% in the EU and Australia, 3% in Japan [47]
Spectrum	Partial UVA2, UVB [25]
Systemic absorption	Low, but possible [261]
Safety in pregnancy	Not recommended [30]
Ecological concerns	Not anticipated [262]
Endocrine disruptor potential	No data [228]
Sensitization potential	Rare [263]
Photostability	Photostable [89], small possibilities of photodegradation [264]
Areas of concern	Difficult to incorporate in water-based formulations [262]

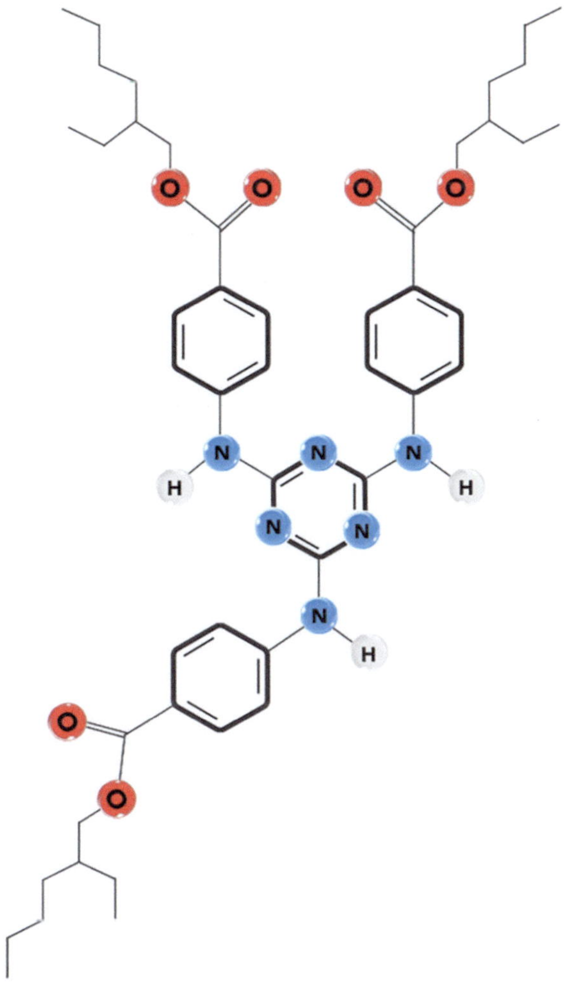

Fig. 8.36 Chemical structure of ethylhexyl triazone

soluble formulations is considered a challenge [262]. It is related to bemotrizinol and iscotrizinol.

The skin penetration is considered to be low, for this filter, due to its high molecular weight [89, 262]. At 823 Daltons, EHT is the second largest UV filter, by molecular weight, after polysilicone 15 [226]. The unencapsulated form demonstrates a diffusion of more than 20% in to the stratum corneum, which is nearly halved with the use of lipid microparticle encapsulation techniques [264]. The filter is considered to be stable itself and also to enhance the photostability of other filters in the formulation [265].

EHT is considered to be reef-safe and ecofriendly. Its oil solubility makes this filter a good candidate for water-resistant sunscreens [262]. EHT is a rare cause of contact dermatitis.

8.2.26 Tris Biphenyl Triazine

TBPT is an insoluble filter with a high absorbance in the UVB and UVA2 spectrum Table 8.28, Fig. 8.37. It is marketed as aqueous nanoparticulate dispersions, where the stipulations for the particles include a 98% purity, no coating, and a size more than 80 nm [89, 266]. Like other particulate filters, inorganic such as zinc or titanium or organic like MBBT, TBPT may also have some level of white cast perception. Accordingly, this filter may be expected to provide some benefit in the visible light spectrum [266]. The mode of preparation of the aqueous nanoparticle dispersions may have some influence on the shifting of the protection range into the longer wavelength regions [267]. Similar to zinc this filter may also produce a drying effect on the skin [268].

The <E11> of TBPT is 581, making it one of the most effective UV filters currently available. For every percentage of the filter, an SPF of 2, and a UVA-PF of 1 is enabled. It is also very photostable, retaining its photoprotection even after 2 h of

Table 8.28 Profile snapshot of Tris-biphenyl triazine

Tris-biphenyl triazine (TBT, TBPT), Fig. 8.37	
Approval status	Approved in the EU, Australia, Japan [25]
Mechanism of photoprotection	UV absorption and scattering [47]
Maximum concentration in a sunscreen	10% in the EU and Australia [25]
Spectrum	UVA2, UVB [25, 30]
Systemic absorption	Expected to be low [89]
Safety in pregnancy	No data [30]
Ecological concerns	No data
Endocrine disruptor potential	No data
Sensitization potential	Not known to possess irritant or allergic potential [47]
Photostability	Photostable [89]
Areas of concern	New filter with relatively less data

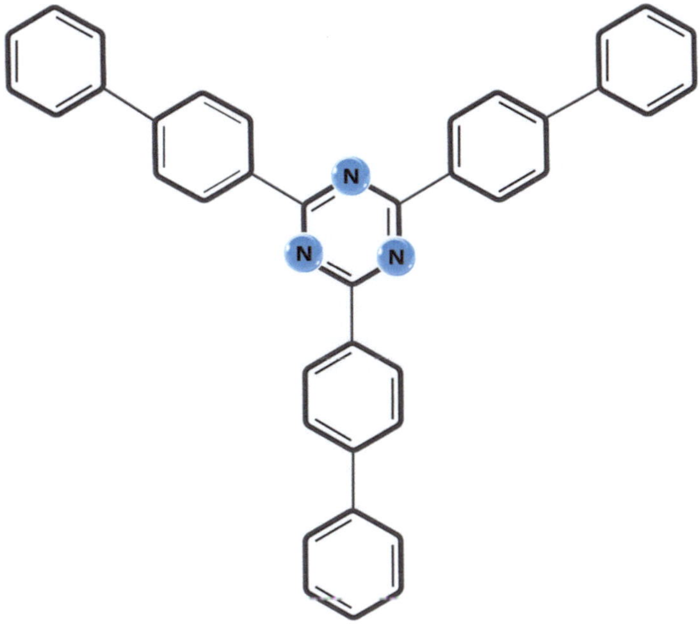

Fig. 8.37 Chemical structure of trisbiphenyl triazine

irradiation. Interestingly, this filter was also known to demonstrate anti-inflammatory benefits, a highly desirable effect in sunscreens, given the negative impact of chronic inflammation attributable to sun exposure [268].
Systemic absorption is expected to be low due to the large particle size and the lack of solubility [89].

8.2.27 *Iscotrizinol*

Iscotrizinol is one of the most photostable filters with a rate constant of decay at 0.00008 k/min Table 8.29, Fig. 8.38 [32]. As a filter with protection mainly in the UVB spectrum, and an absorption peak at 311 nm, iscotrizinol is mostly used in combinations to provide added photostability [269]. Iscotrizinol is expected to have no significant adverse effects on humans or the environment, based on the currently available data. This sunscreen has been noted to possess anti-inflammatory properties [89].

Table 8.29 Profile snapshot of iscotrizinol

Iscotrizinol (iscotriazine, diethylhexyl butamido triazone, DBT), Fig. 8.38	
Approval status	Approved in the EU, Australia, Japan [25]
Mechanism of photoprotection	UV absorption [47]
Maximum concentration in a sunscreen	10% in the EU and Australia, and 5% in Japan [25, 89]
Spectrum	UVB [25, 30, 47]
Systemic absorption	Expected to be low [89]
Safety in pregnancy	No data [30]
Ecological concerns	No data
Endocrine disruptor potential	Considered to have low ED potential [89]
Sensitization potential	Not known to possess irritant or allergic potential [89]
Photostability	Photostable [88, 89]
Areas of concern	Limited spectral coverage

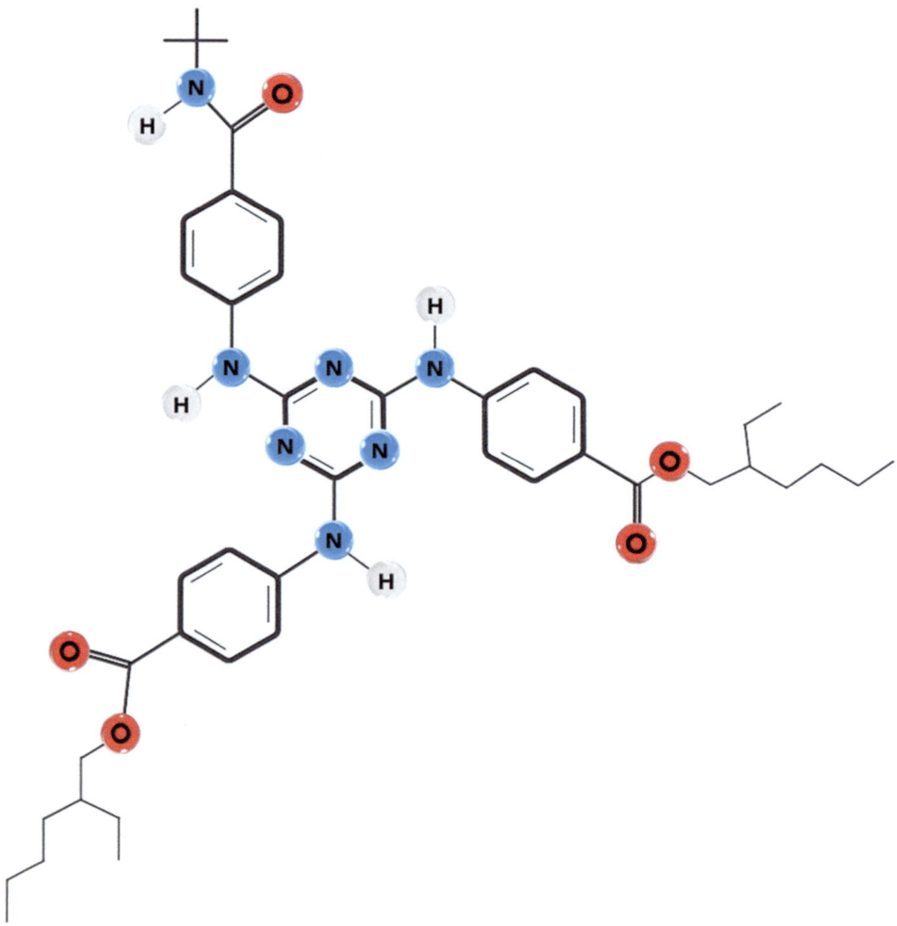

Fig. 8.38 Chemical structure of iscotrizinol

8.2.28 *Polysilicone 15*

Polysilicone 15 is an organic polymeric filter with predominant absorption in the UVB spectrum Table 8.30, Fig. 8.39. As a unique combination of silicones with organic filters, Polysilicone 15 is a liquid material composed of a polysiloxane backbone to which chromophores are attached, resulting in a large molecule of more than 6000 Daltons. The advantage of this larger size is the limited skin penetration, providing a factor of safety against systemic absorption. It has an absorption maximum of 315 nm and therefore must be used in combination with a UVA covering filter such as avobenzone. In such combinations, polysilicone 15 seems to provide photostability to the formulation [89]. Polysilicone is used in hair care products for improved feel and smoothness and can be used in pressurised hairsprays up to a concentration of 0.1%. This filter has been rarely implicated in allergic contact dermatitis, alone in sunscreen lip balms, and along with BEMT in a sunscreen cream [235, 270]. As a relatively new filter, limited data exists about the long term safety of this compound.

Table 8.30 Profile snapshot of polysilicone 15

Polysilicone 15 (dimethicodiethylbenzal, diethyl benzylidene malonate, dimethico diethyl benzalmalonate), Fig. 8.39	
Approval status	Approved in the EU, Australia, Japan [25]
Mechanism of photoprotection	UV absorption [47]
Maximum concentration in a sunscreen	10% in the EU and Australia and Japan [25, 89]
Spectrum	UVB, Partial UVA2 [25, 30, 47]
Systemic absorption	Expected to be low [89]
Safety in pregnancy	No data [30]
Ecological concerns	No data
Endocrine disruptor potential	Limited data
Sensitization potential	Rare
Photostability	Fairly photostable [88, 89]
Areas of concern	Limited spectral coverage

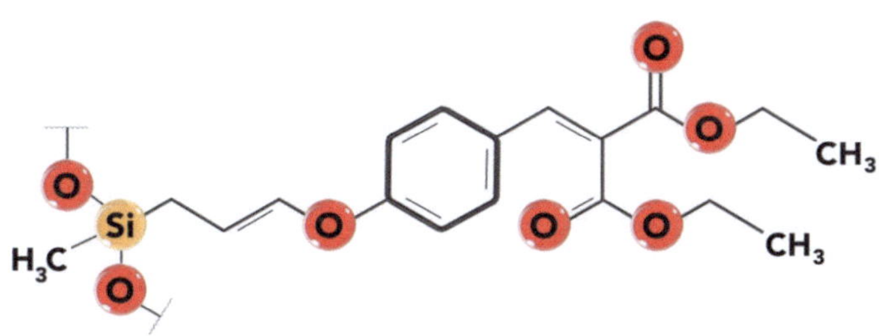

Fig. 8.39 Chemical structure of polysilicone 15

8.2.29 Bis-(Diethylaminohydroxybenzoyl Benzoyl) Piperazine

BDBP is a new chemical filter with specific extinction in the 350–425 nm, protecting against UVA-1, but importantly, the blue light spectrum, Table 8.31, Fig. 8.40 [36]. The efficacy of the protection is proportionate to the size of the particle, with smaller sized particles providing better absorption [89]. Also, neat HAA-299 is difficult to incorporate into formulations, and therefore milling or grinding along with dispersion using other structural ingredients may be required. This filter is considered for use both in its nano and non-nano forms, with a combined maximum concentration in a finished formulation of 10%. In both nano and non nano forms, the filter is considered insoluble, with low chances of skin penetration [89] by UVR at 385 and 405 nm, when combined with other filters [271]. Inhalational toxicity has been considered possible with the nanoform, and hence the product is not intended for applications which have a chance of inhalation [89]. The potential benefits and the possible adverse effect profile will likely be more clear, once the filter is widely available in commercial sunscreen formulation.

Table 8.31 Profile snapshot of Bis-(diethylaminohydroxybenzoyl benzoyl) piperazine

Bis-(diethylaminohydroxybenzoyl benzoyl) piperazine, BDBP, HAA -299, Fig. 8.40	
Approval status	Listed in EU, COMMISSION REGULATION, Annex VI of Regulation No 1223/2009 in 2022, and subsequently amended in COMMISSION REGULATION (EU) 2022/2195 [84, 85]
Mechanism of photoprotection	Absorption [89]
Maximum concentration in a sunscreen	10% in the EU (nano and non-nanoforms) [84, 85]
Spectrum	UVA [84, 85, 89]
Systemic absorption	Early studies show low skin penetration in humans [84]
Safety in pregnancy	No data as yet
Ecological concerns	No data as yet
Endocrine disruptor potential	No data as yet
Sensitization potential	No data as yet
Photostability	Probably stable [84]

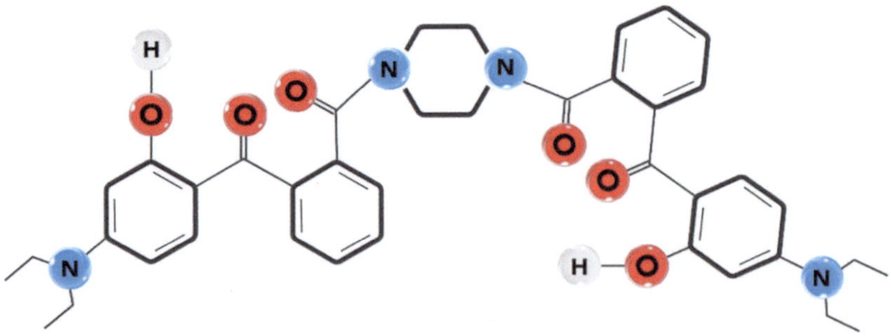

Fig. 8.40 Chemical structure of bis-(diethylaminohydroxybenzoyl bezoyl) piperazine

8.3 Newer Candidates

Sunscreen science is fast evolving, and newer filters are being developed. With safe-by-design and sustainable-by-design concepts in place, the new candidates are being tested for potential endocrine disruption, ecotoxicity, ease of formulation, and oxidation damage, providing hope for obtaining, cleaner and more efficient, safe photo protectors.

Working on 5-arylidene imidazolidine-2,4-dione derivatives, Popiol et al. published the development of two filters, diethyl 2,2′-((*Z*)-4-((*E*)-3-(4-methoxyphenyl) allylidene)-2,5-dioxoimidazolidine-1,3-diyl)diacetate and diethyl 2,2′-((*Z*)-4-(4-methoxybenzylidene) 2,5-dioxoimidazolidine-1,3-diyl)- diacetate, the former with a UVA-PF of 6.83 and the latter with an SPF of 3.07 with good stability and a safe profile [272]. Polonini et al. demonstrated the ability of quinoline derivatives to provide photoprotection with SPF from 2 to 11, and a UVA-PF from 2 to 7, with an ability to provide broad-spectrum protection based on the SPF: UVA-PF ratio [273]. Jesus et al. provide an elegant update of the newer molecules that are under development as potential sunscreen candidates both from synthetics and natural sources [108].

Sinapic acid esters are being looked at as potential replacements for octinoxate, with the sinapoyl malate moiety considered as a plant sunscreen. Compared to the acid, the ester has better photostability because even the cis product obtained from photoirradiation of sinapoyl malate still provides UV protection [274]. Xanthones are another class of chemicals with potential application in sunscreens [275].

Onion peel extracts upcycled from agricultural waste were found to provide UV protection to SPF values of 36.11 and 60.24 in non-encapsulated and microencapsulated versions complexed with cyclodextrin, respectively. While the stability of such formulations over time remains to be established, such eco-friendly options are hoped to replace synthetic UV filters or at least reduce the need for the latter compounds in higher concentration, when used in combination [276].

Another upcycled compound, lignin, is recently coming into importance due to its ability to provide significant photoprotection. Lignin is a natural, biodegradable polyphenolic polymer that binds cellulosic woody cells [277]. While the lignin extracts were found to have an SPF around 7-8, Zhou et al. achieved durable photoprotection with polydopamine grafted lignin (AL-PDA) with SPF values of 195.33 after 8 h of irradiation. Furthermore, these AL-PDA nanocapsules were found to not penetrate into the skin with good water resistance and antioxidant properties [278]. A spiropyran modified lignin variant was found to increase in SPF after 8 h of irradiation, creating a new paradigm concept–radiation-enhanced sunscreen performance [279]. Apart from providing UV protection by itself, lignin nanoparticles have been found to be sustainable carriers and photostabilizers of UV filters, avobenzone and octinoxate [280]. Even though lignins are considered very strong contenders for being considered as natural sunscreens, they have a potential handicap due to their dark colour. Lee et al. proposed overcoming this issue by iterated methods of extraction from specific sources, without losing efficacy [281].

Mycosporines-like amino acids (MAAs) are colourless UV absorbing compounds, produced by marine microorganisms, currently being explored as sustainable sunscreen alternatives. They demonstrate broad-spectrum UV absorption from 310 to 360 nm, but also at lower wavelengths, depending on the amino acid moieties in the MAA. They have significant bioactive capabilities such as anticancer, antioxidant, and anti-inflammatory benefits and are effective scavengers of free radicals [282]. Since the limited natural reserves of these MAAs can be a restraint on their wider application in sunscreens, alternative biosynthetic methods are currently being explored [283].

The skin is prone to oxidative damage, both from endogenous sources and extraneous factors, with outcomes such as photocarcinogenesis, photopigmentation, and photoageing [284]. In protecting against these outcomes, the addition of topical agents which can act against free radical damage is synergistic with the purpose of sunscreen use. In the case of chemical sunscreens which are not particularly photostable and tend to generate reactive photoproducts, the antioxidants may also work to quench the free radicals generated by the UV filter itself. Specifically, for the VL/IR part of the spectrum, which at this point, does not have many options other than pigments for photoprotection, addition of antioxidants to sunscreens may be a very promising strategy. While the inclusion of pigments is limited to 8%, antioxidants may be used in even higher concentrations to prevent free radical-induced damage and bring about measurable improvements in relevant measurements like the radical protection factor (RPF) [18]. Specifically for SOC, antioxidants in sunscreens are an effective way to address the significantly large problems of photopigmentation and aggravation of pigmentary conditions on sun exposure [284].

Several antioxidants have been considered and successfully included in sunscreens providing multifunctional benefits, discussed below. Jesus et al. evaluated the frequency of antioxidants used in sunscreen formulations and noted that Vitamin E, Vitamin C, oxothiazolidine, ferulic acid, ectoine, and niacinamide were the most widely used [285]. Apart from these are the polyphenols which include flavonoids such as silymarin, pycnogenol®, genistein, quercetin, equol, apigenin among other molecules, resveratrol, hydroxycinnamic acids, tea extracts, polypodium, pomegranate extracts, and carotenoids such as astaxanthin and lycopene are popular [269].

8.4 Vitamin E and Related Compounds

A naturally occurring fat soluble vitamin, tocopherol, Fig. 8.41 is well known for its strong antioxidant activity, free radical scavenging potential, and cytoprotective behaviour [285]. Tocopherol functions as a ‘chain breaker’ reducing lipid peroxidation of cellular targets and maintains dermal integrity by countering matrix metalloproteinases. However, this antioxidant is also known for its lack of thermo and photostability, which results in the generation of chromanoxyl radicals. The

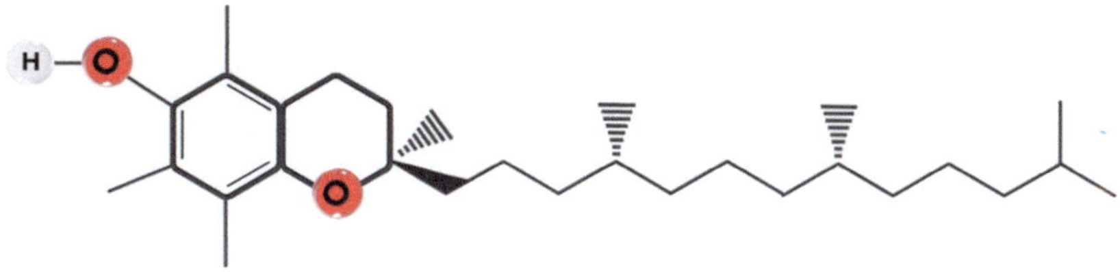

Fig. 8.41 Chemical structure of Vitamin E

provitamin forms possess better stability and solubility and are commonly used in sunscreen formulations. Furthermore, tocopherol exhibits superior performance when combined with synergistic antioxidants like Vitamin C and ferulic acid. On the other hand, pro-oxidant impacts of tocopherol have also been documented. Mixed tocopherols are used for formulation stability, and skin antioxidant benefits, tocopheryl acetate is used commonly in sunscreen products [285]. Addition of antioxidants like alpha tocopherol may help attenuate the ongoing DNA damage that continues in cells even after cessation of UV exposure [23].

8.5 Vitamin C

Vitamin C, Fig. 8.42, is the most abundant antioxidant in the human skin, which has the ability to neutralize free radicals and reduce the production of reactive oxygen species [284]. Despite a lack of stability, vitamin C has been studied to provide a host of benefits to the skin, including widely popular antipigmentation and antiaging benefits [286]. Furthermore, although some studies have established the benefit of oral vitamin C supplementation in protecting against sunburn, when used along with other antioxidants and topical sunscreen, the benefit of topical vitamin C in sunscreen formulations is subject to the stability of the UV filters themselves and other antioxidants in the final mix [287]. Since vitamin C itself is prone to photooxidation and peroxidation [288] either its combinations with other vitamins such as tocopherol or the use of vitamin C in stabilized forms may be considered [289].

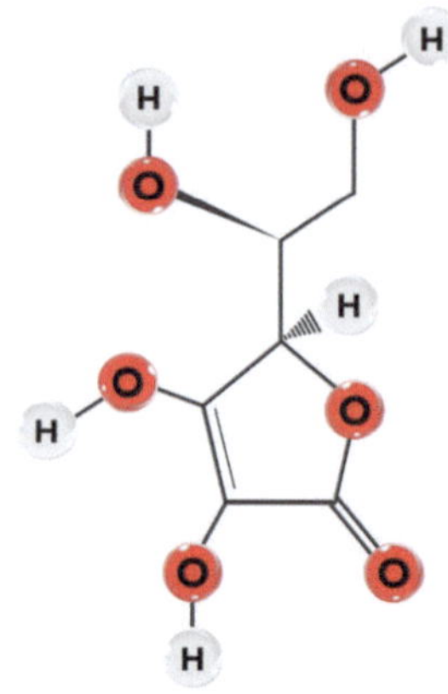

Fig. 8.42 Chemical structure of Vitamin C

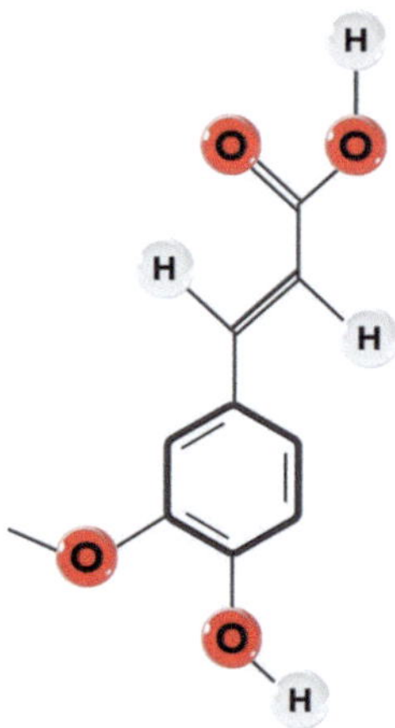

Fig. 8.43 Chemical structure of ferulic acid

8.6 Ferulic Acid

Ferulic acid, Fig. 8.43, is a phenol belonging to the hydroxycinnamic acid family, which occurs naturally in plant cell walls. It is a free radical scavenger, and additionally, inhibits enzymes that promote the generation of free radicals [284]. Ferulic acid has been demonstrated to reduce UV-induced oxidative damage and UV-induced erythema in combination with other antioxidants and UV filters [269]. Acting synergistically with the UV filters such as EHT and BEMT, ferulic acid boosted the SPF by 37% and the UVA-PF by 26% suggesting a broad-spectrum effect for the phenol [290]. Ferulic acid prevents melanogenesis by reducing the activity of tyrosinase, by inhibiting melanocyte proliferation, and by potentially reversing UVA-induced stimulation of pigmentation. Addition of ferulic acid to sunscreen formulations satisfies a multifunctional need for protecting against both sun exposure and the development of pigmentation [284].

Fig. 8.44 Chemical structure of oxothiazolidine

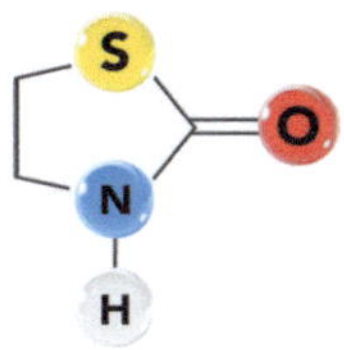

8.7 Oxothiazolidone

Oxothiazolidine, Fig. 8.44, is a novel antioxidant ingredient with an ability to protect the skin from oxidative damage induced by the UVA and IR spectrum of solar radiation, and thereby control cutaneous photodamage. On reaction with ROS, it generates taurine which provides the antioxidant photoprotective benefits. This compound has been documented to protect lipid peroxidation, enhance integrity of the dermo epidermal junction, promote skin barrier health, and prevent the breakdown of dermal collagen. Jesus et al. identified oxothiazolidone to be the third most common antioxidant in sunscreens, after vitamins C and E [285]. Oxothiazolidone is synergistic with delta tocopherol glucoside for photoprotection in sunscreens [291].

8.8 Ectoine

Ectoine, Fig. 8.45, is an amino acid obtained from extremophile marine organisms, with very high antioxidant free radical scavenging capacity [285]. Ectoine containing sunscreens have been studied to provide protection against polymorphic light eruption [292]. The protective action of ectoine has been noted to be effective in the UVA and the visible light spectrum [293]. Addition of ectoine to sunscreens was found to provide higher protection than sunscreen alone, in preventing UV-induced squalene oxidation, catalase activity, and generation of transurocanic acid [294].

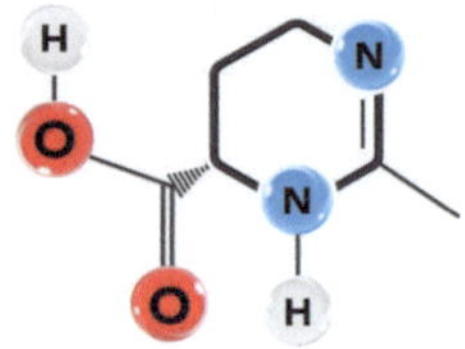

Fig. 8.45 Chemical structure of ectoine

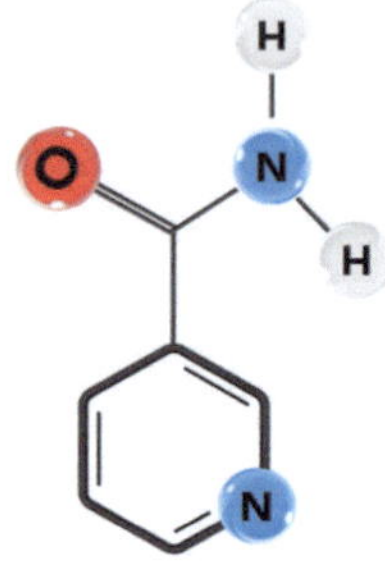

Fig. 8.46 Chemical structure of niacinamide

8.9 Niacinamide

A well-known skin active agent, niacinamide, Fig. 8.46, has been proven to improve dermatological conditions like acne, seborrheic dermatitis, and rosacea and also reduce skin pigmentation by preventing UV-induced melanosome transfer to keratinocytes [295]. Niacinamide has been used in sunscreens that claim to provide skin brightening effects along with other skin lightening agents like 4-n-butylresorcinol and glycyrrhizic acid derivatives and has been found useful to improve pigmentary conditions like melasma [296]. Recently, niacinamide coated zinc incorporated nanogels have been found to be effective in providing enhanced photoprotection [297].

8.10 Polyphenols and Plant Extracts

Polyphenols are plant derived bioactive substances, characterized by the presence of more than one phenol group per molecule, and are known to possess photoprotective properties [269]. Polyphenols include flavonoids, natural plant-based pigmented moieties with UV protection abilities, and which can only be added as supplements since the human body does not synthesize these agents. Incorporating these compounds into sunscreens has been noted to boost SPF, improve photostability, and increase the spectrum of coverage [298].

Different polyphenols absorb UV in different ranges, depending on the number of chromophores they possess. Flavonoids which contain two aromatic rings absorb light in two ranges 240–285 and 300–550 nm and can be valuable additions to sunscreens [298]. Due to their ability to act on sunburnt and photodamaged skin acting through downstream mediators, like in the case of genistein and pycnogenol, they are also an important presence in after-sun products. Genistein is also noted to have antitumourigenic benefits.

Currently quite popular, the flavonoid compound silymarin is obtained from the seeds of the milk thistle. Silymarin has been noted to protect against UV-induced DNA damage and immunosuppression, and therefore has chemoprotective ability, similar to genistein [299]. A 10% formulation of silymarin in an oil in water cream was noted to have an SPF of 9, going up to 14.1, when incorporated as solid lipid nanoparticles (SLN), with good stability [278]. Silymarin is compatible with both the inorganic filters, zinc oxide and titanium dioxide [278].

Similarly, green tea polyphenols have been shown to protect against UVB-induced local and systemic immune suppression in animal studies. Furthermore, the UVB-induced leukocyte infiltration of irradiated skin was also found to be inhibited by green tea polyphenols, along with the prevention of CPD generation [300]. While tea polyphenols, notably EGCG, epigallocatechin-3-gallate, inhibit UV mediated damage, they may not boost SPF significantly [278].

Quercetin is considered the most potent flavonoid in terms of its antioxidant potential. An oil in water sunscreen containing quercetin and hyaluronic acid was found to perform well with complete attenuation of UVB transmission and 85% attenuation of UVA rays [301]. Equol, an isoflavonoid and apigenin, a bioflavonoid, have been found to have potential benefits against the development of photocarcinogenesis [278].

Pycnogenol®, a proprietary extract of the French maritime pine bark, contains a number of phenolic and polyphenolic flavonoids, including monomeric and polymeric procyanidins which provide the compound with UV protection abilities. In aftersun applications, Pycnogenol® was found to reduce UV-induced inflammation, immunosuppression, and tumourigenesis [302]. Explant studies with Pycnogenol® show a protection against UVA, UVB, IR, and VL induced pigmentation [303].

Another potent antioxidant, resveratrol is a polyphenolic phytoalexin that has demonstrated chemopreventive properties in animal studies, with an ability to counter UV-induced tumour promotion and inflammation [278]. In addition to UV-induced oxidation damage, resveratrol also has the potential to counter zinc oxide nanoparticle-induced oxidative damage to aquatic organisms and need further exploration as a means of improving sunscreen performance while mitigating ecotoxicity [304] Along with beta carotene, the trans form of resveratrol was found to both increase the photostability and to decrease cutaneous penetration of sunscreens containing avobenzone among other filters [305] Polonini et al. characterized the photoprotective ability of resveratrol analogues as having a SPF ranging from 2 to 10 and a UVA-PF from 0 to 9 [305].

Polypodium leucotomos extracts which are rich in polyphenols, are used in both oral and topical forms for photoprotection [306] that Improves the UV Barrier Function and Immune Protection Capability of Sunscreen Formulations.). These extracts provide a booster effect in sunscreens and were found to counter UV-induced immunosuppression and barrier dysfunction. Addition of a proprietary *Polypodium leucotomos* extract, Fernblock® to UV filters increased both the SPF and the

UVA-PF levels of the formulations, along with improvement of biological protection factors such as contact hypersensitivity factor (CHF) and human immunoprotection factor (HIF) [307].

Pomegranate extracts have been shown to protect against UVB-induced DNA damage and against UVA-induced cytotoxicity in cell culture studies [269]. The anthocyanins, ellagitannins, and hydrolyzable tannins are considered to contribute to its photoprotective effects [308].

Other plant extracts such as sulphur rich broccoli extracts, caffeine, moss extracts, seaweed extracts, turmeric, sandalwood extracts, and carotenoids like lycopene are capable of significant sun protection in terms of SPF. However, their durability, and photostable protection needs to be further established before becoming mainstream UV filters [309].

8.11 Vegetable Oils with SPF

Vegetable oils have been known to possess some photoprotection effects, with several agents being able to demonstrate some SPF values. Due to the sensationalization on social media, such agents are used by consumers with the erroneous anticipation of ‘natural’ photoprotection. However, some of these agents do have merit and may benefit from incorporation in formulations which are designed to provide photostable protection, with a higher level of naturalness due to the addition of the vegetable agent.

In 2010, Kaur and Saraf evaluated the SPF values of vegetable oils using UV spectrophotometry with the Mansur mathematical model. Accordingly, they found that the SPF value of olive oil and coconut oil to be around 8, with values of 6,5,3, and 2 for castor oil, almond oil, mustard, and chaulmoogra oils and sesame oil, respectively. However, this has been criticized by later studies by Acsova et al. and Couteau et al., who did not concur with the high SPF levels claimed by Kaur et al., and also questioned the methodology that was used to arrive at the SPF, while concluding that fixed oils, essential oils, and related products demonstrate no significant photoprotective benefit in the UV spectrum [310, 311]. Acsova et al. noted that tamanu oil, a dark green vegetable oil rich in oleoresins, xanthones, steroids, and triterpenes may have some UVB protective effect, though there was disparity between the in vitro and in vivo SPF levels [311]. Similarly, Gause et al. noted that while there were some promising candidates like purple carrot extracts when used in high concentration, the UV blocking effect of most natural oils is insufficient to achieve significant photoprotection [312].

8.12 Novel Agents

8.12.1 Melanin

Biomimetic particles such as bacterial and fungal derived melanin are unique in their ability to provide broad-spectrum UV protection, similar to native melanin [306, 313]. Specifically, *Pseudomonas* spp. derived 5,6-dihydroxyindole-2-carboxylic acid (DHICA) melanins were found to behave similarly to eumelanin in terms of protection against UVB [314]. Microbial derived melanins are biocompatible agents with good stability and performance in sunscreen formulations and are specifically able to increase protection in the long UVA and HEVL spectrum, as shown by an increase in the critical wavelength of formulations on addition of melanin [315]. Presence of melanin in sunscreen formulations potentially decreases the amount of UV reaching the epidermal cell nuclei [316].

Melanins are well known free radical scavengers and possess significant anti-inflammatory effect due to their ability to inhibit lipoxygenase and cyclooxygenase pathways [316]. The antioxidant profile of these molecules was found to be similar to that of ascorbic acid, while being higher than that of reduced glutathione [314]. The anticancer benefit of natural melanin is well established for skin cancer, but more recently, biosynthesized melanin has also been found to have a potential role as an antitumour agent for internal malignancies [316].

An extension of the utility of melanin in sunscreens is the application of human hair derived particles, containing melanin. These particles have been known to boost SPF protection either solo or taking advantage of the porous structure of these particles, loaded with antioxidants or sunscreen filters such as octocrylene [317].

8.12.2 Enzymes

The use of DNA repair enzymes in sunscreens is considered as a form of active photoprotection, similar to that of antioxidants. This concept is to be understood in comparison to the passive photoprotection provided by UV filters alone, where there is no further scope for photoprotection after the sun damage has occurred. DNA repair enzymes such as T4 endonuclease, photolyase, and 8-oxoguanine glycosylase have been found to enhance DNA repair mechanisms in the skin resulting in improved tumour surveillance with both reduced tumourigenesis and tumour progression, and reduction of photoageing [80].

Immediately after solar-induced DNA damage, kinases responsive to such damage increase the release of signalling molecules that modulate the immune system, by inducing expression of the appropriate genes. Such alarm responses following repetitive DNA damage result in continued inflammatory responses leading to eventual photoageing and skin cancer. By reducing the cellular damage and mitigating the oxidative distress responses, DNA repair enzymes can promote healthier skin [318].

Photolyases, specifically, are enzymes that are able to repair DNA damage, typically CPD. CPDs are produced by both UVA and UVB and a lack of adequate DNA repair is considered the starting point of long-term UV damage and photocarcinogenesis. As flavoproteins, photolyases absorb UVR and use the energy to break down CPDs, thus adding to the active photoprotective action of sunscreens and antioxidants [24]. Apart from these CPD photolyases, 6-4 photolyases are also exist that are able to repair 6-4 photoproducts [319]. In addition to promoting DNA repair, photolyases are also able to reduce expression of MMP-1 in both the dermis and the epidermis. CPD photolyases have been studied in liposomal encapsulations for delivery of the enzyme into the viable epidermis. Proof of concept studies are available to support the role of photolyases in reducing UVB-induced CPD generation and a few open label studies are available that support a beneficial role of photolyases in a zinc mineral sunscreen along with antioxidants and peptides [318]. After sun lotions containing photolyases obtained from *Anacystis nidulans* and endonucleases obtained from *Micrococcus luteus* were found to be beneficial in preventing PLE when used along with a 30SPF sunscreen [320].

Similar to photolyases, T4 endonucleases act to repair damaged DNA by screening for, and then cleavage of the damaged portion. They also have the ability to promote skin regeneration, reduction of MMP-1 in the skin, maintenance of ECM integrity and skin reconstruction, and thus contribute to the prevention of photoageing. Like photolyases, T4 endonucleases also require a liposome-based drug delivery for optimum performance. Overall, DNA repair enzymes have the potential to protect the skin both against photocarcinogenesis and photoageing [318, 321].

Recently, Alvares et al. compared sunscreens with and without photolyases against the end points of forearm skin ageing and reduction in actinic keratosis and found that there was no difference between the two arms of the study, indicating no potential advantage for the addition of photolyases. Furthermore, this study found that antioxidants could reduce actinic keratosis compared to placebo [322]. This was in agreement with a systematic review by Luze et al. who highlighted the need for further research to demonstrate efficacy before DNA repair enzymes can be considered as mainstream ingredients for functional sunscreens [319]. Interestingly, photolyases may not be effective when combined with sunscreens specifically designed to protect against visible light with inclusion of blue light blocking active agents, since these enzymes are activated to perform by exposure to light [323].

Topical sun protection has evolved significantly over the years, and it could be said that innovations in the last decade have been instrumental in establishing state of the art practices in sunscreen science. As the momentum continues in the direction of safety along with efficacy, the coming years can be said to be the golden era of cutaneous photoprotection.

8.13 Chapter Summary

Several UV filters are currently available to engineer the development of sunscreens with full spectrum coverage. Chemical sunscreens predominantly protect against sunlight by absorbing UV energy, while physical sunscreens are considered to protect by scattering or reflecting light. However, as seen with the detailing for each filter, with smaller particle size, absorption is an important mechanism for UV protection even for mineral filters, and particulate chemical filters are able to scatter light in addition to absorption. This chapter gives an overview of the different UV filters currently in use in sunscreens and provides relevant clinical information on the protection metrics and the impact of the filter on human and environmental health.

References

1. Pirotta G. Sunscreen regulation in the world. In: Handbook of environmental chemistry, vol. 94. Cham: Springer; 2020. p. 15 35.
2. Daly S, Ouyang H, Maitra P. Chemistry of sunscreens. Principles and practice of photoprotection [Internet]. 2016 Jan 1 [cited 2024 Apr 3];159–78. Available from: https://www.researchgate.net/publication/300329558_Chemistry_of_Sunscreens
3. Ruszkiewicz JA, Pinkas A, Ferrer B, Peres T V., Tsatsakis A, Aschner M. Neurotoxic effect of active ingredients in sunscreen products, a contemporary review. Toxicol Rep [Internet]. 2017 [cited 2024 Apr 2];4:245–59. Available from: https://pubmed.ncbi.nlm.nih.gov/28959646/
4. United States Adopted Names naming guidelines | American Medical Association [Internet]. [cited 2024 Apr 2]. Available from: https://www.ama-assn.org/about/united-states-adopted-names/united-states-adopted-names-naming-guidelines
5. https://downloads.regulations.gov/FDA-2021-P-0497-0001/attachment_1.pdf—Google Search [Internet]. [cited 2024 Apr 6]. Available from: https://www.google.com/search?q=https%3A%2F%2Fdownloads.regulations.gov%2FFDA-2021-P-0497-0001%2Fattachment_1.pdf&sca_esv=bb28bdcaf5fa39f0&ei=WyERZtqZMIO5seMPsbGO6AI&ved=0ahUKEwias4uarq2FAxWDXGwGHbGYAy0Q4dUDCBA&uact=5&oq=https%3A%2F%2Fdownloads.regulations.gov%2FFDA-2021-P-0497-0001%2Fattachment_1.pdf&gs_lp=Egxnd3-Mtd2l6LXNlcnAiR2h0dHBzOi8vZG93bmxvYWRzLnJlZ3VsYXRpb25zLmdvdi9GREEtMjAyMS1QLTA0OTctMDAwMS9hdHRhY2htZW50XzEucGRmSABQAFgAcAB4A-JABAJgBAKABAKoBALgBA8gBAPgBAZgCAKACAJgDAJIHAKAHAA&sclient=gws-wiz-serp
6. Nicole W. Skin protection dilemma: testing detects benzene in some sun care products. Environ Health Perspect [Internet]. 2022 May 1 [cited 2024 Apr 2];130(5). Available from: https://www.ncbi.nlm.nih.gov/pmc/articles/PMC9113541/
7. Conte S, Lagacé F, Netchiporouk E, Sasseville D, Litvinov I V. Common personal care products contaminated with benzene, a known human carcinogen, identified recently. J Cutan Med Surg [Internet]. 2022 Jul 1 [cited 2024 Apr 2];26(4):430–1. Available from: https://pubmed.ncbi.nlm.nih.gov/35220803/
8. Yeoman AM, Shaw M, Ward M, Ives L, Andrews SJ, Lewis AC. Gas phase emissions of volatile organic compounds arising from the application of sunscreens. Int J Environ Res Public Health [Internet]. 2023 Jun 1 [cited 2024 Mar 16];20(11):5944. Available from: https://www.mdpi.com/1660-4601/20/11/5944/htm

9. Pal VK, Lee S, Kannan K. Occurrence of and dermal exposure to benzene, toluene and styrene in sunscreen products marketed in the United States. Sci Total Environ [Internet]. 2023 Aug 25 [cited 2024 Apr 2];888. Available from: https://pubmed.ncbi.nlm.nih.gov/37201845/
10. Pal VK, Lee S, Naidu M, Lee C, Kannan K. Occurrence of and dermal exposure to benzene, toluene and styrene found in hand sanitizers from the United States. Environ Int. 2022;167:107449.
11. Hudspeth A, Zenzola N, Kucera K, Wu Q, Light D. Independent sun care product screening for benzene contamination. Environ Health Perspect [Internet]. 2022 Mar 1 [cited 2024 Apr 2];130(3). Available from: https://pubmed.ncbi.nlm.nih.gov/35349356/
12. Shetty N, Schalka S, Lim HW, Mohammad TF. The effects of UV filters on health and the environment. Photochem Photobiol Sci [Internet]. 2023 Oct 1 [cited 2024 Mar 3];22(10):2463–71. Available from: https://pubmed.ncbi.nlm.nih.gov/37344707/
13. Schneider SL, Lim HW. A review of inorganic UV filters zinc oxide and titanium dioxide. Photodermatol Photoimmunol Photomed [Internet]. 2019 Nov 1 [cited 2024 Mar 11];35(6):442–6. Available from: https://pubmed.ncbi.nlm.nih.gov/30444533/
14. Matta MK, Zusterzeel R, Pilli NR, Patel V, Volpe DA, Florian J, et al. Effect of sunscreen application under maximal use conditions on plasma concentration of sunscreen active ingredients: a randomized clinical trial. JAMA—J Am Med Assoc [Internet]. 2019 Jun 4 [cited 2024 Apr 2];321(21):2082–91. Available from: https://www.cosmeticsandtoiletries.com/formulas-products/sun-care/article/21835866/feel-and-function-attuning-attributes-in-mineral-sunscreens
15. Feel and function: attuning attributes in mineral sunscreens | cosmetics & toiletries [Internet]. [cited 2024 Apr 2]. Available from: https://www.cosmeticsandtoiletries.com/formulas-products/sun-care/article/21835866/feel-and-function-attuning-attributes-in-mineral-sunscreens
16. Solish N, Humphrey S, Waller B, Vanderveen S. Photoprotection with mineral-based sunscreens. Dermatol Surg [Internet]. 2020 Dec 1 [cited 2024 Apr 2];46(12):1508–13. Available from: https://pubmed.ncbi.nlm.nih.gov/32541340/
17. Cole C, Shyr T, Ou-Yang H. Metal oxide sunscreens protect skin by absorption, not by reflection or scattering. Photodermatol Photoimmunol Photomed [Internet]. 2016 Jan 1 [cited 2024 Apr 2];32(1):5–10. Available from: https://pubmed.ncbi.nlm.nih.gov/26431814/
18. Zastrow L, Meinke MC, Albrecht S, Patzelt A, Lademann J. From UV protection to protection in the whole spectral range of the solar radiation: new aspects of sunscreen development. Adv Exp Med Biol [Internet]. 2017 [cited 2024 Mar 3];996:311–8. Available from: https://pubmed.ncbi.nlm.nih.gov/29124711/
19. Mascarenhas-Melo F, Mathur A, Murugappan S, Sharma A, Tanwar K, Dua K, et al. Inorganic nanoparticles in dermopharmaceutical and cosmetic products: properties, formulation development, toxicity, and regulatory issues. Eur J Pharm Biopharm [Internet]. 2023 Nov 1 [cited 2024 Apr 2];192:25–40. Available from: https://pubmed.ncbi.nlm.nih.gov/37739239/
20. Wang SQ, Tooley IR. Photoprotection in the era of nanotechnology. Semin Cutan Med Surg [Internet]. 2011 [cited 2024 Apr 2];30(4):210–3. Available from: https://pubmed.ncbi.nlm.nih.gov/22123418/
21. Addor FAS anna, Barcaui CB, Gomes EE, Lupi O, Marçon CR, Miot HA. Sunscreen lotions in the dermatological prescription: review of concepts and controversies. An Bras Dermatol [Internet]. 2022 Mar 1 [cited 2024 Apr 2];97(2):204–22. Available from: https://pubmed.ncbi.nlm.nih.gov/35039207/
22. Nash JF, Tanner PR. Relevance of UV filter/sunscreen product photostability to human safety. Photodermatol Photoimmunol Photomed [Internet]. 2014 [cited 2024 Mar 16];30(2–3):88–95. Available from: https://pubmed.ncbi.nlm.nih.gov/24433498/
23. Cutaneous photoprotection: a review of the current status and evolving strategies—PubMed [Internet]. [cited 2024 Mar 26]. Available from: https://pubmed.ncbi.nlm.nih.gov/32226337/
24. Guan LL, Lim HW, Mohammad TF. Sunscreens and photoaging: a review of current literature. Am J Clin Dermatol [Internet]. 2021 Nov 1 [cited 2024 Mar 16];22(6):819–28. Available from: https://pubmed.ncbi.nlm.nih.gov/34387824/

25. Chavda VP, Acharya D, Hala V, Daware S, Vora LK. Sunscreens: a comprehensive review with the application of nanotechnology. J Drug Deliv Sci Technol. 2023;86:104720.
26. Serpone N. Sunscreens and their usefulness: have we made any progress in the last two decades? Photochem Photobiol Sci 2021 20:2 [Internet]. 2021 Feb 18 [cited 2024 Mar 3];20(2):189–244. Available from: https://link.springer.com/article/10.1007/s43630-021-00013-1
27. Chatzigianni M, Pavlou P, Siamidi A, Vlachou M, Varvaresou A, Papageorgiou S. Environmental impacts due to the use of sunscreen products: a mini-review. Ecotoxicology [Internet]. 2022 Nov 1 [cited 2024 Apr 2];31(9):1331. Available from: https://www.ncbi.nlm.nih.gov/pmc/articles/PMC9652235/
28. Al-Jamal MS, Griffith JL, Lim HW. Photoprotection in ethnic skin. Dermatol Sin. 2014;32(4):217–24.
29. Osterwalder U, Sohn M, Herzog B. Global state of sunscreens. Photodermatol Photoimmunol Photomed [Internet]. 2014 [cited 2024 Mar 22];30(2–3):62–80. Available from: https://pubmed.ncbi.nlm.nih.gov/24734281/
30. Sabzevari N, Qiblawi S, Norton SA, Fivenson D. Sunscreens: UV filters to protect us: part 1: changing regulations and choices for optimal sun protection. Int J Womens Dermatol. 2021;7(1):28–44.
31. Latha MS, Martis J, Shobha V, Shinde RS, Bangera S, Krishnankutty B, et al. Sunscreening agents: a review. J Clin Aesthet Dermatol [Internet]. 2013 Jan [cited 2024 Mar 20];6(1):16. Available from: https://www.ncbi.nlm.nih.gov/pmc/articles/PMC3543289/
32. Krause M, Klit A, Blomberg Jensen M, Søeborg T, Frederiksen H, Schlumpf M, et al. Sunscreens: are they beneficial for health? An overview of endocrine disrupting properties of UV-filters. Int J Androl [Internet]. 2012 Jun [cited 2024 Mar 15];35(3):424–36. Available from: https://pubmed.ncbi.nlm.nih.gov/22612478/
33. Rai R, Shanmuga S, Srinivas CR. Update on photoprotection. Indian J Dermatol [Internet]. 2012 Sep [cited 2024 Mar 3];57(5):335–42. Available from: https://pubmed.ncbi.nlm.nih.gov/23112351/
34. Al-Khafaji Z, Brito S, Bin BH. Zinc and zinc transporters in dermatology. Int J Mol Sci [Internet]. 2022 Dec 18 [cited 2024 Mar 27];23(24):16165. Available from: https://www.mdpi.com/1422-0067/23/24/16165/htm
35. Pawlowski S, Herzog B, Sohn M, Petersen-Thiery M, Acker S. EcoSun Pass: a tool to evaluate the ecofriendliness of UV filters used in sunscreen products. Int J Cosmet Sci [Internet]. 2021 Apr 1 [cited 2024 Mar 16];43(2):201–10. Available from: https://pubmed.ncbi.nlm.nih.gov/33289148/
36. Aguilera J, Gracia-Cazaña T, Gilaberte Y. New developments in sunscreens. Photochem Photobiol Sci [Internet]. 2023 Oct 1 [cited 2024 Mar 3];22(10):2473–82. Available from: https://pubmed.ncbi.nlm.nih.gov/37543534/
37. Gupta M, Mahajan VK, Mehta KS, Chauhan PS. Zinc therapy in dermatology: a review. Dermatol Res Pract [Internet]. 2014 [cited 2024 Apr 2];2014. Available from: https://www.ncbi.nlm.nih.gov/pmc/articles/PMC4120804/
38. Labille J, Catalano R, Slomberg D, Motellier S, Pinsino A, Hennebert P, et al. Assessing sunscreen lifecycle to minimize environmental risk posed by nanoparticulate UV-filters—a review for safer-by-design products. Front Environ Sci. 2020;8:546963.
39. Ginzburg AL, Blackburn RS, Santillan C, Truong L, Tanguay RL, Hutchison JE. Zinc oxide-induced changes to sunscreen ingredient efficacy and toxicity under UV irradiation. Photochem Photobiol Sci [Internet]. 2021 Oct 1 [cited 2024 Mar 27];20(10):1273. Available from: https://www.ncbi.nlm.nih.gov/pmc/articles/PMC8550398/
40. Couteau C, Chammas R, Alami-El Boury S, Choquenet B, Paparis E, Coiffard LJM. Combination of UVA-filters and UVB-filters or inorganic UV filters-influence on the sun protection factor (SPF) and the PF-UVA determined by in vitro method. J Dermatol Sci [Internet]. 2008 May [cited 2024 Mar 27];50(2):159–61. Available from: https://pubmed.ncbi.nlm.nih.gov/18262775/

41. McCormick PG, Tsuzuki T. In vitro testing of zinc oxide sunscreens. Int J Cosmet Sci [Internet]. 2012 Aug [cited 2024 Mar 21];34(4):291–7. Available from: https://pubmed.ncbi.nlm.nih.gov/22591031/
42. Poh Agin P. Measuring ultraviolet A protection in sunscreen products. J Am Acad Dermatol [Internet]. 2017 Sep 1 [cited 2024 Mar 22];77(3):e81. Available from: http://www.jaad.org/article/S0190962217317255/fulltext
43. What's your fav sunscreen? | AnandTech Forums: Technology, Hardware, Software, and Deals [Internet]. [cited 2024 Apr 6]. Available from: https://forums.anandtech.com/threads/whats-your-fav-sunscreen.2320449/
44. Australian regulatory guidelines for sunscreens (ARGS) | Therapeutic Goods Administration (TGA) [Internet]. [cited 2024 Mar 21]. Available from: https://www.tga.gov.au/resources/resource/guidance/australian-regulatory-guidelines-sunscreens-args
45. Federal Register:: Sunscreen drug products for over-the-counter human use [Internet]. [cited 2024 Mar 20]. Available from: https://www.federalregister.gov/documents/2019/02/26/2019-03019/sunscreen-drug-products-for-over-the-counter-human-use
46. Shi J, Han S, Zhang J, Liu Y, Chen Z, Jia G. Advances in genotoxicity of titanium dioxide nanoparticles in vivo and in vitro. NanoImpact [Internet]. 2022 Jan 1 [cited 2024 Apr 4];25. Available from: https://pubmed.ncbi.nlm.nih.gov/35559883/
47. Pantelic MN, Wong N, Kwa M, Lim HW. Ultraviolet filters in the United States and European Union: a review of safety and implications for the future of US sunscreens. J Am Acad Dermatol [Internet]. 2023 Mar 1 [cited 2024 Mar 3];88(3):632–46. Available from: https://pubmed.ncbi.nlm.nih.gov/36442641/
48. Vaudagna MV, Aiassa V, Marcotti A, Pince Beti MF, Constantín MF, Pérez MF, et al. Titanium Dioxide Nanoparticles in sunscreens and skin photo-damage. Development, synthesis and characterization of a novel biocompatible alternative based on their in vitro and in vivo study. J Photochem Photobiol. 2023;15:100173.
49. Smijs TG, Pavel S. Titanium dioxide and zinc oxide nanoparticles in sunscreens: focus on their safety and effectiveness. Nanotechnol Sci Appl [Internet]. 2011 [cited 2024 Apr 4];4(1):95. Available from: https://www.ncbi.nlm.nih.gov/pmc/articles/PMC3781714/
50. Commission Delegated Regulation (EU) 2020/217 of 4 October 2019 amending, for the purposes of its adaptation to technical and scientific progress, Regulation (EC) No 1272/2008 of the European Parliament and of the Council on classification, labelling and packaging of substances and mixtures and correcting that Regulation (Text with EEA relevance). https://webarchive.nationalarchives.gov.uk/eu-exit/https://eur-lex.europa.eu/legal-content/EN/TXT/?uri=CELEX:02020R0217-20200218
51. Titanium, Judgment of the General Court in Joined Cases T-279/20, T-288/20 and T-283/20 | CWS Powder Coatings, https://curia.europa.eu/jcms/upload/docs/application/pdf/2022-11/cp220190en.pdf.—Google Search [Internet]. [cited 2024 Apr 4]. Available from: https://www.google.com/search?q=Titanium%2C+%E2%80%9CJudgment+of+the+General+Court+in+Joined+Cases+T-279%2F20%2C+T-288%2F20+and+T-283%2F20+%7C+CWS+Powder+Coatings%2C%E2%80%9D+https%3A%2F%2Fcuria.europa.eu%2Fjcms%2Fupload%2Fdocs%2Fapplication%2Fpdf%2F2022-11%2Fcp220190en.pdf.&oq=Titanium%2C+%E2%80%9CJudgment+of+the+General+Court+in+Joined+Cases+T-279%2F20%2C+T-288%2F20+and+T-283%2F20+%7C+CWS+Powder+Coatings%2C%-E2%80%9D+https%3A%2F%2Fcuria.europa.eu%2Fjcms%2Fupload%2Fdocs%2Fapplication%2Fpdf%2F2022-11%2Fcp220190en.pdf.+&gs_lcrp=EgZjaHJvbWUyBggAEEUYOTIHCAEQIRiPAjIHCAIQIRiPAjIHCAMQIRiPAtIBCTMwMjJqMGoxNagCCLACAQ&sourceid=chrome&ie=UTF-8
52. Gondikas AP, Von Der Kammer F, Reed RB, Wagner S, Ranville JF, Hofmann T. Release of TiO2 nanoparticles from sunscreens into surface waters: a one-year survey at the old danube recreational lake. Environ Sci Technol [Internet]. 2014 May 20 [cited 2024 Apr 4];48(10):5415–22. Available from: https://pubs.acs.org/doi/abs/10.1021/es405596y
53. Gambardella C, Pinsino A. Nanomaterial ecotoxicology in the terrestrial and aquatic environment: a systematic review. Toxics [Internet]. 2022 Jul 1 [cited 2024 Apr 4];10(7):393. Available from: https://www.mdpi.com/2305-6304/10/7/393/htm

54. Kubáč L, Akrman J, Kejlová K, Bendová H, Klánová K, Hladíková Z, et al. Characteristics of titanium dioxide microdispersions with different photo-activity suitable for sunscreen formulations. Int J Pharm [Internet]. 2015 Mar 15 [cited 2024 Apr 4];481(1–2):91–6. Available from: https://pubmed.ncbi.nlm.nih.gov/25655716/
55. Hoffmann SS, Elberling J, Thyssen JP, Hansen KS, Johansen JD. Does aluminium in sunscreens cause dermatitis in children with aluminium contact allergy: a repeated open application test study. Contact Dermatitis [Internet]. 2022 Jan 1 [cited 2024 Mar 29];86(1):9–14. Available from: https://pubmed.ncbi.nlm.nih.gov/34536036/
56. Commission Regulation (EU) 2016/1143 of 13 July 2016amending Annex VI to Regulation (EC) No 1223/2009 of the European Parliament and of the Council on cosmetic products—Google Search [Internet]. [cited 2024 Apr 4]. Available from: https://www.google.com/search?q=COMMISSION+REGULATION+%28EU%29+2016%2F1143+of+13+July+2016amending+Annex+VI+to+Regulation+%28EC%29+No+1223%2F2009+of+the+European+Parliament+and+of+the+Council+on+cosmetic+products%2C%E2%80%9D+&sca_esv=ba9cb985dba3a779&ei=fE4OZtHWE9S5seMP34e0-AE&ved=0ahUKEwjRhOLo_KeFAxXUXGwGHd8DDR8Q4dUDCBA&uact=5&oq=COMMISSION+REGULATION+%28EU%29+2016%2F1143+of+13+July+2016amending+Annex+VI+to+Regulation+%28EC%29+No+1223%2F2009+of+the+European+Parliament+and+of+the+Council+on+cosmetic+products%2C%E2%80%9D+&gs_lp=E-gxnd3Mtd2l6LXNlcnAirQFDT01NSVNTSU9OIFJFR1VMQVRJT04gKEVVKSAyMDE2LzExNDMgb2YgMTMgSnVseSAyMDE2YW1lbmRpbmcgQW5uZXggVkkgdG8gUmVndWxhdGlvbiAoRUMpIE5vIDEyMjMvMjAwOSBvZiB0aGUgRXVyb3BlY-W4gUGFybGlhbWVudCBhbmQgb2YgdGhlIENvdW5jaWwgb24gY29zbWV0aW-MgcHJvZHVjdHMs4oCdIDIWEAAYAxiPARjlAhjqAhi0AhiMA9gBATIWEAAYAxiPARjlAhjqAhi0AhiMA9gBATIWEAAYAxiPARjlAhjqAhi0AhiMA9gBATIWEAAYAxiPARjlAhjqAhi0AhiMA9gBATIWEAAYAxiPARjlAhjqAhi0AhiMA9gBATIWEAAYAxiPARjlAhjqAhi0AhiMA9gBATIWEAAYAxiPARjlAhjqAhi0AhiMA9gBATIWEAAYAxiPARjlAhjqAhi0AhiMA9gBAUjNLVAAWKYqcAF4AJABAJgBAKABAKoBALgBA8gBAPgBAfgBApgCAaACHqgCCpgDHroGBAgBGAqSBwExoAcA&sclient=gws-wiz-serp
57. Casas-Beltran DA, Hernández-Pedraza M, Alvarado-Flores J. Estimation of the discharge of sunscreens in aquatic environments of the Mexican Caribbean. Environments [Internet]. 2020 Feb 20 [cited 2024 Mar 28];7(2):15. Available from: https://www.mdpi.com/2076-3298/7/2/15/htm
58. Tsalidis GA, Soeteman-Hernández LG, Noorlander CW, Saedy S, Ruud van Ommen J, Vijver MG, et al. Safe-and-sustainable-by-design framework based on a prospective life cycle assessment: lessons learned from a nano-titanium dioxide case study. Int J Environ Res Public Health [Internet]. 2022 Apr 1 [cited 2024 Mar 16];19(7). Available from: https://www.mdpi.com/1660-4601/19/7/4241
59. Campodoni E, Montanari M, Artusi C, Bergamini L, Bassi G, Destro E, et al. Biomineralization: a new tool for developing eco-sustainable Ti-doped hydroxyapatite-based hybrid UV filters. Biomater Adv [Internet]. 2023 Aug 1 [cited 2024 Apr 4];151. Available from: https://pubmed.ncbi.nlm.nih.gov/37207586/
60. Pinnell SR, Fairhurst D, Gillies R, Mitchnick MA, Kollias N. Microfine zinc oxide is a superior sunscreen ingredient to microfine titanium dioxide. Dermatol Surg [Internet]. 2000 [cited 2024 Apr 4];26(4):309–14. Available from: https://pubmed.ncbi.nlm.nih.gov/10759815/
61. Maier T, Korting HC. Sunscreens—which and what for? Skin Pharmacol Physiol [Internet]. 2005 Nov [cited 2024 Mar 3];18(6):253–62. Available from: https://pubmed.ncbi.nlm.nih.gov/16113595/
62. Mineral filters in sunscreen products--comparison of the efficacy of zinc oxide and titanium dioxide by in vitro method—PubMed [Internet]. [cited 2024 Apr 4]. Available from: https://pubmed.ncbi.nlm.nih.gov/18271305/

63. D'Souza G, Evans GRD. Mexoryl: a review of an ultraviolet a filter. Plast Reconstr Surg [Internet]. 2007 Sep [cited 2024 Apr 4];120(4):1071–5. Available from: https://pubmed.ncbi.nlm.nih.gov/17805138/
64. Beasley DG, Meyer TA. Characterization of the UVA protection provided by avobenzone, zinc oxide, and titanium dioxide in broad-spectrum sunscreen products. Am J Clin Dermatol [Internet]. 2010 [cited 2024 Mar 27];11(6):413–21. Available from: https://pubmed.ncbi.nlm.nih.gov/20806994/
65. Moyal D. Need for a well-balanced sunscreen to protect human skin from both Ultraviolet A and Ultraviolet B damage. Indian J Dermatol Venereol Leprol [Internet]. 2012 Jun 1 [cited 2024 Mar 22];78(SUPPL.1):24. Available from: https://ijdvl.com/need-for-a-well-balanced-sunscreen-to-protect-human-skin-from-both-ultraviolet-a-and-ultraviolet-b-damage/
66. Keyes E, Werth VP, Brod B. Potential allergenicity of commonly sold high SPF broad spectrum sunscreens in the United States; from the perspective of patients with autoimmune skin disease. Int J Womens Dermatol [Internet]. 2019 Sep 1 [cited 2024 Mar 29];5(4):227. Available from: https://www.ncbi.nlm.nih.gov/pmc/articles/PMC6831754/
67. Bernerd F, Marionnet C, Duval C. Solar ultraviolet radiation induces biological alterations in human skin in vitro: relevance of a well-balanced UVA/UVB protection. Indian J Dermatol Venereol Leprol [Internet]. 2012 Jan 1 [cited 2024 Mar 25];78(SUPPL.1):15–23. Available from: https://www.researchgate.net/publication/227706545_Solar_ultraviolet_radiation_induces_biological_alterations_in_human_skin_in_vitro_Relevance_of_a_well-balanced_UVAUVB_protection
68. Cole Y, Ilyas AM, Ilyas EN. Availability of adequate photoprotection for skin of color. Cureus. 2023;15(8):e42794.
69. Zhou C, Lee C, Salas J, Luke J. Guide to tinted sunscreens in skin of color. Int J Dermatol [Internet]. 2024 Mar 1 [cited 2024 Apr 4];63(3):272–6. Available from: https://pubmed.ncbi.nlm.nih.gov/38073075/
70. Comparatively speaking: natural- vs. mineral-based colorants | cosmetics & toiletries [Internet]. [cited 2024 Apr 4]. Available from: https://www.cosmeticsandtoiletries.com/cosmetic-ingredients/colorant/article/21834695/comparatively-speaking-natural-vs-mineral-based-colorants
71. Dumbuya H, Grimes PE, Lynch S, Ji K, Brahmachary M, Zheng Q, et al. Impact of iron-oxide containing formulations against visible light-induced skin pigmentation in skin of color individuals. J Drugs Dermatol [Internet]. 2020 Jul 1 [cited 2024 Apr 4];19(7):712–7. Available from: https://pubmed.ncbi.nlm.nih.gov/32726103/
72. Banerjee T, Samanta A. Metal oxides for cosmetics and sunscreens. In: Metal oxides for biomedical and biosensor applications. Amsterdam: Elsevier; 2021. p. 119–35.
73. Kam O, Na S, Guo W, Tejeda CI, Kaufmann T. Frontal fibrosing alopecia and personal care product use: a systematic review and meta-analysis. Arch Dermatol Res [Internet]. 2023 Oct 1 [cited 2024 Mar 30];315(8):2313–31. Available from: https://pubmed.ncbi.nlm.nih.gov/37014396/
74. Nery ÉM, Martinez RM, Velasco MVR, Baby AR. A short review of alternative ingredients and technologies of inorganic UV filters. J Cosmet Dermatol [Internet]. 2021 Apr 1 [cited 2024 Apr 4];20(4):1061–5. Available from: https://onlinelibrary.wiley.com/doi/full/10.1111/jocd.13694
75. Seixas VC, Serra OA. Stability of sunscreens containing CePO4: proposal for a new inorganic UV filter. Molecules [Internet]. 2014 [cited 2024 Mar 16];19(7):9907–25. Available from: https://pubmed.ncbi.nlm.nih.gov/25010465/
76. Miri A, Akbarpour Birjandi S, Sarani M. Survey of cytotoxic and UV protection effects of biosynthesized cerium oxide nanoparticles. J Biochem Mol Toxicol [Internet]. 2020 Jun 1 [cited 2024 Apr 4];34(6). Available from: https://pubmed.ncbi.nlm.nih.gov/32053270/
77. Verma S, Bamzai KK. Preparation of cerium orthophosphate nanosphere by coprecipitation route and its structural, thermal, optical, and electrical characterization. J Nanoparticles. 2014;2014:1–12.

78. Agarwal T, Komini Babu S, Sievert A, Mary Peter A, Kailasnath M. Investigation of intensity dependent nonlinear absorption in cerium phosphate nanorods. J Phys Conf Ser [Internet]. 2022 Oct 1 [cited 2024 Apr 4];2357(1):012013. Available from: https://iopscience.iop.org/article/10.1088/1742-6596/2357/1/012013
79. Caputo F, De Nicola M, Sienkiewicz A, Giovanetti A, Bejarano I, Licoccia S, et al. Cerium oxide nanoparticles, combining antioxidant and UV shielding properties, prevent UV-induced cell damage and mutagenesis. Nanoscale [Internet]. 2015 Oct 14 [cited 2024 Apr 4];7(38):15643–56. Available from: https://pubmed.ncbi.nlm.nih.gov/26349675/
80. Ngoc LTN, Bui VKH, Moon JY, Lee YC. In-vitro cytotoxicity and oxidative stress induced by cerium aminoclay and cerium oxide nanoparticles in human skin keratinocyte cells. J Nanosci Nanotechnol [Internet]. 2019 Apr 26 [cited 2024 Mar 20];19(10):6369–75. Available from: https://pubmed.ncbi.nlm.nih.gov/31026963/
81. Dhillon B, Singh S, Keifer J, Kumar U, Shaikh S, Ho S, et al. Ameliorating hydroxychloroquine induced retinal toxicity through cerium oxide nanoparticle treatments. J Biomater Appl [Internet]. 2022 Jan 1 [cited 2024 Apr 4];36(6):1033–41. Available from: https://pubmed.ncbi.nlm.nih.gov/34210196/
82. EU Cosmetics Regulation [Regulation (EC) No. 1223/2009]—Google Search [Internet]. [cited 2024 Apr 2]. Available from: https://www.google.com/search?q=EU+Cosmetics+Regulation+%5BRegulation+(EC)+No.+1223%2F2009%5D&oq=EU+Cosmetics+Regulation+%5BRegulation+(EC)+No.+1223%2F2009%5D&gs_lcrp=EgZjaHJvbWUyBggAEEUYOdIBBzg2MWowajSoAgiwAgE&sourceid=chrome&ie=UTF-8
83. Study of the efficacy of 18 sun filters authorized in European Union tested in vitro—PubMed [Internet]. [cited 2024 Apr 4]. Available from: https://pubmed.ncbi.nlm.nih.gov/17663193/
84. Scientific Committee on Consumer Safety SCCS OPINION ON HAA299 (nano).
85. COMMISSION REGULATION (EU) 2022/2195 of 10 November 2022 amending Regulation (EC) No 1223/2009 of the European Parliament and of the Council as regards the use of Butylated Hydroxytoluene, Acid Yellow 3, Homosalate and HAA299 in cosmetic products and correcting that Regulation as regards the use of Resorcinol in cosmetic products [Internet]. [cited 2024 Apr 5]. Available from: https://eur-lex.europa.eu/legal-content/EN/TXT/HTML/?uri=CELEX%3A32022R2195
86. Federal Register:: Amending over-the-counter monograph M020: sunscreen drug products for over-the-counter human use; over the counter monograph proposed order; Availability [Internet]. [cited 2024 Mar 20]. Available from: https://www.federalregister.gov/documents/2021/09/27/2021-20780/amending-over-the-counter-monograph-m020-sunscreen-drug-products-for-over-the-counter-human-use-over
87. Regulation (EC) No 1223/2009 of the European Parliament and of the Council of 30 November 2009 on cosmetic products (recast) (Text with EEA relevance). 2009;
88. Sunscreen photostability, in Principles and practice of photoprotection, Springer International Publishing Switzerland 2016, p. 247.—Google Search [Internet]. [cited 2024 Apr 4]. Available from: https://www.google.com/search?q=Sunscreen+Photostability%2C%E2%80%9D+in+Principles+and+Practice+of+Photoprotection%2C+Springer+International+Publishing+Switzerland+2016%2C+p.+247.&sca_esv=6b393546f34dc1ef&ei=9oAOZvikBMLg4-EPpL-X4A4&ved=0ahUKEwj496r6rKiFAxVC8DgGHaTfBewQ4dUDCBA&uact=5&oq=Sunscreen+Photostability%2C%E2%80%9D+in+Principles+and+Practice+of+Photoprotection%2C+Springer+International+Publishing+Switzerland+2016%2C+p.+247.&gs_lp=Egxnd3Mt-d2l6LXNlcnAihwFTdW5zY3JlZW4gUGhvdG9zdGFiaWxpdHks4oCdIGluIFByaW5jaXBsZXMgYW5kIFByYWN0aWNlIG9mIFBob3RvcHJvdGVjdGlvbiwgU3ByaW5nZXIgSW50ZX-JuYXRpb25hbCBQdWJsaXNoaW5nIFN3aXR6ZXJsYW5kIDIwMTYsIHAuIDI0Ny4yFhAAGAMYjwEY5QIY6gIYtAIYjAPYAQEyFhAAGAMYjwEY5QIY6gIYtAIYjAPYAQEyFhAAGAMYjwEY5QIY6gIYtAIYjAPYAQEyFhAAGAMYjwEY5QIY6gIYtAIYjAPYAQEyFhAAGAMYjwEY5QIY6gIYtAIYjAPYAQEyFhAAGAMYjwEY5QI-Y6gIYtAIYjAPYAQEyFhAAGAMYjwEY5QIY6gIYtAIYjAPYAQEyFhAAGAMYjwEY5QIY6gIYtAIYjAPYAQEyFhAuGAMYjwEY5QIY6gIYtAIYjAPYAQFItA1Q4AlY4AlwAXgAkAEAmAEAoAEAqgEAuAEDy

AEA-AEB-AECmAIBoAIPqAIKmAMPugYECAEYCpIHATGgBwA&sclient=gws-wiz-serp
89. Nitulescu G, Lupuliasa D, Adam-Dima I, Nitulescu GM. Ultraviolet filters for cosmetic applications. Cosmetics [Internet]. 2023 Jul 12 [cited 2024 Apr 4];10(4):101. Available from: https://www.mdpi.com/2079-9284/10/4/101/htm
90. Matta MK, Florian J, Zusterzeel R, Pilli NR, Patel V, Volpe DA, et al. Effect of sunscreen application on plasma concentration of sunscreen active ingredients: a randomized clinical trial. JAMA [Internet]. 2020 Jan 21 [cited 2024 Mar 27];323(3):256–67. Available from: https://jamanetwork.com/journals/jama/fullarticle/2759002
91. Registration dossier—ECHA [Internet]. [cited 2024 Apr 4]. Available from: https://echa.europa.eu/de/registration-dossier/-/registered-dossier/31837/6/1
92. Schmidt T, Ring J, Abeck D. Photoallergic contact dermatitis due to combined UVB (4-methylbenzylidene camphor/octyl methoxycinnamate) and UVA (benzophenone-3/butyl methoxydibenzoylmethane) absorber sensitization. Dermatology [Internet]. 1998 [cited 2024 Apr 4];196(3):354–7. Available from: https://pubmed.ncbi.nlm.nih.gov/9621150/
93. Fourtanier A, Labat-Robert J, Kern P, Berrebi C, Gracia AM, Boyer B. In vivo evaluation of photoprotection against chronic ultraviolet-A irradiation by a new sunscreen Mexoryl SX. Photochem Photobiol [Internet]. 1992 [cited 2024 Apr 4];55(4):549–60. Available from: https://pubmed.ncbi.nlm.nih.gov/1320278/
94. Fourtanier A. Mexoryl SX protects against solar-simulated UVR-induced photocarcinogenesis in mice. Photochem Photobiol [Internet]. 1996 [cited 2024 Apr 4];64(4):688–93. Available from: https://pubmed.ncbi.nlm.nih.gov/8863475/
95. An in vitro strategy to evaluate the phototoxicity of solar UV at the molecular and cellular level: application to photoprotection assessment—PubMed [Internet]. [cited 2024 Apr 4]. Available from: https://pubmed.ncbi.nlm.nih.gov/9729050/
96. Séite S, Moyal D, Richard S, De Rigal J, Lévêque JL, Hourseau C, et al. Mexoryl® SX: a broad absorption UVA filter protects human skin from the effects of repeated suberythemal doses of UVA. J Photochem Photobiol B [Internet]. 1998 Jun 15 [cited 2024 Apr 4];44(1):69–76. Available from: https://pubmed.ncbi.nlm.nih.gov/9745729/
97. Evaluation of the protective effect of sunscreens on in vitro reconstructed human skin exposed to UVB or UVA irradiation—PubMed [Internet]. [cited 2024 Apr 4]. Available from: https://pubmed.ncbi.nlm.nih.gov/10732449/
98. Seité S, Colige A, Piquemal-Vivenot P, Montastier C, Fourtanier A, Lapière C, et al. A full-UV spectrum absorbing daily use cream protects human skin against biological changes occurring in photoaging. Photodermatol Photoimmunol Photomed [Internet]. 2000 [cited 2024 Apr 4];16(4):147–55. Available from: https://pubmed.ncbi.nlm.nih.gov/11019938/
99. Moyal D. Prevention of ultraviolet-induced skin pigmentation. Photodermatol Photoimmunol Photomed [Internet]. 2004 Oct [cited 2024 Mar 4];20(5):243–7. Available from: https://pubmed.ncbi.nlm.nih.gov/15379874/
100. Fourtanier A, Moyal D, Seité S. Sunscreens containing the broad-spectrum UVA absorber, Mexoryl SX, prevent the cutaneous detrimental effects of UV exposure: a review of clinical study results. Photodermatol Photoimmunol Photomed [Internet]. 2008 Aug [cited 2024 Apr 4];24(4):164–74. Available from: https://pubmed.ncbi.nlm.nih.gov/18717957/
101. Benech-Kieffer F, Meuling WJA, Leclerc C, Roza L, Leclaire J, Nohynek G. Percutaneous absorption of Mexoryl SX in human volunteers: comparison with in vitro data. Skin Pharmacol Appl Skin Physiol [Internet]. 2003 [cited 2024 Apr 4];16(6):343–55. Available from: https://pubmed.ncbi.nlm.nih.gov/14528058/
102. A new ecamsule-containing SPF 40 sunscreen cream for the prevention of polymorphous light eruption: a double-blind, randomized, controlled study in maximized outdoor conditions—PubMed [Internet]. [cited 2024 Mar 14]. Available from: https://pubmed.ncbi.nlm.nih.gov/19326695/
103. Yang Y, Ako-Adounvo AM, Wang J, Coelho SG, Adah SA, Matta MK, et al. In vitro testing of sunscreens for dermal absorption: method comparison and rank order correlation with in vivo

absorption. AAPS PharmSciTech [Internet]. 2022 Jul 1 [cited 2024 Mar 27];23(5). Available from: https://pubmed.ncbi.nlm.nih.gov/35459978/

104. Clergeaud F, Giraudo M, Rodrigues AMS, Thorel E, Lebaron P, Stien D. On the fate of butyl methoxydibenzoylmethane (avobenzone) in coral tissue and its effect on coral metabolome. Metabolites [Internet]. 2023 Apr 1 [cited 2024 Apr 4];13(4):533. Available from: https://www.mdpi.com/2218-1989/13/4/533/htm
105. Kwon B, Choi K. Occurrence of major organic UV filters in aquatic environments and their endocrine disruption potentials: a mini-review. Integr Environ Assess Manag [Internet]. 2021 Sep 1 [cited 2024 Apr 4];17(5):940–50. Available from: https://pubmed.ncbi.nlm.nih.gov/33991024/
106. da Silva ACP, Santos BAMC, Castro HC, Rodrigues CR. Ethylhexyl methoxycinnamate and butyl methoxydibenzoylmethane: toxicological effects on marine biota and human concerns. J Appl Toxicol [Internet]. 2022 Jan 1 [cited 2024 Apr 4];42(1):73–86. Available from: https://pubmed.ncbi.nlm.nih.gov/34101210/
107. Ekstein SF, Hylwa S. Sunscreens: a review of UV filters and their allergic potential. https://home.liebertpub.com/derm [Internet]. 2023 May 17 [cited 2024 Apr 4];34(3):176–90. Available from: https://www.liebertpub.com/doi/10.1097/DER.0000000000000963
108. Jesus A, Sousa E, Cruz MT, Cidade H, Lobo JMS, Almeida IF. UV filters: challenges and prospects. Pharmaceuticals [Internet]. 2022 Mar 1 [cited 2024 Mar 3];15(3). Available from: https://www.ncbi.nlm.nih.gov/pmc/articles/PMC8955451/
109. Wang SQ, Stanfield JW, Osterwalder U. In vitro assessments of UVA protection by popular sunscreens available in the United States. J Am Acad Dermatol [Internet]. 2008 Dec [cited 2024 Mar 21];59(6):934–42. Available from: https://pubmed.ncbi.nlm.nih.gov/18835064/
110. Sohn M, Krus S, Jung K, Seifert M, Schnyder M. Impact of photostability and UVA/UVA-blue light protection on free radical generation. 2019.
111. Dondi D, Albini A, Serpone N. Interactions between different solar UVB/UVA filters contained in commercial suncreams and consequent loss of UV protection. Photochem Photobiol Sci [Internet]. 2006 Aug 29 [cited 2024 Mar 27];5(9):835–43. Available from: https://pubmed.ncbi.nlm.nih.gov/17047836/
112. Afonso S, Horita K, Sousa E Silva JP, Almeida IF, Amaral MH, Lobão PA, et al. Photodegradation of avobenzone: stabilization effect of antioxidants. J Photochem Photobiol B [Internet]. 2014 [cited 2024 Mar 27];140:36–40. Available from: https://pubmed.ncbi.nlm.nih.gov/25086322/
113. Ahn S, An S, Lee M, Lee E, Pyo JJ, Kim JH, et al. A long-wave UVA filter avobenzone induces obesogenic phenotypes in normal human epidermal keratinocytes and mesenchymal stem cells. Arch Toxicol [Internet]. 2019 Jul 1 [cited 2024 Apr 4];93(7):1903–15. Available from: https://pubmed.ncbi.nlm.nih.gov/31016361/
114. Chamorro-Garcia R, Veiga-Lopez A. The new kids on the block: emerging obesogens. Adv Pharmacol [Internet]. 2021 Jan 1 [cited 2024 Apr 4];92:457. Available from: https://www.ncbi.nlm.nih.gov/pmc/articles/PMC8941623/
115. Janjua NR, Mogensen B, Andersson AM, Petersen JH, Henriksen M, Skakkebæk NE, et al. Systemic absorption of the sunscreens benzophenone-3, octyl-methoxycinnamate, and 3-(4-methyl-benzylidene) camphor after whole-body topical application and reproductive hormone levels in humans. J Invest Dermatol [Internet]. 2004 [cited 2024 Mar 30];123(1):57–61. Available from: https://pubmed.ncbi.nlm.nih.gov/15191542/
116. Schlumpf M, Cotton B, Conscience M, Haller V, Steinmann B, Lichtensteiger W. In vitro and in vivo estrogenicity of UV screens. Environ Health Perspect [Internet]. 2001 [cited 2024 Apr 4];109(3):239. Available from: https://www.ncbi.nlm.nih.gov/pmc/articles/PMC1240241/
117. National Academies of Sciences, Engineering, and Medicine. Review of fate, exposure, and effects of Sunscreens in aquatic environments and implications for sunscreen usage and human health. Washington, DC: The National Academies Press; 2022. p. 1–409.
118. Herzog B, Amorós-Galicia L, Sohn M, Hofer M, Quass K, Giesinger J. Analysis of photokinetics of 2'-ethylhexyl-4-methoxycinnamate in sunscreens. Photochem Photobiol Sci

[Internet]. 2019 [cited 2024 Apr 4];18(7):1773–81. Available from: https://pubmed.ncbi.nlm.nih.gov/31112187/

119. Lorigo M, Mangana C, Cairrao E. Disrupting effects of the emerging contaminant octylmethoxycinnamate (OMC) on human umbilical artery relaxation. Environ Pollut [Internet]. 2023 Oct 15 [cited 2024 Mar 27];335. Available from: https://pubmed.ncbi.nlm.nih.gov/37536478/
120. Lorigo M, Quintaneiro C, Maia CJ, Breitenfeld L, Cairrao E. UV-B filter octylmethoxycinnamate impaired the main vasorelaxant mechanism of human umbilical artery. Chemosphere [Internet]. 2021 Aug 1 [cited 2024 Apr 4];277. Available from: https://pubmed.ncbi.nlm.nih.gov/33789217/
121. Sunscreen allergy in Singapore—PubMed [Internet]. [cited 2024 Mar 29]. Available from: https://pubmed.ncbi.nlm.nih.gov/9471986/
122. Chuah SY, Leow YH, Goon ATJ, Theng CTS, Chong WS. Photopatch testing in Asians: a 5-year experience in Singapore. Photodermatol Photoimmunol Photomed [Internet]. 2013 Jun [cited 2024 Mar 29];29(3):116–20. Available from: https://pubmed.ncbi.nlm.nih.gov/23651271/
123. Lim SYD, Goon ATJ, Leow YH, Chong TYR, Tan EST, Cheng WNS. Photopatch testing in Singapore: a 10-year retrospective study. Photodermatol Photoimmunol Photomed [Internet]. 2023 Nov 1 [cited 2024 Mar 29];39(6):642–7. Available from: https://pubmed.ncbi.nlm.nih.gov/37749909/
124. Lorigo M, Quintaneiro C, Breitenfeld L, Cairrao E. UV-B filter octylmethoxycinnamate is a modulator of the serotonin and histamine receptors in human umbilical arteries. Biomedicines [Internet]. 2022 May 1 [cited 2024 Apr 4];10(5). Available from: https://pubmed.ncbi.nlm.nih.gov/35625791/
125. Huang Y, Wang P, Law JCF, Zhao Y, Wei Q, Zhou Y, et al. Organic UV filter exposure and pubertal development: a prospective follow-up study of urban Chinese adolescents. Environ Int [Internet]. 2020 Oct 1 [cited 2024 Apr 4];143. Available from: https://pubmed.ncbi.nlm.nih.gov/32679395/
126. Wang B, Jin Y, Li J, Yang F, Lu H, Zhou J, et al. Exploring environmental obesogenous effects of organic ultraviolet filters on children from a case-control study. Chemosphere [Internet]. 2023 Nov 1 [cited 2024 Apr 4];341. Available from: https://pubmed.ncbi.nlm.nih.gov/37672813/
127. Onyango DO, Selman BG, Rose JL, Ellison CA, Nash JF. Comparison between endocrine activity assessed using ToxCast/Tox21 database and human plasma concentration of sunscreen active ingredients/UV filters. Toxicol Sci [Internet]. 2023 Oct 30 [cited 2024 Mar 15];196(1):25–37. Available from: https://doi.org/10.1093/toxsci/kfad082
128. Lorigo M, Mariana M, Cairrao E. Photoprotection of ultraviolet-B filters: updated review of endocrine disrupting properties. Steroids [Internet]. 2018 Mar 1 [cited 2024 Apr 4];131:46–58. Available from: https://pubmed.ncbi.nlm.nih.gov/29360537/
129. Liu Y, Gao L, Ai Q, Qiao L, Li J, Lyu B, et al. Concentrations, profiles, and health risks of organic ultraviolet filters in eight food categories determined through the sixth Chinese Total diet study. Environ Sci Technol [Internet]. 2023 Sep 12 [cited 2024 Mar 27];57(36):13366–74. Available from: https://pubs.acs.org/doi/abs/10.1021/acs.est.3c03888
130. elstant. Opinion of the Scientific Committee on Consumer Safety on Octocrylene.
131. Huang Y, Law JCF, Lam TK, Leung KSY. Risks of organic UV filters: a review of environmental and human health concern studies. Sci Total Environ [Internet]. 2021 Feb 10 [cited 2024 Apr 4];755(Pt 1). Available from: https://pubmed.ncbi.nlm.nih.gov/33038838/
132. Gu J, Yuan T, Ni N, Ma Y, Shen Z, Yu X, et al. Urinary concentration of personal care products and polycystic ovary syndrome: a case-control study. Environ Res [Internet]. 2019 Jan 1 [cited 2024 Apr 4];168:48–53. Available from: https://pubmed.ncbi.nlm.nih.gov/30265948/
133. Downs CA, Dinardo JC, Stien D, Rodrigues AMS, Lebaron P. Benzophenone accumulates over time from the degradation of octocrylene in commercial sunscreen products. Chem Res Toxicol [Internet]. 2021 Apr 19 [cited 2024 Apr 4];34(4):1046–54. Available from: https://pubmed.ncbi.nlm.nih.gov/33682414/

134. Berardesca E, Zuberbier T, Sanchez Viera M, Marinovich M. Review of the safety of octocrylene used as an ultraviolet filter in cosmetics. J Eur Acad Dermatol Venereol [Internet]. 2019 Nov 1 [cited 2024 Apr 4];33 Suppl 7(S7):25–33. Available from: https://pubmed.ncbi.nlm.nih.gov/31588614/
135. Commission Regulation (EU) 2022/1176 of 7 July 2022 amending Regulation (EC) No 1223/2009 of the European Parliament and of the Council as regards the use of certain UV filters in cosmetic products (Text with EEA relevance). [cited 2024 Apr 4]; Available from: https://ec.europa.eu/health/sites/default/files/
136. Gaspar LR, Maia Campos PMBG. Evaluation of the photostability of different UV filter combinations in a sunscreen. Int J Pharm [Internet]. 2006 Jan 13 [cited 2024 Apr 4];307(2):123–8. Available from: https://pubmed.ncbi.nlm.nih.gov/16289662/
137. Subiabre-Ferrer D, Esteve-Martínez A, Blasco-Encinas R, Sierra-Talamantes C, Pérez-Ferriols A, Zaragoza-Ninet V. European photopatch test baseline series: a 3-year experience. Contact Dermatitis [Internet]. 2019 Jan 1 [cited 2024 Mar 29];80(1):5–8. Available from: https://pubmed.ncbi.nlm.nih.gov/30221361/
138. Foubert K, Dendooven E, Theunis M, Naessens T, Ivanova B, Pieters L, et al. The presence of benzophenone in sunscreens and cosmetics containing the organic UV filter octocrylene: a laboratory study. Contact Dermatitis [Internet]. 2021 Jul 1 [cited 2024 Apr 4];85(1):69–77. Available from: https://pubmed.ncbi.nlm.nih.gov/33763894/
139. Avenel-Audran M, Dutartre H, Goossens A, Jeanmougin M, Comte C, Bernier C, et al. Octocrylene, an emerging photoallergen. Arch Dermatol [Internet]. 2010 [cited 2024 Apr 2];146(7):753–7. Available from: https://pubmed.ncbi.nlm.nih.gov/20644036/
140. Karlsson I, Vanden Broecke K, Mårtensson J, Goossens A, Börje A. Clinical and experimental studies of octocrylene's allergenic potency. Contact Dermatitis [Internet]. 2011 Jun [cited 2024 Apr 4];64(6):343–52. Available from: https://pubmed.ncbi.nlm.nih.gov/21504434/
141. Meng Q, Yeung K, Chan KM. Toxic effects of octocrylene on zebrafish larvae and liver cell line (ZFL). Aquat Toxicol [Internet]. 2021 Jul 1 [cited 2024 Apr 4];236. Available from: https://pubmed.ncbi.nlm.nih.gov/34010734/
142. Yan S, Liang M, Chen R, Hong X, Zha J. Reproductive toxicity and estrogen activity in Japanese medaka (Oryzias latipes) exposed to environmentally relevant concentrations of octocrylene. Environ Pollut [Internet]. 2020 Jun 1 [cited 2024 Apr 4];261. Available from: https://pubmed.ncbi.nlm.nih.gov/32045793/
143. Shin JC, Lee E, An S, Jin SH, Ha J, Choi WJ, et al. Benzophenone-3 and benzophenone-8 exhibit obesogenic activity via peroxisome proliferator-activated receptor γ pathway. Toxicol In Vitro [Internet]. 2020 Sep 1 [cited 2024 Apr 4];67. Available from: https://pubmed.ncbi.nlm.nih.gov/32407875/
144. Ko H, An S, Ahn S, Park IG, Gong J, Hwang SY, et al. Sunscreen filter octocrylene is a potential obesogen by acting as a PPARγ partial agonist. Toxicol Lett [Internet]. 2022 Feb 1 [cited 2024 Apr 4];355:141–9. Available from: https://pubmed.ncbi.nlm.nih.gov/34864131/
145. Mizukawa A, Molins-Delgado D, de Azevedo JCR, Fernandes CVS, Díaz-Cruz S, Barceló D. Sediments as a sink for UV filters and benzotriazoles: the case study of Upper Iguaçu watershed, Curitiba (Brazil). Environ Sci Pollut Res Int [Internet]. 2017 Aug 1 [cited 2024 Apr 4];24(22):18284–94. Available from: https://pubmed.ncbi.nlm.nih.gov/28639014/
146. Couselo-Rodríguez C, González-Esteban PC, Diéguez Montes MP, Flórez Á. Environmental impact of UV filters. Actas Dermosifiliogr [Internet]. 2022 Sep [cited 2024 Apr 4];113(8):792–803. Available from: https://pubmed.ncbi.nlm.nih.gov/35508210/
147. Saunders LJ, Hoffman AD, Nichols JW, Gobas FAPC. Dietary bioaccumulation and biotransformation of hydrophobic organic sunscreen agents in rainbow trout. Environ Toxicol Chem [Internet]. 2020 Mar 1 [cited 2024 Apr 4];39(3):574–86. Available from: https://pubmed.ncbi.nlm.nih.gov/31749247/
148. Pawlowski S, Lanzinger AC, Dolich T, Füßl S, Salinas ER, Zok S, et al. Evaluation of the bioaccumulation of octocrylene after dietary and aqueous exposure. Sci Total Environ [Internet]. 2019 Jul 1 [cited 2024 Apr 4];672:669–79. Available from: https://pubmed.ncbi.nlm.nih.gov/30974358/

149. Bury D, Weber T, Ebert KE, Zülz S, Brüning T, Koch HM, et al. Increasing exposure to the UV filters octocrylene and 2-ethylhexyl salicylate in Germany from 1996 to 2020: human biomonitoring in 24-h urine samples of the German Environmental Specimen Bank (ESB). Environ Int [Internet]. 2023 Dec 1 [cited 2024 Apr 4];182. Available from: https://pubmed.ncbi.nlm.nih.gov/38029623/
150. Duis K, Junker T, Coors A. Review of the environmental fate and effects of two UV filter substances used in cosmetic products. Sci Total Environ. 2022;808:151931.
151. Wnuk W, Michalska K, Krupa A, Pawlak K. Benzophenone-3, a chemical UV-filter in cosmetics: is it really safe for children and pregnant women? Postepy Dermatol Alergol [Internet]. 2022 [cited 2024 Mar 27];39(1):26–33. Available from: https://www.researchgate.net/publication/358904304_Benzophenone-3_a_chemical_UV-filter_in_cosmetics_is_it_really_safe_for_children_and_pregnant_women
152. Mustieles V, Balogh RK, Axelstad M, Montazeri P, Márquez S, Vrijheid M, et al. Benzophenone-3: comprehensive review of the toxicological and human evidence with meta-analysis of human biomonitoring studies. Environ Int [Internet]. 2023 Mar 1 [cited 2024 Mar 15];173. Available from: https://pubmed.ncbi.nlm.nih.gov/36805158/
153. Hofer S, Stonig M, Wally V, Hartmann A, Fuchs D, Hermann M, et al. Contradictory effects of chemical filters in UV/ROS-stressed human keratinocyte and fibroblast cells. ALTEX [Internet]. 2019 [cited 2024 Mar 11];36(2):231–44. Available from: https://pubmed.ncbi.nlm.nih.gov/30488083/
154. Heurung AR, Raju SI, Warshaw EM. Benzophenones. Dermatitis [Internet]. 2014 [cited 2024 Apr 5];25(1):3–10. Available from: https://pubmed.ncbi.nlm.nih.gov/24407064/
155. Samaran Q, Raison-Peyron N, Clark E, Svedman C, Dahlin J, Dereure O, et al. A new case of photoallergic contact dermatitis caused by benzophenones in magazine covers. Contact Dermatitis [Internet]. 2022 Apr 1 [cited 2024 Apr 5];86(4):300–7. Available from: https://pubmed.ncbi.nlm.nih.gov/35089601/
156. Liu R, Mabury SA. Printing ink related chemicals, including synthetic phenolic antioxidants, organophosphite antioxidants, and photoinitiators, in printing paper products and implications for human exposure. Environ Int [Internet]. 2021 Apr 1 [cited 2024 Apr 5];149. Available from: https://pubmed.ncbi.nlm.nih.gov/33548846/
157. Calafat AM, Wong LY, Ye X, Reidy JA, Needham LL. Concentrations of the sunscreen agent benzophenone-3 in residents of the United States: National Health and Nutrition Examination Survey 2003–2004. Environ Health Perspect [Internet]. 2008 Jul [cited 2024 Apr 5];116(7):893. Available from: https://www.ncbi.nlm.nih.gov/pmc/articles/PMC2453157/
158. Zamoiski RD, Cahoon EK, Michal Freedman D, Linet MS. Self-reported sunscreen use and urinary benzophenone-3 concentrations in the United States: NHANES 2003–2006 and 2009–2012. Environ Res [Internet]. 2015 Oct 1 [cited 2024 Apr 5];142:563. Available from: https://www.ncbi.nlm.nih.gov/pmc/articles/PMC4609273/
159. Li AJ, Kannan K. Elevated concentrations of bisphenols, benzophenones, and antimicrobials in pantyhose collected from six countries. Environ Sci Technol [Internet]. 2018 Sep 18 [cited 2024 Apr 5];52(18):10812–9. Available from: https://pubmed.ncbi.nlm.nih.gov/30137966/
160. Iribarne-Durán LM, Serrano L, Peinado FM, Peña-Caballero M, Hurtado JA, Vela-Soria F, et al. Biomonitoring bisphenols, parabens, and benzophenones in breast milk from a human milk bank in Southern Spain. Sci Total Environ [Internet]. 2022 Jul 15 [cited 2024 Apr 5];830. Available from: https://pubmed.ncbi.nlm.nih.gov/35337871/
161. Krause M, Frederiksen H, Sundberg K, Jørgensen FS, Jensen LN, Nørgaard P, et al. Presence of benzophenones commonly used as UV filters and absorbers in paired maternal and fetal samples. Environ Int [Internet]. 2018 Jan 1 [cited 2024 Mar 15];110:51–60. Available from: https://pubmed.ncbi.nlm.nih.gov/29100749/
162. Joensen UN, Jørgensen N, Thyssen JP, Szecsi PB, Stender S, Petersen JH, et al. Urinary excretion of phenols, parabens and benzophenones in young men: associations to reproductive hormones and semen quality are modified by mutations in the Filaggrin gene. Environ Int [Internet]. 2018 Dec 1 [cited 2024 Apr 5];121(Pt 1):365–74. Available from: https://pubmed.ncbi.nlm.nih.gov/30245359/

163. Wang SQ, Burnett ME, Lim HW. Safety of oxybenzone: putting numbers into perspective. Arch Dermatol [Internet]. 2011 Jul 1 [cited 2024 Mar 15];147(7):865–6. Available from: https://jamanetwork.com/journals/jamadermatology/fullarticle/1105240
164. Kim S, Choi K. Occurrences, toxicities, and ecological risks of benzophenone-3, a common component of organic sunscreen products: a mini-review. Environ Int [Internet]. 2014 [cited 2024 Apr 5];70:143–57. Available from: https://pubmed.ncbi.nlm.nih.gov/24934855/
165. Peinado FM, Ocón-Hernández O, Iribarne-Durán LM, Vela-Soria F, Ubiña A, Padilla C, et al. Cosmetic and personal care product use, urinary levels of parabens and benzophenones, and risk of endometriosis: results from the EndEA study. Environ Res [Internet]. 2021 May 1 [cited 2024 Apr 5];196. Available from: https://pubmed.ncbi.nlm.nih.gov/33069703/
166. Wieczorek K, Szczęsna D, Jurewicz J. Environmental exposure to non-persistent endocrine disrupting chemicals and endometriosis: a systematic review. Int J Environ Res Public Health [Internet]. 2022 May 1 [cited 2024 Apr 5];19(9). Available from: https://pubmed.ncbi.nlm.nih.gov/35565013/
167. Pollack AZ, Buck Louis GM, Chen Z, Sun L, Trabert B, Guo Y, et al. Bisphenol A, benzophenone-type ultraviolet filters, and phthalates in relation to uterine leiomyoma. Environ Res [Internet]. 2015 Feb 1 [cited 2024 Apr 5];137:101–7. Available from: https://pubmed.ncbi.nlm.nih.gov/25531814/
168. Lee AW, Eata V. Association of environmental phenols with endometriosis and uterine leiomyoma: an analysis of NHANES, 2003–2006. Reprod Toxicol [Internet]. 2022 Oct 1 [cited 2024 Apr 5];113:30–4. Available from: https://pubmed.ncbi.nlm.nih.gov/35948171/
169. Huo W, Cai P, Chen M, Li H, Tang J, Xu C, et al. The relationship between prenatal exposure to BP-3 and Hirschsprung's disease. Chemosphere [Internet]. 2016 Feb 1 [cited 2024 Apr 5];144:1091–7. Available from: https://pubmed.ncbi.nlm.nih.gov/26454118/
170. DiNardo JC, Downs CA. Dermatological and environmental toxicological impact of the sunscreen ingredient oxybenzone/benzophenone-3. J Cosmet Dermatol [Internet]. 2018 Feb 1 [cited 2024 Apr 5];17(1):15–9. Available from: https://pubmed.ncbi.nlm.nih.gov/29086472/
171. DiNardo JC, Downs CA. Can oxybenzone cause Hirschsprung's disease? Reprod Toxicol [Internet]. 2019 Jun 1 [cited 2024 Apr 5];86:98–100. Available from: https://pubmed.ncbi.nlm.nih.gov/30831214/
172. Frederiksen H, Krause M, Jørgensen N, Rehfeld A, Skakkebæk NE, Andersson AM. UV filters in matched seminal fluid-, urine-, and serum samples from young men. J Expo Sci Environ Epidemiol [Internet]. 2021 Mar 1 [cited 2024 Apr 5];31(2):345–55. Available from: https://pubmed.ncbi.nlm.nih.gov/32051500/
173. Kim S, Kim S, Won S, Choi K. Considering common sources of exposure in association studies—Urinary benzophenone-3 and DEHP metabolites are associated with altered thyroid hormone balance in the NHANES 2007-2008. Environ Int [Internet]. 2017 [cited 2024 Apr 5];107:25–32. Available from: https://pubmed.ncbi.nlm.nih.gov/28651165/
174. Almstrup K, Frederiksen H, Andersson AM, Juul A. Levels of endocrine-disrupting chemicals are associated with changes in the peri-pubertal epigenome. Endocr Connect [Internet]. 2020 [cited 2024 Apr 5];9(8):845. Available from: https://www.ncbi.nlm.nih.gov/pmc/articles/PMC7487188/
175. Krause M, Frederiksen H, Sundberg K, Jørgensen FS, Jensen LN, Nørgaard P, et al. Maternal exposure to UV filters: associations with maternal thyroid hormones, IGF-I/IGFBP3 and birth outcomes. Endocr Connect [Internet]. 2018 Feb 1 [cited 2024 Apr 5];7(2):334–46. Available from: https://pubmed.ncbi.nlm.nih.gov/29362228/
176. Yan Y, Guo F, Liu K, Ding R, Wang Y. The effect of endocrine-disrupting chemicals on placental development. Front Endocrinol (Lausanne) [Internet]. 2023 [cited 2024 Apr 5];14. Available from: https://pubmed.ncbi.nlm.nih.gov/36896182/
177. Scheele A, Sutter K, Karatum O, Danley-Thomson AA, Redfern LK. Environmental impacts of the ultraviolet filter oxybenzone. Sci Total Environ [Internet]. 2023 Mar 10 [cited 2024 Apr 5];863. Available from: https://pubmed.ncbi.nlm.nih.gov/36535482/
178. González-Bareiro E, Montesdeoca-Esponda S, De la Fuente J, Sosa-Ferrera Z, Arbelo M, Fernández A, et al. Assessment of the presence of UV filters and UV stabilizers in stranded dolphin blubber. Sci Total Environ. 2023;895:165041.

179. Narla S, Lim HW. Sunscreen: FDA regulation, and environmental and health impact. Photochem Photobiol Sci [Internet]. 2020 Jan 21 [cited 2024 Apr 5];19(1):66–70. Available from: https://pubs.rsc.org/en/content/articlehtml/2020/pp/c9pp00366e
180. Bury D, Brüning T, Koch HM. Determination of metabolites of the UV filter 2-ethylhexyl salicylate in human urine by online-SPE-LC-MS/MS. J Chromatogr B Analyt Technol Biomed Life Sci [Internet]. 2019 Mar 15 [cited 2024 Apr 5];1110–1111:59–66. Available from: https://pubmed.ncbi.nlm.nih.gov/30780012/
181. SCCS. Scientific Advice on the safety of Homosalate (CAS No 118-56-9, EC No 204-260-8) as a UV-filter in cosmetic products.
182. Christiansen S, Petersen MA, Boberg J. Faglig vurdering af foreløbig SCCS vurdering for Homosalat [Internet]. Citation. APA; 2020 [cited 2024 Apr 5]. Available from: https://orbit.dtu.dk/en/publications/faglig-vurdering-af-forel%C3%B8big-sccs-vurdering-for-homosalat
183. Original: Japanese Provisional Translation Standards for Cosmetics.
184. Hayden CGJ, Cross SE, Anderson C, Saunders NA, Roberts MS. Sunscreen penetration of human skin and related keratinocyte toxicity after topical application. Skin Pharmacol Physiol [Internet]. 2005 Jul [cited 2024 Apr 5];18(4):170–4. Available from: https://pubmed.ncbi.nlm.nih.gov/15908756/
185. Sung CR, Kim KB, Lee JY, Lee BM, Kwack SJ. Risk assessment of ethylhexyl dimethyl PABA in cosmetics. Toxicol Res [Internet]. 2019 [cited 2024 Apr 5];35(2):131–6. Available from: https://pubmed.ncbi.nlm.nih.gov/31015895/
186. Carve M, Nugegoda D, Allinson G, Shimeta J. A systematic review and ecological risk assessment for organic ultraviolet filters in aquatic environments. Environ Pollut [Internet]. 2021 Jan 1 [cited 2024 Apr 5];268(Pt B). Available from: https://pubmed.ncbi.nlm.nih.gov/33120145/
187. UV-filters in cosmetics-prioritisation for environmental assessment. 2008 [cited 2024 Apr 5]; Available from: www.environment-agency.gov.uk
188. Scalia S, Molinari A, Casolari A, Maldotti A. Complexation of the sunscreen agent, phenylbenzimidazole sulphonic acid with cyclodextrins: effect on stability and photo-induced free radical formation. Eur J Pharm Sci [Internet]. 2004 Jul [cited 2024 Apr 5];22(4):241–9. Available from: https://pubmed.ncbi.nlm.nih.gov/15196580/
189. Melánová K, Kopecká K, Beneš L, Kutálek P, Knotek P, Zmrhalová Z, et al. Functionalization of ZnAl-layered double hydroxide with ensulizole and its application as a UV-protective agent in a transparent polymer coating. Molecules [Internet]. 2023 Sep 1 [cited 2024 Apr 5];28(17):6262. Available from: https://www.mdpi.com/1420-3049/28/17/6262/htm
190. Abdelraheem WHM, He X, Duan X, Dionysiou DD. Degradation and mineralization of organic UV absorber compound 2-phenylbenzimidazole-5-sulfonic acid (PBSA) using UV-254nm/H2O2. J Hazard Mater [Internet]. 2015 [cited 2024 Apr 5];282:233–40. Available from: https://pubmed.ncbi.nlm.nih.gov/25123523/
191. Lee JK, Kim KB, Lee JD, Shin CY, Kwack SJ, Lee BM, et al. Risk assessment of drometrizole, a cosmetic ingredient used as an ultraviolet light absorber. Toxicol Res [Internet]. 2019 [cited 2024 Apr 5];35(2):119–29. Available from: https://pubmed.ncbi.nlm.nih.gov/31015894/
192. Burnett CL. Amended final report of the safety assessment of Drometrizole as used in cosmetics. Int J Toxicol [Internet]. 2008 [cited 2024 Apr 5];27 Suppl 1(SUPPL. 1):63–75. Available from: https://pubmed.ncbi.nlm.nih.gov/18569163/
193. Cadena-Aizaga MI, Montesdeoca-Esponda S, Sosa-Ferrera Z, Santana-Rodríguez JJ. Occurrence and environmental hazard of organic UV filters in seawater and wastewater from Gran Canaria Island (Canary Islands, Spain). Environ Pollut. 2022;300:118843.
194. Rehfeld A, Dissing S, Skakkebæk NE. Chemical UV filters mimic the effect of progesterone on Ca2+ signaling in human sperm cells. Endocrinology [Internet]. 2016 Nov 1 [cited 2024 Apr 5];157(11):4297–308. Available from: https://doi.org/10.1210/en.2016-1473
195. Pastor-Nieto MA, Gatica-Ortega ME. Allergic contact dermatitis to drometrizole trisiloxane in a woman thereafter diagnosed with frontal fibrosing alopecia. Contact Dermatitis

[Internet]. 2023 Sep 1 [cited 2024 Apr 5];89(3):215–7. Available from: https://pubmed.ncbi.nlm.nih.gov/37386688/

196. Hughes TM, Martin JA, Lewis VJ, Stone NM. Allergic contact dermatitis to drometrizole trisiloxane in a sunscreen with concomitant sensitivities to other sun screens. Contact Dermatitis [Internet]. 2005 Apr [cited 2024 Apr 5];52(4):226–7. Available from: https://pubmed.ncbi.nlm.nih.gov/15859995/
197. Stege H, Budde MA, Grether-Beck S, Krutmann J. Evaluation of the capacity of sunscreens to photoprotect lupus erythematosus patients by employing the photoprovocation test. Photodermatol Photoimmunol Photomed [Internet]. 2000 [cited 2024 Apr 5];16(6):256–9. Available from: https://pubmed.ncbi.nlm.nih.gov/11132128/
198. Wang Y, Jiang S, Chen X, Liu X, Li N, Nie Y, et al. Comparison of developmental toxicity of benzophenone-3 and its metabolite benzophenone-8 in zebrafish. Aquat Toxicol [Internet]. 2023 May 1 [cited 2024 Apr 5];258. Available from: https://pubmed.ncbi.nlm.nih.gov/37011548/
199. Mao JF, Li W, Ong CN, He Y, Jong MC, Gin KYH. Assessment of human exposure to benzophenone-type UV filters: a review. Environ Int [Internet]. 2022 Sep 1 [cited 2024 Apr 5];167. Available from: https://pubmed.ncbi.nlm.nih.gov/35843073/
200. Kumar M, Silori R, Mazumder P, Tauseef SM. Screening of pharmaceutical and personal care products (PPCPs) along wastewater treatment system equipped with root zone treatment: a potential model for domestic waste leachate management. J Environ Manage [Internet]. 2023 Jun 1 [cited 2024 Apr 5];335. Available from: https://pubmed.ncbi.nlm.nih.gov/36871357/
201. Rodrigues N d. N, Cebrián J, Montané A, Mendez S. Intermolecular Interactions and In Vitro Performance of Methyl Anthranilate in Commercial Sunscreen Formulations. AppliedChem [Internet]. 2021 Aug 24 [cited 2024 Apr 5];1(1):50–61. Available from: https://www.mdpi.com/2673-9623/1/1/5/htm
202. Rodrigues N d. N, Cole-Filipiak NC, Blodgett KN, Abeysekera C, Zwier TS, Stavros VG. Wavepacket insights into the photoprotection mechanism of the UV filter methyl anthranilate. Nat Commun [Internet]. 2018 Dec 1 [cited 2024 Apr 5];9(1). Available from: https://pubmed.ncbi.nlm.nih.gov/30518753/
203. Kitasaka S, Yagi M, Kikuchi A. Suppression of menthyl anthranilate (UV-A sunscreen)-sensitized singlet oxygen generation by Trolox and α-tocopherol. Photochem Photobiol Sci [Internet]. 2020 Jul 14 [cited 2024 Apr 5];19(7):913–9. Available from: https://pubs.rsc.org/en/content/articlehtml/2020/pp/d0pp00023j
204. Battis N, Ekstein SF, Neeley AB. Photoallergic contact dermatitis to menthyl anthranilate (meradimate). Dermatitis [Internet]. 2023 Mar 1 [cited 2024 Apr 5];34(2):153–4. Available from: https://pubmed.ncbi.nlm.nih.gov/36917525/
205. Marionnet C, de Dormael R, Marat X, Roudot A, Gizard J, Planel E, et al. Sunscreens with the new MCE filter cover the whole UV spectrum: improved UVA1 photoprotection in vitro and in a randomized controlled trial. JID Innov [Internet]. 2021 Jan 1 [cited 2024 Mar 3];2(1). Available from: https://pubmed.ncbi.nlm.nih.gov/35072138/
206. Opinion on methoxypropylamino cyclohexenylidene ethoxyethylcyanoacetate (S87)-submission II-final opinion opinion on methoxypropylamino cyclohexenylidene ethoxyethylcyanoacetate (S87)-submission II ____ 2 Acknowledgments. [cited 2024 Apr 5]; Available from: http://ec.europa.eu/health/scientific_committees/experts/declarations/sccs_en.htm
207. Flament F, Mercurio DG, Muller B, Li J, Tricaud C, Bernerd F, et al. The impact of methoxypropylamino cyclohexenylidene ethoxyethylcyanoacetate (MCE) UVA1 filter on pigmentary and ageing signs: an outdoor prospective 8-week randomized, intra-individual comparative study in two populations of different genetic background. J Eur Acad Dermatol Venereol [Internet]. 2024 Jan 1 [cited 2024 Apr 5];38(1):214–22. Available from: https://pubmed.ncbi.nlm.nih.gov/37655436/

208. Bernerd F, Passeron T, Castiel I, Marionnet C. The damaging effects of long UVA (UVA1) rays: a major challenge to preserve skin health and integrity. Int J Mol Sci [Internet]. 2022 Aug 1 [cited 2024 Apr 5];23(15). Available from: https://www.ncbi.nlm.nih.gov/pmc/articles/PMC9368482/
209. de Dormael R, Tricaud C, Bastien P, Candau D, Roudot A, Bernerd F. Gain of photoprotection afforded by the cyclic merocyanine UVA1 absorber MCE® in sunscreen formulae: a dose effect in vivo clinical trial. J Cosmet Dermatol [Internet]. 2023 Jun 1 [cited 2024 Apr 5];22(6):1929–31. Available from: https://pubmed.ncbi.nlm.nih.gov/36701164/
210. Valle-Sistac J, Molins-Delgado D, Díaz M, Ibáñez L, Barceló D, Silvia Díaz-Cruz M. Determination of parabens and benzophenone-type UV filters in human placenta. First description of the existence of benzyl paraben and benzophenone-4. Environ Int [Internet]. 2016 Mar 1 [cited 2024 Apr 5];88:243–9. Available from: https://pubmed.ncbi.nlm.nih.gov/26773395/
211. Molins-Delgado D, Díaz-Cruz MS, Barceló D. Ecological risk assessment associated to the removal of endocrine-disrupting parabens and benzophenone-4 in wastewater treatment. J Hazard Mater [Internet]. 2016 Jun 5 [cited 2024 Apr 5];310:143–51. Available from: https://pubmed.ncbi.nlm.nih.gov/26905612/
212. Gavrila AA, Dasteridis IS, Tzimas AA, Chatzimitakos TG, Stalikas CD. Benzophenones in the environment: occurrence, fate and sample preparation in the analysis. Molecules [Internet]. 2023 Jan 27 [cited 2024 Apr 5];28(3):1229. Available from: https://www.mdpi.com/1420-3049/28/3/1229/htm
213. Chen Q, Chen Q, Su G, Chen D, Ding Z, Sun H. The associations between high-levels of urine benzophenone-type UV filters (BPs) and changes in serum lipid concentrations. Chemosphere [Internet]. 2024 Jan 1 [cited 2024 Apr 5];346. Available from: https://pubmed.ncbi.nlm.nih.gov/37898463/
214. Warshaw EM, Xiong M, Belsito D V., Adler BL, Atwater AR, Dekoven JG, et al. Patch testing with benzophenone-3 and -4: the North American Contact Dermatitis Group Experience, 2013–2020. Dermatitis [Internet]. 2023 Mar 1 [cited 2024 Apr 5];34(2):105–12. Available from: https://pubmed.ncbi.nlm.nih.gov/36917534/
215. Cuccaro A, Freitas R, De Marchi L, Oliva M, Pretti C. UV-filters in marine environments: a review of research trends, meta-analysis, and ecotoxicological impacts of 4-methylbenzylidene-camphor and benzophenone-3 on marine invertebrate communities. Environ Sci Pollut Res Int [Internet]. 2022 Sep 1 [cited 2024 Apr 5];29(43):64370–91. Available from: https://pubmed.ncbi.nlm.nih.gov/35852751/
216. Zhang J, Pei ZT, Zhao YN, Zhang M, Zhang LL, Wang WQ, et al. Mutagenicity evaluation to UV filters of benzophenone-6, benzophenone-8, and 4-methylbenzylidene camphor by Ames test. PLoS One [Internet]. 2021 Sep 1 [cited 2024 Apr 5];16(9). Available from: https://pubmed.ncbi.nlm.nih.gov/34473729/
217. Søeborg T, Basse LH, Halling-Sørensen B. Risk assessment of topically applied products. Toxicology [Internet]. 2007 Jul 1 [cited 2024 Apr 5];236(1–2):140–8. Available from: https://pubmed.ncbi.nlm.nih.gov/17499903/
218. Journe F, Marguery MC, Rakotondrazafy J, El Sayed FE, Bazex J. Sunscreen sensitization: a 5-year study. Acta Derm Venereol [Internet]. 1999 [cited 2024 Apr 5];79(3):211–3. Available from: https://pubmed.ncbi.nlm.nih.gov/10384919/
219. Marguery MC, Rakotondrazafy J, Sayed F El, Bayle-Lebey P, Journe F, Bazex J. Contact allergy to 3-(4' methylbenzylidene) camphor and contact and photocontact allergy to 4-isopropyl dibenzoylmethane. Photodermatol Photoimmunol Photomed [Internet]. 1995 [cited 2024 Apr 5];11(5–6):209–12. Available from: https://pubmed.ncbi.nlm.nih.gov/8738716/
220. Buckley DA, O'sullivan D, Murphy GM. Contact and photocontact allergy to dibenzoylmethanes and contact allergy to methylbenzylidene camphor. Contact Dermatitis [Internet]. 1993 [cited 2024 Apr 5];29(1):47–47. Available from: https://pubmed.ncbi.nlm.nih.gov/8365160/
221. de Groot AC, van der Walle HB, Jagtman BA, Weyland JW. Contact allergy to 4-isopropyl-dibenzoylmethane and 3-(4'-methylbenzylidene) camphor in the sunscreen Eusolex 8021.

Contact Dermatitis [Internet]. 1987 [cited 2024 Apr 5];16(5):249–54. Available from: https://pubmed.ncbi.nlm.nih.gov/3621925/

222. Rubio-González B, Ortiz-De Frutos FJ. Allergic contact dermatitis to hexyl cinnamaldehyde, cinnamaldehyde, and 3,4 methylbenzylidene camphor in a patient with previous photoallergic contact dermatitis to dexketoprofen. Actas Dermosifiliogr [Internet]. 2015 Mar 1 [cited 2024 Apr 5];106(2):146–8. Available from: https://pubmed.ncbi.nlm.nih.gov/25109769/
223. Egambaram OP, Kesavan Pillai S, Ray SS. Materials science challenges in skin UV protection: a review. Photochem Photobiol [Internet]. 2020 Jul 1 [cited 2024 Mar 3];96(4):779–97. Available from: https://pubmed.ncbi.nlm.nih.gov/31886889/
224. Balaguer A, Chisvert A, Salvador A. Sequential-injection determination of traces of disodium phenyl dibenzimidazole tetrasulphonate in urine from users of sunscreens by on-line solid-phase extraction coupled with a fluorimetric detector. J Pharm Biomed Anal [Internet]. 2006 Mar 3 [cited 2024 Apr 5];40(4):922–7. Available from: https://pubmed.ncbi.nlm.nih.gov/16242289/
225. Balaguer A, Salvador A, Chisvert A, Meliá M, Herráez M, Díez O. A liquid chromatography-fluorimetric method for the in vitro estimation of the skin penetration of disodium phenyldibenzimidazole tetrasulfonate from sunscreen formulations through human skin. Anal Bioanal Chem [Internet]. 2006 Aug [cited 2024 Apr 5];385(7):1225–32. Available from: https://pubmed.ncbi.nlm.nih.gov/16550422/
226. Shaath NA. The chemistry of ultraviolet filters. In: Principles and practice of photoprotection. Cham: Adis; 2016. p. 143–57.
227. Lange-Asschenfeldt B, Huegel R, Brasch J. Anaphylactic reaction caused by the UVA absorber disodium phenyl dibenzimidazole tetrasulfonate. Acta Derm Venereol [Internet]. 2005 [cited 2024 Apr 5];85(3):280–1. Available from: https://pubmed.ncbi.nlm.nih.gov/16040428/
228. Axelstad M, Hass U, Kinnberg KL, Bjerregaard P. Assessment of the endocrine disrupting potential of 23 UV-filters (j.no. MST-656-00150) Danish Centre for Endocrine Disrupters.
229. Fivenson D, Sabzevari N, Qiblawi S, Blitz J, Norton BB, Norton SA. Sunscreens: UV filters to protect us: part 2-increasing awareness of UV filters and their potential toxicities to us and our environment. Int J Womens Dermatol [Internet]. 2021 Jan 1 [cited 2024 Mar 15];7(1):45. Available from: https://www.ncbi.nlm.nih.gov/pmc/articles/PMC7838327/
230. Haque T, Crowther JM, Lane ME, Moore DJ. Chemical ultraviolet absorbers topically applied in a skin barrier mimetic formulation remain in the outer stratum corneum of porcine skin. Int J Pharm [Internet]. 2016 Aug 20 [cited 2024 Apr 5];510(1):250–4. Available from: https://pubmed.ncbi.nlm.nih.gov/27321112/
231. Santander Ballestín S, Luesma Bartolomé MJ. Toxicity of different chemical components in sun cream filters and their impact on human health: a review. Appl Sci [Internet]. 2023 Jan 4 [cited 2024 Apr 5];13(2):712. Available from: https://www.mdpi.com/2076-3417/13/2/712/htm
232. D'Ruiz CD, Plautz JR, Schuetz R, Sanabria C, Hammonds J, Erato C, et al. Preliminary clinical pharmacokinetic evaluation of bemotrizinol—a new sunscreen active ingredient being considered for inclusion under FDA's over-the-counter (OTC) sunscreen monograph. Regul Toxicol Pharmacol [Internet]. 2023 Mar 1 [cited 2024 Mar 15];139. Available from: https://pubmed.ncbi.nlm.nih.gov/36738872/
233. Varrella S, Danovaro R, Corinaldesi C. Assessing the eco-compatibility of new generation sunscreen products through a combined microscopic-molecular approach. Environ Pollut. 2022;314:120212.
234. Luna-Bastante L, Gatica-Ortega ME, Pastor-Nieto MA, Vergara-de-la-Campa L, Gómez-Dorado BA, Alonso-Naranjo L, et al. Allergic contact dermatitis to Tinosorb S, Scutellaria baicalensis, and other emerging allergens in cosmetics. Contact Dermatitis [Internet]. 2020 May 1 [cited 2024 Apr 5];82(5):307–9. Available from: https://pubmed.ncbi.nlm.nih.gov/31879957/
235. Suzuki K, Futamura K, Sugiyama M, Matsunaga K, Yagami A. Allergic contact dermatitis caused by dimethicodiethylbenzalmalonate (polysilicone-15, Parsol SLX) and bis-ethylhexyloxyphenol methoxyphenyl triazine (Tinosorb S) in sunscreen cream. Contact

Dermatitis [Internet]. 2022 Jul 1 [cited 2024 Mar 29];87(1):108–10. Available from: https://pubmed.ncbi.nlm.nih.gov/35306675/

236. Benjatikul K, Mahamongkol H, Wongtrakul P. Sunscreen properties of marl. J Oleo Sci [Internet]. 2020 [cited 2024 Mar 27];69(1):73–82. Available from: https://pubmed.ncbi.nlm.nih.gov/31902898/
237. Benevenuto CG, Guerra LO, Gaspar LR. Combination of retinyl palmitate and UV-filters: phototoxic risk assessment based on photostability and in vitro and in vivo phototoxicity assays. Eur J Pharm Sci [Internet]. 2015 Feb 20 [cited 2024 Apr 5];68:127–36. Available from: https://pubmed.ncbi.nlm.nih.gov/25533240/
238. Durand L, Habran N, Henschel V, Amighi K. In vitro evaluation of the cutaneous penetration of sprayable sunscreen emulsions with high concentrations of UV filters. Int J Cosmet Sci [Internet]. 2009 Aug [cited 2024 Apr 5];31(4):279–92. Available from: https://pubmed.ncbi.nlm.nih.gov/19496837/
239. Stien D, Suzuki M, Rodrigues AMS, Yvin M, Clergeaud F, Thorel E, et al. A unique approach to monitor stress in coral exposed to emerging pollutants. Sci Rep 2020 10:1 [Internet]. 2020 Jun 15 [cited 2024 Apr 5];10(1):1–11. Available from: https://www.nature.com/articles/s41598-020-66117-3
240. Thorel E, Clergeaud F, Jaugeon L, Rodrigues AMS, Lucas J, Stien D, et al. Effect of 10 UV filters on the brine shrimp Artemia salina and the marine microalga Tetraselmis sp. Toxics [Internet]. 2020 Jun 1 [cited 2024 Apr 2];8(2). Available from: https://pubmed.ncbi.nlm.nih.gov/32290111/
241. González-Pérez R, Trébol I, García-Río I, Arregui MA, Soloeta R. Allergic contact dermatitis from methylene-bis-benzotriazolyl tetramethylbutylphenol (Tinosorb M). Contact Dermatitis [Internet]. 2007 Feb [cited 2024 Mar 29];56(2):121. Available from: https://pubmed.ncbi.nlm.nih.gov/17244092/
242. De Groot AC, Van Zuuren EJ, Hissink D. Contact allergy to Tinosorb® M: recommendations for diagnostic improvement. Contact Dermatitis [Internet]. 2014 [cited 2024 Mar 29];70(4):251–4. Available from: https://www.researchgate.net/publication/260802511_Contact_allergy_to_TinosorbR_M_Recommendations_for_diagnostic_improvement
243. (PDF) Prediction of sun protection factors by calculation of transmissions with a calibrated step film model [Internet]. [cited 2024 Apr 5]. Available from: https://www.researchgate.net/publication/11447897_Prediction_of_sun_protection_factors_by_calculation_of_transmissions_with_a_calibrated_step_film_model
244. Herzog B, Quass K, Schmidt E, Müller S, Luther H. Physical properties of organic particulate UV absorbers used in sunscreens: II. UV-attenuating efficiency as function of particle size. J Colloid Interface Sci [Internet]. 2004 Aug 15 [cited 2024 Apr 5];276(2):354–63. Available from: https://pubmed.ncbi.nlm.nih.gov/15271563/
245. Adlhart C, Baschong W. Surface distribution and depths profiling of particulate organic UV absorbers by Raman imaging and tape stripping. Int J Cosmet Sci [Internet]. 2011 Dec [cited 2024 Apr 5];33(6):527–34. Available from: https://pubmed.ncbi.nlm.nih.gov/21692815/
246. Zgadzaj A, Skrzypczak A, Welenc I, Ługowska A, Parzonko A, Siedlecka E, et al. Evaluation of photodegradation, phototoxicity and photogenotoxicity of ofloxacin in ointments with sunscreens and in solutions. J Photochem Photobiol B [Internet]. 2015 [cited 2024 Apr 5];144:76–84. Available from: https://pubmed.ncbi.nlm.nih.gov/25728226/
247. Positive patch- and photopatch-test reactions to methylene bis-benzotriazolyl tetramethylbutylphenol in patients with both atopic dermatitis and chronic actinic dermatitis—PubMed [Internet]. [cited 2024 Apr 5]. Available from: https://pubmed.ncbi.nlm.nih.gov/21504696/
248. Liuti F, Borrego L. Contact dermatitis caused by Tinosorb® M: the importance of pach testing with pure methylene bis-benzotriazolyl tetramethylbutylphenol. Contact Dermatitis [Internet]. 2015 Sep 1 [cited 2024 Mar 29];73(3):192–3. Available from: https://pubmed.ncbi.nlm.nih.gov/25962512/
249. Apel C, Joerss H, Ebinghaus R. Environmental occurrence and hazard of organic UV stabilizers and UV filters in the sediment of European North and Baltic Seas. Chemosphere

[Internet]. 2018 Dec 1 [cited 2024 Apr 5];212:254–61. Available from: https://pubmed.ncbi.nlm.nih.gov/30145417/
250. Opinion on the safety of cosmetic ingredients Phenylene Bis-Diphenyltriazine (CAS No 55514-22-2)—S86—submission II. [cited 2024 Apr 5]; Available from: http://ec.europa.eu/health/scientific_committees/experts/declarations/sccs_en.htm
251. Bacqueville D, Jacques-Jamin C, Lapalud P, Douki T, Roullet N, Sereno J, et al. Formulation of a new broad-spectrum UVB + UVA and blue light SPF50+ sunscreen containing Phenylene Bis-Diphenyltriazine (TriAsorB), an innovative sun filter with unique optical properties. J Eur Acad Dermatol Venereol [Internet]. 2022 Jun 1 [cited 2024 Mar 15];36 Suppl 6(S6):29–37. Available from: https://pubmed.ncbi.nlm.nih.gov/35738811/
252. Bacqueville D, Jacques-Jamin C, Dromigny H, Boyer F, Brunel Y, Ferret PJ, et al. Phenylene Bis-Diphenyltriazine (TriAsorB), a new sunfilter protecting the skin against both UVB + UVA and blue light radiations. Photochem Photobiol Sci [Internet]. 2021 Nov 1 [cited 2024 Apr 5];20(11):1475–86. Available from: https://pubmed.ncbi.nlm.nih.gov/34643936/
253. Boyer F, Delsol C, Ribet V, Lapalud P. Broad-spectrum sunscreens containing the TriAsorB™ filter: in vitro photoprotection and clinical evaluation of blue light-induced skin pigmentation. J Eur Acad Dermatol Venereol [Internet]. 2023 Oct 1 [cited 2024 Apr 5];37 Suppl 6(S6):12–21. Available from: https://pubmed.ncbi.nlm.nih.gov/37671996/
254. Le Digabel J, Filiol J, Lauze C, Redoulès D, Josse G. In vivo method for evaluating sunscreen protection against high-energy visible light. J Eur Acad Dermatol Venereol [Internet]. 2023 Oct 1 [cited 2024 Mar 14];37 Suppl 6(S6):6–11. Available from: https://pubmed.ncbi.nlm.nih.gov/37671998/
255. Souza C, Maia Campos PMBG. Development of a HPLC method for determination of four UV filters in sunscreen and its application to skin penetration studies. Biomed Chromatogr [Internet]. 2017 Dec 1 [cited 2024 Apr 5];31(12). Available from: https://pubmed.ncbi.nlm.nih.gov/28623841/
256. Gatica-Ortega ME, Vergara-de-la-Campa L, Alonso-Naranjo L, Pastor-Nieto MA. Relevant sensitization to diethylamino hydroxybenzoyl hexyl benzoate and fragrances in a patient with frontal fibrosing alopecia and acquired dermal macular hyperpigmentation. Contact Dermatitis [Internet]. 2022 Sep 1 [cited 2024 Apr 5];87(3):287–9. Available from: https://pubmed.ncbi.nlm.nih.gov/35506507/
257. Santos AJM, da Silva JCGE. Degradation studies of UV filter hexyl 2-[4-(diethylamino)-2-hydroxybenzoyl]-benzoate (DHHB) in aqueous solution. J Contam Hydrol [Internet]. 2021 Jan 1 [cited 2024 Apr 5];236. Available from: https://pubmed.ncbi.nlm.nih.gov/33271496/
258. Shan P, Lin J, Zhai Y, Dong S, How ZT, Qin R. Transformation and toxicity studies of UV filter diethylamino hydroxybenzoyl hexyl benzoate in the swimming pools. Sci Total Environ [Internet]. 2023 Jul 10 [cited 2024 Apr 5];881. Available from: https://pubmed.ncbi.nlm.nih.gov/37068670/
259. Ye F, Chen W, Deng Z, Chen SL, Dong Z, Dang L, et al. Ultrafast excited-state energy dissipation pathway of diethylamino hydroxybenzoyl hexyl benzoate (DHHB) via the nanoparticles. Photochem Photobiol Sci [Internet]. 2023 Sep 1 [cited 2024 Apr 6];22(9):2133–42. Available from: https://pubmed.ncbi.nlm.nih.gov/37195390/
260. Ma Q, Zhang Y, Huangfu Y, Gao S, Zhou C, Rong H, et al. Solid SiO2-sealed mesoporous silica for synergistically combined use of inorganic and organic filters to achieve safe and effective skin protection from all-band UV radiation. ACS Appl Mater Interfaces [Internet]. 2023 Mar 8 [cited 2024 Apr 6];15(9):12209–20. Available from: https://pubmed.ncbi.nlm.nih.gov/36846915/
261. Hojerová J, Peráčková Z, Beránková M. Margin of safety for two UV filters estimated by in vitro permeation studies mimicking consumer habits: effects of skin shaving and sunscreen reapplication. Food Chem Toxicol [Internet]. 2017 May 1 [cited 2024 Apr 6];103:66–78. Available from: https://pubmed.ncbi.nlm.nih.gov/28216167/
262. Tampucci S, Tofani G, Chetoni P, Di Gangi M, Mezzetta A, Paganini V, et al. Sporopollenin microcapsule: sunscreen delivery system with photoprotective properties. Pharmaceutics

2022 [Internet]. 2022 Sep 24 [cited 2024 Apr 6];14(10):2041. Available from: https://www.mdpi.com/1999-4923/14/10/2041/htm

263. Bryden AM, Moseley H, Ibbotson SH, Chowdhury MMU, Beck MH, Bourke J, et al. Photopatch testing of 1155 patients: results of the U.K. multicentre photopatch study group. Br J Dermatol [Internet]. 2006 Oct [cited 2024 Mar 29];155(4):737–47. Available from: https://pubmed.ncbi.nlm.nih.gov/16965423/
264. Scalia S, Battaglioli S, Bianchi A. In vivo human skin penetration of the UV filter ethylhexyl triazone: effect of lipid microparticle encapsulation. Skin Pharmacol Physiol [Internet]. 2019 Dec 1 [cited 2024 Apr 6];32(1):22–31. Available from: https://pubmed.ncbi.nlm.nih.gov/30380536/
265. Baker LA, Clark SL, Habershon S, Stavros VG. Ultrafast transient absorption spectroscopy of the sunscreen constituent ethylhexyl triazone. J Phys Chem Lett [Internet]. 2017 May 18 [cited 2024 Apr 6];8(10):2113–8. Available from: https://pubmed.ncbi.nlm.nih.gov/28437110/
266. Hewitt JP. Sunscreen formulation: optimising aesthetic elements for twenty-first-century consumers. Principles and practice of photoprotection [Internet]. 2016 Jan 1 [cited 2024 Apr 6];289–302. Available from: https://www.researchgate.net/publication/300329561_Sunscreen_Formulation_Optimising_Aesthetic_Elements_for_Twenty-First-Century_Consumers
267. Naumov S, Herzog B, Abel B. Spectra and photorelaxation of tris-biphenyl-triazine-type UV absorbers: from monomers to nanoparticles. Photochem Photobiol Sci [Internet]. 2023 Sep 1 [cited 2024 Apr 6];22(9):2143–51. Available from: https://pubmed.ncbi.nlm.nih.gov/37277672/
268. Couteau C, Paparis E, Chauvet C, Coiffard L. Tris-biphenyl triazine, a new ultraviolet filter studied in terms of photoprotective efficacy. Int J Pharm [Internet]. 2015 Jun 20 [cited 2024 Apr 6];487(1–2):120–3. Available from: https://pubmed.ncbi.nlm.nih.gov/25843762/
269. Gilaberte Y, González S. Update on photoprotection. Actas Dermosifiliogr (Engl Ed). 2010;101(8):659–72.
270. Sarre ME, Guérin-Moreau M, Lepoittevin JP, Martin L, Avenel-Audran M. Allergic contact cheilitis caused by polysilicone-15 (Parsol® SLX) in a lipcare balm. Contact Dermatitis [Internet]. 2014 Feb [cited 2024 Mar 29];70(2):119–21. Available from: https://pubmed.ncbi.nlm.nih.gov/24450826/
271. Lawrence KP, Sarkany RPE, Acker S, Herzog B, Young AR. A new visible light absorbing organic filter offers superior protection against pigmentation by wavelengths at the UVR-visible boundary region. J Photochem Photobiol B. 2022;227:112372.
272. Słoczyńska K, Popiół J, Gunia-Krzyżak A, Koczurkiewicz-Adamczyk P, Żmudzki P, Pękala E. Evaluation of two novel hydantoin derivatives using reconstructed human skin model Episkin™: perspectives for application as potential sunscreen agents. Molecules [Internet]. 2022 Mar 1 [cited 2024 Apr 6];27(6). Available from: https://www.ncbi.nlm.nih.gov/pmc/articles/PMC8949075/
273. Polonini HC, Dias RMP, Souza IO, Gonçalves KM, Gomes TBB, Raposo NRB, et al. Quinolines derivatives as novel sunscreening agents. Bioorg Med Chem Lett [Internet]. 2013 Aug 15 [cited 2024 Apr 6];23(16):4506–10. Available from: https://pubmed.ncbi.nlm.nih.gov/23856048/
274. Baker LA, Horbury MD, Greenough SE, Allais F, Walsh PS, Habershon S, et al. Ultrafast photoprotecting sunscreens in natural plants. J Phys Chem Lett [Internet]. 2016 Jan 7 [cited 2024 Apr 6];7(1):56–61. Available from: https://pubmed.ncbi.nlm.nih.gov/26654715/
275. Popiół J, Gunia-Krzyżak A, Słoczyńska K, Koczurkiewicz-Adamczyk P, Piska K, Wójcik-Pszczoła K, et al. The involvement of xanthone and (E)-cinnamoyl chromophores for the design and synthesis of novel sunscreening agents. Int J Mol Sci [Internet]. 2020 Jan 1 [cited 2024 Apr 6];22(1):1–23. Available from: https://pubmed.ncbi.nlm.nih.gov/33375127/
276. Messias MA, Ferreira SM, Tavares L, Santos L. A comparative study between onion peel extracts, free and complexed with β-cyclodextrin, as a natural UV filter to cosmetic formula-

tions. Int J Mol Sci [Internet]. 2023 Nov 1 [cited 2024 Apr 2];24(21):15854. Available from: https://www.mdpi.com/1422-0067/24/21/15854/htm

277. Widsten P. Lignin-based sunscreens—state-of-the-art, prospects and challenges. Cosmetics [Internet]. 2020 Nov 6 [cited 2024 Apr 6];7(4):85. Available from: https://www.mdpi.com/2079-9284/7/4/85/htm
278. He hailun, Li anqi, Li shiqin, Tang jie, Li li, Xiong lidan. Natural components in sunscreens: topical formulations with sun protection factor (SPF). Biomed Pharmacother [Internet]. 2021 Feb 1 [cited 2024 Apr 6];134. Available from: https://pubmed.ncbi.nlm.nih.gov/33360043/
279. Wu Y, Gao J, Li JH, Chen BK. Construction of photo-responsive lignin as a broad-spectrum sunscreen agent. Int J Biol Macromol [Internet]. 2023 Dec 31 [cited 2024 Apr 6];253(Pt 6). Available from: https://pubmed.ncbi.nlm.nih.gov/37806425/
280. Piccinino D, Capecchi E, Trifero V, Tomaino E, Marconi C, Del Giudice A, et al. Lignin nanoparticles as sustainable photoprotective carriers for sunscreen filters. ACS Omega [Internet]. 2022 Oct 25 [cited 2024 Apr 6];7(42):37070–7. Available from: https://pubmed.ncbi.nlm.nih.gov/36312404/
281. Lee SC, Yoo E, Lee SH, Won K. Preparation and application of light-colored lignin nanoparticles for broad-spectrum sunscreens. Polymers (Basel) [Internet]. 2020 Mar 1 [cited 2024 Apr 6];12(3). Available from: https://pubmed.ncbi.nlm.nih.gov/32245174/
282. Singh A, Čížková M, Bišová K, Vítová M. Exploring mycosporine-like amino acids (MAAs) as safe and natural protective agents against uv-induced skin damage. Antioxidants (Basel) [Internet]. 2021 May 1 [cited 2024 Apr 6];10(5). Available from: https://pubmed.ncbi.nlm.nih.gov/33925517/
283. Chen M, Jiang Y, Ding Y. Recent progress in unraveling the biosynthesis of natural sunscreens mycosporine-like amino acids. J Ind Microbiol Biotechnol [Internet]. 2023 [cited 2024 Apr 6];50(1). Available from: https://pubmed.ncbi.nlm.nih.gov/37950572/
284. Chen J, Liu Y, Zhao Z, Qiu J. Oxidative stress in the skin: impact and related protection. Int J Cosmet Sci [Internet]. 2021 Oct 1 [cited 2024 Apr 6];43(5):495–509. Available from: https://pubmed.ncbi.nlm.nih.gov/34312881/
285. Jesus A, Mota S, Torres A, Cruz MT, Sousa E, Almeida IF, et al. Antioxidants in sunscreens: which and what for? Antioxidants [Internet]. 2023 Jan 1 [cited 2024 Mar 26];12(1). Available from: https://www.ncbi.nlm.nih.gov/pmc/articles/PMC9854756/
286. Pullar JM, Carr AC, Vissers MCM. The roles of vitamin C in skin health. Nutrients [Internet]. 2017 Aug 12 [cited 2024 Apr 6];9(8). Available from: https://www.ncbi.nlm.nih.gov/pmc/articles/PMC5579659/
287. Gaspar LR, Campos PMBGM. Photostability and efficacy studies of topical formulations containing UV-filters combination and vitamins A, C and E. Int J Pharm [Internet]. 2007 Oct 1 [cited 2024 Mar 27];343(1–2):181–9. Available from: https://pubmed.ncbi.nlm.nih.gov/17614223/
288. Molecular analysis of the chemoprotective effects of topical sunscreen and vitamin C in preventing UV-induced and reactive oxygen species-induced DNA damage, respectively, using the PCR inhibition methodology—PubMed [Internet]. [cited 2024 Apr 6]. Available from: https://pubmed.ncbi.nlm.nih.gov/12553007/
289. Eberlein-Konig B, Placzek M, Przybilla B. Protective effect against sunburn of combined systemic ascorbic acid (vitamin C) and d-alpha-tocopherol (vitamin E). J Am Acad Dermatol [Internet]. 1998 [cited 2024 Apr 6];38(1):45–8. Available from: https://pubmed.ncbi.nlm.nih.gov/9448204/
290. Peres DDA, Sarruf FD, de Oliveira CA, Velasco MVR, Baby AR. Ferulic acid photoprotective properties in association with UV filters: multifunctional sunscreen with improved SPF and UVA-PF. J Photochem Photobiol B [Internet]. 2018 Aug 1 [cited 2024 Apr 6];185:46–9. Available from: https://pubmed.ncbi.nlm.nih.gov/29864725/
291. Jacques C, Bacqueville D, Jeanjean-Miquel C, Génies C, Noizet M, Tourette A, et al. Sustained effect of two antioxidants (oxothiazolidine and δ-tocopheryl glucoside) for immediate and long-term sun protection in a sunscreen emulsion based on their different penetrat-

ing properties. Int J Cosmet Sci [Internet]. 2021 Aug 1 [cited 2024 Apr 6];43(4):391–404. Available from: https://pubmed.ncbi.nlm.nih.gov/33848378/
292. Duteil L, Queille-Roussel C, Aladren S, Bustos X, Trullas C, Granger C, et al. Prevention of polymorphic light eruption afforded by a very high broad-spectrum protection sunscreen containing ectoin. Dermatol Ther (Heidelb) [Internet]. 2022 Jul 1 [cited 2024 Mar 14];12(7):1603–13. Available from: https://pubmed.ncbi.nlm.nih.gov/35716331/
293. Botta C, Di Giorgio C, Sabatier AS, De Méo M. Genotoxicity of visible light (400-800 nm) and photoprotection assessment of ectoin, L-ergothioneine and mannitol and four sunscreens. J Photochem Photobiol B [Internet]. 2008 Apr 25 [cited 2024 Apr 6];91(1):24–34. Available from: https://pubmed.ncbi.nlm.nih.gov/18325778/
294. Fontbonne A, Teme B, Abric E, Lecerf G, Callejon S, Moga A, et al. Positive and ecobiological contribution in skin photoprotection of ectoine and mannitol combined in vivo with UV filters. J Cosmet Dermatol [Internet]. 2024 Jan 1 [cited 2024 Apr 6];23(1):308–15. Available from: https://pubmed.ncbi.nlm.nih.gov/37539499/
295. Fabbrocini G, Cantelli M, Monfrecola G. Topical nicotinamide for seborrheic dermatitis: an open randomized study. J Dermatolog Treat [Internet]. 2014 Jun [cited 2024 Apr 6];25(3):241–5. Available from: https://pubmed.ncbi.nlm.nih.gov/23763270/
296. Cantelli M, Ferrillo M, Granger C, Fabbrocini G. An open-label, investigator-initiated, single-center, prospective, pilot clinical study to evaluate the efficacy of a skin whitening serum applied twice daily combined with a spot-preventing SPF50+ sunscreen in healthy female subjects with melasma hyperpigmentation. J Cosmet Dermatol [Internet]. 2022 Apr 1 [cited 2024 Apr 6];21(4):1523–32. Available from: https://pubmed.ncbi.nlm.nih.gov/34087055/
297. Jo HJ, Joo SM, Kim JY, Yu KH, Kim SW, Peng B. Development of a hybrid chitosan- a nd niacinamide-coupled ZnO nanoparticle composite for sun protection application. J Nanomater 2019;2019.
298. Morocho-Jácome AL, Freire TB, de Oliveira AC, de Almeida TS, Rosado C, Velasco MVR, et al. In vivo SPF from multifunctional sunscreen systems developed with natural compounds-A review. J Cosmet Dermatol [Internet]. 2021 Mar 1 [cited 2024 Apr 6];20(3):729–37. Available from: https://pubmed.ncbi.nlm.nih.gov/32649016/
299. Silymarin and skin cancer prevention: anti-inflammatory, antioxidant and immunomodulatory effects (Review)—PubMed [Internet]. [cited 2024 Apr 6]. Available from: https://pubmed.ncbi.nlm.nih.gov/15586237/
300. Katiyar SK. Skin photoprotection by green tea: antioxidant and immunomodulatory effects. Curr Drug Targets Immune Endocr Metabol Disord [Internet]. 2003 [cited 2024 Apr 6];3(3):234–42. Available from: https://pubmed.ncbi.nlm.nih.gov/12871030/
301. Lee SJ, Lee D, Park SA, Park JJ, Park WH. Hyaluronic acid/polyphenol sunscreens with broad-spectrum UV protection properties from tannic acid and quercetin. Int J Biol Macromol [Internet]. 2024 Feb 1 [cited 2024 Apr 6];257(Pt 1). Available from: https://pubmed.ncbi.nlm.nih.gov/38056734/
302. Protection from inflammation, immunosuppression and carcinogenesis induced by UV radiation in mice by topical Pycnogenol—PubMed [Internet]. [cited 2024 Apr 6]. Available from: https://pubmed.ncbi.nlm.nih.gov/15068032/
303. (PDF) Ex vivo study for evaluating the whitening activity of Pycnogenol® after exposure to ultraviolet and infrared radiations, and visible light [Internet]. [cited 2024 Apr 6]. Available from: https://www.researchgate.net/publication/294733560_Ex_vivo_study_for_evaluating_the_whitening_activity_of_PycnogenolR_after_exposure_to_ultraviolet_and_infrared_radiations_and_visible_light
304. Abdel-Daim MM, Eissa IAM, Abdeen A, Abdel-Latif HMR, Ismail M, Dawood MAO, et al. Lycopene and resveratrol ameliorate zinc oxide nanoparticles-induced oxidative stress in Nile tilapia, Oreochromis niloticus. Environ Toxicol Pharmacol [Internet]. 2019 Jul 1 [cited 2024 Apr 6];69:44–50. Available from: https://pubmed.ncbi.nlm.nih.gov/30953933/
305. Polonini HC, Lima LL, Gonçalves KM, Do Carmo AMR, Da Silva AD, Raposo NRB. Photoprotective activity of resveratrol analogues. Bioorg Med Chem [Internet].

2013 Feb 15 [cited 2024 Apr 6];21(4):964–8. Available from: https://pubmed.ncbi.nlm.nih.gov/23321013/

306. Aguilera J, Vicente-Manzanares M, de Gálvez MV, Herrera-Ceballos E, Rodríguez-Luna A, González S. Booster effect of a natural extract of Polypodium leucotomos (Fernblock®) that improves the UV barrier function and immune protection capability of sunscreen formulations. Front Med (Lausanne) [Internet]. 2021 Jun 2 [cited 2024 Mar 26];8. Available from: https://pubmed.ncbi.nlm.nih.gov/34150816/
307. Pourang A, Dourra M, Ezekwe N, Kohli I, Hamzavi I, Lim HW. The potential effect of Polypodium leucotomos extract on ultraviolet- and visible light-induced photoaging. Photochem Photobiol Sci [Internet]. 2021 Sep 1 [cited 2024 Apr 6];20(9):1229–38. Available from: https://pubmed.ncbi.nlm.nih.gov/34449075/
308. Bosch R, Philips N, Suárez-Pérez JA, Juarranz A, Devmurari A, Chalensouk-Khaosaat J, et al. Mechanisms of photoaging and cutaneous photocarcinogenesis, and photoprotective strategies with phytochemicals. Antioxidants [Internet]. 2015 Jun 1 [cited 2024 Apr 6];4(2):248. Available from: https://www.ncbi.nlm.nih.gov/pmc/articles/PMC4665475/
309. Ganesan P, Choi DK. Current application of phytocompound-based nanocosmeceuticals for beauty and skin therapy. Int J Nanomedicine [Internet]. 2016 May 11 [cited 2024 Apr 6];11:1987–2007. Available from: https://pubmed.ncbi.nlm.nih.gov/27274231/
310. Couteau CAC, Paparis E, Coiffard LJM. An in vitro study of fixed and essential oils claimed to have photoprotective properties. J Photochem Photobiol A Chem. 2022;426:113743.
311. Ácsová A, Hojerová J, Janotková L, Bendová H, Jedličková L, Hamranová V, et al. The real UVB photoprotective efficacy of vegetable oils: in vitro and in vivo studies. Photochem Photobiol Sci [Internet]. 2021 Jan 1 [cited 2024 Apr 6];20(1):139–51. Available from: https://pubmed.ncbi.nlm.nih.gov/33721242/
312. Gause S, Chauhan A. UV-blocking potential of oils and juices. Int J Cosmet Sci [Internet]. 2016 Aug 1 [cited 2024 Apr 6];38(4):354–63. Available from: https://pubmed.ncbi.nlm.nih.gov/26610885/
313. Suwannarach N, Kumla J, Watanabe B, Matsui K, Lumyong S. Characterization of melanin and optimal conditions for pigment production by an endophytic fungus, Spissiomyces endophytica SDBR-CMU319. PLoS One [Internet]. 2019 Sep 1 [cited 2024 Apr 6];14(9):e0222187. Available from: https://journals.plos.org/plosone/article?id=10.1371/journal.pone.0222187
314. Seelam SD, Agsar D, Halmuthur M. SK, Reddy Shetty P, Vemireddy S, Reddy KM, et al. Characterization and photoprotective potentiality of lime dwelling Pseudomonas mediated melanin as sunscreen agent against UV-B radiations. J Photochem Photobiol B [Internet]. 2021 Mar 1 [cited 2024 Apr 6];216. Available from: https://pubmed.ncbi.nlm.nih.gov/33516151/
315. Kurian NK, Bhat SG. Food, cosmetic and biological applications of characterized DOPA-melanin from Vibrio alginolyticus strain BTKKS3. Appl Biol Chem [Internet]. 2018 Apr 1 [cited 2024 Apr 6];61(2):163–71. Available from: https://applbiolchem.springeropen.com/articles/10.1007/s13765-018-0343-y
316. El-Naggar NEA, Saber WIA. Natural melanin: current trends, and future approaches, with especial reference to microbial source. Polymers [Internet]. 2022 Mar 25 [cited 2024 Apr 6];14(7):1339. Available from: https://www.mdpi.com/2073-4360/14/7/1339/htm
317. Hong S, Peng Z, Wu M, Nie Y, Yi Y, Cai H, et al. Human-hair-derived natural particles as multifunctional sunscreen for effective UV protection. ACS Nano [Internet]. 2023 Aug 8 [cited 2024 Apr 6];17(15):14943–53. Available from: https://pubs.acs.org/doi/abs/10.1021/acsnano.3c03504
318. Yarosh DB, Rosenthal A, Moy R. Six critical questions for DNA repair enzymes in skincare products: a review in dialog. Clin Cosmet Investig Dermatol [Internet]. 2019 [cited 2024 Apr 6];12:617–24. Available from: https://pubmed.ncbi.nlm.nih.gov/31695467/
319. Luze H, Nischwitz SP, Zalaudek I, Müllegger R, Kamolz LP. DNA repair enzymes in sunscreens and their impact on photoageing-A systematic review. Photodermatol Photoimmunol Photomed [Internet]. 2020 Nov 1 [cited 2024 Apr 6];36(6):424–32. Available from: https://pubmed.ncbi.nlm.nih.gov/32772409/

320. Hofer A, Legat FJ, Gruber-Wackernagel A, Quehenberger F, Wolf P. Topical liposomal DNA-repair enzymes in polymorphic light eruption. Photochem Photobiol Sci [Internet]. 2011 [cited 2024 Apr 6];10(7):1118–28. Available from: https://pubmed.ncbi.nlm.nih.gov/21437317/
321. Ramírez-Gamboa D, Díaz-Zamorano AL, Meléndez-Sánchez ER, Reyes-Pardo H, Villaseñor-Zepeda KR, López-Arellanes ME, et al. Photolyase production and current applications: a review. Molecules [Internet]. 2022 Sep 1 [cited 2024 Apr 6];27(18). Available from: https://www.ncbi.nlm.nih.gov/pmc/articles/PMC9505440/
322. Alvares BA, Miola AC, Schimitt JV, Miot HA, Abbade LPF. Efficacy of sunscreen with photolyase or regular sunscreen associated with topical antioxidants in treating advanced photodamage and cutaneous field cancerization: a randomized clinical trial. An Bras Dermatol [Internet]. 2022 Mar 1 [cited 2024 Apr 6];97(2):157–65. Available from: https://pubmed.ncbi.nlm.nih.gov/35039206/
323. Geisler AN, Austin E, Nguyen J, Hamzavi I, Jagdeo J, Lim HW. Visible light. Part II: photoprotection against visible and ultraviolet light. J Am Acad Dermatol [Internet]. 2021 May 1 [cited 2024 Mar 20];84(5):1233–44. Available from: https://pubmed.ncbi.nlm.nih.gov/33640513/

Chapter 9
Oral Photoprotective Agents

Abbreviations

AP -1	Activator protein 1
COX-2	Cyclooxygenases-2
DFMO	Difluoromethylornithine
EC	Epicatechin
ECG	Epicatechin 3 gallate
EGC	Epigallocatechin
EGCG	Epigallocatechin-3-gallate
GTE	Green tea extract
MED	Minimal erythemal dose
MITF	Microphthalmia-associated transcription factor
MMP-1	Matrix metalloproteinases-1
NF-κB	Nuclear factor kappa B
NOs	Nitrous oxides species
NRF-2	Nuclear factor erythroid 2 related protein
NSAID	Nonsteroidal anti-inflammatory drugs
PGE2	Prostaglandin E2
PM	Particulate matter
PMLE	Polymorphous light eruption
SCC	Squamous cell carcinoma
SOC	Skin of colour
SPF	Sun protection factor
TF3'G	Theaflavin-3'-gallate
TNF	Tumour necrosis factor
TRP	Tyrosine-related protein
UVA	Ultraviolet-A
UVA-PF	Ultraviolet A-protection factor
UVB	Ultraviolet-B
UVR	Ultraviolet radiation

R. Rajan, *Sunscreens for Skin of Color*,
https://doi.org/10.1007/978-981-97-3195-4_9

Key Objectives

- Oral antioxidants have been proven to provide significant UV protection abilities.
- The advantages of oral photoprotection agents are that they are easy to use, and also provide holistic benefits in addition to UV protection, many of them being antioxidants and free radical scavengers. However, the exact reliability and repeatability of the protection they provide remains to be established.
- Vitamin D, carotenoids, astaxanthin, extracts of green tea, polypodium and pine bark, resveratrol, niacinamide, and vitamin C, among other agents, demonstrate UV photoprotection abilities.
- Topical sunscreens cannot be replaced by oral sunscreens, despite their holistic benefits on other organ systems in addition to photoprotection.

9.1 Systemic Photoprotective Agents for Prevention of Skin Cancer

Oral supplements that provide some protection against the effects of UV radiation on the skin have been popularly called internal sunscreens or oral sunscreens, or even more colloquially, as 'sunscreen pills'. However, the loose usage of this terminology has been criticized, as consumers often consider such sunscreen pills as equivalent to topical sunscreen, preferring the simpler act of swallowing a pill. Comparatively, a topical sunscreen looks messier especially when there is a need for periodic reapplication. So, it is recommended to consider oral photoprotective agents as photoprotective supplements that cannot be considered a replacement for topical sunscreens, which are supported by a larger body of research and evidence. However, research on oral photo protecting supplements has been significant in the last few decades and adds an important tool in providing/achieving holistic sun protection. Furthermore, since many of these supplements are, in essence, strong antioxidants, a case for holistic health and successful ageing, can also be made.

The main advantages of systemic photoprotection agents are the ease of use and lesser dependence on external conditions. Furthermore, it is possible to clearly elucidate half-lives and bioavailability and establish systemic safety and toxicity parameters, which remain fairly uniform across different climates and environments. However, it is very crucial that systemic sun protection agents have cutaneous affinity and are graded by responses which make sense to skin health. Otherwise, the lack of selectivity in terms of reducing solar induced skin changes such as sunburn and tanning may make some of these agents less than optimal for long-term use [1]. Overall, most of these antioxidants, even those with demonstrated protective effects, may need to be used in conjunction with conventional therapies for clinical benefit when treating pigmentation and photoageing [2].

9.1.1 Vitamin D

Though often not listed as a typical systemic photoprotective agent, optimal levels of vitamin D3 are considered important for maintaining antioxidant levels which may be protective against cancer. The structure of Vitamin D3 is depicted in Fig. 9.1. The total antioxidant capacity was found to be low in individuals with skin cancer, who also had vitamin D deficiencies [3]. While larger studies found no significant benefit for vitamin D3 supplementation for the prevention of melanoma or non-melanoma skin cancers, very low vitamin D levels were observed in cases with distant metastasis. Also, a small protective benefit for vitamin D3 in prevention of malignant melanoma was noted in women with a known history of nonmelanoma skin cancer [4]. The optimal recommended vitamin D3 level is 50–60 ng/ml and it may be advisable to stay within this narrow zone to balance vitamin D requirement for the body and toxic and/or pro-oxidant effects [5]. For a detailed discussion on the subject of topical sunscreen use and vitamin D deficiency, visit the section in Chap. 12.

Fig. 9.1 Chemical structure of Vitamin D

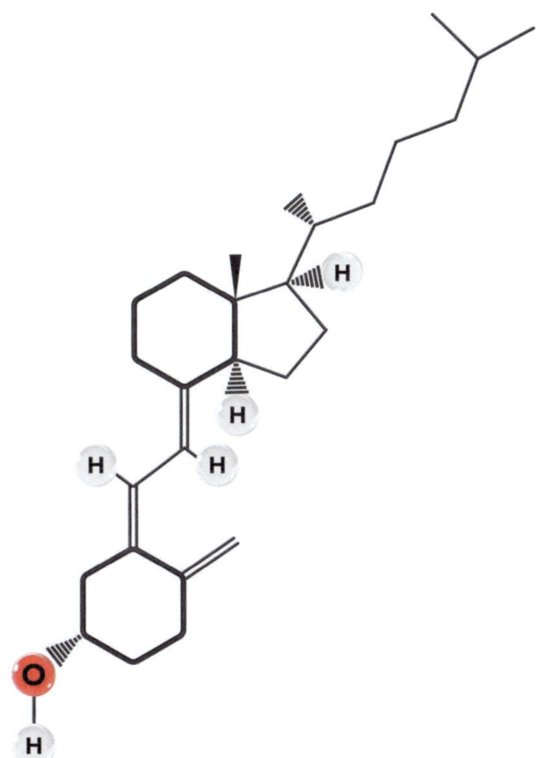

9.1.2 Carotenoids

Carotenoids are present abundantly in diet, in over 50 varieties. They have the potential to reduce ultraviolet A (UVA) and ultraviolet B (UVB) induced free radical generation, and thereby boost antioxidant reserves in skin, preventing lipid peroxidation and DNA damage. Among carotenoids, lycopenes are considered to have the most potent antioxidant effect. Lycopene intake, either as supplements or in diet, was found to improve skin biophysical parameters, mainly acting through suppression of UVB-induced free radical generation and Matrix metalloproteinases-1 (MMP -1) with a resultant decrease in collagen breakdown and skin photoageing. A tumour suppression effect was also noted with lycopene supplementation, through inhibition of recruitment of inflammatory mediators to sites of ultraviolet (UV) induced damage. The interesting aspect about photoprotection from antioxidants like lycopene is that while supplementation reduces UV-induced erythema by 37%, there was a total inhibition of free radical driven UVA induced gene transcription, which is very encouraging [6].

Still, the ideal dose for photoprotection, and any advantage of proprietary supplements over increase intake of lycopene in diet, is unknown [1]. As a dietary source, sun dried tomatoes contain up to 4–6 times more lycopene than fresh tomatoes [7].

The role of beta-carotene, another potent carotenoid, in cutaneous photoprotection, seems to be dose dependent, with higher doses demonstrating pro-oxidant behaviour, structure in Fig. 9.2. Despite a lack of benefit against cancer as demonstrated in the Nambour studies [8], and being implicated as displaying a potential risk for increased occurrence of lung and gastrointestinal malignancies [9], beta-carotenes continue to be used as a photoprotection agent, due to their ability to reduce photosensitivity in up to 80% of patients with erythropoietic porphyria. More recently, beta-carotene supplementation was found to protect against sunburn [10]. No increased risk for melanoma was noted [11]. However, recommendations for long-term supplementation with beta-carotene for cancer chemoprevention remains controversial [12].

9.1.3 Tea

Green tea extracts from Camellia species have been known to have anti-inflammatory, antioxidant, photoprotective, and chemopreventive benefits on oral intake. Four specific flavonoid catechins are responsible for these effects. These are (−)-epigallocatechin-3-gallate (EGCG), (−)-epigallocatechin (EGC), (−)-epicatechin-3-gallate (ECG), and (−)-epicatechin (EC) [13]. In a double-blind placebo controlled study, 250 mg daily supplementation of green tea extract (GTE) was found to lessen brown spots and UV spots on the skin, at 1 year of supplementation. Consumption of a larger volume of green tea up to 1 litre was found to be

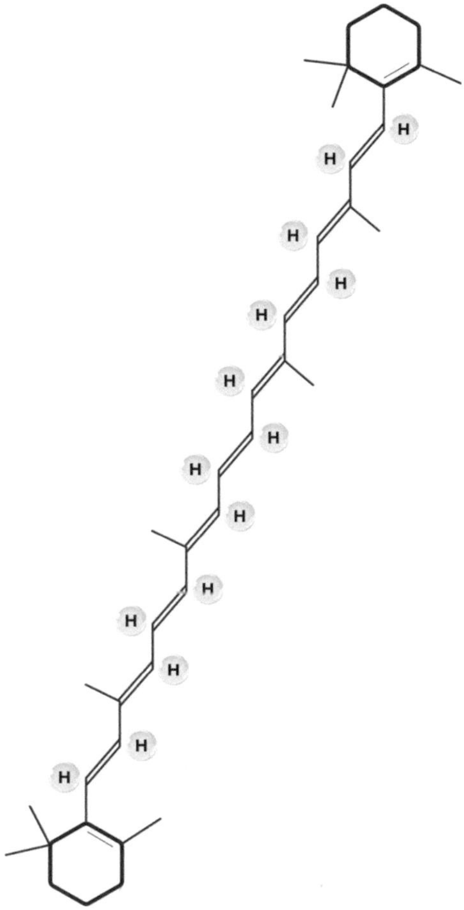

Fig. 9.2 Chemical structure of beta-carotene

associated with skin antiageing parameters such as increased skin hydration and elasticity, but the practicality and safety of such large volume consumption remains to be seen [14].

Green tea catechins have been studied to provide systemic photoprotection, evidenced as reduction of UV-induced erythema. This effect is attributed to the ability of green tea catechins to counter cyclooxygenase pathways, where UV induced erythema is dependent on prostaglandin E2 (PGE2) among other inflammatory mediators [13]. EGCG is able to counter tumourigenesis and oxidative stress, in the initiation phase, Fig. 9.3. When compared to placebo, green tea oral catechin intake was found to protect against ultraviolet radiation (UVR) induced erythema in the minimal erythemal dose (MED) range of 1.25–1.3 [15]. Catechin extracts from other tea species such as 2S,3R-6-methoxycarbonyl gallocatechin and theaflavin-3'-gallate (TF3'G) have also been studied to protect against UVB-induced inflammatory changes [16, 17]. However, Farrar et al. observed no benefit from oral supplementation of green tea catechins in preventing UV-induced damage through

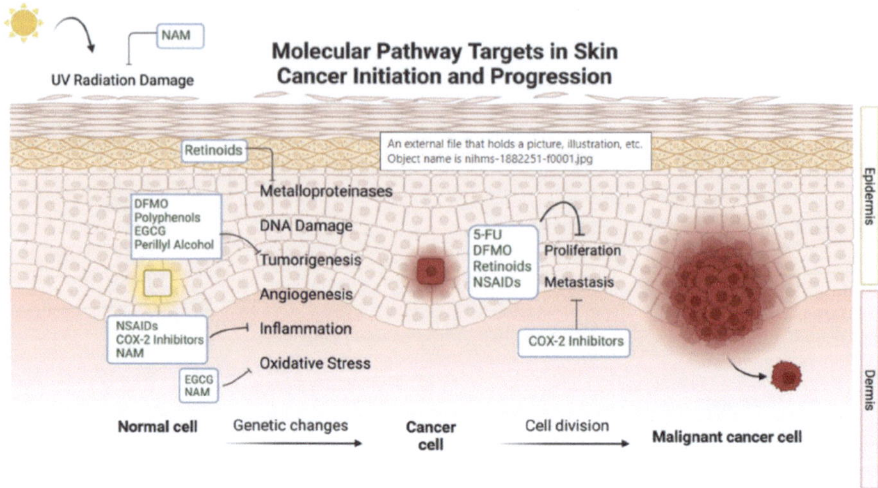

Fig. 9.3 Molecular pathway targets in skin cancer initiation and progression. NAM nicotinamide, DFMO difluoromethylornithine, 5-FU 5-fluorouracil, COX cyclooxygenase, NSAID non-steroidal anti-inflammatory drugs, EGCG epigallocatechin-3-gallate. (Obtained from Jiminez and Yusuf, under a Creative Commons Attribution 4.0 International License (https://creativecommons.org/licenses/by/4.0/) [56])

protection from pro-inflammatory processes or cellular chemotaxis [18, 19]. More data is required to use this dietary antioxidant for measurable and reliable photoprotection.

9.1.4 *Polypodium*

Polypodium is a plant extract, obtained from the fern *Polypodium leucotomos*, traditionally known for its medicinal potential in Central and South America. A proprietary standardized aqueous extract obtained from the plant, as Fernblock®, is used as a photoprotective agent, in both topical formulations and as oral supplements. Caffeic and ferulic acid are the most notable and principal phenolic antioxidants in this extract, and along with vanillic, p-coumaric, and chlorogenic acid among other polyphenols, said to be responsible for the photoprotective effects attributed to this phytoactive. Specifically, as a proprietary ingredient, Fernblock® has been compared to other polypodium extracts, and claimed to provide superior photoprotection properties owing to a controlled ratio of the different polyphenol components [20].

The mechanism of action of polypodium is centred around its antioxidant ability to reduce lipid peroxidation and quenching of reactive oxygen species and downstream free radicals. This action is said to be more comprehensive in comparison to the antioxidant vitamins, A, C, and E, which are said to act predominantly against singlet oxygen. Polypodium also exhibits photoprotective activity against inflammatory mediators and inflammation related transcriptional factors such as cyclooxygenases-2 (COX2), PGE2, tumour necrosis factor-α (TNF-α), nitrous oxide species (NOs), nuclear factor κ-B (NF-κB), AP-1 (activator protein 1), NRF 2 (nuclear factor erythroid 2 related protein). In topical sunscreen formulations, addition of 1% polypodium was found to be synergistic with UV filters, both chemical and mineral, and significantly attenuated UVR on the skin. Furthermore, sunscreen performance in terms of standard metrics like sun protection factor (SPF) and ultraviolet protection factor (UVA-PF) was found to be boosted by the addition of polypodium to sunscreen formulations. Specifically, biological protection factors such as contact hypersensitivity factors and human immunoprotective factors were also noted to be increased by polypodium supplementation in these sunscreens providing benefit against solar induced immunosuppression [21, 22]. Used in topical sunscreen formulations along with oral supplementation and sun protection behaviour, polypodium was found to reduce the risk of new lesions in patients with xeroderma pigmentosum [23]. An additive photoprotective effect of the oral polypodium supplement was noted in patients with actinic keratosis over a 12-month study period [24]. The protective action potentially stems from the antioxidant ability of polypodium to restore optimal expression of p53, reduce cell proliferation, and inhibit UV induced cyclooxygenase-2 in skin cells [25]. Attenuation of the UVB-induced erythema was noted within 2 h of ingestion of a 240 mg dose of polypodium, in light-skinned individuals [26].

Polypodium supplements have been evaluated as part of a combination approach for melasma in Asian skin. A double-blind, placebo controlled trial compared the additional benefit of polypodium supplement in patients who were treated for melasma with sunscreens and topical 4% hydroquinone and found that the addition of oral polypodium supplement accelerated the clinical response, compared to placebo [27]. Polypodium oral supplementation in combination with pomegranate extracts was found to increase skin hydration, elasticity, and reduce skin sebum and melanin index, over a 3-month period [28].

Furthermore, polypodium has been considered beneficial in a host of other photoaggravated conditions such as polymorphous light eruption (PMLE), actinic prurigo, solar urticaria, chronic actinic dermatosis, photosensitive lupus lesions, and rosacea [22]. Interestingly, polypodium leucotomos supplements have also been used in vitiligo, potentially to address Astaxanthin, a xanthophyll the oxidative stress hypothesis where an impaired melanocyte redox homeostasis initiates the onset of vitiligo [29].

9.1.5 Astaxanthin

Astaxanthin, a xanthophyll carotenoid, has been observed to have photoprotective properties when taken orally, Fig. 9.4 [30, 31]. Astaxanthin is naturally found in the marine and aquatic environment, biosynthesized by microalgae and phytoplankton [32]. Progressive accumulation occurs up the food chain through zooplankton,

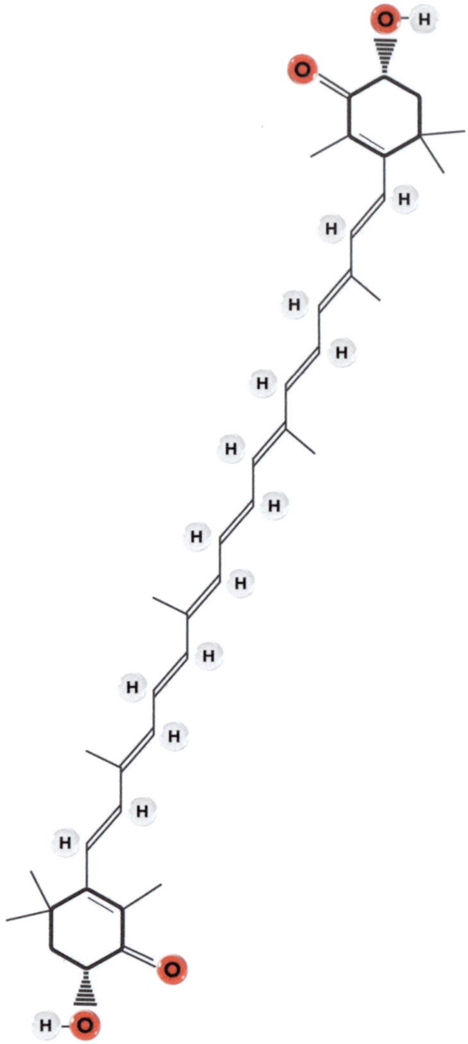

Fig. 9.4 Chemical structure of astaxanthin

crustaceans, and fish, like salmonids, shrimp, crayfish, and further to higher organisms, typically flamingo, giving these organisms their characteristic red-orange hue. In these organisms, astaxanthin regulates several important biological functions, such as pigmentation, UV protection, biocommunication, immune responses, reproduction, stress tolerance, and protection against oxidation. For applications in well regulated human cosmeceuticals and nutraceuticals, astaxanthin is predominantly obtained from the microalgae *Haematococcus pluvialis,* though synthetic forms are also in the market [33].

Though astaxanthin is structurally related to other carotenoids, it does not get converted to vitamin A. The bioactivity of astaxanthin is also much higher than beta-carotene, lutein and zeaxanthin, with very efficient free radical scavenging properties, mitochondrial protection, restoration of redox balance, and preservation of cell membrane integrity. Astaxanthin has both lipophilic and hydrophilic domains, resulting in effective free radical scavenging both at the cell surface and at the phospholipid bilayer of the cellular membranes. In addition to cutaneous UV protection in humans, astaxanthin potentially also has other multifunctional benefits such as anticancer, anti-inflammatory, antioxidant function with cardio and neuro protective behaviour [4, 33]. The anti-inflammatory properties of astaxanthin protect against UV-induced reactive nitrogen species generation, expression of inflammatory cytokines, and modulate apoptosis in DNA damaged keratinocytes in addition to countering UV-induced immunosuppression. In humans, dietary astaxanthin supplementation reduced UV-induced erythema and skin dryness [32]. Astaxanthin has been considered for cancer chemoprevention of skin cancers, though limited data exists [4]. In the domain of photoageing, the benefits of astaxanthin supplementation are related to its ability to suppress hyperpigmentation and melanin synthesis and to reduce signs of photoageing by inhibiting matrix metalloproteinases. This leads to a prevention of collagen breakdown and an increase in skin collagen levels. An enhanced wound repairing ability attributed to astaxanthin also prevents photoageing. Combining astaxanthin with oral collagen peptides was found to be synergistic for prevention of skin ageing [33]. Astaxanthin has been used in clinical studies at 12 mg per day for up to a year in renal transplant patients and is considered safe at a daily intake of 2–4 mg [34].

More recently, the ability of topical astaxanthin to act as an antioxidant in sunscreens has been explored. Astaxanthin acts by reducing redness and oedema associated with sun exposure in addition to being protective against UV light [35]. Liposomal formulations of astaxanthin have been shown to reduce UV induced skin thickening and collagen breakdown, with more potent free radical scavenging capacity than alpha tocopherol [36, 37]. Interestingly, astaxanthin topical eye drops have been found to reduce UV induced corneal damage [38].

9.1.6 Pycnogenol®

Pycnogenol® is a standardized procyanidin rich proprietary compound obtained from the bark of *Pinus pinaster*, the French maritime pine tree. The other active antioxidant moieties in Pycnogenol® include bioflavonoids, catechins, and phenolic acids [39].

Saliou et al. found that oral supplementation of Pycnogenol® increased the UVR dose required to achieve 1MED, indicating an ability to reduce UV induced erythema, potentially acting through inhibition of NF-κB-dependant gene expression [40]. Relevant to skin of colour (SOC), Pycnogenol® was found to significantly inhibit UV radiation induced upregulation of microphthalmia-associated transcription factor (MITF) and tyrosinase-related protein (TRP-1), key molecules involved in photopigmentation and pigmentary conditions like melasma. Another potential pathway is through the aryl hydrocarbon receptor which is involved in UV induced cutaneous pigmentation [39]. Pycnogenol® was found to decrease particulate pollution induced skin pigmentation in women exposed to particulate matter (PM), typically PM2.5 pollution in hot climates, compared to placebo. This is advantageous, considering the facilitation of photopigmentation by air pollution [41].

9.1.7 Nicotinamide

Nicotinamide acts by enhancing local production of adenosine triphosphate in the skin, to counter an energy crisis that occurs following UV irradiation with cellular depletion and reduced production of ATP, structure in Fig. 9.5. This results in cellular protection from the effects of UV induced immunosuppression and promotes enhanced DNA repair resulting in reduction of cutaneous photocarcinogenesis, Fig. 9.6. Oral supplementation of nicotinamide was found to reduce the progression of precancerous lesions, to malignant tumours, specifically actinic keratosis, in a high risk population [42]. This agent has been considered to be of benefit in preventing distant spread and/or recurrence of squamous cell carcinoma (SCC) [4]. Nicotinamide also enhances immune function, which plays a key role in preventing photocarcinogenesis [43]. Nicotinamide is easily obtained from natural sources such as potatoes, banana, grains, turkey, and tuna [44]. The daily recommended intake of this water soluble vitamin varies by age, gender, pregnancy, and lactation status [43]. Diarrhoea may be a side effect with oral supplementation at higher doses [4].

9.1.8 Vitamin C

Contrary to expectations, the role of vitamin C supplementation for cutaneous photoprotection is controversial. The structure of L-ascorbic acid is shown in Fig. 9.7. in Serge et al. found an increase in the risk of skin cancers for women, on

Fig. 9.5 Chemical structure of nicotinamide

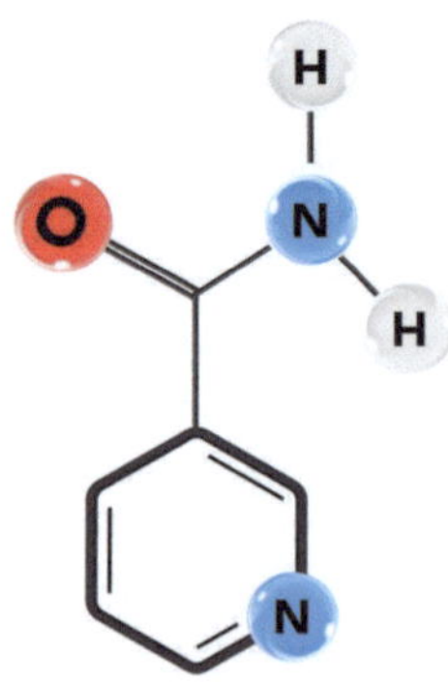

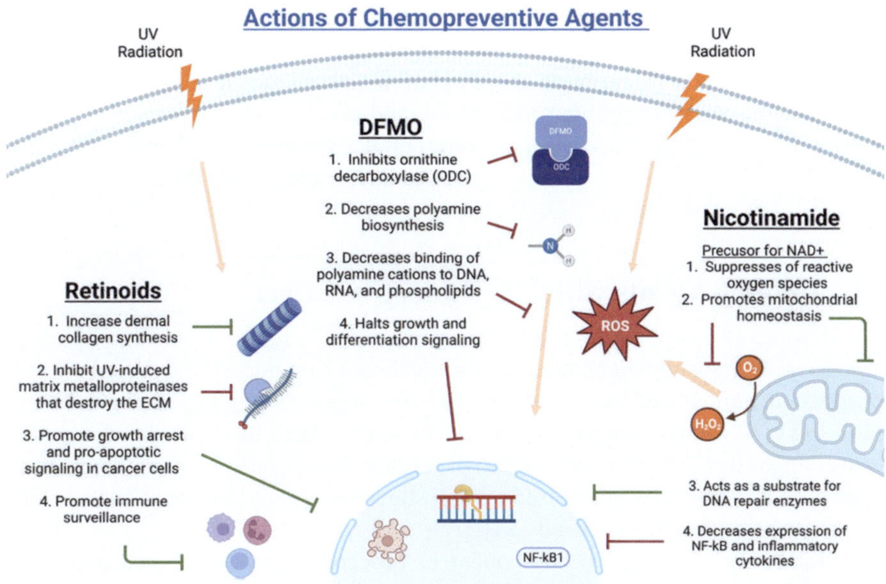

Fig. 9.6 Detailed Mechanisms of Retinoids, DFMO, and Nicotinamide Chemoprevention. (Obtained from Jiminez and Yusuf [56], under a Creative Commons Attribution 4.0 International License (https://creativecommons.org/licenses/by/4.0/) [56]

Fig. 9.7 Chemical structure of Vitamin C

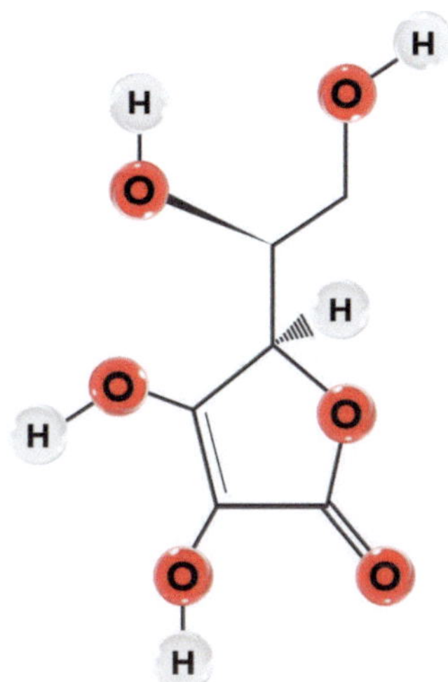

antioxidant supplements which included vitamin C, while Kashif et al. found that vitamin C, and also vitamin A, at doses that lower free radical generation, accelerate the metastasis of malignant melanoma [45, 46]. Furthermore, stopping the supplements was found to reduce the risk of skin cancer [47]. Interestingly, the adverse effects of these antioxidants were noted more commonly in women. The increased risk of melanoma was considered relevant even for intake of vitamin C for dietary sources such as orange juice [48]. However, researchers have noted that high concentrations of vitamin C promote apoptosis of malignant melanoma cells, while low concentrations may act counterproductively and promote tumour growth [49, 50]. Wang et al. suggest that there may be differential responses to oral and intravenous supplementation, with only the latter being toxic to cancer cells [50].

9.2 Dietary Agents with UV Protective Effect

Mangifera indica supplementation has been shown to reduce UV induced wrinkle formation in animal studies, and wrinkling as a component of photoageing in human studies [51, 52]. Interestingly, in the human study where the benefits of mangoes were compared at different daily doses, the higher dosage failed to show a beneficial effect probably due to the increased overall sugar content in the diet resulting from, precisely, the higher dosage itself [53].

Sulforaphane, a bioactive component in broccoli, has been known to protect against UV induced erythema and free radical damage with a potential for chemoprevention of skin cancer, structure shown in Fig. 9.8. Cucumber, kale, and tomato are other dietary supplements rich in lycopene and related compounds, with possible benefits for the prevention of photoageing and photopigmentation as well [54].

There exists a significant perception gap among consumers regarding the amount of dietary agents that needs to be taken to achieve significant benefits as had been demonstrated in clinical studies and trials which mostly employ highly concentrated forms of the phytochemicals [55] For example, to achieve a therapeutic dose of 1 g of resveratrol, a person may need to consume more than 30,000 kg of peanuts in a day! (Fig. 9.9).

9.2.1 Drugs for Systemic Photoprotection

Retinoids like isotretinoin and anti-inflammatory agents like non-steroidal anti-inflammatory drugs (NSAIDs) have been used to protect against photocarcinogenesis in select groups of predisposed individuals such as solid organ transplant recipients, but the utility of these agents for general photoprotection is not clear [56, 57]. Difluoromethylornithine (DFMO), a novel molecule, reduces polyamine generation as an inhibitor of ornithine decarboxylase and has been associated with

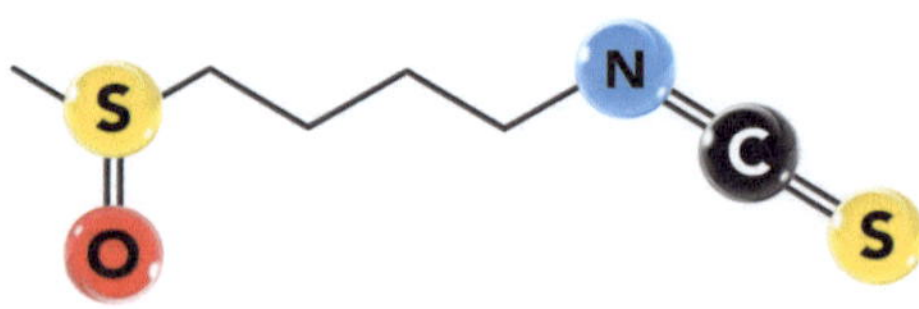

Fig. 9.8 Chemical structure of sulforaphane

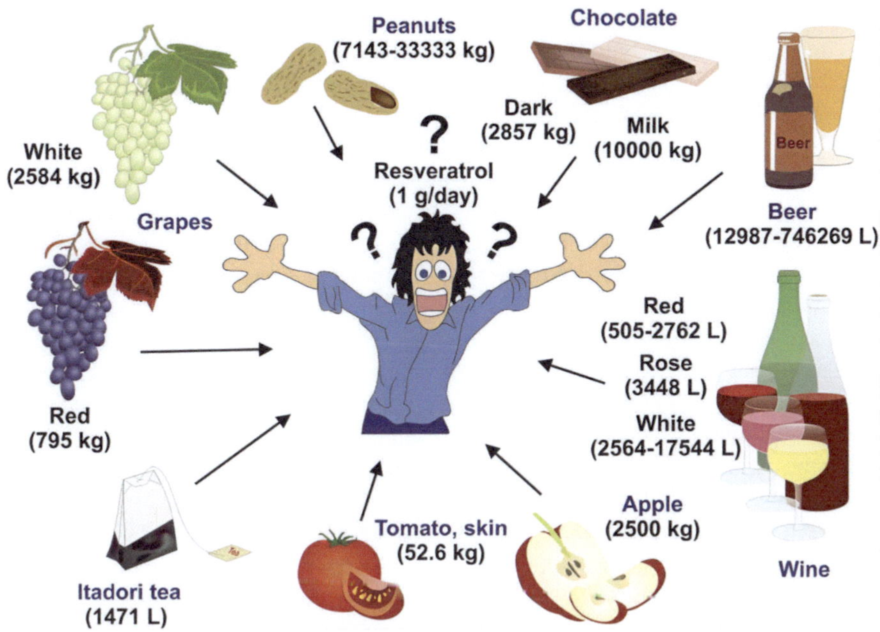

Fig. 9.9 Quantities of food and beverages that must be consumed to reach therapeutic doses. Based on animal studies, daily resveratrol doses in the range of hundreds of milligrams to several grams for therapeutic intervention have been proposed. If a person intends to ingest 1 g resveratrol each day, this would require consuming the depicted quantities of foods or beverages. The calculation is based on typical resveratrol contents found in peanuts without seed coats (0.03–0.14 μg/g), red wine (Pinot noir from France, 0.362–1.979 mg/L) (127), white wine (Riesling from Spain, 0.057–0.390 mg/L), rosé wine from Serbia (0.29 mg/L), beer (1.34–77.0 μg/L), skin of tomato (~19 μg/g dry weight), dark chocolate (350 μg/kg), milk chocolate (100 μg/kg), Itadori tea (68 μg/100 mL, when prepared by infusing 1 g of the commercial root prepared with 100 mL of boiling water for 5 min), red Merlot grapes from Japan (1259 μg/kg fresh weight), white Riesling grapes from Japan (387 μg/kg fresh weight), and cultivated apples (estimating a mean total content of 400 μg/kg fresh weight found in 150 different cultivars). (Obtained with permission from Weiskirchen and Weiskirchen [55]. Copyright Clearance Center, Inc. [55])

reduction of tumourigenesis in early studies, Figs. 9.3 and 9.6. Since such drugs have to be used for prolonged periods of time to achieve a meaningful reduction in cancer burden, the side effect profile merits scrutiny. DFMO, for example, was reported to be associated with dose-dependent hearing loss [43, 58]. However, as an evolving science, chemoprevention for both photocarcinogenesis and for photoageing and photopigmentation are interesting avenues for further research [57].

Many other agents are now being explored to have UV protecting properties such as oral fish collagen supplements [59, 60], apigenin, equine placental extracts, red paprika supplements, and milk ferments among others. As an attractive prospect for providing holistic health benefits, oral photoprotection agents are increasing in popularity.

The Antioxidant Paradox!

While antioxidants have a definite place in photoprotection, there is the question of the antioxidant paradox. Though antioxidants are protective against tumour genesis, they may also promote tumour development once the tumour is established, by reducing the oxidative stress on the tumour cells. Antioxidant substances that can be sustainably used over time need to offer differential impact to host cells and tumour cells, an area that needs further research [42]. Furthermore, the response to different antioxidants across different routes of administration and different substrates of evaluation has thrown up conflicting conclusions. Ascorbic acid and beta carotene were found to reduce protective responses to UVR, while tocopherol analogues enhance protection in an in vitro study [61]. In contrast, in an animal study, topical tocopherol alone enhanced tumourigenesis but tocopherol in combination with vitamin C and ferulic acid, reduced tumourigenesis [62]. Beta-carotene, which has been found to be effective for certain types of porphyria, has been documented to have a pro-oxidant role [12]. Furthermore, the role of antioxidants can vary from protective to promoting, depending on the types of systemic malignancy [63–65]. This demonstrates a very nuanced interplay of various cell signals modulated by these vitamins [66]. Much more research is needed in this domain, before concluding all vitamins or antioxidants as 'must have' supplements.

9.3 Chapter Summary

Photoprotection approaches in best practice are a composite strategy anchored on topical sunscreens, physical sun protection methods, and oral sunscreens. Several antioxidants have been demonstrated to have photoprotection benefits, mostly studied in the UV domain. The endpoints for clinical benefit of these oral agents studied range from UV induced erythema to biological endpoints like UV induced immunosuppression, much like the clinical outcomes studied when evaluating the efficacy of topical sunscreens.

References

1. Parrado C, Philips N, Gilaberte Y, Juarranz A, González S. Oral photoprotection: effective agents and potential candidates. Front Med (Lausanne) [Internet]. 2018 Jun 1 [cited 2024 Mar 26];5(JUN). Available from: https://pubmed.ncbi.nlm.nih.gov/29998107/
2. Searle T, Ali FR, Al-Niaimi F. Systemic photoprotection in 2021. Clin Exp Dermatol [Internet]. 2021 Oct 1 [cited 2024 Mar 26];46(7):1189–204. Available from: https://pubmed.ncbi.nlm.nih.gov/33872410/

3. Karampinis E, Aloizou AM, Zafiriou E, Bargiota A, Skaperda Z, Kouretas D, et al. Non-melanoma skin cancer and vitamin D: the "lost sunlight" paradox and the oxidative stress explanation. Antioxidants (Basel) [Internet]. 2023 May 1 [cited 2024 Mar 26];12(5). Available from: https://pubmed.ncbi.nlm.nih.gov/37237973/
4. Hyeraci M, Papanikolau ES, Grimaldi M, Ricci F, Pallotta S, Monetta R, et al. Systemic photoprotection in melanoma and non-melanoma skin cancer. Biomolecules [Internet]. 2023 Jul 1 [cited 2024 Mar 26];13(7). Available from: https://pubmed.ncbi.nlm.nih.gov/37509103/
5. Schagen SK, Zampeli VA, Makrantonaki E, Zouboulis CC. Discovering the link between nutrition and skin aging. Dermatoendocrinol [Internet]. 2012 Jul 7 [cited 2024 Mar 26];4(3):298. Available from: https://www.ncbi.nlm.nih.gov/pmc/articles/PMC3583891/
6. Heinrich U, Gärtner C, Wiebusch M, Eichler O, Sies H, Tronnier H, et al. Supplementation with β-carotene or a similar amount of mixed carotenoids protects humans from UV-induced erythema. J Nutr. 2003;133(1):98–101.
7. Karakaya S, Yilmaz N. Lycopene content and antioxidant activity of fresh and processed tomatoes and in vitro bioavailability of lycopene. J Sci Food Agric [Internet]. 2007 Sep 1 [cited 2024 Mar 26];87(12):2342–7. Available from: https://onlinelibrary.wiley.com/doi/full/10.1002/jsfa.2998
8. Green A, Williams G, Neale R, Hart V, Leslie D, Parsons P, et al. Daily sunscreen application and betacarotene supplementation in prevention of basal-cell and squamous-cell carcinomas of the skin: a randomised controlled trial. Lancet [Internet]. 1999 Aug 28 [cited 2024 Mar 3];354(9180):723–9. Available from: https://pubmed.ncbi.nlm.nih.gov/10475183/
9. Druesne-Pecollo N, Latino-Martel P, Norat T, Barrandon E, Bertrais S, Galan P, et al. Beta-carotene supplementation and cancer risk: a systematic review and metaanalysis of randomized controlled trials. Int J Cancer [Internet]. 2010 Jul 1 [cited 2024 Mar 26];127(1):172–84. Available from: https://pubmed.ncbi.nlm.nih.gov/19876916/
10. Köpcke W, Krutmann J. Protection from sunburn with beta-Carotene--a meta-analysis. Photochem Photobiol [Internet]. 2008 Mar [cited 2024 Mar 26];84(2):284–8. Available from: https://pubmed.ncbi.nlm.nih.gov/18086246/
11. Asgari MM, Maruti SS, Kushi LH, White E. Antioxidant supplementation and risk of incident melanomas: results of a large prospective cohort study. Arch Dermatol [Internet]. 2009 Aug [cited 2024 Mar 26];145(8):879–82. Available from: https://pubmed.ncbi.nlm.nih.gov/19687417/
12. Black HS. Pro-carcinogenic activity of beta-carotene, a putative systemic photoprotectant. Photochem Photobiol Sci [Internet]. 2004 Aug 4 [cited 2024 Mar 26];3(8):753–8. Available from: https://pubmed.ncbi.nlm.nih.gov/15295631/
13. Kapoor MP, Sugita M, Fukuzawa Y, Timm D, Ozeki M, Okubo T. Green tea catechin association with ultraviolet radiation-induced erythema: a systematic review and meta-analysis. Molecules [Internet]. 2021 Jun 17 [cited 2024 Mar 26];26(12). Available from: https://pubmed.ncbi.nlm.nih.gov/34204433/
14. Rabinovich L, Kazlouskaya V. Herbal sun protection agents: human studies. Clin Dermatol [Internet]. 2018 May 1 [cited 2024 Mar 26];36(3):369–75. Available from: https://pubmed.ncbi.nlm.nih.gov/29908579/
15. Heinrich U, Moore CE, De Spirt S, Tronnier H, Stahl W. Green tea polyphenols provide photoprotection, increase microcirculation, and modulate skin properties of women. J Nutr [Internet]. 2011 Jun 1 [cited 2024 Mar 26];141(6):1202–8. Available from: https://pubmed.ncbi.nlm.nih.gov/21525260/
16. Kim D, Hu R, Fan Y, Xu YN, Park HJ, Lee SK. Photoprotective effects of 2S,3R-6-methoxycarbonylgallocatechin isolated from Anhua dark tea on UVB-induced inflammatory responses in human keratinocytes. J Photochem Photobiol B [Internet]. 2020 Jan 1 [cited 2024 Mar 26];202. Available from: https://pubmed.ncbi.nlm.nih.gov/31743829/
17. Zheng X, Feng M, Wan J, Shi Y, Xie X, Pan W, et al. Anti-damage effect of theaflavin-3'-gallate from black tea on UVB-irradiated HaCaT cells by photoprotection and maintaining cell homeostasis. J Photochem Photobiol B [Internet]. 2021 Nov 1 [cited 2024 Mar 26];224. Available from: https://pubmed.ncbi.nlm.nih.gov/34536907/

18. Farrar MD, Nicolaou A, Clarke KA, Mason S, Massey KA, Dew TP, et al. A randomized controlled trial of green tea catechins in protection against ultraviolet radiation-induced cutaneous inflammation. Am J Clin Nutr [Internet]. 2015 Sep 1 [cited 2024 Mar 26];102(3):608–15. Available from: https://pubmed.ncbi.nlm.nih.gov/26178731/
19. Farrar MD, Huq R, Mason S, Nicolaou A, Clarke KA, Dew TP, et al. Oral green tea catechins do not provide photoprotection from direct DNA damage induced by higher dose solar simulated radiation: a randomized controlled trial. J Am Acad Dermatol [Internet]. 2018 Feb 1 [cited 2024 Mar 26];78(2):414–6. Available from: https://pubmed.ncbi.nlm.nih.gov/29332714/
20. Polypodium Leucotomos Extract (PLE): new study gives evidence-based insight into "Ain't nothing like the real thing"—PubMed [Internet]. [cited 2024 Mar 26]. Available from: https://pubmed.ncbi.nlm.nih.gov/31531171/
21. Aguilera J, Vicente-Manzanares M, de Gálvez MV, Herrera-Ceballos E, Rodríguez-Luna A, González S. Booster Effect of a Natural Extract of Polypodium leucotomos (Fernblock®) That Improves the UV Barrier Function and Immune Protection Capability of Sunscreen Formulations. Front Med (Lausanne) [Internet]. 2021 Jun 2 [cited 2024 Mar 26];8. Available from: https://pubmed.ncbi.nlm.nih.gov/34150816/
22. Rodríguez-Luna A, Zamarrón A, Juarranz Á, González S. Clinical applications of Polypodium leucotomos (Fernblock®): an update. Life (Basel) [Internet]. 2023 Jul 1 [cited 2024 Mar 26];13(7). Available from: https://pubmed.ncbi.nlm.nih.gov/37511888/
23. El Mansouri M, Essaddouki S, Mouradi M, Oukerroum A, El Fatoiki FZ, Truchuelo MT, et al. Evaluation of the effectiveness and safety of combined oral and topical photoprotection with a standardized extract of Polypodium leucotomos (Fernblock®) in a Moroccan population with xeroderma pigmentosum. Photodermatol Photoimmunol Photomed [Internet]. 2023 Nov 1 [cited 2024 Mar 26];39(6):607–12. Available from: https://pubmed.ncbi.nlm.nih.gov/37584519/
24. Pellacani G, Peris K, Ciardo S, Pezzini C, Tambone S, Farnetani F, et al. The combination of oral and topical photoprotection with a standardized Polypodium leucotomos extract is beneficial against actinic keratosis. Photodermatol Photoimmunol Photomed [Internet]. 2023 Jul 1 [cited 2024 Mar 26];39(4):384–91. Available from: https://pubmed.ncbi.nlm.nih.gov/36892441/
25. Parrado C, Nicolas J, Juarranz A, Gonzalez S. The role of the aqueous extract Polypodium leucotomos in photoprotection. Photochem Photobiol Sci [Internet]. 2020 Jun 1 [cited 2024 Mar 26];19(6):831–43. Available from: https://pubmed.ncbi.nlm.nih.gov/33856681/
26. Kohli I, Shafi R, Isedeh P, Griffith JL, Al-Jamal MS, Silpa-archa N, et al. The impact of oral Polypodium leucotomos extract on ultraviolet B response: a human clinical study. J Am Acad Dermatol [Internet]. 2017 Jul 1 [cited 2024 Mar 26];77(1):33–41.e1. Available from: https://pubmed.ncbi.nlm.nih.gov/28341348/
27. Double-blind, placebo-controlled trial to evaluate the effectiveness of Polypodium Leucotomos extract in the treatment of melasma in Asian skin: a pilot study—PubMed [Internet]. [cited 2024 Mar 26]. Available from: https://pubmed.ncbi.nlm.nih.gov/29606995/
28. Comparative effects of a fixed Polypodium leucotomos/Pomegranate combination versus Polypodium leucotomos alone on skin biophysical parameters—PubMed [Internet]. [cited 2024 Mar 26]. Available from: https://pubmed.ncbi.nlm.nih.gov/28456146/
29. Xuan Y, Yang Y, Xiang L, Zhang C. The role of oxidative stress in the pathogenesis of vitiligo: a culprit for melanocyte death. Oxid Med Cell Longev [Internet]. 2022 [cited 2024 Mar 26];2022. Available from: https://pubmed.ncbi.nlm.nih.gov/35103096/
30. Yoshihisa Y, Rehman M ur, Shimizu T. Astaxanthin, a xanthophyll carotenoid, inhibits ultraviolet-induced apoptosis in keratinocytes. Exp Dermatol [Internet]. 2014 [cited 2024 Mar 26];23(3):178–83. Available from: https://pubmed.ncbi.nlm.nih.gov/24521161/
31. Imokawa G. The xanthophyll carotenoid astaxanthin has distinct biological effects to prevent the photoaging of the skin even by its postirradiation treatment. Photochem Photobiol [Internet]. 2019 Mar 1 [cited 2024 Apr 8];95(2):490–500. Available from: https://pubmed.ncbi.nlm.nih.gov/30338860/

32. Ito N, Seki S, Ueda F. The protective role of astaxanthin for UV-induced skin deterioration in healthy people-a randomized, double-blind, placebo-controlled trial. Nutrients [Internet]. 2018 Jul 1 [cited 2024 Mar 26];10(7). Available from: https://pubmed.ncbi.nlm.nih.gov/29941810/
33. Davinelli S, Nielsen ME, Scapagnini G. Astaxanthin in skin health, repair, and disease: a comprehensive review. Nutrients [Internet]. 2018 Apr 22 [cited 2024 Mar 26];10(4). Available from: https://www.ncbi.nlm.nih.gov/pmc/articles/PMC5946307/
34. Visioli F, Artaria C. Astaxanthin in cardiovascular health and disease: mechanisms of action, therapeutic merits, and knowledge gaps. Food Funct [Internet]. 2017 Jan 1 [cited 2024 Mar 26];8(1):39–63. Available from: https://pubmed.ncbi.nlm.nih.gov/27924978/
35. The history of sunscreen. J Am Acad Dermatol [Internet]. 2013 Apr 1 [cited 2024 Mar 26];68(4):AB34. Available from: http://www.jaad.org/article/S0190962212014223/fulltext
36. Hama S, Takahashi K, Inai Y, Shiota K, Sakamoto R, Yamada A, et al. Protective effects of topical application of a poorly soluble antioxidant astaxanthin liposomal formulation on ultraviolet-induced skin damage. J Pharm Sci [Internet]. 2012 [cited 2024 Mar 26];101(8):2909–16. Available from: https://pubmed.ncbi.nlm.nih.gov/22628205/
37. Hama S, Uenishi S, Yamada A, Ohgita T, Tsuchiya H, Yamashita E, et al. Scavenging of hydroxyl radicals in aqueous solution by astaxanthin encapsulated in liposomes. Biol Pharm Bull [Internet]. 2012 Dec [cited 2024 Mar 26];35(12):2238–42. Available from: https://pubmed.ncbi.nlm.nih.gov/23207776/
38. Amelioration of ultraviolet-induced photokeratitis in mice treated with astaxanthin eye drops—PubMed [Internet]. [cited 2024 Mar 26]. Available from: https://pubmed.ncbi.nlm.nih.gov/22393271/
39. Grether-Beck S, Marini A, Jaenicke T, Krutmann J. French maritime pine bark extract (Pycnogenol®) effects on human skin: clinical and molecular evidence. Skin Pharmacol Physiol [Internet]. 2016 Feb 1 [cited 2024 Mar 26];29(1):13–7. Available from: https://pubmed.ncbi.nlm.nih.gov/26492562/
40. Saliou C, Rimbach G, Moini H, McLaughlin L, Hosseini S, Lee J, et al. Solar ultraviolet-induced erythema in human skin and nuclear factor-kappa-B-dependent gene expression in keratinocytes are modulated by a French maritime pine bark extract. Free Radic Biol Med [Internet]. 2001 Jan 15 [cited 2024 Mar 26];30(2):154–60. Available from: https://pubmed.ncbi.nlm.nih.gov/11163532/
41. Zhao H, Wu J, Wang N, Grether-Beck S, Krutmann J, Wei L. Oral Pycnogenol® intake benefits the skin in urban chinese outdoor workers: a randomized, placebo-controlled, double-blind, and crossover intervention study. Skin Pharmacol Physiol [Internet]. 2021 Apr 1 [cited 2024 Mar 26];34(3):135–45. Available from: https://pubmed.ncbi.nlm.nih.gov/33789311/
42. Cutaneous photoprotection: a review of the current status and evolving strategies—PubMed [Internet]. [cited 2024 Mar 26]. Available from: https://pubmed.ncbi.nlm.nih.gov/32226337/
43. Chen AC, Damian DL, Halliday GM. Oral and systemic photoprotection. Photodermatol Photoimmunol Photomed [Internet]. 2014 [cited 2024 Mar 26];30(2–3):102–11. Available from: https://pubmed.ncbi.nlm.nih.gov/24313740/
44. Jesus A, Mota S, Torres A, Cruz MT, Sousa E, Almeida IF, et al. Antioxidants in sunscreens: which and what for? Antioxidants [Internet]. 2023 Jan 1 [cited 2024 Mar 26];12(1). Available from: https://www.ncbi.nlm.nih.gov/pmc/articles/PMC9854756/
45. Kashif M, Yao H, Schmidt S, Chen X, Truong M, Tüksammel E, et al. ROS-lowering doses of vitamins C and A accelerate malignant melanoma metastasis. Redox Biol [Internet]. 2023 Apr 1 [cited 2024 Mar 26];60. Available from: https://pubmed.ncbi.nlm.nih.gov/36774779/
46. Hercberg S, Ezzedine K, Guinot C, Preziosi P, Galan P, Bertrais S, et al. Antioxidant supplementation increases the risk of skin cancers in women but not in men. J Nutr [Internet]. 2007 [cited 2024 Mar 26];137(9):2098–105. Available from: https://pubmed.ncbi.nlm.nih.gov/17709449/
47. Ezzedine K, Latreille J, Kesse-Guyot E, Galan P, Hercberg S, Guinot C, et al. Incidence of skin cancers during 5-year follow-up after stopping antioxidant vitamins and mineral supplementation. Eur J Cancer [Internet]. 2010 [cited 2024 Mar 26];46(18):3316–22. Available from: https://pubmed.ncbi.nlm.nih.gov/20605091/

48. Feskanich D, Willett WC, Hunter DJ, Colditz GA. Dietary intakes of vitamins A, C, and E and risk of melanoma in two cohorts of women. Br J Cancer [Internet]. 2003 May 6 [cited 2024 Mar 26];88(9):1381–7. Available from: https://pubmed.ncbi.nlm.nih.gov/12778065/
49. Yang G, Yan Y, Ma Y, Yang Y. Vitamin C at high concentrations induces cytotoxicity in malignant melanoma but promotes tumor growth at low concentrations. Mol Carcinog [Internet]. 2017 Aug 1 [cited 2024 Mar 26];56(8):1965–76. Available from: https://pubmed.ncbi.nlm.nih.gov/28370562/
50. Wang K, Jiang H, Li W, Qiang M, Dong T, Li H. role of vitamin C in skin diseases. Front Physiol [Internet]. 2018 Jul 4 [cited 2024 Mar 26];9(JUL). Available from: https://pubmed.ncbi.nlm.nih.gov/30022952/
51. Song JH, Bae EY, Choi G, Hyun JW, Lee MY, Lee HW, et al. Protective effect of mango (Mangifera indica L.) against UVB-induced skin aging in hairless mice. Photodermatol Photoimmunol Photomed [Internet]. 2013 Apr [cited 2024 Mar 26];29(2):84–9. Available from: https://pubmed.ncbi.nlm.nih.gov/23458392/
52. Fam VW, Holt RR, Keen CL, Sivamani RK, Hackman RM. Prospective evaluation of mango fruit intake on facial wrinkles and erythema in postmenopausal women: a randomized clinical pilot study. Nutrients [Internet]. 2020 Nov 1 [cited 2024 Mar 26];12(11):1–11. Available from: https://pubmed.ncbi.nlm.nih.gov/33158079/
53. Flores-Balderas X, Peña-Peña M, Rada KM, Alvarez-Alvarez YQ, Guzmán-Martín CA, Sánchez-Gloria JL, et al. Beneficial effects of plant-based diets on skin health and inflammatory skin diseases. Nutrients [Internet]. 2023 Jul 1 [cited 2024 Mar 26];15(13). Available from: https://pubmed.ncbi.nlm.nih.gov/37447169/
54. Moskwa J, Bronikowska M, Socha K, Markiewicz-Żukowska R. Vegetable as a source of bioactive compounds with photoprotective properties: implication in the aging process. Nutrients 2023, Vol 15, Page 3594 [Internet]. 2023 Aug 16 [cited 2024 Mar 26];15(16):3594. Available from: https://www.mdpi.com/2072-6643/15/16/3594/htm
55. Weiskirchen S, Weiskirchen R. Resveratrol: how much wine do you have to drink to stay healthy? Adv Nutr [Internet]. 2016 Jul 1 [cited 2024 Mar 26];7(4):706. Available from: https://www.ncbi.nlm.nih.gov/pmc/articles/PMC4942868/
56. Jiminez V, Yusuf N. An update on clinical trials for chemoprevention of human skin cancer. J Cancer Metastasis Treat [Internet]. 2023 [cited 2024 Mar 26];9(1). Available from: https://www.ncbi.nlm.nih.gov/pmc/articles/PMC10544834/
57. Mounessa J, Qin R, Dunnick CA, Dellavalle RP. Chemoprevention of keratinocyte carcinomas: an updated review. Am J Clin Dermatol [Internet] 2016 Oct 1 [cited 2024 Mar 26];17(5):475–84. Available from: https://pubmed.ncbi.nlm.nih.gov/27372106/
58. Chow CL, Havighurst T, Lozar T, Jones TD, Kim KM, Bailey HH. Ototoxicity of long-term α-difluoromethylornithine for skin cancer prevention. Laryngoscope [Internet]. 2023 Mar 1 [cited 2024 Mar 26];133(3):676–82. Available from: https://pubmed.ncbi.nlm.nih.gov/35620919/
59. Aguirre-Cruz G, León-López A, Cruz-Gómez V, Jiménez-Alvarado R, Aguirre-Álvarez G. Collagen hydrolysates for skin protection: oral administration and topical formulation. Antioxidants (Basel) [Internet]. 2020 Feb 1 [cited 2024 Apr 8];9(2). Available from: https://pubmed.ncbi.nlm.nih.gov/32098294/
60. Majma Sanaye P, Mojaveri MR, Ahmadian R, Sabet Jahromi M, Bahramsoltani R. Apigenin and its dermatological applications: a comprehensive review. Phytochemistry [Internet]. 2022 Nov 1 [cited 2024 Apr 8];203. Available from: https://pubmed.ncbi.nlm.nih.gov/35998830/
61. Jones SA, McArdle F, Jack CIA, Jackson MJ. Effect of antioxidant supplementation on the adaptive response of human skin fibroblasts to UV-induced oxidative stress. Redox Rep [Internet]. 1999 [cited 2024 Mar 26];4(6):291–9. Available from: https://pubmed.ncbi.nlm.nih.gov/10772068/
62. Burns EM, Tober KL, Riggenbach JA, Kusewitt DF, Young GS, Oberyszyn TM. Differential effects of topical vitamin E and C E Ferulic® treatments on ultraviolet light B-induced cutane-

ous tumor development in Skh-1 mice. PLoS One [Internet]. 2013 May 14 [cited 2024 Mar 26];8(5). Available from: https://pubmed.ncbi.nlm.nih.gov/23691100/

63. Loh WQ, Yin X, Kishida R, Chia SE, Ong CN, Seow WJ. Association between vitamin A and E forms and prostate cancer risk in the singapore prostate cancer study. Nutrients [Internet]. 2023 Jun 1 [cited 2024 Mar 26];15(12). Available from: https://pubmed.ncbi.nlm.nih.gov/37375581/
64. Loh WQ, Youn J, Seow WJ. Vitamin E intake and risk of prostate cancer: a meta-analysis. Nutrients [Internet]. 2022 Jan 1 [cited 2024 Mar 26];15(1). Available from: https://pubmed.ncbi.nlm.nih.gov/36615673/
65. Zhang Y, Yang J, Na X, Zhao A. Association between β-carotene supplementation and risk of cancer: a meta-analysis of randomized controlled trials. Nutr Rev [Internet]. 2023 Sep 1 [cited 2024 Mar 26];81(9):1118–30. Available from: https://pubmed.ncbi.nlm.nih.gov/36715090/
66. Black HS. Interaction of ascorbic acid and tocopherol on beta-carotene modulated carcinogenesis. Hemoglobin [Internet]. 2010 Jun [cited 2024 Mar 26];34(3):284–90. Available from: https://pubmed.ncbi.nlm.nih.gov/20524818/

Chapter 10
Physical Photoprotection

Abbreviations

ASTM	American Society for Testing and Materials
CW	Critical wavelength
SOC	Skin of colour
SPF	Sun protection factor
UPF	Ultraviolet protection factor
UV	Ultraviolet
UVA	Ultraviolet-A
UVB	Ultraviolet-B
UVR	Ultraviolet radiation

Key Objectives

- Shade seeking behaviour, usage of hat and sunglasses, and sun protective clothing with appropriate UPF are all options available for holistic sun protection.
- The UPF of a fabric is influenced by several factors such as porosity, stretch, wetness, and fabric type. Colour and design are also additional factors that influence the overall sun protection afforded by the fabric.
- Personal wear sunglasses may also be used as photoprotective agents, and rating methodologies are available to help the consumer choose the product as per their requirement.
- It is important to factor in the sunlight albedo, reflected by water and sand, as additional to direct sunlight, to arrive at the levels of exposure, and accordingly, methods of protection.

Skin cancers in vulnerable populations are on the increase, despite growing use of sunscreens. In skin of colour (SOC), the ability of the sunscreen to reduce skin pigmentation and provide an overall lighter complexion are inherent drivers for sunscreen use, while the prevention of photocarcinogenesis is the goal for lighter-skinned populations, at risk of skin cancer.

R. Rajan, *Sunscreens for Skin of Color*,
https://doi.org/10.1007/978-981-97-3195-4_10

However, sunscreen is only one of several tools available for sun protection, though disproportionately, the most widely used. Sunscreen use was reported by over 30% of white Americans when they anticipated to stay in the sun for more than an hour. This was followed by shade seeking behaviour in 25%, usage of a hat by 16%, with only 6% using full sleeved clothing. Interestingly, sunburns were most common in those who reported frequent sunscreen use, while usage of hats was protective against multiple sunburns. The increase in frequency of sunscreen usage may reflect the longer hours spent under the sun, with resultant sunburn, as compared to sun avoidance and use of long sleeves, which were protective against solar skin damage [1]. Seeking shade as a sun protection method is known to protect against UVA, preferentially, than against UVB [2]. Combined with the above information that shade protects against sunburn, shade seeking may be an ideal sun safe behaviour to balance sunburn prevention and vitamin D production in lighter-skinned individuals. Sun protection behaviour was also found to be dependent on age and level of education, though overall, it is encouraging to know that sun protection awareness reflected in practical behaviour, is indeed increasing [3]. Gender and skin type were also important parameters that influenced the effectiveness of safe sun awareness campaigns [4].

10.1 Sun Protection by Textiles

Clothing is an eco-friendly, reusable, universally applicable way of effective sun protection. Sun protective clothing [5] with ultraviolet protection factor (UPF) rating is available as a sustainable alternative to sunscreens, Table 10.1. Though not new by any means, the evolution of sun protection clothing [6] enables the achievement of holistic sun safe behaviour instead of relying only on sunscreens. Similar to sun protection factor (SPF) for sunscreens, textiles are rated using UPF based on their ability to filter out ultraviolet (UV) radiation. Defined as the ratio of average effective UV irradiance through air and through fabric, UPF is rated as per the American Society for Testing and Materials (ASTM) guidelines [7], shown in Table 10.1.

Depending on the fabric, UPF can range from 2 to several thousand, the higher ranges being regularly achieved by fabrics like denim [8]. Much like the SPF, the UPF also considers the erythema response as a biological end point to sun exposure and does not account for the impact of non erythemogenic wavelengths on the skin. The additional use of critical wavelength in measuring sun protection ability helps

Table 10.1 UPF rating of fabrics [5–7]

Grade	UPF	Percentage of UV blocked
Good protection	15–24	93.3–95.9
Very good protection	25–39	96.0–97.4
Excellent protection	40 to 50+	97.5–98+

circumvent this issue. Interpreted together with the UPF, the critical wavelength can potentially ensure coverage across the entire UV spectrum. However, in some countries, the % blocking ability of a sunscreen in the UVA and UVB spectra, namely a measure of transmittance through the fabric, is used in preference to critical wavelength for garments [9].

Several factors determine the level of protection provided by clothing, namely porosity and weave, fabric type, stretch, wetness, colour, and finally, design as shown in Fig. 10.1 [10].

Firstly, the UPF is strongly influenced by the porosity of the material [11]. Heavier fabric with less porosity provides better sun protection compared to lighter, loosely woven material [9, 11]. Lycra, spandex, polyester, and nylon, all with thicker weaves provide better sun protection [12]. Synthetic fabrics have been able to achieve higher UPF ratings compared to natural fibres [6]. Denim seems to be able to provide an almost 100% protection against both Ultraviolet-A (UVA) and Ultraviolet-B (UVB), achieving an UPF of 2000, a critical wavelength (CW) of 389 nm, achieving 100% blockage of UVB and 99% of UVA. Following denim, polyester has an UPF of 721, with a slightly lower CW at 387 nm [9, 13]. Blended fabrics were found to provide better sun protection and have higher UPF ratings, compared to 100% cotton fabrics, when evaluating children's summer clothing [14].

The UPF is impacted by wetness and stretch—both reduce UPF. For the minimum UPF of 15, the gap between the fibres of the fabric, called interstices, should occupy no more than 6% of the total surface area of the fabric [5, 6]. Stretch increases the size of the interstices and contributes to lowered performance. Preferably, fabrics with a rating of 30+ may be considered to provide better protection with some resistance to wetting, stretch and environmental stresses [6].

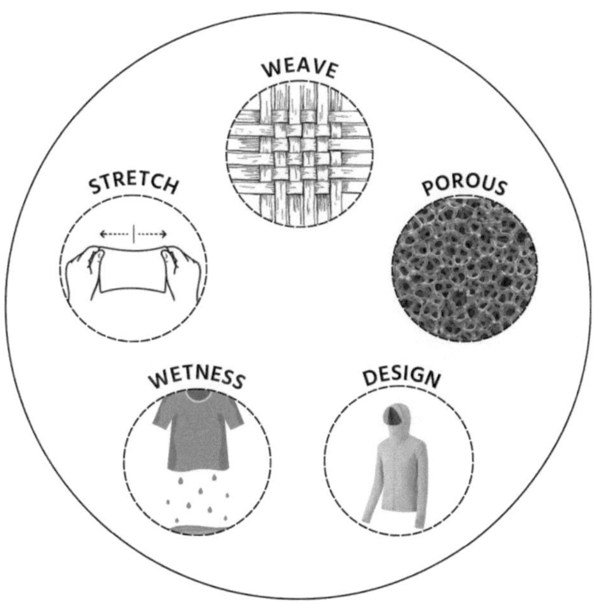

Fig. 10.1 UV protecting fabrics

A lesser determinant is the colour of the fabric, with black, navy-blue, white, green, and beige colours achieving higher UPF ratings [6]. White cotton has a UPF of 9, blocking close to 90% of UVA and UVB, while dark grey cotton has a UPF of 98, providing about 99% blockage of UV. Repeated use and loss of colour from bleaching during laundry decrease the UPF. UPF boosting detergent additives, clothing dyes, and formic acid pretreatment of natural fibre derived fabrics have been studied to boost UPF [7].

Finally, the design of the clothing also contributes to the sun protective efficacy of the fabric. The standard requirements require the clothing to provide coverage from the base of the neck all the way down to the knees and to cover three quarters of the upper arm. For protective clothing, a 30+ labelling is typical. For summer clothing, a value of 20+ is considered sufficient [6].

Berry et al. assessed the sun protective efficacy of two sunscreens at SPF 30 and 50, and compared them to off white coloured sun protective textiles, made of nylon and polyester, the latter having three different knit structures–a pique, an interlock, and an interlock with a titanium dioxide dot printing covering 30% of the surface. The researchers found the fabrics to outperform the sunscreens across all measured parameters—SPF, UPF, critical wavelength, % blocking of UVA and UVB. Based on the current data, clothing outperforms sunscreen in all aspects of solar protection, and therefore should be considered the cornerstone of sun protection [9] with sunscreen usage for areas that cannot be reliably protected using clothing.

While clothing is considered one of the most durable, eco-friendly, easy to adapt means of photoprotection, addition of molecules or dyes meant to enhance sun protection, may inadvertently lead to instances of photosensitization, or offer inadequate protection against phototoxicity, due to the presence of intrinsic or extrinsic absorbing molecules [8].

Interestingly and paradoxically, clothing may also reduce sun protection from applied sunscreens if the clothing is worn too soon after applying sunscreen. Beyer et al. recommend waiting for a minimum of 8 min, and an ideal time of 20 min, between applying sunscreen on the skin, and wearing clothes, to reduce loss of efficacy from product rub off [15].

Using sun protective clothing has ecological advantages of reducing the burden of personal care product release into the environment, reduction of potential absorption of endocrine disrupting chemicals in sun care products, reduced packaging related environmental burden and has provided a significant cost advantage to the consumer, over time.

10.2 Sun Protection by Hats

Diffey et al. suggest using hats with a brim of at least 7.5 cm to protect the nose and ears reliably, stating that flat caps and peaked baseball style caps do not offer adequate protection [16]. Accordingly, some of the styles recommended by the Australian SUNSMART educational literature include the broad brimmed hat,

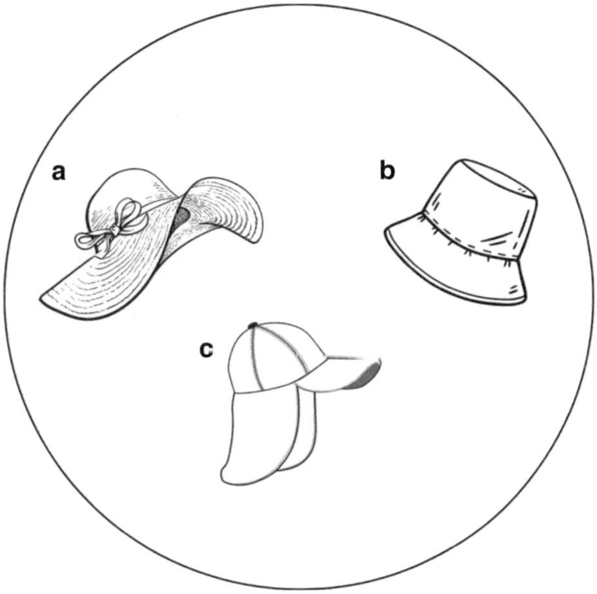

Fig. 10.2 Sun protection hat (**a**) broad brimmed hat (**b**) bucket hat (**c**) legionnaire hat

bucket hat, and the legionnaire hat, Fig. 10.2. Considering that topical sunscreen usage is not recommended for babies less than 6 months of age, physical protection including for the head may need to be achieved using these types of apparel. A bucket hat may be most comfortable for babies and young children [17].

10.3 Sun Protection by Glass

UV protection obtained from tinted or laminated glass, used in applications such as windows and car windshields, is significant. UVB is filtered by clear glass while allowing around 30% of UVA to pass through. Up to 90% of UVA, and more than 99% of UVB, is filtered by most types of laminated glass. Tinted glass provides additional sun protection and is able to block up to 99% of wavelengths less than 380 nm. Glass substitutes like polycarbonate plastics are also able to offer similar filtering of UV rays [10].

For personal wear like sunglasses, UV protection ratings are offered by professional agencies, set to standards similar to that of sunscreens [18]. The Australian standard updated in 2017 is widely used and requires that the sunglasses must offer significant protection within the range of 280–400 nm, Table 10.2 [19]. Lenses may be further categorized by the level of tints from light to darkest, by both Australian and the United States of America (USA) standards.

Table 10.2 Sun protection grading of eyewear [19]

Category	Class	Blocks light by
0	Fashion spectacles, providing no to some protection from UVR, but no reduction in sunglare	0–20%
1	Fashion spectacles, providing protection from ultraviolet radiation (UVR), and limited reduction in sunglare, not suitable for driving at night	20–40%
2	Sunglasses for everyday use, providing medium protection from UVR and sunglare	40–65%
3	Sunglasses providing good protection from UVR and able to reduce sunglare	65–90%
4	Sunglasses providing high level of protection from UVR and able to reduce sunglare well, but not suited for driving	90–97%

10.4 Sun Protection by Shade

Multiple sun protection measures are required for providing optimal cutaneous protection. While shade is a strong protection factor, not all shade can be considered adequate. Ou-Yang et al. evaluated the shade provided by a beach umbrella alone, compared to the combination of a beach umbrella and sunscreen usage in beach goers, and found that the latter was significantly more effective in sun protection [20]. Structures that provide shade, typically like gazebos at the beach, varied in their level of protection based on the angle of incident light, design of the shade, and UV albedo from reflective structures like sand [21]. Shade seeking behaviour was found to be significantly more prevalent in 2020 compared to a decade earlier [3].

Sun protection strategy has to be holistic to be effective. Though sunscreens form the bulk of the conversation around sun protection, they need to be complemented with highly effective and more eco-friendly measures such as protective clothing. Furthermore, lifestyle changes such as sun avoidance behaviours, including shade seeking behaviour, and dietary plans which include UV protecting, antioxidant foods, provide a well-rounded, sustainable way of sun protection.

10.5 Chapter Summary

This chapter gives a brief overview of the tools available for physical sun protection. The UPF rating for clothing has become more popularly used in recent years. Clothing and hats, seeking shade and using UV rated sunglasses are all ways to increase the overall sun protection, without increasing the environmental footprint of repetitive sunscreen use over areas which can indeed be protected by physical measures.

References

1. Linos E, Keiser E, Fu T, Colditz G, Chen S, Tang JY. Hat, shade, long sleeves, or sunscreen? Rethinking US sun protection messages based on their relative effectiveness. Cancer Causes Control [Internet]. 2011 Jul [cited 2024 Mar 27];22(7):1067–71. Available from: https://www.researchgate.net/publication/51188374_Hat_shade_long_sleeves_or_sunscreen_Rethinking_US_sun_protection_messages_based_on_their_relative_effectiveness
2. Turnbull DJ, Parisi A V. Latitudinal variations over Australia of the solar UV-radiation exposures for vitamin D3 in shade compared to full sun. Radiat Res [Internet]. 2010 Mar 1 [cited 2024 Mar 27];173(3):373–9. Available from: https://pubmed.ncbi.nlm.nih.gov/20199222/
3. McKenzie C, Nahm WJ, Kearney CA, Zampella JG. Sun-protective behaviors and sunburn among US adults. Arch Dermatol Res [Internet]. 2023 Aug 1 [cited 2024 Mar 27];315(6):1665–74. Available from: https://link.springer.com/article/10.1007/s00403-023-02547-z
4. Pettigrew S, Jongenelis M, Strickland M, Minto C, Slevin T, Jalleh G, et al. Predictors of sun protection behaviours and sunburn among Australian adolescents. BMC Public Health [Internet]. 2016 Jul 13 [cited 2024 Mar 27];16(1):1–8. Available from: https://link.springer.com/articles/10.1186/s12889-016-3197-4
5. Cutaneous photoprotection: a review of the current status and evolving strategies—PubMed [Internet]. [cited 2024 Mar 26]. Available from: https://pubmed.ncbi.nlm.nih.gov/32226337/
6. Gambichler T, Rotterdam S, Altmeyer P, Hoffmann K. Protection against ultraviolet radiation by commercial summer clothing: need for standardised testing and labelling. BMC Dermatol [Internet]. 2001 Oct 25 [cited 2024 Mar 27];1. Available from: https://pubmed.ncbi.nlm.nih.gov/11710968/
7. (PDF) Assessment of anti-bacterial effect, anti- odoureffect, uv-protection factor and xrd on formic acid treated modal and cotton fabric [Internet]. [cited 2024 Mar 3]. Available from: https://www.researchgate.net/publication/333419423_Assessment_of_anti-bacterial_effect_anti-_odoureffect_uv-protection_factor_and_xrd_on_formic_acid_treated_modal_and_cotton_fabric
8. Menter JM, Hatch KL. Clothing as solar radiation protection. Curr Probl Dermatol [Internet]. 2003 [cited 2024 Mar 27];31:50–63. Available from: https://pubmed.ncbi.nlm.nih.gov/12882019/
9. Berry EG, Bezecny J, Acton M, Sulmonetti TP, Anderson DM, Beckham HW, et al. Slip versus slop: a head-to-head comparison of UV-protective clothing to sunscreen. Cancers (Basel) [Internet]. 2022 Feb 1 [cited 2024 Mar 3];14(3):542. Available from: https://www.mdpi.com/2072-6694/14/3/542/htm
10. Al-Jamal MS, Griffith JL, Lim HW. Photoprotection in ethnic skin. Dermatol Sin. 2014;32(4):217–24.
11. Kan CW. A study on ultraviolet protection of 100% cotton knitted fabric: effect of fabric parameters. Sci World J. 2014;2014:1.
12. Sander M, Sander M, Burbidge T, Beecker J. The efficacy and safety of sunscreen use for the prevention of skin cancer. CMAJ [Internet]. 2020 Dec 14 [cited 2024 Mar 27];192(50):E1802–8. Available from: https://www.ncbi.nlm.nih.gov/pmc/articles/PMC7759112/
13. Coyne EQ, Lichtman MK, Simons J, Sarkar AK, Rünger TM. In vitro assessment of the broad-spectrum ultraviolet protection of clothing. J Am Acad Dermatol [Internet]. 2018 Aug 1 [cited 2024 Mar 27];79(2):373–5. Available from: https://pubmed.ncbi.nlm.nih.gov/29317283/
14. Cole Y, Ilyas AM, Ilyas EN. Assessment of UV Protection for Children's Summer Clothing. Cureus [Internet]. 2023 Aug 26 [cited 2024 Mar 27];15(8). Available from: https://pubmed.ncbi.nlm.nih.gov/37753032/
15. Beyer DM, Faurschou A, Hædersdal M, Wulf HC. Clothing reduces the sun protection factor of sunscreens. Br J Dermatol [Internet]. 2010 Feb [cited 2024 Mar 27];162(2):415–9. Available from: https://pubmed.ncbi.nlm.nih.gov/19845666/

16. Diffey BL, Cheeseman J. Sun protection with hats. Br J Dermatol [Internet]. 1992 [cited 2024 Mar 27];127(1):10–2. Available from: https://pubmed.ncbi.nlm.nih.gov/1637687/
17. When choosing a hat look at.
18. Donglikar M, Deore S, Deore S, Deore S. Sunscreens: a review. Pharm J. 2016;8(3):171–9.
19. Sunglasses & fashion spectacles | Product Safety Australia [Internet]. [cited 2024 Mar 27]. Available from: https://www.productsafety.gov.au/product-safety-laws/safety-standards-bans/mandatory-standards/sunglasses-fashion-spectacles#toc-about-the-mandatory-standard
20. Hao OY, Jiang LI, Meyer K, Wang SQ, Farberg AS, Rigel DS. Sun protection by beach umbrella vs sunscreen with a high sun protection factor: a randomized clinical trial. JAMA Dermatol [Internet]. 2017 Mar 1 [cited 2024 Mar 27];153(3):304–8. Available from: https://pubmed.ncbi.nlm.nih.gov/28114650/
21. Grifoni D, Betti G, Bogi A, Bramanti L, Chiarugi A, Gozzini B, et al. Protective measures from solar ultraviolet radiation for beach lifeguards in Tuscany (Italy): shade and clothing strategies. Saf Health Work [Internet]. 2022 Dec 1 [cited 2024 Mar 27];13(4):421–8. Available from: https://pubmed.ncbi.nlm.nih.gov/36579014/

Chapter 11
Sunscreen Challenges: Stability, Systemic Absorption, and Environmental Concerns

Abbreviations

BEMT	Bis-ethylhexyloxyphenol methoxyphenyl triazine
BP -3	Benzophenone -3
CPD	Cyclobutane pyrimidine dimers
DBT	Diethylhexyl butamido triazone
DESM	Diethyl hexyl syringylidenemalonate
DHHB	Diethylaminohydroxybenzoyl hexylbenzoate
DTU	Technical University of Denmark
ECHA	European Chemicals Agency
EFSA	European Food Safety Authority
EHT	Ethylhexyl triazone
ENM	Engineered nanomaterials
ERA	Ecological risk assessments
ES	Ethylhexyl salicylate
HSE	Heat separated human epidermis
IVPT	In vitro permeation test
MBBT	Methylene bis-benzotriazolyl tetramethylbutylphenol
MeO-MBM	Methoxy-monobenzoyl methane
MoS	Margin of safety
NOAEL	No observed adverse effect level
OTC	Over the counter
PABA	Paramino benzoic acid
PAH	Polycyclic aromatic hydrocarbons
PSLTs	Poorly soluble particles
TEAS	Transient electronic absorption spectroscopy
US FDA	United States Food and Drug Administration
USA	United States of America
UV	Ultraviolet
UVR	Ultraviolet radiation

R. Rajan, *Sunscreens for Skin of Color*,
https://doi.org/10.1007/978-981-97-3195-4_11

Key Objectives

- Photostability of sunscreens decides the ultimate outcome of sunscreen use in clinical terms. Use of photo unstable sunscreens may have contributed to the lack of a decisive impact of sunscreens in preventing skin cancer.
- Sunscreen particles can penetrate into the skin through transcellular, intercellular, or appendageal pathways. Cutaneous penetration seems to be a function of size and lipophilicity among other factors. The inorganic sunscreens are not noted to penetrate the viable epidermis to any significant level.
- Sunscreen filters have been detected both in remote seas and proximal waterways, in coral and in much larger mammals, and also recently in the food chain with the human being as the end consumer.
- Durable sunscreens with a higher efficacy at a lower concentration, a judicious revisit of the frequency of sunscreen reapplication, avoiding sunscreens when the risk of UV exposure is low typically in latitudes above 40N, and use of physical protection over areas which can indeed by covered, are all ways to explore to reduce the growing sunscreen burden on the planet.

There are three main challenges that sunscreens pose, Fig. 11.1. The first is potential human toxicity from systemic absorption. Next is the issue of ecotoxicity,

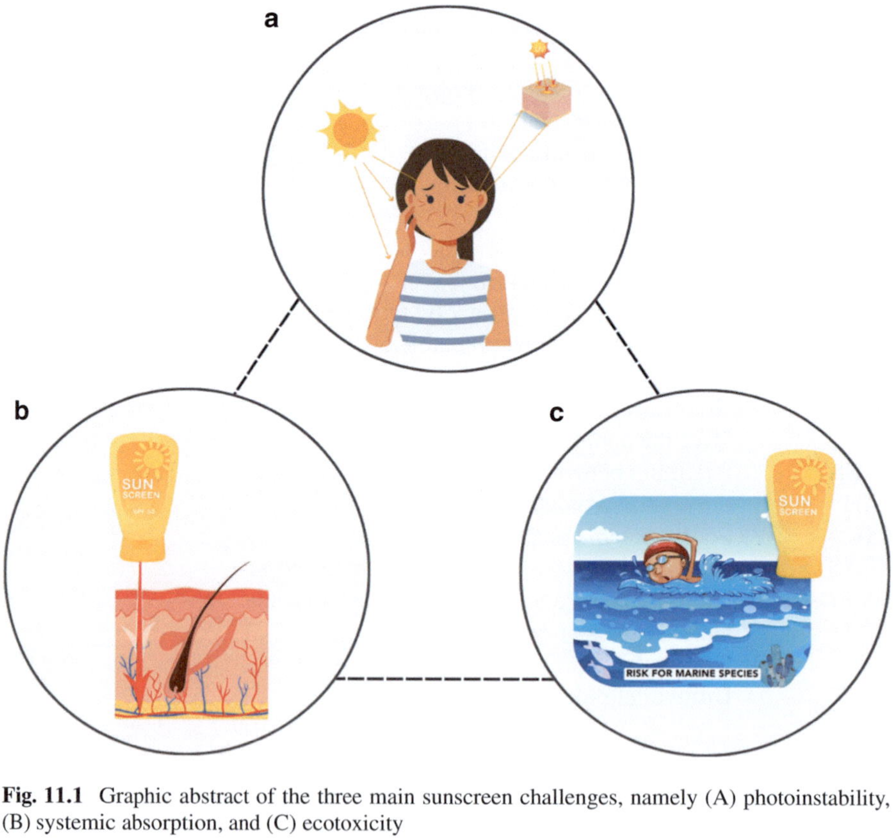

Fig. 11.1 Graphic abstract of the three main sunscreen challenges, namely (A) photoinstability, (B) systemic absorption, and (C) ecotoxicity

potentially for the long term due to UV filter persistence in the environment. The third area to address is photo instability, resulting either in inadequate protection that fails to prevent photocarcinogenesis or worse, pro-oxidant behaviour [1].

11.1 Photostability of Sunscreens

Photoinstability in organic sunscreens is almost a by-product of their mechanism of sun protection. Chemical sunscreens act by absorbing ultraviolet radiation (UVR). The mostly aromatic structure of organic sunscreens features functional groups, which act as electron donors and electron acceptors. On ultraviolet irradiation, the electron transfer shifts the molecule into a preferred, higher energy state [2]. Then with the release of the energy, the molecule returns to its original state, but not always. The process can also lead to irreversible photodegradation or photoisomerization. As long as the photoisomer has a similar photoprotective action and is able to absorb UV in the same way as the original unaltered molecule, the UV filter is deemed stable [1]. A typical example would be 4MBC. On the other hand, photoproducts that form post-UV exposure may generate free radicals with pro-oxidant effects that negatively interact with cellular components including DNA. They may also interact with other ingredients in the formulation, making the sunscreen unstable. This is evident with PABA (para amino benzoic acid), the prototype UV filter, where photodegradation leads to the generation of reactive nitroso compounds with carcinogenic potential [3]. More recently, octocrylene was found to undergo a UV mediated condensation into a benzophenone derivative with potential phototoxic effects [1]. Most commonly, photodegradation reduces the sun protection capacity of the sunscreen.

Photodegradation includes processes such as photoisomerization, producing molecules which could be both less effective and potentially toxic, and photofragmentation which causes the sunscreen filter molecule to break down into reactive fragments including free radicals. These breakdown products may then interact with cellular targets and accelerate UV-induced DNA damage, including generation of cyclobutane pyrimidine dimers (CPDs). For a detailed discussion on UV induced CPDs, please see Chap. 2.

Cutaneous phototoxicity due to the generation of photoproducts from sunscreens has been likened to that arising from pollutants such as polycyclic aromatic hydrocarbons (PAH). PAHs, typified by molecules such as benza(o)pyrene and benzanthracene, are by-products of incomplete combustion and occur as air pollutants in industrial regions, as components of cigarette smoke, and also as a result of innocuous human activities like grilling of meat. Photoexcitation of PAHs which have structures similar to the aromatic hydrocarbons that make up most chemical sunscreens, generate free radicals which damage the cell and the cellular DNA. Photoinstability of a sunscreen filter can contribute to a primary loss of sun protection, pro-oxidative damage to cells, and impact other sunscreen components negatively. This can lead to downstream problems spanning the spectrum from skin cancer to photoageing, Fig. 11.2.

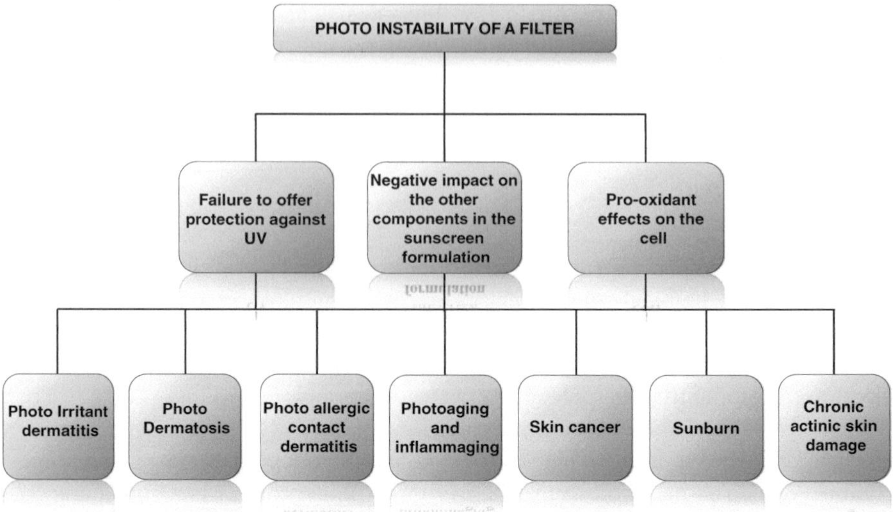

Fig. 11.2 Photoinstability of a sunscreen filter can contribute to a primary loss of sun protection, pro-oxidative damage to cells, and impact other sunscreen components negatively. This can lead to downstream problems spanning the spectrum from skin cancer to photoageing

A currently widely used filter that is considered to be particularly photounstable is avobenzone, which has one of the most photoprotective profiles, yet capable of generating the highest number of photodegradation end products [1]. After 8 h of UVB irradiation of avobenzone, around ten photodegradation products were generated, as identified by Schwack and Rudolph, with ongoing discovery of newer degradation products by other workers [4]. On UVR exposure, avobenzone undergoes a keto-enol isomerization and fragmentation into phenacyl and benzoyl radicals which further generate oxidative photoproducts [1]. Photoisomerization and downstream regulation of reactive by-products is also noted with octinoxate. Padimate O, interestingly, is stable in the UVB spectrum, and unstable in the UVA region.

Photoinstability as evidenced by the detection of photodegradation by-products on UV irradiation of the sunscreen is influenced by a number of factors, including the nature of the formulation, pH, combination of the UV filters, solvent used, duration of exposure, and availability of oxidation quenchers in the product [1, 5]. Filter combinations may impact photostability in specific mechanisms related to relaxation pathways, which may render originally photostable filters, prone to generation of reactive photoproducts when in combination [6]. Avobenzone and octinoxate were found to undergo irreversible photochemical reactions when combined together in any form—neat raw materials, in apolar solvents and in commercial sunscreen formulations, with eventual loss of performance [7]. This combination is not approved in the United States of America (USA). Photostability is also impacted by concomitant use of other supportive ingredients as well as other UV filters in the sunscreen formulation. For example, naringenin, a flavonoid present in bergamot extracts, and retinoids can compound the photodegradation of avobenzone [8]. Similarly, zinc oxide was found to cause photodegradation of certain chemical sunscreens containing avobenzone in addition to other organic filters [9].

Considering the broad-spectrum coverage of avobenzone, several methods have been tried to photo stabilize this filter. These include addition of antioxidants like vitamin C, E, ubiquinone, and resveratrol, but also the synergistic combination of avobenzone with other more stable UV filters, typically 4-Methylbenzylidene camphor (4-MBC), bis-ethylhexyloxyphenol methoxyphenyl triazine (BEMT) and octocrylene [10, 11]. Structural manipulations like encapsulation in microsized alginate particles or stabilizing the filter in nano and microspheres, were found to enhance photostability, and additionally these manipulations also translated into clinically appreciable outcomes such as an improved skin compatibility. Lignin nanoparticles are a recent attempt at ecosustainably enhancing the half-life stability of avobenzone and octinoxate. Notable about this work is the use of upcycled olive waste derivatives as encapsulation material [12]. Quenchers that are photostable by themselves such as diethylhexyl syringylidene malonate (DESM) were found to enhance the stability of avobenzone, and also that of homosalate and octisalate [13]. Considering the inherent ability of avobenzone to undergo rapid photoisomerization between the keto and the enol forms, with resultant photoinstability, chemical modification of the structure by methylation to withdraw the electrons, resulted in better photostability [14], conversely deuterization resulted in more photodegradation [15]. An interesting update is the exploration of methoxy monobenzoylmethane (MeO-MBM), an antioxidant. While not an inherent UVA or UVB filter, MeO-MBM converts into avobenzone on UV exposure, the conversion process itself providing antioxidant effects [16]. In early human studies, MeO-MBM demonstrated anti-inflammatory benefits and improved skin barrier function, probably acting through the retinoid gamma receptor. In contrast to avobenzone, whose photodegradation is deemed irreversible, Meo-MBM is said to have photo antioxidative properties, as the intermediaries produced by UV irradiation here, have free radical neutralizing abilities [16]. Marl, an upcycled ingredient obtained from marble industry waste, contains more than 95% calcium carbonate. Addition of marl to a photounstable sunscreen formulation containing octinoxate and avobenzone was found to stabilize the product, much like bemotrizinol and octocrylene [17].

Despite evidently recognizing avobenzone as photounstable, the amount of research that is being carried out to stabilize this filter is due to the lack of many other alternatives that are active in the UVA spectrum, the only other stable alternative being zinc oxide [18–20]. With so much work in this domain, it would seem that stabilized delivery of avobenzone in the sunscreen formulation to the skin is almost akin to a drug delivery process, quite removed from the perception of sunscreens predominantly as cosmetics [14]. In the future, the use of advanced evaluation photophysics techniques like transient electronic absorption spectroscopy (TEAS) which can depict the hours-long photodegradation process in seconds, translates into time efficient development of more photostable commercial sunscreens [18].

Methods to Increase Photostability

- Structural modifications including physical measures such as encapsulation and chemical process like methylation
- Use of synergistic and stabilizing UV filters
- Addition of antioxidants and free radicals quenchers

Despite the large body of work on increasing sunscreen stability, the clinical impact of such unstable behaviour seems equivocal, at least as per a review by Nash et al. [21]. The authors here acknowledge the propensity of certain sunscreens like Paramino benzoic acid (PABA) and avobenzone to undergo photodegradation but argue that this has not reduced clinical performance in terms of preventing photocarcinogenesis, citing the Nambour skin cancer prevention study [22]. The Nambour cohort demonstrated a significant reduction in squamous cell carcinomas and invasive melanomas in study participants, during the study and on follow-up [23]. However, it must be remembered that this study demonstrated no significant reduction of basal cell carcinomas or noninvasive melanomas between sunscreen users and nonusers that were followed up in the study for 4.5 years. This is significant considering basal cell carcinoma is the most common type of skin cancer world over [24, 25]. The longer latency period to the development of basal cell carcinoma, about 10–40 years, and the lack of precursor lesions, make shorter term follow-up studies difficult to interpret with regard to the effectiveness of sunscreen use.

In contrast to the chemical sunscreens, mineral sunscreen filters like zinc and titanium, and newer chemical filters like bemotrizinol and bisoctrizole are considered photostable, i.e., have the same UV absorption spectrum before and after irradiation [21].

11.2 Sunscreens and Systemic Absorption

Apart from the blood and the urine, sunscreens have been identified in other body fluids such as breast milk, semen, and in foetal tissues such as the amniotic fluid and the placenta [26]. The significance of such systemic absorption has gained interest in the last few years, driven by a few salient factors. The first one is new research that demonstrated that even a single application of sunscreen can result in systemic absorption of UV filters resulting in blood levels above expected threshold levels [27]. The second reason for the increased interest, at times coupled with social panic, is the growing body of research that suggests that this systemic absorption likely has human medical impact, in contrast to what was assumed this far, related particularly to the endocrine, reproductive, and genotoxicity domains [28]. Furthermore, the extrapolation continues into the ecosystem, not just with an impact on marine animals but also water sources that could be accessed by humans for various purposes. Finally, the sheer magnitude of global sunscreen usage in thousands of tons, boosted by the increase in the number of consumers who use sunscreen, now for anti-ageing purposes in addition to prevention of photocarcinogenesis. Sadly, systemic exposure may soon no longer be just about topical application of sunscreens, with UV filters being detected in waterways and in the food chain [26, 29–31].

UV filters in their functional role of sun protection are ideally expected to work at the surface of the skin, absorbing or reflecting incident solar light. Mineral sunscreens both nano and non-nano forms are not expected to cross the stratum corneum significantly. For chemical sunscreens like benzophenone, the smaller particle size facilitates absorption through the dermal layer and into the bloodstream. To begin with, the lipophilic nature of chemical filters makes it easier for them to the dermis by passing between the lamellae of the keratinocytes, aided by a concentration gradient [32]. Water resistant sunscreens are more lipid based, and therefore more likely to be absorbed into the dermis [2]. The lipophilicity is also likely to make the product more stable and persistent in the marine ecosystem and has even been considered to promote global warming [33].

Systemic absorption begins with movement of filters into the viable part of the epidermis and then onward and deeper. Cutaneous absorption of organic sunscreens is understood as a three-stage process—penetration, permeation, and resorption [34]. Penetration involves the passage of the UV filter across the layers of stratum corneum, mostly travelling between the lamellae, but also through hair follicle and eccrine openings [35]. Permeation involves further movement of the molecule down the dermis, hypodermis, and subcutis to eventually get reabsorbed into the bloodstream. Systemic absorption through cutaneous penetration, increases with prolonged exposure times, for certain filters like oxybenzone, suggesting a continuous influx with repeated applications, Fig. 11.3 [35, 36].

UV radiation itself seems to play a differential role in percutaneous absorption of sunscreen filters in experimental models, by interfering with the skin surface characteristics and barrier function, with an added weightage for lipophilicity versus hydrophilicity of formulations [37].

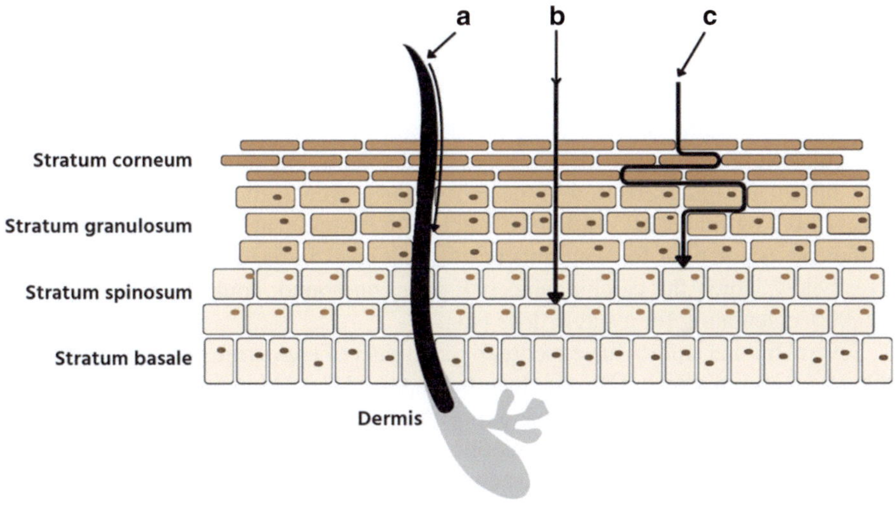

Fig. 11.3 The viable epidermis, underlying the SC, contains three layers, the stratum basal, the stratum spinosum, and the stratum granulosum. The SC consists of approximately 15 layers of corneocytes. The main cell type in the viable epidermis is the keratinocyte. Pathways for cutaneous penetration include the transappendageal (a), transcellular (b), and intercellular (c). (Modified from Nanotechnology, Science and Applications 2011 4 95–112' Originally published by and used with permission from Dove Medical Press Ltd. [35])

The most widely researched UV filter in terms of systemic absorption is Benzophenone-3 (BP-3). Up to 0.5% of a topically applied dosage of Benzophenone (BP) was identified in urine, the main elimination pathway of this compound, for up to 48 h [2, 28]. Up to 10% of applied BP-3 was found to penetrate the skin of children, raising concerns about the applicability of this filter in products meant for children, considering the greater skin surface area to body weight in this group [38]. Benzophenone-3 has also been identified in the human amniotic fluid, found to be excreted into breast milk, and detected in human placenta [39]. The importance of the detection of this lipophilic filter in these fluids is underlined by the ability of BP-3 to cross the blood–brain barrier [2, 32]. While Benzophenone-3 is widely understood by consumers only as being present in sunscreens, it is also present in several personal care products such as body washes, soaps and bath oils, makeup cosmetics, hair care products, fragrances, and anti-ageing creams. In addition, benzophenones are also found in the material exposome around us, having been used in plastic materials and containers, either as precursors or as additives to prevent UV induced degradation. In this context, adding further exposure to benzophenones in the form of sunscreens lowers the threshold limits for human toxicity [39].

The Official Journal of the European Union carried a Commission Regulation in 2022, on the permissible levels of benzophenone 2 and octocrylene in sunscreens. While acknowledging the potential health risks to consumers from the use of these two filters in cosmetic products including sunscreens, the Scientific Committee on Consumer Safety (SCCS) proposed to reduce the maximum allowed concentration of benzophenone-3 to 2.2%, for use in body creams, propellant sprays, and pump sprays, from the earlier allowed level of 6% [40]. This is the second reduction in 5 years, with an earlier drop in 2017, from 10% to 6% as the permissible limit for benzophenone in sunscreens [32].

Studies by Matta et al. identified that highly lipophilic UV filters with lower molecular weight, typically BP-3 demonstrate a depot effect on prolonged contact, with significant filter retention in the skin, up to 3 weeks after the application [27, 40]. The 0.5 ng/ml cut off used in the studies for systemic absorption limit is meant to indicate a potential for carcinogenesis. This level indicates the highest plasma level below which the carcinogenic risk of a compound would be less than 1 in 100,000, calculating for a single dose [41].

Several human studies have recorded the impact of endocrine disruption attributable to sunscreen filters. These include the reported links between polycystic ovary syndrome (PCOS) and octocrylene exposure, benzophenone and autism spectrum disorder, prenatal exposure to benzophenone and markers of male reproductive behaviour in adulthood, BP-3 levels, and infertility in women, among other emerging data [42–45]. Paradoxically, Wang et al. observed a decreased risk of pubertal childhood overweight and obesity by 55% and 29%, respectively, related to exposure of organic UV filters [46]. Several arguments against a human impact from systemic absorption of sunscreen ingredients are directed at the inferences having been made predominantly from animal studies with tests done employing much higher doses than clinically relevant [28].

The SCCS assumes a utilization of about 18 g per day in humans, for calculations to arrive at the margin of safety (MoS) [47]. This is based on actual average sunscreen utilization of up to 8.5 g per day based on pooled data, and the added possibility of sun filters being present in other personal care products including after sun creams. It may be argued that the amount of sunscreen used in other populations than those cited for this calculation, is lesser. The variability in absorption is significantly influenced by the formulation in addition to the molecular structure of the filter.

The Technical University of Denmark (DTU) has evaluated the threshold values used by the European Chemicals Agency (ECHA)/European Food Safety Authority (EFSA) guidelines to arrive at SCCS opinions as not accurate, and as discrepant in evaluating endocrine disruption. Specifically, the DTU notes that while the ECHA guidelines proposed to include an equal sensitivity of thyroid hormone disruption across human and rodent studies where liver enzyme induction causes increased thyroid hormone clearance, this was not followed in arriving at the safety limits for octocrylene. Octocrylene potentially causes endocrine disruption acting through liver enzyme induction, and therefore should have been evaluated at a higher level of safety to arrive at the NOAEL level (no observed adverse effect level), than presently [48].

The newer testing protocols which include a preliminary in vitro permeation test (IVPT) and subsequent maximum usage trial (MUsT) testing at maximal dosing offer a way to correlate the NOAEL in animal studies to clinically relevant plasma concentrations [49]. In these studies, the systemic absorption of the UV filter is studied at the maximum allowed concentrations, in formulations that have the highest potential for skin penetration, at usage volumes relevant to the consumer. Since skin penetration is altered by the type of the emulsion, presence, or absence of penetration enhancers, and the nature of the excipients, the pilot MUsT is preceded by the IVPT which helps identify formulations that are likely to be absorbed systemically, and only these formulations are then used in the MUsT studies. Designed as a Phase I Pilot and Phase III pivotal trial, the MUsT pharmacokinetic assessments are now mandatory for sunscreen filters, in potential consideration for inclusion in the over the counter (OTC) sunscreen monograph of the United States Food and Drug Administration (US FDA). Bemotrizinol is the first UV filter to be evaluated using the MUsT protocol ahead of approval [50]. In early studies, BEMT has been shown to have no adverse impact on certain aquatic species compared to homosalate and octocrylene which exhibited significant toxicity towards the tested species [50].

IVPT is a useful tool which helps to understand the variability in permeability of different formulations and can be therefore used to guide product development. Maximal dosing in the MUsT protocol is comparable to an infinite dosing protocol in the IVPT, while detection of the filter after a single dermal application is comparable to IVPT finite dosing [40]. Dermatomed human skin and heat separated human epidermis (HSE) are used as substrates used for IVPT testing. The latter is preferred for sunscreen testing due to lesser variability and the shorter duration of testing, typically less than 24 h [40].

As a corollary to IVPT being a precedent to identifying the best formulation for demonstrating absorption by MUsT, the potential plasma levels of reformulations can be arrived upon by comparing the IVPT to that of the reference formula. Yang et al. demonstrated that the skin permeability of oxybenzone and octinoxate containing formulations correlated with the plasma levels seen in observations of Matta et al., while this was not the case for avobenzone, octinoxate, homosalate, and octisalate containing sunscreens [40].

To address the depot effect of certain sunscreens to accumulate in the skin, IVPT can be used noninvasively to predict UV filter retention in the skin, through further refinements in protocols for better fidelity. Larger phase 3 pivotal MUsT studies may provide a way to reduce variability by formulation type and skin thickness in addition to differences in real-life use cases [40].

The systemic absorption of mineral sunscreens has been evaluated to be negligible, based on several studies. At best, zinc nanoparticles were found to penetrate into the epidermis only slightly without permeating the stratum corneum, while titanium particles reached the upper dermis [51]. Neither was found to penetrate any deeper [52]. Information is also limited by the inability of assays to completely differentiate between mineral ions attributable to sunscreens, to those absorbed from other sources, including and especially dietary [52, 53].

In contrast to the topical routes of absorption from sunscreen lotions and creams, sunscreen sprays are associated with a possible inhalational risk. Potential bloodstream absorption can occur as the nanoparticles are not adequately cleared from the alveoli. Furthermore, titanium was as a carcinogen by the International Agency for Research on Carcinogens based on inhalational toxicity, a decision that has recently been annulled [53, 54].

Titanium particles are considered as PSLTs—poorly soluble particles and have been postulated to provoke lung carcinogenesis in animal studies through pathways of chronic inflammation, cell proliferation, and oxidative stress. In contrast to titanium nanoparticles, coated zinc particles were rapidly eliminated after inhalational exposure, within a day [55]. Considering that the inhalation route of systemic absorption is significant even with mineral UV filters as it is with chemical sunscreens, it seems prudent to recommend that spray sunscreens only be used in well ventilated surroundings [55].

The <E11> or the average specific extinction of a sunscreen is an important factor in determining the amount of filter that is available to be absorbed systemically from the sunscreen application. High efficacy sunscreen filters are likely to be present in lower concentrations within a formula, and therefore be less available for absorption, compared to filters which must be employed in large volumes for optimal sun screening benefits [56]. Homosalate is the least efficient UV filter while tris-biphenyl triazine is the most powerful chemical sun filter. Among the mineral sunscreens, titanium dioxide has an <E11> that is four times higher than the other mineral sunscreen, zinc oxide.

Apart from the concentration of a filter required in a formulation, molecular size of the UV filter and formulation strategies seem to be key areas of preventing systemic absorption. Avobenzone with octocrylene in a sol-gel silica capsule was found to be absorbed less from the final sunscreen product than when these two filters were used in an unencapsulated format [57]. Furthermore, the encapsulation enhanced the safety of the final formulation. Sunscreen penetration is also a function of molecular size, with penetration potential decreasing with increasing molecular size [58]. Diagram of molecular size of sunscreen filters is illustrated below, Fig. 11.4 [59–83].

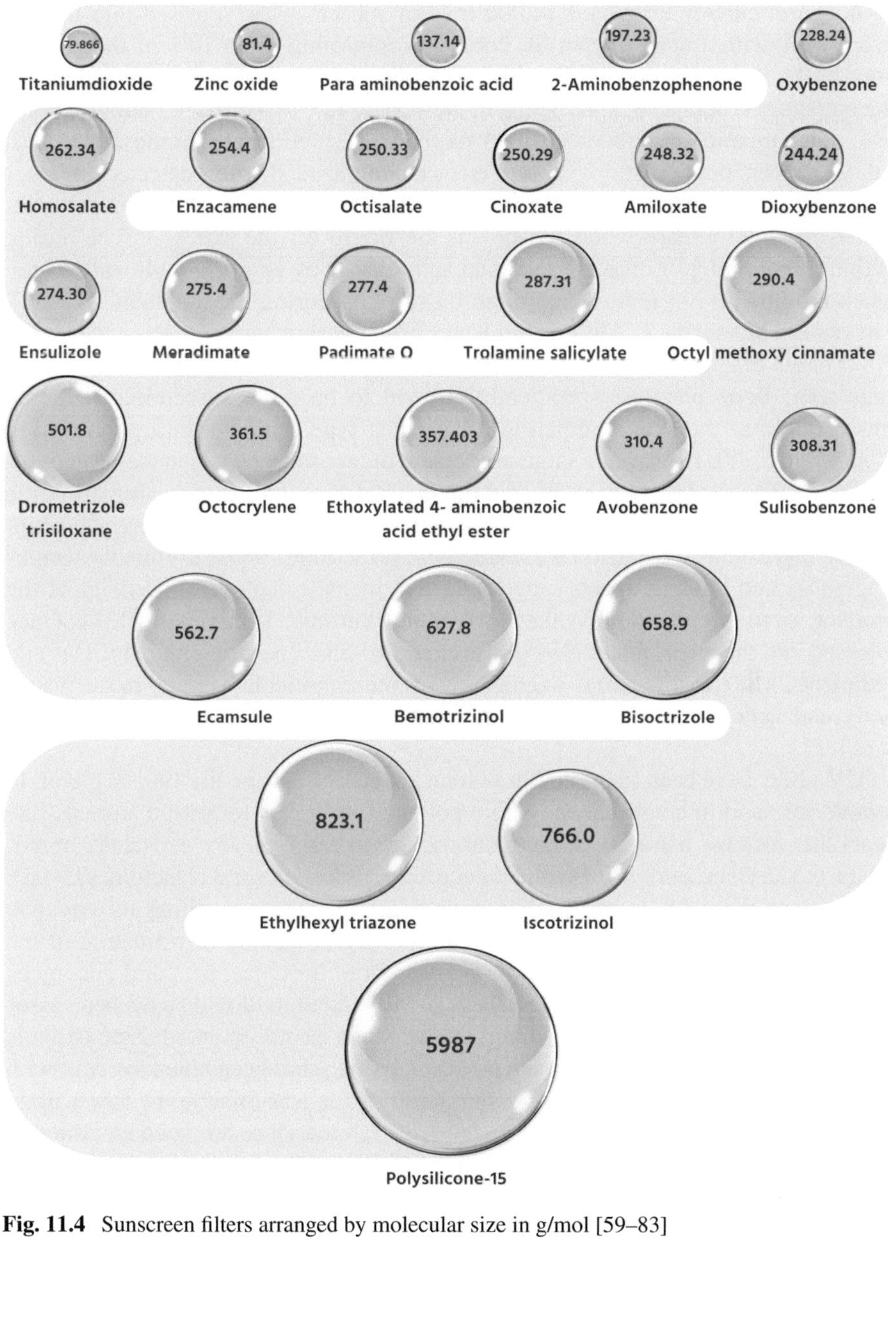

Fig. 11.4 Sunscreen filters arranged by molecular size in g/mol [59–83]

11.3 Sunscreens and the Ecosystem

Despite short half lives in the environment, a constant introduction of progressively increasing levels of sunscreens into the oceans endangers an ecosystem that already faces multiple threats such as global warming, increasing human traffic for energy generation and recreational purposes, overfishing, dumping of sewage, effluent, and plastic [26].

A conservatively estimated 14,000 tons of sunscreen are released into the sea every year, with a huge impact for coral life, impacting up to 10% of the world's coral reefs, and along the coasts, up to 40% of coastal reefs may be affected due to the increased effluence of sunscreens in these areas due to increased human activity [84, 85]. Organic sunscreens such as oxybenzone, octinoxate, homosalate, octisalate, avobenzone, octocrylene, and enzacamene have all been detected in water bodies in various locations in the world [86]. UV filters may enter water bodies either by direct release when sunscreens are rinsed off the skin's surface during bathing, swimming or other recreational activities or by entry through wastewater, when the filter is not removed through biosorption during the treatment [87, 88]. The elution of specific UV filters into water from the skin has been demonstrated to differ based on the composition, application rate as well as the physical form of the sunscreen. Benzophenone specifically seemed to be more susceptible to being rinsed off from the skin, comparing for product type (lotions), in a porcine skin model study [89]. However, a large proportion of any sunscreen is made of ingredients other than the UV filter itself, and the specific contribution to rinsing off of the final sunscreen product, from this component of excipients, preservatives and supportive ingredients must also be considered. Furthermore, some excipients such as fragrances and binding agents may interact to increase the overall toxicity of the product, even if individually, they may not contribute significantly [33]. Once released into the environment, lipophilic chemical filters partition into particles and sediments. Mineral filters may aggregate with other particulate matter in the waterbody and accumulate. Zinc oxide may further break down into its constituent ions [85].

UV filters have been identified in several species of marine life [90, 91], both in remote seas and in coastal areas with a potential to impact terrestrial animals like bears that feed off fish [92]. Among corals, UV filters, typically octisalate, homosalate, octocrylene, and oxybenzone induce a change called coral bleaching [93–95]. Exposure to these filters causes activation of coral viruses resulting in oxidative stress. This leads to extrusion of the symbiotic algae, leading to whitening of the coral or bleaching. Without the symbiotic support of the algae, the coral undergoes extinction [96]. While mineral sunscreens such as titanium dioxide have been associated with significant coral bleaching, recovery has also been noted. Zinc oxide is considered to have a lowered impact; however, damage has been noted to occur with the nanomineral forms [86]. Non-nano titanium oxide was found to be less acutely toxic to clownfish compared to oxybenzone [97]. Octocrylene has been identified in adipose tissue of stranded dolphins, along with BP-3 [98], and is considered as an emerging pollutant [99], alongside other ingredients of personal care products,

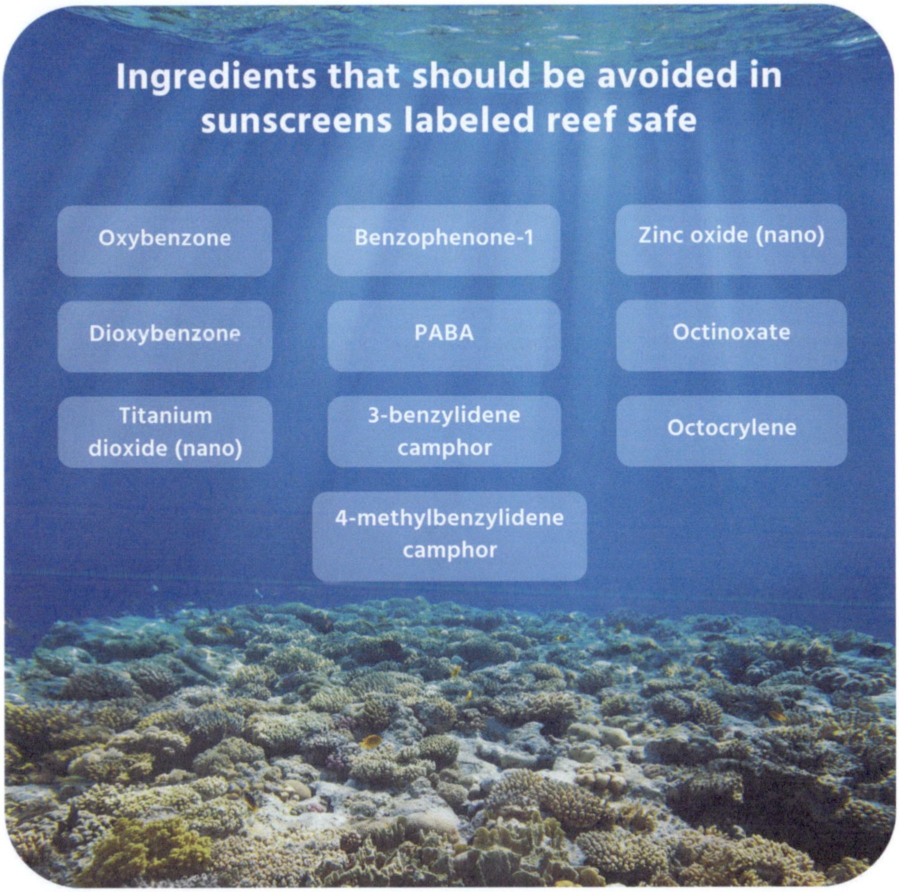

Fig. 11.5 Filters to be avoided in sunscreens designated as Reef Safe [101]

typified in the exposome of coastal tourism [100]. Several studies have recorded the detection of organic UV filters in many organisms such as white fish, cod, rainbow trout, mussels, roach, perch, chub, and barb, Figs. 11.5 and 11.6 [86].

The identification of the impact of UV filters on coral bleaching led to a legislative ban on oxybenzone and octinoxate in Hawaii [87]. This started the wave of popularity for reef safe sunscreens. The National Oceanic and Atmospheric Administration came out with a list of sunscreen filters that must be avoided for the sunscreen formulation to be considered as 'reef-safe', Fig. 11.5 [101]. Accordingly, these ingredients in a sunscreen would render it unfriendly to aquatic life. Though this is perceived as pertaining only to sunscreens that are used by the sea or the beach, even sunscreens used at other locations eventually would find their way to the sea through the wastewater runoffs. Aquatic species identified to be impacted by sunscreen filters, based on currently available data [50, 90, 91, 102–118] and detection UV filters from natural sources, around the world [119–153] are illustrated in Figs. 11.6 and 11.7.

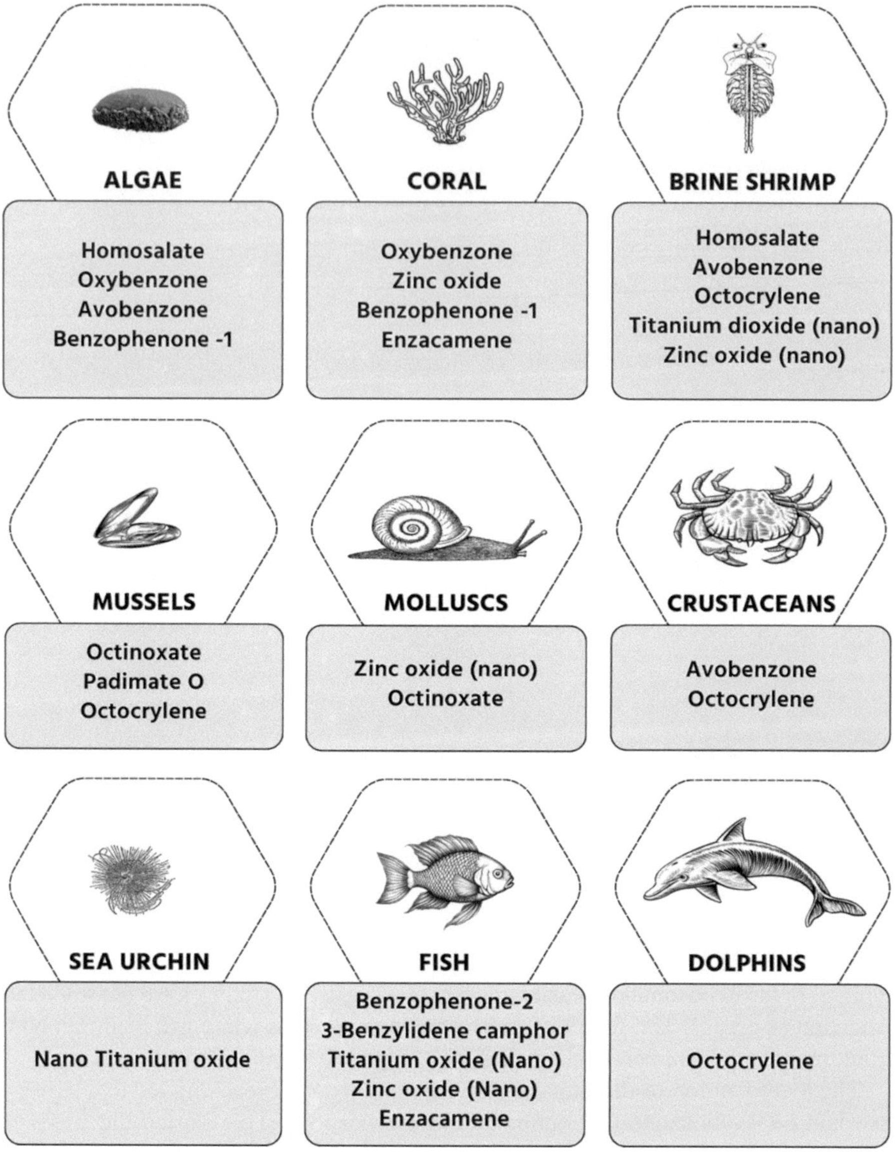

Fig. 11.6 Infographic of aquatic species identified to be impacted by sunscreen filters, based on the currently available data [50, 90, 91, 102–118]

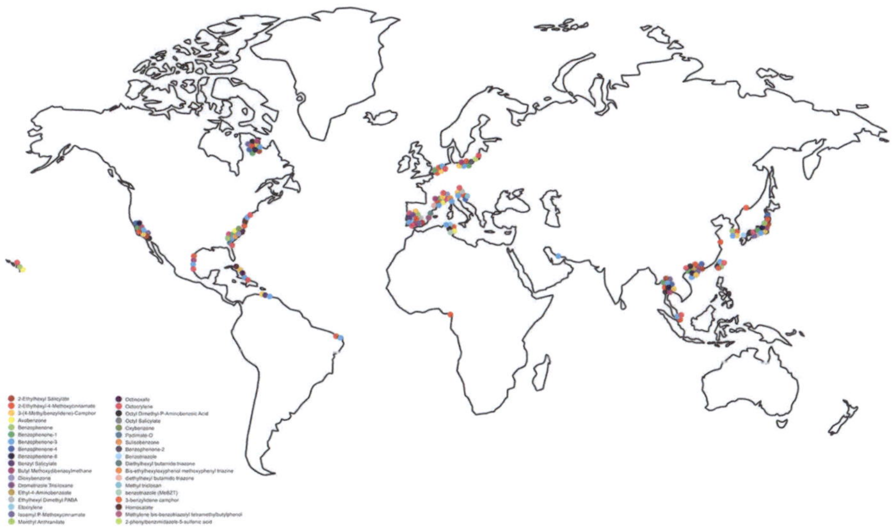

Fig. 11.7 Map depicting detection of UV filters from natural sources, around the world [119–153]

While the ecological impact of individual UV filters has been characterized, impact as seen with final sunscreen formulations which carry more than one UV filter, has more real world implications. This also reflects the potential interactions in final effluents where UV filters have been shown to interact with each other on wastewater treatment. Inorganic sunscreens in the form of nanoparticles have been known to aggravate the photocatalytic behaviour of organic sunscreens, resulting in an overall increase in the generation of toxic free radicals in the environment. Organic sunscreen filters also behave similarly. Lee et al. confirmed the anti-androgenic/estrogenic behaviour of homosalate acting alone on male zebrafish. In addition, they highlighted the potentiation of this endocrine disruption effect, when avobenzone was also added to homosalate [154]. A combination of these two filters is not unusual in the marketplace today, however. In a study by Thorel et al. on brine shrimp and microalgae, homosalate and octocrylene were found to exert significant toxicity on these two aquatic species. BEMT, diethylhexyl butamido triazone (DBT), ethylhexyl triazone (ET), methylene bis-benzotriazolyl tetramethylbutyl-phenol (MBBT) were found to be harmless to both species even at high concentrations, while ethylhexyl salicylate (ES), BP-3, and diethylaminohydroxybenzoyl hexylbenzoate (DHHB) showed some inhibitory behaviour towards the algae [50]. Among engineered nanomaterials (ENM), zinc and titanium nanoparticles are considered the most intensively active, contributing to 94% of the ENMs in personal care products [155].

With such large volumes of sunscreen usage, the impact extends beyond marine life and into food chain relevant to humans. Bioaccumulation of sunscreens has been documented, where the UV filters accumulate in an organism through any means of exposure. Subsequent bioconcentration is said to occur when the concentration of the filter is higher in the organism than in the surrounding medium. An increase in concentration of the chemical at the next higher trophic level is called biomagnification or trophic magnification [92].

Bioaccumulation and biomagnification of sunscreens and their entry into the human food chain, and subsequent detection in biological fluids, outside of direct systemic absorption has been demonstrated. Chemical filters such as avobenzone, octocrylene, octinoxate, oxybenzone, homosalate, padimate O, and the inorganic filter, titanium dioxide have been shown to have a low to moderate bioaccumulation potential. Octocrylene and oxybenzone were commonly noted to bioaccumulate in cod liver, raising concerns for human consumption [155]. Liu et al. found that the presence of certain UV filters in diet correlated with the levels of these filters secreted in breast milk [31]. In this context, the slow biodegradability or the lack of biodegradability of sunscreens has become a concern. Some sunscreens such as BP-3, BEMT, MBBT, DBT, ethylhexyl triazone (EHT), DHHB have been noted to have lesser biodegradability [156].

Cognisant of the huge environmental impact of sunscreen related ingredient pollution, several stakeholders have been working to mitigate the damage.

Newer sunscreens in development are put through safe by design and sustainable by design processes, which aim to protect against eco-damage from the level of product concept ideation [157]. Processes such as ecological risk assessments (ERA) help identify specific ecological settings in which a UV filter may cause an adverse impact, and this information can be proactively factored in, during the sunscreen development stage [87]. Passivization of inorganic mineral filters, using specialized coatings, is an example [158].

The prevention of damage must begin with reproducible measurements to assess the potential of different UV filters for ecotoxicity. Grading systems such as the The Ecosun Pass, that considers the multiple aspects of ecological impact of a sunscreen and assigns a score that globally, are useful [56]. The domains evaluated are biodegradation, bioaccumulation, acute and chronic aquatic toxicity, chronic terrestrial toxicity, and sediment toxicity. Impact in each of these domains is weighted to arrive at a score which can then be understood as a measure of ecological impact. The uniqueness of this grading system is that it allows for the accounting of sunscreens as mixtures of UV filters. It also acknowledges the potential ecological impact of the supportive ingredients/excipients used in the formulation, and which by themselves may be contributing to ecotoxicity [159], additively or individually. Creating compartments within the grading system, for example, bioaccumulation versus biodegradability, provides an idea of where action must be directed for a higher level of ecofriendliness of the product.

The recent suggestion by Diffey on reducing sunscreen usage in conditions where it may be unnecessary and the increasing data on durable sunscreens with retained protection for up to 8 h, may all work towards decreasing the global burden of sunscreens [160, 161].

11.4 Chapter Summary

For many dermatological conditions and procedural treatments, the use of sunscreens is essential for preventive and therapeutic purposes. Despite their prominence, it becomes increasingly clear that that exposure to sunscreens themselves has potential downsides to it. Problems mainly arise from the photo instability of a sunscreen, leading to inadequate protection despite and otherwise perception. Systemic absorption and sunscreen filter presence in the ecosystem creates problems for human, animal, and plant health, the consequences of which may be far reaching given the quantum of sunscreen use, globally. A better understanding of the hows and whys of sunscreen photostability, has encouraged the development of newer technologies to create stable sunscreens with reliable benefit. Revisiting the quantity of usage, need for use, frequency of reapplication, combination of filters, and the behaviour of UV filters in the environment, are all hot areas of research with a focus to make sunscreen usage safer and sustainable, for people and the environment.

References

1. Jesus A, Sousa E, Cruz MT, Cidade H, Lobo JMS, Almeida IF. UV filters: challenges and prospects. Pharmaceuticals [Internet]. 2022 Mar 1 [cited 2024 Mar 3];15(3). Available from: https://www.ncbi.nlm.nih.gov/pmc/articles/PMC8955451/
2. Maier T, Korting HC. Sunscreens—which and what for? Skin Pharmacol Physiol [Internet]. 2005 Nov [cited 2024 Mar 3];18(6):253–62. Available from: https://pubmed.ncbi.nlm.nih.gov/16113595/
3. Drissi M, Carr E, Housewright C. Sunscreen: a brief walk through history. Proc (Bayl Univ Med Cent) [Internet]. 2022 [cited 2024 Mar 15];35(1):121. Available from: https://www.ncbi.nlm.nih.gov/pmc/articles/PMC8682817/
4. Berenbeim JA, Wong NGK, Cockett MCR, Berden G, Oomens J, Rijs AM, et al. Unravelling the keto-enol tautomer dependent photochemistry and degradation pathways of the protonated UVA filter avobenzone. J Phys Chem A [Internet]. 2020 Apr 16 [cited 2024 Mar 27];124(15):2919–30. Available from: https://pubmed.ncbi.nlm.nih.gov/32208697/
5. Wong NGK, Berenbeim JA, Hawkridge M, Matthews E, Dessent CEH. Mapping the intrinsic absorption properties and photodegradation pathways of the protonated and deprotonated forms of the sunscreen oxybenzone. Phys Chem Chem Phys [Internet]. 2019 Jul 3 [cited 2024 Mar 27];21(26):14311–21. Available from: https://pubs.rsc.org/en/content/articlehtml/2019/cp/c8cp06794e
6. Berenbeim JA, Wong NGK, Cockett MCR, Berden G, Oomens J, Rijs AM, et al. Sodium cationization can disrupt the intramolecular hydrogen bond that mediates the sunscreen activity of oxybenzone. Phys Chem Chem Phys [Internet]. 2020 Sep 16 [cited 2024 Mar 27];22(35):19522–31. Available from: https://pubs.rsc.org/en/content/articlehtml/2020/cp/d0cp03152f
7. Dondi D, Albini A, Serpone N. Interactions between different solar UVB/UVA filters contained in commercial suncreams and consequent loss of UV protection. Photochem Photobiol Sci [Internet]. 2006 Aug 29 [cited 2024 Mar 27];5(9):835–43. Available from: https://pubmed.ncbi.nlm.nih.gov/17047836/

8. Kawakami CM, Gaspar LR. Mangiferin and naringenin affect the photostability and phototoxicity of sunscreens containing avobenzone. J Photochem Photobiol B [Internet]. 2015 Oct 1 [cited 2024 Mar 27];151:239–47. Available from: https://pubmed.ncbi.nlm.nih.gov/26318281/
9. Ginzburg AL, Blackburn RS, Santillan C, Truong L, Tanguay RL, Hutchison JE. Zinc oxide-induced changes to sunscreen ingredient efficacy and toxicity under UV irradiation. Photochem Photobiol Sci [Internet]. 2021 Oct 1 [cited 2024 Apr 6];20(10):1273. Available from: https://www.ncbi.nlm.nih.gov/pmc/articles/PMC8550398/
10. Afonso S, Horita K, Sousa E Silva JP, Almeida IF, Amaral MH, Lobão PA, et al. Photodegradation of avobenzone: stabilization effect of antioxidants. J Photochem Photobiol B [Internet]. 2014 [cited 2024 Mar 27];140:36–40. Available from: https://pubmed.ncbi.nlm.nih.gov/25086322/
11. Gaspar LR, Campos PMBGM. Photostability and efficacy studies of topical formulations containing UV-filters combination and vitamins A, C and E. Int J Pharm [Internet]. 2007 Oct 1 [cited 2024 Mar 27];343(1–2):181–9. Available from: https://pubmed.ncbi.nlm.nih.gov/17614223/
12. Piccinino D, Capecchi E, Trifero V, Tomaino E, Marconi C, Del Giudice A, et al. Lignin nanoparticles as sustainable photoprotective carriers for sunscreen filters. ACS Omega [Internet]. 2022 Oct 25 [cited 2024 Apr 6];7(42):37070–7. Available from: https://pubmed.ncbi.nlm.nih.gov/36312404/
13. Chaudhuri RK, Lascu Z, Puccetti G, Deshpande AA, Paknikar SK. Design of a photostabilizer having built-in antioxidant functionality and its utility in obtaining broad-spectrum sunscreen formulations. Photochem Photobiol [Internet]. 2006 May [cited 2024 Mar 27];82(3):823–8. Available from: https://pubmed.ncbi.nlm.nih.gov/16492073/
14. Gholap AD, Sayyad SF, Hatvate NT, Dhumal V V., Pardeshi SR, Chavda VP, et al. Drug delivery strategies for avobenzone: a case study of photostabilization. pharmaceutics [Internet]. 2023 Mar 21 [cited 2024 Mar 11];15(3):1008. Available from: https://www.mdpi.com/1999-4923/15/3/1008/htm
15. Murphy RB, Staton J, Rawal A, Darwish TA. The effect of deuteration on the keto–enol equilibrium and photostability of the sunscreen agent avobenzone. Photochem Photobiol Sci [Internet]. 2020 Oct 13 [cited 2024 Mar 27];19(10):1410–22. Available from: https://pubs.rsc.org/en/content/articlehtml/2020/pp/d0pp00265h
16. Termer M, Jaeger A, Carola C, Salazar A, Keck CM, Kolmar H, et al. Methoxy-monobenzoylmethane protects skin from UV-induced damages in a randomized, placebo controlled, double-blinded human in vivo study and prevents signs of inflammation while improving the skin barrier. Dermatol Ther (Heidelb) [Internet]. 2022 Feb 1 [cited 2024 Mar 27];12(2):435–49. Available from: https://pubmed.ncbi.nlm.nih.gov/34939179/
17. Benjatikul K, Mahamongkol H, Wongtrakul P. Sunscreen properties of marl. J Oleo Sci [Internet]. 2020 [cited 2024 Mar 27];69(1):73–82. Available from: https://pubmed.ncbi.nlm.nih.gov/31902898/
18. Holt EL, Rodrigues N d. N, Cebrián J, Stavros VG. Determining the photostability of avobenzone in sunscreen formulation models using ultrafast spectroscopy. Phys Chem Chem Phys [Internet]. 2021 Nov 14 [cited 2024 Mar 15];23(42):24439–48. Available from: https://pubmed.ncbi.nlm.nih.gov/34694312/
19. Beasley DG, Meyer TA. Characterization of the UVA protection provided by avobenzone, zinc oxide, and titanium dioxide in broad-spectrum sunscreen products. Am J Clin Dermatol [Internet]. 2010 [cited 2024 Mar 27];11(6):413–21. Available from: https://pubmed.ncbi.nlm.nih.gov/20806994/
20. Ginzburg AL, Blackburn RS, Santillan C, Truong L, Tanguay RL, Hutchison JE. Zinc oxide-induced changes to sunscreen ingredient efficacy and toxicity under UV irradiation. Photochem Photobiol Sci [Internet]. 2021 Oct 1 [cited 2024 Mar 11];20(10):1273–85. Available from: https://pubmed.ncbi.nlm.nih.gov/34647278/

21. Nash JF, Tanner PR. Relevance of UV filter/sunscreen product photostability to human safety. Photodermatol Photoimmunol Photomed [Internet]. 2014 [cited 2024 Mar 16];30(2–3):88–95. Available from: https://pubmed.ncbi.nlm.nih.gov/24433498/
22. Green A, Williams G, Neale R, Hart V, Leslie D, Parsons P, et al. Daily sunscreen application and betacarotene supplementation in prevention of basal-cell and squamous-cell carcinomas of the skin: a randomised controlled trial. Lancet [Internet]. 1999 Aug 28 [cited 2024 Mar 3];354(9180):723–9. Available from: https://pubmed.ncbi.nlm.nih.gov/10475183/
23. Green AC, Williams GM, Logan V, Strutton GM. Reduced melanoma after regular sunscreen use: randomized trial follow-up. J Clin Oncol [Internet]. 2011 Jan 20 [cited 2024 Mar 11];29(3):257–63. Available from: https://pubmed.ncbi.nlm.nih.gov/21135266/
24. Lal ST, Banipal RPS, Bhatti DJ, Yadav HP. Changing trends of skin cancer: a tertiary care hospital study in Malwa Region of Punjab. J Clin Diagn Res [Internet]. 2016 Jun 1 [cited 2024 Mar 11];10(6):PC12–5. Available from: https://pubmed.ncbi.nlm.nih.gov/27504344/
25. Harken EBO, Fazio J. Basal cell carcinoma. Atlas of dermatologic diseases in solid organ transplant recipients [Internet]. 2022 Sep 19 [cited 2024 Mar 27];331–46. Available from: https://www.ncbi.nlm.nih.gov/books/NBK482439/
26. (PDF) Cutaneous photoprotection: a review of the current status and evolving strategies [Internet]. [cited 2024 Mar 3]. Available from: https://www.researchgate.net/publication/340352263_Cutaneous_Photoprotection_A_Review_of_the_Current_Status_and_Evolving_Strategies
27. Matta MK, Florian J, Zusterzeel R, Pilli NR, Patel V, Volpe DA, et al. Effect of sunscreen application on plasma concentration of sunscreen active ingredients: a randomized clinical trial. JAMA [Internet]. 2020 Jan 21 [cited 2024 Mar 27];323(3):256–67. Available from: https://jamanetwork.com/journals/jama/fullarticle/2759002
28. Wang SQ, Burnett ME, Lim HW. Safety of oxybenzone: putting numbers into perspective. Arch Dermatol [Internet]. 2011 Jul 1 [cited 2024 Mar 15];147(7):865–6. Available from: https://jamanetwork.com/journals/jamadermatology/fullarticle/1105240
29. Sunscreen fountain of youth: use of sunscreen for anti-aging purposes increased 25% from 2021-22 | Mintel [Internet]. [cited 2024 Mar 27]. Available from: https://www.mintel.com/press-centre/sunscreen-fountain-of-youth-use-of-sunscreen-for-anti-aging-purposes-increased-25-from-2021-22/
30. Osterwalder U, Sohn M, Herzog B. Global state of sunscreens. Photodermatol Photoimmunol Photomed [Internet]. 2014 [cited 2024 Mar 22];30(2–3):62–80. Available from: https://pubmed.ncbi.nlm.nih.gov/24734281/
31. Liu Y, Gao L, Ai Q, Qiao L, Li J, Lyu B, et al. Concentrations, profiles, and health risks of organic ultraviolet filters in eight food categories determined through the sixth Chinese total diet study. Environ Sci Technol [Internet]. 2023 Sep 12 [cited 2024 Mar 27];57(36):13366–74. Available from: https://pubs.acs.org/doi/abs/10.1021/acs.est.3c03888
32. Wnuk W, Michalska K, Krupa A, Pawlak K. Benzophenone-3, a chemical UV-filter in cosmetics: is it really safe for children and pregnant women? Postepy Dermatol Alergol [Internet]. 2022 [cited 2024 Mar 27];39(1):26–33. Available from: https://www.researchgate.net/publication/358904304_Benzophenone-3_a_chemical_UV-filter_in_cosmetics_is_it_really_safe_for_children_and_pregnant_women
33. Varrella S, Danovaro R, Corinaldesi C. Assessing the eco-compatibility of new generation sunscreen products through a combined microscopic-molecular approach. Environ Pollut. 2022;314:120212.
34. Egambaram OP, Kesavan Pillai S, Ray SS. Materials science challenges in skin UV protection: a review. Photochem Photobiol [Internet]. 2020 Jul 1 [cited 2024 Mar 3];96(4):779–97. Available from: https://pubmed.ncbi.nlm.nih.gov/31886889/
35. Smijs TG, Pavel S. Titanium dioxide and zinc oxide nanoparticles in sunscreens: focus on their safety and effectiveness. Nanotechnol Sci Appl [Internet]. 2011 [cited 2024 Apr 4];4(1):95. Available from: https://www.ncbi.nlm.nih.gov/pmc/articles/PMC3781714/

36. Wang M, Tan J, Qi Z, Ge X, Li G, Yu Y. A combined study of skin penetration by confocal Raman spectroscopy and human metabolism: a case of benzophenone-3 in sunscreen. Environ Pollut [Internet]. 2024 Jan 1 [cited 2024 Mar 27];340(Pt 1). Available from: https://pubmed.ncbi.nlm.nih.gov/37926406/
37. Duracher L, Blasco L, Abdel Jaoued A, Vian L, Marti-Mestres G. Irradiation of skin and contrasting effects on absorption of hydrophilic and lipophilic compounds. Photochem Photobiol [Internet]. 2009 [cited 2024 Mar 27];85(6):1459–67. Available from: https://pubmed.ncbi.nlm.nih.gov/19656323/
38. Jiang R, Roberts MS, Collins DM, Benson HAE. Absorption of sunscreens across human skin: an evaluation of commercial products for children and adults. Br J Clin Pharmacol [Internet]. 1999 [cited 2024 Mar 27];48(4):635. Available from: https://www.ncbi.nlm.nih.gov/pmc/articles/PMC2014387/
39. Molins-Delgado D, Olmo-Campos M del M, Valeta-Juan G, Pleguezuelos-Hernández V, Barceló D, Díaz-Cruz MS. Determination of UV filters in human breast milk using turbulent flow chromatography and babies' daily intake estimation. Environ Res [Internet]. 2018 Feb 1 [cited 2024 Mar 27];161:532–9. Available from: https://pubmed.ncbi.nlm.nih.gov/29232646/
40. Yang Y, Ako-Adounvo AM, Wang J, Coelho SG, Adah SA, Matta MK, et al. In vitro testing of sunscreens for dermal absorption: method comparison and rank order correlation with in vivo absorption. AAPS PharmSciTech [Internet]. 2022 Jul 1 [cited 2024 Mar 27];23(5). Available from: https://pubmed.ncbi.nlm.nih.gov/35459978/
41. Serpone N. Sunscreens and their usefulness: have we made any progress in the last two decades? Photochem Photobiol Sci 2021 20:2 [Internet]. 2021 Feb 18 [cited 2024 Mar 3];20(2):189–244. Available from: https://link.springer.com/article/10.1007/s43630-021-00013-1
42. Holmboe SA, Scheutz Henriksen L, Frederiksen H, Andersson AM, Priskorn L, Jørgensen N, et al. Prenatal exposure to phenols and benzophenones in relation to markers of male reproductive function in adulthood. Front Endocrinol (Lausanne) [Internet]. 2022 Dec 9 [cited 2024 Mar 27];13. Available from: https://pubmed.ncbi.nlm.nih.gov/36568115/
43. Arya S, Dwivedi AK, Alvarado L, Kupesic-Plavsic S. Exposure of U.S. population to endocrine disruptive chemicals (Parabens, Benzophenone-3, Bisphenol-A and Triclosan) and their associations with female infertility. Environ Pollut [Internet]. 2020 Oct 1 [cited 2024 Mar 27];265(Pt A). Available from: https://pubmed.ncbi.nlm.nih.gov/32806428/
44. Gao CJ, Yang F, Wu B, Liang Y, Qin YY, Guo Y. A pilot study of several environmental endocrine disrupting chemicals in children with autism spectrum disorder in south China. Environ Monit Assess [Internet]. 2023 Aug 1 [cited 2024 Mar 27];195(8). Available from: https://pubmed.ncbi.nlm.nih.gov/37462787/
45. Lorigo M, Mangana C, Cairrao E. Disrupting effects of the emerging contaminant octylmethoxycinnamate (OMC) on human umbilical artery relaxation. Environ Pollut [Internet]. 2023 Oct 15 [cited 2024 Mar 27];335. Available from: https://pubmed.ncbi.nlm.nih.gov/37536478/
46. Wang P, Huang Y, Zhao Y, Zhou Y, Wang H, Zhang L, et al. Organic UV filters mixture exposure and childhood adiposity: a prospective follow-up study in China. Environ Int [Internet]. 2022 Jan 1 [cited 2024 Mar 27];158. Available from: https://pubmed.ncbi.nlm.nih.gov/34619533/
47. Scientific Committee on Consumer Safety SCCS the SCCS notes of guidance for the testing of cosmetic ingredients and their safety evaluation 12 th revision.
48. Christiansen S, Petersen MA, Boberg J. Faglig vurdering af foreløbig SCCS vurdering for Homosalat [Internet]. Citation. APA; 2020 [cited 2024 Apr 5]. Available from: https://orbit.dtu.dk/en/publications/faglig-vurdering-af-forel%C3%B8big-sccs-vurdering-for-homosalat
49. D'Ruiz CD, Plautz JR, Schuetz R, Sanabria C, Hammonds J, Erato C, et al. Preliminary clinical pharmacokinetic evaluation of bemotrizinol—a new sunscreen active ingredient being considered for inclusion under FDA's over-the-counter (OTC) sunscreen monograph. Regul Toxicol Pharmacol [Internet]. 2023 Mar 1 [cited 2024 Mar 15];139. Available from: https://pubmed.ncbi.nlm.nih.gov/36738872/
50. Thorel E, Clergeaud F, Jaugeon L, Rodrigues AMS, Lucas J, Stien D, et al. Effect of 10 UV filters on the brine shrimp Artemia salina and the marine microalga Tetraselmis sp. Toxics

[Internet]. 2020 Jun 1 [cited 2024 Apr 2];8(2). Available from: https://pubmed.ncbi.nlm.nih.gov/32290111/

51. Al-Khafaji Z, Brito S, Bin BH. Zinc and zinc transporters in dermatology. Int J Mol Sci [Internet]. 2022 Dec 18 [cited 2024 Mar 27];23(24):16165. Available from: https://www.mdpi.com/1422-0067/23/24/16165/htm
52. Schneider SL, Lim HW. A review of inorganic UV filters zinc oxide and titanium dioxide. Photodermatol Photoimmunol Photomed [Internet]. 2019 Nov 1 [cited 2024 Mar 11];35(6):442–6. Available from: https://pubmed.ncbi.nlm.nih.gov/30444533/
53. Grande F, Tucci P. Titanium dioxide nanoparticles: a risk for human health? Mini Rev Med Chem [Internet]. 2016 Apr 18 [cited 2024 Mar 27];16(9):762–9. Available from: https://pubmed.ncbi.nlm.nih.gov/26996620/
54. https://curia.europa.eu/jcms/upload/docs/application/pdf/2022-11/cp220190en.pdf.—Google Search [Internet]. [cited 2024 Mar 28]. Available from: https://www.google.com/search?q=https%3A%2F%2Fcuria.europa.eu%2Fjcms%2Fupload%2Fdocs%2Fapplication%2Fpdf%2F2022-11%2Fcp220190en.pdf.&sca_esv=44539afece030e85&ei=RfEEZpO8Laew4-EPoM-w6A8&ved=0ahUKEwjT8pnUjpaFAxUn2DgGHaAnDP0Q4dUDCBA&uact=5&oq=https%3A%2F%2Fcuria.europa.eu%2Fjcms%2Fupload%2Fdocs%2Fapplication%2Fpdf%2F2022-11%2Fcp220190en.pdf.&gs_lp=Egxnd3Mtd2l6LXNlcnAiUGh0dHBzOi8vY3VyaWEuZXVyb3BhLmV1L2pjbXMvdXBsb2FkL2RvY3MvYXBwbGljYXRpb24vcGRmLzIwMjItMTEvY3AyMjAxOTBlbi5wZGYuMhYQABgDGI8BGOUCGOoCGLQCGIwD2AEBMhYQABgDGI8BGOUCGOoCGLQCGIwD2AEBMhYQABgDGI8BGOUCGOoCGLQCGIwD2AEBMhYQABgDGI8BGOUCGOoCGLQCGIwD2AEBMhYQABgDGI8BGOUCGOoCGLQCGIwD2AEBMhYQABgDGI8BGOUCGOoCGLQCGIwD2AEBMhYQABgDGI8BGOUCGOoCGLQCGIwD2AEBMhYQABgDGI8BGOUCGOoCGLQCGIwD2AEBMhYQABgDGI8BGOUCGOoCGLQCGIwD2AEBSKsNUMAHWMAHcAF4AJABAJgBAKABAKoBALgBA8gBAPgBAfgBApgCAaACDagCCpgDDboGBAgBGAqSBwExoAcA&sclient=gws-wiz-serp
55. Creutzenberg O, Pohlmann G, Schaudien D, Kock H. Toxicokinetics of nanoparticles deposited in lungs using occupational exposure scenarios. Front Public Health [Internet]. 2022 [cited 2024 Mar 28];10:909247. Available from: https://pubmed.ncbi.nlm.nih.gov/35801236/
56. Pawlowski S, Herzog B, Sohn M, Petersen-Thiery M, Acker S. EcoSun Pass: atool to evaluate the ecofriendliness of UV filters used in sunscreen products. Int J Cosmet Sci [Internet]. 2021 Apr 1 [cited 2024 Mar 16];43(2):201–10. Available from: https://pubmed.ncbi.nlm.nih.gov/33289148/
57. Cozzi AC, Perugini P, Gourion-Arsiquaud S. Comparative behavior between sunscreens based on free or encapsulated UV filters in term of skin penetration, retention and photostability. Eur J Pharm Sci [Internet]. 2018 Aug 30 [cited 2024 Mar 16];121:309–18. Available from: https://pubmed.ncbi.nlm.nih.gov/29874551/
58. Shaath NA. The chemistry of ultraviolet filters. In: Principles and practice of photoprotection. Cham: Adis; 2016. p. 143–57.
59. Polysilicone-15 | Socosur [Internet]. [cited 2024 Mar 28]. Available from: https://www.toxby.design/toxicology-by-design/pde/details/polysilicone-15-2898
60. muyldjn. Scientific Committee on Consumer Safety SCCS opinion on polysilicone-15 COLIPA n° S74. 2010 [cited 2024 Mar 28]; Available from: http://ec.europa.eu/health/scientific_committees/consumer_safety/index_en.htm
61. 2-Aminobenzophenone | C13H11NO | CID 76080—PubChem [Internet]. [cited 2024 Apr 2]. Available from: https://pubchem.ncbi.nlm.nih.gov/compound/2-Aminobenzophenone
62. Oxybenzone | C14H12O3 | CID 4632—PubChem [Internet]. [cited 2024 Apr 2]. Available from: https://pubchem.ncbi.nlm.nih.gov/compound/Oxybenzone
63. Cinoxate | C14H18O4 | CID 5373773—PubChem [Internet]. [cited 2024 Apr 2]. Available from: https://pubchem.ncbi.nlm.nih.gov/compound/Cinoxate

64. Octyl salicylate | C15H22O3 | CID 62624—PubChem [Internet]. [cited 2024 Apr 2]. Available from: https://pubchem.ncbi.nlm.nih.gov/compound/octyl%20o-hydroxybenzoate
65. 3-(4-Methylbenzylidene)camphor | C18H22O | CID 7019255—PubChem [Internet]. [cited 2024 Apr 2]. Available from: https://pubchem.ncbi.nlm.nih.gov/compound/3-_4-Methylbenzylidene_camphor
66. Homosalate | C16H22O3 | CID 8362—PubChem [Internet]. [cited 2024 Apr 2]. Available from: https://pubchem.ncbi.nlm.nih.gov/compound/Homosalate
67. Trolamine Salicylate | C13H21NO6 | CID 25213—PubChem [Internet]. [cited 2024 Apr 2]. Available from: https://pubchem.ncbi.nlm.nih.gov/compound/Trolamine-Salicylate
68. Sulisobenzone | C14H12O6S | CID 19988—PubChem [Internet]. [cited 2024 Apr 2]. Available from: https://pubchem.ncbi.nlm.nih.gov/compound/Sulisobenzone
69. Avobenzone | C20H22O3 | CID 51040—PubChem [Internet]. [cited 2024 Apr 2]. Available from: https://pubchem.ncbi.nlm.nih.gov/compound/Avobenzone
70. Octocrylene | C24H27NO2 | CID 22571—PubChem [Internet]. [cited 2024 Apr 2]. Available from: https://pubchem.ncbi.nlm.nih.gov/compound/Octocrylene
71. Drometrizole trisiloxane | C24H39N3O3Si3 | CID 9848888—PubChem [Internet]. [cited 2024 Apr 2]. Available from: https://pubchem.ncbi.nlm.nih.gov/compound/Drometrizole-trisiloxane
72. Terephthalylidene dicamphor sulfonic acid | C28H34O8S2 | CID 6439900—PubChem [Internet]. [cited 2024 Apr 2]. Available from: https://pubchem.ncbi.nlm.nih.gov/compound/Terephthalylidene-dicamphor-sulfonic-acid
73. Bisoctrizole | C41H50N6O2 | CID 3571576—PubChem [Internet]. [cited 2024 Apr 2]. Available from: https://pubchem.ncbi.nlm.nih.gov/compound/Bisoctrizole
74. Iscotrizinol | C44H59N7O5 | CID 9810816—PubChem [Internet]. [cited 2024 Apr 2]. Available from: https://pubchem.ncbi.nlm.nih.gov/compound/Iscotrizinol
75. 4-Aminobenzoic acid | C7H7NO2 | CID 978—PubChem [Internet]. [cited 2024 Apr 2]. Available from: https://pubchem.ncbi.nlm.nih.gov/compound/4-Aminobenzoic-acid
76. Dioxybenzone | C14H12O4 | CID 8569—PubChem [Internet]. [cited 2024 Apr 2]. Available from: https://pubchem.ncbi.nlm.nih.gov/compound/Dioxybenzone
77. Ensulizole | C13H10N2O3S | CID 33919—PubChem [Internet]. [cited 2024 Apr 2]. Available from: https://pubchem.ncbi.nlm.nih.gov/compound/2-phenylbenzimidazole-5-sulfonic%20 acid
78. Menthyl anthranilate | C17H25NO2 | CID 8633—PubChem [Internet]. [cited 2024 Apr 2]. Available from: https://pubchem.ncbi.nlm.nih.gov/compound/8633
79. Padimate O | C17H27NO2 | CID 30541—PubChem [Internet]. [cited 2024 Apr 2]. Available from: https://pubchem.ncbi.nlm.nih.gov/compound/Escalol%20507
80. Octinoxate | C18H26O3 | CID 5355130—PubChem [Internet]. [cited 2024 Apr 2]. Available from: https://pubchem.ncbi.nlm.nih.gov/compound/Octinoxate
81. Titanium Dioxide | TiO2 | CID 26042—PubChem [Internet]. [cited 2024 Apr 2]. Available from: https://pubchem.ncbi.nlm.nih.gov/compound/Titanium-Dioxide
82. Zinc Oxide | OZn | CID 3007857—PubChem [Internet]. [cited 2024 Apr 2]. Available from: https://pubchem.ncbi.nlm.nih.gov/compound/Zinc-Oxide
83. Ethylhexyl triazone | C48H66N6O6 | CID 159201—PubChem [Internet]. [cited 2024 Apr 2]. Available from: https://pubchem.ncbi.nlm.nih.gov/compound/Ethylhexyl-triazone
84. Casas-Beltran DA, Hernández-Pedraza M, Alvarado-Flores J. Estimation of the discharge of sunscreens in aquatic environments of the Mexican Caribbean. Environments [Internet]. 2020 Feb 20 [cited 2024 Mar 28];7(2):15. Available from: https://www.mdpi.com/2076-3298/7/2/15/htm
85. Fivenson D, Sabzevari N, Qiblawi S, Blitz J, Norton BB, Norton SA. Sunscreens: UV filters to protect us: part 2-increasing awareness of UV filters and their potential toxicities to us and our environment. Int J Womens Dermatol [Internet]. 2021 Jan 1 [cited 2024 Mar 15];7(1):45. Available from: https://www.ncbi.nlm.nih.gov/pmc/articles/PMC7838327/
86. Ouchene L, Litvinov I V., Netchiporouk E. Hawaii and other jurisdictions ban oxybenzone or octinoxate sunscreens based on the confirmed adverse environmental effects of sunscreen

ingredients on aquatic environments. J Cutan Med Surg [Internet]. 2019 Nov 1 [cited 2024 Mar 16];23(6):648–9. Available from: https://pubmed.ncbi.nlm.nih.gov/31729915/

87. National Academies of Sciences, Engineering, and Medicine. Review of fate, exposure, and effects of sunscreens in aquatic environments and implications for sunscreen usage and human health. Washington, DC: National Academies Press; 2022. p. 1–409.
88. Langford KH, Thomas K V. Inputs of chemicals from recreational activities into the Norwegian coastal zone. J Environ Monit [Internet]. 2008 [cited 2024 Mar 28];10(7):894–8. Available from: https://pubmed.ncbi.nlm.nih.gov/18688459/
89. Saxe JK, Dean S, Jones RL, Mullins LA, Reynertson KA. Development of a novel rinse-off method for improved sunscreen exposure assessment. Integr Environ Assess Manag [Internet]. 2021 Sep 1 [cited 2024 Mar 28];17(5):961–6. Available from: https://pubmed.ncbi.nlm.nih.gov/34002489/
90. Tsui MMP, Lam JCW, Ng TY, Ang PO, Murphy MB, Lam PKS. Occurrence, distribution, and fate of organic UV filters in coral communities. Environ Sci Technol [Internet]. 2017 Apr 18 [cited 2024 Apr 2];51(8):4182–90. Available from: https://pubmed.ncbi.nlm.nih.gov/28351139/
91. Corinaldesi C, Marcellini F, Nepote E, Damiani E, Danovaro R. Impact of inorganic UV filters contained in sunscreen products on tropical stony corals (Acropora spp.). Sci Total Environ [Internet]. 2018 Oct 1 [cited 2024 Apr 2];637–638:1279–85. Available from: https://pubmed.ncbi.nlm.nih.gov/29801220/
92. Bioaccumulation and measured concentrations of UV filters in biota, in Review of fate, exposure, and effects of sunscreens in aquatic environments and implications for sunscreen usage and human health. Available from: https://www.ncbi.nlm.nih.gov/books/NBK587278/, Washington (DC): National Academies Press (US); 2022 Aug 9. 5.—Google Search [Internet]. [cited 2024 Mar 28]. Available from: https://www.google.com/search?q=Bioaccumulation+and+Measured+Concentrations+of+UV+Filters+in+Biota%2C%E2%80%9D+in+Review+of+Fate%2C+Exposure%2C+and+Effects+of+Sunscreens+in+Aquatic+Environments+and+Implications+for+Sunscreen+Usage+and+Human+Health.+%2C+Available+from%3A+https%3A%2F%2Fwww.ncbi.nlm.nih.gov%2Fbooks%2FNBK587278%2F%2C+Washington+(DC)%3A+National+Academies+Press+(US)%3B+2022+Aug+9.+5.&oq=Bioaccumulation+and+Measured+Concentrations+of+UV+Filters+in+Biota%2C%E2%80%9D+in+Review+of+Fate%2C+Exposure%2C+and+Effects+of+Sunscreens+in+Aquatic+Environments+and+Implications+for+Sunscreen+Usage+and+Human+Health.+%2C+Available+from%3A+https%3A%2F%2Fwww.ncbi.nlm.nih.gov%2Fbooks%2FNBK587278%2F%2C+Washington+(DC)%3A+National+Academies+Press+(US)%3B+2022+Aug+9.+5.&gs_lcrp=EgZjaHJvbWUyBggAEEUYOdIBCDEwNTJqMGo0qAIAsAIB&sourceid=chrome&ie=UTF-8
93. Conway AJ, Gonsior M, Clark C, Heyes A, Mitchelmore CL. Acute toxicity of the UV filter oxybenzone to the coral Galaxea fascicularis. Sci Total Environ [Internet]. 2021 Nov 20 [cited 2024 Mar 28];796. Available from: https://pubmed.ncbi.nlm.nih.gov/34273823/
94. Mitchelmore CL, Burns EE, Conway A, Heyes A, Davies IA. A critical review of organic ultraviolet filter exposure, hazard, and risk to corals. Environ Toxicol Chem [Internet]. 2021 Apr 1 [cited 2024 Mar 28];40(4):967–88. Available from: https://pubmed.ncbi.nlm.nih.gov/33528837/
95. Mitchelmore CL, He K, Gonsior M, Hain E, Heyes A, Clark C, et al. Occurrence and distribution of UV-filters and other anthropogenic contaminants in coastal surface water, sediment, and coral tissue from Hawaii. Sci Total Environ [Internet]. 2019 Jun 20 [cited 2024 Mar 28];670:398–410. Available from: https://pubmed.ncbi.nlm.nih.gov/30904653/
96. Danovaro R, Bongiorni L, Corinaldesi C, Giovannelli D, Damiani E, Astolfi P, et al. Sunscreens cause coral bleaching by promoting viral infections. Environ Health Perspect [Internet]. 2008 Apr [cited 2024 Mar 28];116(4):441. Available from: https://www.ncbi.nlm.nih.gov/pmc/articles/PMC2291018/

97. Barone AN, Hayes CE, Kerr JJ, Lee RC, Flaherty DB. Acute toxicity testing of TiO2-based vs. oxybenzone-based sunscreens on clownfish (Amphiprion ocellaris). Environ Sci Pollut Res Int [Internet]. 2019 [cited 2024 Mar 28];26(14). Available from: https://pubmed.ncbi.nlm.nih.gov/30875073/
98. González-Bareiro E, Montesdeoca-Esponda S, De la Fuente J, Sosa-Ferrera Z, Arbelo M, Fernández A, et al. Assessment of the presence of UV filters and UV stabilizers in stranded dolphin blubber. Sci Total Environ. 2023;895:165041.
99. Tovar-Sánchez A, Sánchez-Quiles D, Basterretxea G, Benedé JL, Chisvert A, Salvador A, et al. Sunscreen products as emerging pollutants to coastal waters. PLoS One [Internet]. 2013 Jun 5 [cited 2024 Mar 28];8(6):e65451. Available from: https://journals.plos.org/plosone/article?id=10.1371/journal.pone.0065451
100. Sánchez-Quiles D, Tovar-Sánchez A. Are sunscreens a new environmental risk associated with coastal tourism? Environ Int [Internet]. 2015 Jul 4 [cited 2024 Mar 28];83:158–70. Available from: https://pubmed.ncbi.nlm.nih.gov/26142925/
101. Guan LL, Lim HW, Mohammad TF. Sunscreens and photoaging: a review of current literature. Am J Clin Dermatol [Internet]. 2021 Nov 1 [cited 2024 Mar 16];22(6):819–28. Available from: https://pubmed.ncbi.nlm.nih.gov/34387824/
102. He T, Tsui MMP, Tan CJ, Ng KY, Guo FW, Wang LH, et al. Comparative toxicities of four benzophenone ultraviolet filters to two life stages of two coral species. Sci Total Environ. 2019;651:2391–9.
103. Araújo MJ, Rocha RJM, Soares AMVM, Benedé JL, Chisvert A, Monteiro MS. Effects of UV filter 4-methylbenzylidene camphor during early development of Solea senegalensis Kaup, 1858. Sci Total Environ. 2018;628–629:1395–404.
104. Mao F, He Y, Gin KYH. Evaluating the joint toxicity of two benzophenone-type UV filters on the green alga Chlamydomonas reinhardtii with response surface methodology. Toxics [Internet]. 2018 Jan 10 [cited 2024 Apr 2];6(1). Available from: https://pubmed.ncbi.nlm.nih.gov/29320457/
105. Araújo CVM, Rodríguez-Romero A, Fernández M, Sparaventi E, Medina MM, Tovar-Sánchez A. Repellency and mortality effects of sunscreens on the shrimp Palaemon varians: toxicity dependent on exposure method. Chemosphere [Internet]. 2020 Oct 1 [cited 2024 Apr 2];257. Available from: https://pubmed.ncbi.nlm.nih.gov/32480091/
106. Boyd A, Stewart CB, Philibert DA, How ZT, El-Din MG, Tierney KB, et al. A burning issue: the effect of organic ultraviolet filter exposure on the behaviour and physiology of Daphnia magna. Sci Total Environ [Internet]. 2021 Jan 1 [cited 2024 Apr 2];750. Available from: https://pubmed.ncbi.nlm.nih.gov/33182172/
107. Gago-Ferrero P, Alonso MB, Bertozzi CP, Marigo J, Barbosa L, Cremer M, et al. First determination of UV filters in marine mammals. Octocrylene levels in Franciscana dolphins. Environ Sci Technol [Internet]. 2013 Jun 4 [cited 2024 Apr 2];47(11):5619–25. Available from: https://pubmed.ncbi.nlm.nih.gov/23627728/
108. Chatzigianni M, Pavlou P, Siamidi A, Vlachou M, Varvaresou A, Papageorgiou S. Environmental impacts due to the use of sunscreen products: a mini-review. Ecotoxicology [Internet]. 2022 Nov 1 [cited 2024 Apr 2];31(9):1331. Available from: https://www.ncbi.nlm.nih.gov/pmc/articles/PMC9652235/
109. Cahova J, Blahova J, Marsalek P, Doubkova V, Franc A, Garajová M, et al. The biological activity of the organic UV filter ethylhexyl methoxycinnamate in rainbow trout (Oncorhynchus mykiss). Sci Total Environ [Internet]. 2021 Jun 20 [cited 2024 Apr 2];774. Available from: https://pubmed.ncbi.nlm.nih.gov/33609814/
110. Quintaneiro C, Teixeira B, Benedé JL, Chisvert A, Soares AMVM, Monteiro MS. Toxicity effects of the organic UV-filter 4-Methylbenzylidene camphor in zebrafish embryos. Chemosphere [Internet]. 2019 Mar 1 [cited 2024 Apr 2];218:273–81. Available from: https://pubmed.ncbi.nlm.nih.gov/30472611/
111. Picot Groz M, Martinez Bueno MJ, Rosain D, Fenet H, Casellas C, Pereira C, et al. Detection of emerging contaminants (UV filters, UV stabilizers and musks) in marine mussels from Portuguese coast by QuEChERS extraction and GC-MS/MS. Sci Total Environ [Internet].

2014 Sep 15 [cited 2024 Apr 2];493:162–9. Available from: https://pubmed.ncbi.nlm.nih.gov/24946029/

112. Bachelot M, Li Z, Munaron D, Le Gall P, Casellas C, Fenet H, et al. Organic UV filter concentrations in marine mussels from French coastal regions. Sci Total Environ [Internet]. 2012 Mar 15 [cited 2024 Apr 2];420:273–9. Available from: https://pubmed.ncbi.nlm.nih.gov/22330425/
113. Shi W, Guan X, Sun S, Han Y, Du X, Tang Y, et al. Nanoparticles decrease the byssal attachment strength of the thick shell mussel Mytilus coruscus. Chemosphere [Internet]. 2020 Oct 1 [cited 2024 Apr 2];257. Available from: https://pubmed.ncbi.nlm.nih.gov/32473408/
114. Tsui MMP, Leung HW, Kwan BKY, Ng KY, Yamashita N, Taniyasu S, et al. Occurrence, distribution and ecological risk assessment of multiple classes of UV filters in marine sediments in Hong Kong and Japan. J Hazard Mater [Internet]. 2015 Jul 5 [cited 2024 Apr 2];292:180–7. Available from: https://pubmed.ncbi.nlm.nih.gov/25804793/
115. Corinaldesi C, Damiani E, Marcellini F, Falugi C, Tiano L, Brugè F, et al. Sunscreen products impair the early developmental stages of the sea urchin Paracentrotus lividus. Sci Rep [Internet]. 2017 Dec 1 [cited 2024 Apr 2];7(1). Available from: https://pubmed.ncbi.nlm.nih.gov/28798318/
116. Chen L, Li X, Hong H, Shi D. Multigenerational effects of 4-methylbenzylidene camphor (4-MBC) on the survival, development and reproduction of the marine copepod Tigriopus japonicus. Aquat Toxicol [Internet]. 2018 Jan 1 [cited 2024 Apr 2];194:94–102. Available from: https://pubmed.ncbi.nlm.nih.gov/29172130/
117. Cunningham B, Torres-Duarte C, Cherr G, Adams N. Effects of three zinc-containing sunscreens on development of purple sea urchin (Strongylocentrotus purpuratus) embryos. Aquat Toxicol [Internet]. 2020 Jan 1 [cited 2024 Apr 2];218. Available from: https://pubmed.ncbi.nlm.nih.gov/31790937/
118. Gambardella C, Aluigi MG, Ferrando S, Gallus L, Ramoino P, Gatti AM, et al. Developmental abnormalities and changes in cholinesterase activity in sea urchin embryos and larvae from sperm exposed to engineered nanoparticles. Aquat Toxicol [Internet]. 2013 Apr 5 [cited 2024 Apr 2];130–131:77–85. Available from: https://pubmed.ncbi.nlm.nih.gov/23376697/
119. Li AJ, Sang Z, Chow CH, Law JCF, Guo Y, Leung KSY. Environmental behavior of 12 UV filters and photocatalytic profile of ethyl-4-aminobenzoate. J Hazard Mater. 2017;337:115–25.
120. Sankoda K, Murata K, Tanihata M, Suzuki K, Nomiyama K, Shinohara R. Seasonal and diurnal variation of organic ultraviolet filters from personal care products used along the Japanese coast. Arch Environ Contam Toxicol [Internet]. 2015 Jan 20 [cited 2024 Apr 2];68(2):217–24. Available from: https://link.springer.com/article/10.1007/s00244-014-0106-7
121. Kim KY, Ekpeghere KI, Jeong HJ, Oh JE. Effects of the summer holiday season on UV filter and illicit drug concentrations in the Korean wastewater system and aquatic environment. Environ Pollut. 2017;227:587–95.
122. Downs CA, Kramarsky-Winter E, Segal R, Fauth J, Knutson S, Bronstein O, et al. Toxicopathological effects of the sunscreen UV filter, oxybenzone (benzophenone-3), on coral planulae and cultured primary cells and its environmental contamination in Hawaii and the U.S. Virgin Islands. Arch Environ Contam Toxicol [Internet]. 2015 Oct 20 [cited 2024 Apr 2];70(2):265–88. Available from: https://link.springer.com/article/10.1007/s00244-015-0227-7
123. Bratkovics S, Sapozhnikova Y. Determination of seven commonly used organic UV filters in fresh and saline waters by liquid chromatography-tandem mass spectrometry. Analytical Methods [Internet]. 2011 Dec 1 [cited 2024 Apr 2];3(12):2943–50. Available from: https://pubs.rsc.org/en/content/articlehtml/2011/ay/c1ay05390f
124. Bratkovics S, Wirth E, Sapozhnikova Y, Pennington P, Sanger D. Baseline monitoring of organic sunscreen compounds along South Carolina's coastal marine environment. Mar Pollut Bull. 2015;101(1):370–7.
125. Vila M, Pablo Lamas J, Garcia-Jares C, Dagnac T, Llompart M. Ultrasound-assisted emulsification microextraction followed by gas chromatography–mass spectrometry and gas chro-

matography–tandem mass spectrometry for the analysis of UV filters in water. Microchem J. 2016;124:530–9.
126. Vila M, Celeiro M, Lamas JP, Dagnac T, Llompart M, Garcia-Jares C. Determination of fourteen UV filters in bathing water by headspace solid-phase microextraction and gas chromatography-tandem mass spectrometry. Anal Methods [Internet]. 2016 Oct 6 [cited 2024 Apr 2];8(39):7069–79. Available from: https://pubs.rsc.org/en/content/articlehtml/2016/ay/c6ay01787h
127. Schaap I, Slijkerman DME. An environmental risk assessment of three organic UV-filters at Lac Bay, Bonaire, Southern Caribbean. Mar Pollut Bull. 2018;135:490–5.
128. Kung TA, Lee SH, Yang TC, Wang WH. Survey of selected personal care products in surface water of coral reefs in Kenting National Park, Taiwan. Sci Total Environ. 2018;635:1302–7.
129. Tashiro Y, Kameda Y. Concentration of organic sun-blocking agents in seawater of beaches and coral reefs of Okinawa Island, Japan. Mar Pollut Bull. 2013;77(1–2):333–40.
130. Astel A, Stec M, Rykowska I. Occurrence and distribution of UV filters in beach sediments of the southern Baltic Sea coast. Water (Switzerland) [Internet]. 2020 Nov 1 [cited 2024 Apr 2];12(11):3024. Available from: https://openurl.ebsco.com/contentitem/doi:10.3390%2Fw12113024?sid=ebsco:plink:crawler&id=ebsco:doi:10.3390%2Fw12113024
131. Manasfi T, Coulomb B, Ravier S, Boudenne JL. Degradation of organic UV filters in chlorinated seawater swimming pools: transformation pathways and bromoform formation. Environ Sci Technol [Internet]. 2017 Nov 21 [cited 2024 Apr 2];51(23):13580–91. Available from: https://hal.science/hal-01656941
132. Takahashi S, Nakata H, Murata S, Shinohara R, Filatreau J, Isobe T, et al. Occurrence and concentrations of persistent personal care products, organic UV filters, in the marine environment. 2009 [cited 2024 Apr 2]; Available from: https://www.researchgate.net/publication/228652572
133. Fagervold SK, Rodrigues AS, Rohée C, Roe R, Bourrain M, Stien D, et al. Occurrence and environmental distribution of 5 UV filters during the summer season in different water bodies. Water Air Soil Pollut [Internet]. 2019 Jul 1 [cited 2024 Apr 2];230(7):1–13. Available from: https://link.springer.com/article/10.1007/s11270-019-4217-7
134. Arpin-Pont L, Martínez-Bueno MJ, Gomez E, Fenet H. Occurrence of PPCPs in the marine environment: a review. Environ Sci Pollut Res Int [Internet]. 2016 Mar 1 [cited 2024 Apr 2];23(6):4978–91. Available from: https://pubmed.ncbi.nlm.nih.gov/25253059/
135. Amine H, Gomez E, Halwani J, Casellas C, Fenet H. UV filters, ethylhexyl methoxycinnamate, octocrylene and ethylhexyl dimethyl PABA from untreated wastewater in sediment from eastern Mediterranean river transition and coastal zones. Mar Pollut Bull. 2012;64(11):2435–42.
136. Balmer ME, Buser HR, Müller MD, Poiger T. Occurrence of some organic UV filters in wastewater, in surface waters, and in fish from Swiss Lakes. Environ Sci Technol [Internet]. 2005 Feb 15 [cited 2024 Apr 2];39(4):953–62. Available from: https://pubs.acs.org/doi/abs/10.1021/es040055r
137. Fent K, Zenker A, Rapp M. Widespread occurrence of estrogenic UV-filters in aquatic ecosystems in Switzerland. Environ Pollut. 2010;158(5):1817–24.
138. Kaiser D, Wappelhorst O, Oetken M, Oehlmann J. Occurrence of widely used organic UV filters in lake and river sediments. Environ Chem [Internet]. 2012 Apr 23 [cited 2024 Apr 2];9(2):139–47. Available from: https://www.publish.csiro.au/en/EN11076
139. Molins-Delgado D, Távora J, Silvia Díaz-Cruz M, Barceló D. UV filters and benzotriazoles in urban aquatic ecosystems: the footprint of daily use products. Sci Total Environ. 2017;601–602:975–86.
140. He K, Hain E, Timm A, Tarnowski M, Blaney L. Occurrence of antibiotics, estrogenic hormones, and UV-filters in water, sediment, and oyster tissue from the Chesapeake Bay. Sci Total Environ. 2019;650:3101–9.
141. Ekpeghere KI, Kim UJ, O SH, Kim HY, Oh JE. Distribution and seasonal occurrence of UV filters in rivers and wastewater treatment plants in Korea. Sci Total Environ. 2016;542:121–8.

142. Labille J, Slomberg D, Catalano R, Robert S, Apers-Tremelo ML, Boudenne JL, et al. Assessing UV filter inputs into beach waters during recreational activity: a field study of three French Mediterranean beaches from consumer survey to water analysis. Sci Total Environ. 2020;706:136010.
143. Downs CA, Diaz-Cruz MS, White WT, Rice M, Jim L, Punihaole C, et al. Beach showers as sources of contamination for sunscreen pollution in marine protected areas and areas of intensive beach tourism in Hawaii, USA. J Hazard Mater. 2022;438:129546.
144. Sharifan H, Klein D, Morse AN. UV filters are an environmental threat in the Gulf of Mexico: a case study of Texas coastal zones. Oceanologia. 2016;58(4):327–35.
145. Gago-Ferrero P, Díaz-Cruz MS, Barceló D. UV filters bioaccumulation in fish from Iberian river basins. Sci Total Environ. 2015:518, 518–9, 525.
146. da Silva CP, Emídio ES, de Marchi MRR. The occurrence of UV filters in natural and drinking water in São Paulo State (Brazil). Environ Sci Pollut Res Int [Internet]. 2015 Dec 1 [cited 2024 Apr 2];22(24):19706–15. Available from: https://pubmed.ncbi.nlm.nih.gov/26278906/
147. Giokas DL, Sakkas VA, Albanis TA. Determination of residues of UV filters in natural waters by solid-phase extraction coupled to liquid chromatography–photodiode array detection and gas chromatography–mass spectrometry. J Chromatogr A. 2004;1026(1–2):289–93.
148. Magi E, Di Carro M, Scapolla C, Nguyen KTN. Stir bar sorptive extraction and LC-MS/MS for trace analysis of UV filters in different water matrices. Chromatographia [Internet]. 2012 Sep 19 [cited 2024 Apr 2];75(17–18):973–82. Available from: https://link.springer.com/article/10.1007/s10337-012-2202-z
149. Cuderman P, Heath E. Determination of UV filters and antimicrobial agents in environmental water samples. Anal Bioanal Chem [Internet]. 2007 Feb [cited 2024 Apr 2];387(4):1343–50. Available from: https://pubmed.ncbi.nlm.nih.gov/17136341/
150. Vosough M, Hassanbeigi Z, Salemi A. Determination of ultraviolet filter compounds in environmental water samples using membrane-protected micro-solid-phase extraction. J Sep Sci [Internet]. 2018 Jun 1 [cited 2024 Apr 2];41(11):2401–10. Available from: https://onlinelibrary.wiley.com/doi/full/10.1002/jssc.201701082
151. Bargar TA, Alvarez DA, Garrison VH. Synthetic ultraviolet light filtering chemical contamination of coastal waters of Virgin Islands national park, St. John, U.S. Virgin Islands. Mar Pollut Bull. 2015;101(1):193–9.
152. Fisch K, Waniek JJ, Schulz-Bull DE. Occurrence of pharmaceuticals and UV-filters in riverine run-offs and waters of the German Baltic Sea. Mar Pollut Bull. 2017;124(1):388–99.
153. Cadena-Aizaga MI, Montesdeoca-Esponda S, Sosa-Ferrera Z, Santana-Rodríguez JJ. Occurrence and environmental hazard of organic UV filters in seawater and wastewater from Gran Canaria Island (Canary Islands, Spain). Environ Pollut. 2022;300:118843.
154. Lee S, Ka Y, Lee B, Lee I, Seo YE, Shin H, et al. Single and mixture toxicity evaluation of avobenzone and homosalate to male zebrafish and H295R cells. Chemosphere [Internet]. 2023 Dec 1 [cited 2024 Mar 28];343. Available from: https://pubmed.ncbi.nlm.nih.gov/37758070/
155. Langford KH, Reid MJ, Fjeld E, Øxnevad S, Thomas K V. Environmental occurrence and risk of organic UV filters and stabilizers in multiple matrices in Norway. Environ Int [Internet]. 2015 Jul 1 [cited 2024 Mar 28];80:1–7. Available from: https://pubmed.ncbi.nlm.nih.gov/25827264/
156. Fagervold SK, Rohée C, Lebaron P. Microbial consortia degrade several widely used organic UV filters, but a number of hydrophobic filters remain recalcitrant to biodegradation. Environ Sci Pollut Res Int [Internet]. 2023 Dec 1 [cited 2024 Mar 28];30(60):125931–46. Available from: https://pubmed.ncbi.nlm.nih.gov/38010544/
157. Battistin M, Pascalicchio P, Tabaro B, Hasa D, Bonetto A, Manfredini S, et al. A safe-by-design approach to "reef safe" sunscreens based on ZnO and organic UV filters. Antioxidants (Basel) [Internet]. 2022 Nov 1 [cited 2024 Mar 28];11(11). Available from: https://pubmed.ncbi.nlm.nih.gov/36358585/

158. Labille J, Catalano R, Slomberg D, Motellier S, Pinsino A, Hennebert P, et al. Assessing sunscreen lifecycle to minimize environmental risk posed by nanoparticulate UV-filters—a review for safer-by-design products. Front Environ Sci. 2020;8:546963.
159. Penrose MT, Cobb GP. Identifying potential paraben transformation products and evaluating changes in toxicity as a result of transformation. Water Environ Res [Internet]. 2022 Apr 1 [cited 2024 Mar 28];94(4). Available from: https://pubmed.ncbi.nlm.nih.gov/35415920/
160. Diffey B. When should sunscreen be applied: the balance between health benefit and adverse consequences to humans and the environment. Int J Cosmet Sci [Internet]. 2023 Oct 1 [cited 2024 Mar 28];45 Suppl 1(S1):45–51. Available from: https://pubmed.ncbi.nlm.nih.gov/37799082/
161. Li H, Colantonio S, Dawson A, Lin X, Beecker J. Sunscreen application, safety, and sun protection: the evidence. J Cutan Med Surg [Internet]. 2019 Jul 1 [cited 2024 Mar 28];23(4):357–69. Available from: https://pubmed.ncbi.nlm.nih.gov/31219707/

Chapter 12
Clinical Considerations in Sunscreen Use

Abbreviations

ACD	Allergic contact dermatitis
BP-3	Benzophenone-3
CPDs	Cyclobutane pyrimidine dimers
DHHB	Diethylamino hydroxybenzoyl hexyl benzoate
EDTA	Ethylenediaminetetraacetic acid
EU	European Union
FFA	Frontal fibrosing alopecia
HDRS	Hybrid diffuse reflectance spectroscopy
HRIPT	Human repeated insult patch test
LLP	Lichen planus pigmentosus
MASI	Melasma area and severity index
MED	Minimal erythemal dose
MMP	Matrix metalloproteinases
NSAID	Non-steroidal anti-inflammatory drugs
OCP	Oral contraceptive pills
OD PABA	Octyl dimethyl para amino benzoic acid
OTC	Over the counter
PA+++	Protection grade of UVA
PACD	Photoallergic contact dermatitis
PBSA	Phenylbenzimidazole sulfonic acid
PCP	Personal care products
PHL	Pattern hair loss
PIH	Postinflammatory hyperpigmentation
RDA	Recommended daily allowance
ROAT	Repeat open allergen testing
SED	Standard erythemal dose
SOC	Skin of colour
TEWL	Trans epidermal water loss
UK	United Kingdom

R. Rajan, *Sunscreens for Skin of Color*,
https://doi.org/10.1007/978-981-97-3195-4_12

UPF	Ultraviolet protection factor
US FDA	United States Food and Drug Administration
UVA	Ultraviolet-A
UVA-PF	Ultraviolet-A protection factor
UVB	Ultraviolet-B
UV-PF	Ultraviolet protection factor
UVR	Ultraviolet radiation
WHO	World Health Organization

Key Objectives

- Understanding the selection of sunscreens to suit specific contexts such as pregnancy and lactation, use in children, and use in special populations such as sensitive skin, relies on understanding the guidelines around which filters are recommended in these use cases.
- The impact of sunscreens on vitamin D deficiency is a hotly debated topic. However, studies show that routine use of sunscreens may not cause any meaningful levels of vitamin D deficiency. Supplementation seems the most effective way to manage vitamin D deficiency, which is more common in skin of colour, due to the inherent higher levels of skin melanin acting as an inbuilt sunscreen.
- Frontal fibrosing alopecia is a recent controversy, which may be related to sunscreen use. Specific chemical sunscreens and nanoparticles may play a role in facilitating the development of FFA in predisposed individuals.
- Overall, sensitivity to UV filters is considered to be low. Benzophenone-3 is the most implicated filter in allergic contact dermatitis to sunscreens but is also widely present in multiple personal care products, other than sunscreens.
- New data on sunscreen durability on the skin challenges the existing recommendation to reapply sunscreen every 2 h.

From its origins as a non-aesthetic, prescription product that must be worn to prevent sunburn and skin cancer, the sunscreen has now come to be one of the most prominent personal care products, and the trends show that sunscreen use is set to only increase in the future. Despite differing regulations in different countries, the majority of sunscreens are available as over the counter (OTC) products for consumers to select and use. Several practical questions exist about the use, safety, efficacy, and side effect profile of sunscreens, which are brought to physicians, at times, and more commonly into the domain of public discourse. Accordingly, concerns regarding vitamin D deficiency and sunscreen use, benzene in sunscreens and endocrine disruption from some of the older chemical sunscreens, are common questions that physicians need to be aware of, to effectively counsel their patients and clients. The section below deals with some of these clinical considerations.

12.1 Sunscreens and Vitamin D

Vitamin D is a key regulator of multiple metabolic pathways in the human body, particularly for mineral homeostasis and skeletal system integrity [1], though originally in evolution, vitamin D may have been more relevant to maintaining a functional immune system [2]. In recent times, vitamin D has been studied to be central to several protective functions for the human body from cardiovascular to neurocognitive domains [3, 4].

From an evolutionary point of view, vitamin D may have well played a key role in the regulation, synthesis, and distribution of melanin in the skin, and contributed significantly to the skin colour of races as perceived today, as proposed by Jablonksi et al. almost 20 years ago, and since, supported by biophysical evidence for the vitamin D-folate hypothesis [5]. However, a more recent commentary by Hanel and Carlsten argue against the evolutionary pressure of vitamin D as a significant determinant of skin lightening [6].

The skin is both a site of synthesis of 1,25(OH)2 vitamin D3 (1,25(OH)2D3) and as well, a target organ for this most biologically active form of vitamin D. Ultraviolet-B (UVB) exposure facilitates the conversion of 7 dehydrocholesterol, present in the keratinocyte membrane to cholecalciferol on sunlight exposure [7]. Vitamin D synthesis begins as a photochemical reaction triggered by UVB light around 297 nm, the site of action being the basal and the suprabasal layers of the skin. Previtamin D, 7 dehydrocholesterol generates provitamin D, which then undergoes isomerization to vitamin D. Hydroxyl groups are added in the liver and kidney at positions 25 and 1, respectively, to reach the final form, 1, 25 dihydroxy cholecalciferol or calcitriol, that in the circulation, is used by most of the organs for various processes. However, it seems to be that the serum levels of calcitriol are unable to reach the surface keratinocytes or their vitamin D receptors in any significant quantum. Rather, an autonomous process of calcitriol synthesis occurs in the skin, from generation of vitamin D to its hydroxylation to active calcitriol to eventual catabolism, making keratinocytes the only cells in the body to do so [1]. Considering that the keratinocytes also contain receptors for Vitamin D, they are well able to function as autocrine and paracrine organs, to modify or modulate processes in the vicinity, unrelated to the calcitriol in circulation. While the complete effects of this modulation have not been fully elucidated, this may explain at least in some part, the beneficial effect of UVB on psoriatic keratinocytes. Calcitriol interaction with the keratinocyte may proceed through genomic or nongenomic pathways, resulting in antiproliferative, immunomodulatory, and cytoprotective effects, the extent of which are yet to be fully understood. With regard to the antiproliferative effects, a significant body of evidence exists to the utility of topical vitamin D analogues in psoriasis, with epidermal immunohistochemistry markers from lesional skin turning similar to those of non lesional skin on treatment with topical calcitriol [8]. A smaller impact was noted on the dermal components of psoriasis, considering the lesser bioavailability of vitamin D at the dermal level. The immunomodulatory effects of calcitriol are said to play a role in conditions like atopic dermatitis and allergic contact dermatitis. The photoprotective effects of 1,25 dihydroxy cholecalciferol against UV-induced mitochondrial damage, apoptosis, and induction of cyclobutane pyrimidine dimers (CPDs) due to mutations from incorrectly repaired DNA photoproducts may suggest a unique feedback mechanism to protect the skin from UV damage, considering that UV induces the formation of vitamin D in the first place! In addition to the main site of action in basal and suprabasal epidermis as above, dermal fibroblasts may also contribute to the vitamin D levels, both in the epidermis and in the bloodstream, with hydroxylation at C25. 1,25(OH)2 D3 protects the skin against UVB induced damage and photocarcinogenesis by modulating the synthesis and activity of stress induced protein kinases and interleukins and cell apoptosis [7]. Vitamin D contributes to skin anti-ageing, but this effect may be tempered by innate genetic differences in the pace of ageing, across populations. The vitamin D3 produced in the skin modulates the absorption of calcium in the small intestine, eventually supporting the musculoskeletal system [9].

Vitamin D deficiency is fairly rampant in most geographies and more noticeably among skin of colour [10–14]. It is estimated that up to 1 billion people are vitamin D deficient [15] An increasing lack of sun exposure, with resultant lowered skin production of vitamin D, and an inherent low dietary intake contributes to the global deficiency states observed for this multitasking vitamin, to the extent that this has been labelled a silent epidemic [9, 14]. Dietary sources of vitamin D like oily fish, milk, and egg yolk, contribute in a small way to the overall vitamin D supply, the bulk of vitamin D that is needed for the body is synthesized by the human skin [7]. However, the ability of UV to initiate vitamin D synthesis is modulated by the melanin content of the skin. Skin pigmentation negatively influences cutaneous vitamin D synthesis [16, 17]. Skin of colour filters out close to 75% of UVB compared to lighter skin types. Vitamin D production in the skin is also a function of ageing, due to the progressive decline of the precursor moiety, 7-dehydrocholesterol levels in the skin. These levels were studied to fall almost by 50% from age 20 to age 80 [18]. In India, Vitamin D deficiency has been noted in 88.5% of the study population, with no significant difference between those in indoor or outdoor occupations [19].

The recommended daily allowance (RDA) of vitamin D, to achieve optimal levels in dark-skinned individuals is 1000 IU/day for adults, as compared to 400–600 IU for Caucasians. The higher RDA also holds good for individuals with limited sun exposure and those with photosensitivity disorders who need to avoid the sun [7]. This difference in daily dose recommendation is due to the fact that skin of colour produces vitamin D on sun exposure less effectively. This has been demonstrated in multiple studies, world over. Vitamin D production in the skin decreases progressively on moving from skin type I to VI, with dark skin requiring higher doses of ultraviolet radiation (UVR) and longer durations of exposure for achieving similar levels of vitamin D output. This has been attributed to melanin competing with 7-dehydrocholesterol for absorbing incoming UVB, seemingly as an evolutionary choice to prevent skin cancer than achieve vitamin D sufficiency. Furthermore, it takes about 2 h of sun exposure on darker skin, compared to 25% of that time, 30 min, for lighter coloured skin to achieve vitamin D levels of 50 nmol/L. It is important to note that such a prolonged duration of sun exposure is likely to induce increased levels of melanin synthesis in darker skin types, with further attenuation of vitamin D synthesis over time. Furthermore, this level of sun exposure creates persistent and delayed pigment darkening, if not, long lasting pigmentation, all of which phenomena aggravate or induce pigmentary conditions, specifically bothersome in skin of colour [20, 21]. Interestingly, darker skin colour as a result of increased sun exposure was found to be associated with higher vitamin D levels in Thai patients [22].

Neonatal cord blood of dark-skinned babies was found to have significantly lesser levels of vitamin D, in correlation with maternal vitamin D deficiency, as compared to cord blood for lighter skinned babies [23]. Children of higher skin types needed higher doses of vitamin D supplementation to maintain optimal vitamin D levels, compared to fair skinned children [24]. The latter were able to achieve vitamin D adequacy of 30 ng/ml with daily supplementation of 6mcg/day or 240 IU vitamin D. For darker skinned children, the requirement of vitamin D to reach the same serum levels of vitamin D, 14 mcg, i.e., 560 IU was required. To achieve the optimal values of 50 ng/ml, the dark skin group required 28 mcg supplementation per day, compared to 20 mcg for the fair skinned cohort. Even for response to oral vitamin D correction, post-menopausal women with a fair skin type had a better response compared to higher skin types [11]. Ethnicity as a construct of skin colour plays a significant role in vitamin D deficiency [25].

A further recommendation even within the normal range of 30–100 ng/ml is a consideration to maintain vitamin D levels between 40 and 60 ng/ml. While levels below 40 ng/ml may not confer the anticipated benefits of vitamin D in reducing all cause mortality, cardiovascular events and cancer, levels higher than 60 ng/mL may be associated with higher adverse effects [7].

Sunscreen use was noted to be associated with reduced serum vitamin D levels in some studies [26]. This led to significant concern among people and medical practitioners and created a social media buzz promoting sun exposure and avoiding sunscreen use. Tran et al. noted that in Australia where the incidence of skin cancer is high, about 25% of survey participants were concerned about sunscreen induced vitamin D deficiency [27].

Multiple studies have now demonstrated that routine sunscreen use does not aggravate vitamin D deficiency [28, 29]. An elegant study by Singh et al. in Indian women with melasma demonstrated a lack of significant changes in vitamin D levels in those who used sunscreen versus those who did not. This study applied the common use case of sunscreens at a maximum of once to twice daily in hot and humid climates, where reapplication and heavy sunscreen use is uncomfortable at best, and triggers acne at worst [19, 30]. In Turkey, sunscreen use was noted to be a significant factor for vitamin D deficiency in girls and adolescents, compared to younger children and boys. However, this study also noted an impact of age, sex, and traditional clothing styles on vitamin D levels [26]. As an outcome of optimal skeletal health, bone mineral density or risk of osteoporotic fractures were not found to be negatively influenced by the use of sun protective behaviour, including sunscreen use [31].

In lighter skin types where vitamin D production on sun exposure is more robust, compared to darker skin types where majority of UVB is filtered out by melanin in the skin, lesser sunscreen use may be associated with higher serum vitamin D levels [32]. Libon et al. noted that sunscreen induced reduction in cutaneous vitamin D production did not translate into a corresponding reduction in circulating vitamin D3 levels. Rather, there was only a minimal reduction in serum vit D3 levels, though this study specifically evaluated short-term sunscreen use [33]. Sunscreen application thickness and layering may impact the level of attenuation of vitamin D synthesis [34, 35].

Hoesl et al. calculated that even when all methods of skin protection were considered, to result in a meaningful reduction in vitamin D serum levels, the most rigid UV protection regime would be expected to be applied for at least 30 years [36]. Divyalakshmi et al. noted that sunscreen use was not found to significantly influence vitamin D deficiency, considering the real life use cases of sunscreens in Indian patients [19]. Raymond-Lezman et al. concluded that, at best, sunscreen use only minimally lowers vitamin D levels, and there may be other factors at play, in agreement with other recent work in this domain [20, 37–39]. Passeron et al. concluded that the use of broad spectrum sunscreens even when used optimally is unlikely to impact vitamin D status negatively [40]. Screening in susceptible populations, which may be most people in skin of colour (SOC), and appropriate supplementation is recommended.

The role of sun in stimulation of conditions like melasma, very commonly noted in skin of colour, and therefore of sun protection in the alleviation of such conditions is well established. Sarkar et al. demonstrated a reduction in disease burden using the melasma area and severity index (MASI) score in women with melasma along with an improvement in quality-of-life scores, with the solo use of sunscreens, noting that sun protection should be the starting point of treating such pigmentary conditions [41]. Specifically, the newer generation of sunscreens focus on UVA protection and blue light protection for SOC, both of which domains do not influence vitamin D synthesis, but both of which are implicated in photopigmentation in SOC [40].

Since the majority of evidence points to the fact that sunscreen use may not be associated with vitamin D deficiency and considering the innately high levels of this deficiency in skin of colour, the directive should be to support oral supplementation of vitamin D, along with use of sunscreens to prevent and/or treat photoaggravated pigmentary skin conditions.

12.2 Allergies to Sunscreens

It is often said in humour, that everything under the sun, including the sun, can cause allergies. With the advent of common use of sunscreens, it may be safe to add that agents that protect against sun allergy, may also cause allergies themselves!

Despite common perception, a true contact allergy to sunscreens was considered to be fairly low [42, 43]. However, the trend seems to be changing, illustrated by photopatch testing research reported from Singapore over the years. In 1998, Ang et al. reported a total of 61 suspected cases of sunscreen allergy. Using photopatch testing, only five of these cases were found to have positive reactions, with only 3 out of the 5, known to be specifically allergic to active ingredients in sunscreens. The filters implicated were octinoxate and oxybenzone [43]. This was followed through in 2013, where more than 45% of those who underwent photopatch testing, were found to have positive reactions, notably to the active filters belonging to the benzophenone group, oxybenzone and mexenone, and to octyl dimethyl para amino benzoic acid (OD PABA). This study noted sunscreens to be the most common photo allergens, replacing musk ambrette, based on data up until then [44]. This was also reflected in studies by the European Multicentre Photopatch Study, published around the same time. Ten years later in 2023, benzophenone and mexenone still remained the most relevant photo allergens, in a follow-up study from Singapore [45].

Sunscreen ingredients have been implicated in both allergic contact dermatitis (ACD) and in photoallergic contact dermatitis (PACD). The former is induced by an allergen mediated type IV hypersensitivity reaction. Photoallergic contact dermatitis occurs as a result of UV induced modification of a chemical ingredient into an allergen. Allergic contact dermatitis and photoallergic contact dermatitis can occur 1–4 days after exposure to the allergen. Clinical features notably include pruritus with dermatitis extending outwards from the site of contact. In incidences of irritant dermatitis or phototoxic reactions, pain and blistering localized to the site of contact may act as a differentiating feature to aid diagnosis [46].

Thus far, only chemical UV filters have been implicated in contact/photocontact dermatitis. Inorganic filters, namely, titanium and zinc oxides have not been reported to cause allergic contact dermatitis [47]. So, while chemical sunscreen agents may be high or low prevalence allergens, physical sunscreens are considered as nonallergens [48]. However, titanium dioxide has been known to cause release of gold ions from jewellery and may facilitate the occurrence of an allergic reaction, potentially at distant sites, which may make the diagnosis difficult [47].

The most common allergens according to recent reviews are oxybenzone, which causes PACD almost thrice as commonly as it causes ACD and OD-PABA, where ACD is more common than PACD. Avobenzone behaves like oxybenzone with more instances of PACD than ACD, while sulisobenzone follows OD-PABA with a higher propensity to ACD. The photoallergic behaviour of the inherently photo unstable avobenzone is potentially due to its photodegradation products, such as benzyls and arylglyoxals [46]. Octinoxate is as likely to cause ACD as it is to cause PACD, though the overall allergenic potential was lesser than the above chemical filters. Oxybenzone caused almost ten times as much PACD as octinoxate, as reported in the elegant compilation by Ekstein et al., published recently [47].

The rising incidence of photopatch tests to sunscreen active ingredients, likely represents an increase in overall sun care product use by people, than a specific increase by ingredient type, as seen in the series of photopatch test studies from Singapore [45]. Similar trends are being reported from other countries as well.

Among individuals with photoallergic contact dermatitis in Columbia, positive patch test responses were noted commonly to UV filters. In descending order, the implicated sunscreen active ingredients included oxybenzone, octinoxate, benzophenone-4, mexenone, phenylbenzimidazole sulfonic acid (PBSA), methylbenzylidene camphor, and OD- PABA. The authors confirmed sunscreens to be the most common photo allergens in the Columbian population [49]. The findings were similar in a later study from Bogota, Columbia which reported that 95% of positive photo patch test reactions were attributable to sunscreen filters, most commonly to oxybenzone. The authors recommend extending the follow-up of the photopatch testing to 96 h after irradiation to avoid missing out the delayed positive reactions, which were seen in up to 50% of cases in this study [50]. A similar recommendation is also made by the United Kingdom (UK) multicentre photopatch study group, where standard readings at 48 h, may still need to be augmented by readings after 96 h [51]. This study identified octyl triazone as a new allergen, while oxybenzone remained the most implicated photo allergen. The Skin Allergy group, Spain, found sun filters to be the third most commonly identified allergens, next to topical non-steroidal anti-inflammatory drugs (NSAIDs), typically ketoprofen and fragrances [52], while a 20-year follow-up of photopatch tests identified benzophenone 3, and fragrances as the main reactive agents [53].

Ketoprofen, which is associated with the most number of positive patch test reactions in multiple settings, exhibits cross reactivity with benzophenone, possibly due to the structural similarity of the two molecules [54]. However, even with a less similar structure, cross reactivity exists between ketoprofen and octocrylene [55].

Newer filters introduced more recently have not been known to be associated with significant instances of contact dermatitis according to the European photopatch test baseline series study which analysed positive patch reactions between 2014 and 2016, while finding benzophenone and octocrylene to be significant allergens [56]. It could also be related to the less wide usage, considering the increasing use of these filters only in the last decade or so, and the recent availability of European Union (EU) only approved sun filters in the USA. The low reactivity of the newer filters was also highlighted in a recent Portuguese study which also noticed a downtrend in the overall positive photopatch test reactions attributable to sun filters. Classical UV filters were twice as likely to results in positive patch test reactions, compared to the newer filters, while still being a low occurrence compared to other allergens in the study, led by topical drugs such as ketoprofen and promethazine in addition to systemic diuretics and lipid lowering agents. Interestingly, in this study, Tinosorb-M produced positive patch test reactions, despite being in the newer filter group [57]. Recently, allergic reactions to polysilicone 15 (Parsol SLX) and Tinosorb S (bemotrizinol) [58] have been reported. Polysilicone S has also been implicated in allergic contact cheilitis, as an ingredient in a lip balm [59].

Contact dermatitis due to Tinosorb M merits a closer look. Tinosorb M is a proprietary UV filter from BASF, which contains bisoctrizole as the principal UV filter. Tinosorb M contains, in addition to Bisoctrizole, water, decyl glucoside, propylene glycol, and xanthan gum as other ingredients. Allergic contact dermatitis has been reported to the decyl glucoside moiety of Tinosorb M, by multiple researchers, and less commonly, to xanthan gum in the composite product [60–64]. Testing of the sun filter in isolation, in this case, bisoctrizole, may prove helpful in identifying the true origin of the allergic contact dermatitis [46, 61, 65]. This highlights the fact that, in addition to sunscreen active ingredients, namely the UV filters, allergic contact dermatitis can also arise to other structural and/or support agents contained in sunscreens.

In children known to be allergic to aluminium, presence of this moiety in sunscreens may trigger an allergic response to the sunscreen, as evidenced by ROAT—repeat open allergen testing [66]. This observation gains significance due to inorganic sunscreen filters like titanium dioxide often being coated with aluminium oxide to reduce reactivity.

In mineral sunscreens, ethylenediaminetetraacetic acid (EDTA) is added to perform as a chelating agent and helps reduce aggregation of metal ions. Contact allergy to the tetrasodium EDTA moiety in sunscreens has been reported. Commonly used preservatives like methylisothiazolinone have a potential to induce allergic contact dermatitis, mimicking photoallergic contact dermatitis, when present in sunscreens. The persistence of symptoms even after cessation of product use was likely due to the ability of this preservative to induce photoaggravated contact dermatitis, prompting a ban on use of this agent in personal care products in Europe and Canada [67].

Other than agents like EDTA and/or preservatives which are required for functional performance, agents with other intended purposes such as antioxidants, anti-acne, and skin lightening benefits are often added to sunscreens. Contact dermatitis to phenylethyl resorcinol added to a skin lightening sunscreen has been reported [68]. Owing to the complex nature of the interactions between different ingredients in a sunscreen, it is best to patch test using the patient's own sunscreen where possible [46].

Sunscreen sensitization can also occur as a result of product contact on compromised epidermis, typically as what happens after fractional laser resurfacing. Using a human repeated insult patch test (HRIPT), Boonchai et al. identified a higher level of sensitization to the UV filter, octocrylene in this study, in subjects who had undergone fractional laser resurfacing and who applies sunscreen from the very first day, versus those who applies sunscreen on intact skin. Based on these observations, the authors recommend that sunscreens be started from the third day after fractional resurfacing [69]. However, another group demonstrated that using sunscreens from the very first day after ablative fractional laser resurfacing reduced the incidence of postinflammatory hyperpigmentation (PIH) [70]. It may be left to the dermatologist's prudence to adapt these clinical observations into everyday practice, to look for and select sunscreens with lower sensitization potential, and to devise a case by case plan for restarting sunscreen after fractional ablative procedures depending on the risk of PIH for the given individual.

In contrast to allergic contact dermatitis, irritant reactions to sunscreen products are usually related to the inactive ingredients. Irritant response to sunscreen filters themselves are considered to be very infrequent, at less than 0.6% according to the estimate by the European Multicentre Photopatch Test Study Taskforce [46]. A rare case of a phototoxic reaction to octinoxate has been reported.

12.3 Sunscreen Application

Sunscreens can be considered as functional cosmetics—where a balance of both form and function is required. The requirements of a sunscreen differ depending on the user and the environment in which they use this personal care product. Typically, sunscreen requirements for those who work outdoors are significantly different from those who spend most of their time indoors. Apart from performance metrics related to sun protection, user dependent secondary performance attributes also play a role in optimal sunscreen use. Factors such as biostability on the skin in terms of sweat or water resistance, eye irritation characterized by a burning sensation, especially worsening with sweating, absorption, and settling into the skin, grip and subjective skin feel, whitening effect, compatibility with textiles, and dust and dirt absorption were considered as important secondary performance parameters in a German study by Rocholl et al. [71]. While some of these attributes are relatively easy to measure, such as eye irritation and whitening effect, more subjective measures like skin feel and skin grip may be more difficult to quantify.

Simply put, the efficacy of a sunscreen product is largely dependent on the way it is used, with the human factor playing a very important role even given the newer advances in sunscreen science. Most people do not use sunscreen regularly, or if they use it regularly, not adequately [72].

12.3.1 How Much Sunscreen to Apply?

Balancing human behaviour and sunscreen performance is tricky but necessary, since sun protection is related to quantitative measures of sunscreen application. The United States Food and Drug Administration (US FDA) recommends an application density of 2 mg/cm^2 to achieve optimal sun protection factor (SPF), as claimed on the label. However, in view of the ‘real-world’ incidences of lesser sunscreen usage, the International Organization for Standardization (ISO) 24443 guidelines use a sunscreen application density of 1.3 mg/cm^2 to calculate SPF. But sunscreen usage in practice falls significantly below at very low levels of usage, Kim et al. observed that it was not possible to reliably predict SPF on skin, and the actual protection obtained [73].

The Nambour study found that people on an average use less than half the recommended dose of sunscreen, which may be a key factor that confounds evaluations related to the utility of sunscreens in preventing skin cancer [74]. Further studies around the world found that even with proper education, the application of sunscreens was below the levels required to achieve the SPF on the product label.

That is not to say that awareness measures were not successful, but the success was suboptimal. In a Polish study, subjects who had been primed with educational instructions used 43% of a recommended dose of sunscreen, compared to 34.9% usage by those who received no priming instructions. This is still less than half the intended amount of usage [75]. It is not uncommon for studies to report usage levels as low as 0.2 mg/ml, with even patients with known photosensitivity using sunscreens at densities of 0.5 mg/ml [76].

Application density is said to have a linear relationship with the amount of SPF achieved relative to the label claim [73, 77]. However, this relationship seems to be exponential, according to newer research. Application of twice the recommended density provides a square of the SPF. Similarly halving the application, or applying 0.5 mg/cm^2, reduces the SPF by a square root or a fourth root [78]. A similar non linear observation was seen in the study by Ferrero et al., where a sharp increase in SPF was noted only after the increase in application density beyond 1.5 mg/cm^2 [79].

This problem of application of inadequate quantity of sunscreen may be overcome to some extent with the use of high SPF sunscreens. Only recently have such high SPF sunscreens become mainstream globally, though high SPF sunscreens arrived in markets like Japan, as early as the 90s. The US FDA revised the level of maximum SPF claim in the latest monograph to 60+, in 2019, up from 30+ in 1999, and 50+ in 2011 [80]. Higher SPF sunscreens compensate for the reduced quantity of application to a fair extent. Young et al. found that an SPF 50 sunscreen provides overall protection with reduced epidermal damage, when used at the real-world density of 0.75 mg/cm^2, however, the protection at recommended densities of 1.3 mg and 2 mg/cm^2 were significantly more effective [81].

Furthermore, higher SPF sunscreen also provides a higher level of protection, as has been demonstrated in split face studies comparing products with 50 and 85 SPF, with latter providing a significantly higher protection against sunburn [82]. Ou-Yang et al. compared the performance of an SPF 70 and an SPF 100 sunscreen at various application densities and found that even when applied at the minimum density of 0.5 mg/cm^2, the SPF 100 sunscreen provided 42% higher actual SPF value compared to the SPF 70 sunscreen giving a final SPF of 27 and 19, respectively [83].

Considering the impact of photoirradiation on the skin such as sunburn cells, thymine dimers, p53, and matrix metalloproteinases (MMP) markers, Cole et al. found that a 55 SPF sunscreen with a ultraviolet-A protection factor (UVA-PF) of 22, was found to protect the skin against a radiation dose of 55 minimal erythemal dose (MED), with lesser reactive changes in the skin than what was observed with a dose of 1 MED on unprotected skin. The combination of photostability, and adequate coverage in the ultraviolet-A (UVA) and UVB spectra, accounts for the near complete attenuation of markers of photodamage even with a significantly high dose of UVR [84].

Application density seems to be more significant than actual SPF itself, if not equal, with early reapplication of sunscreen resulting in increased application thickness and therefore coverage and protection [76]. Reapplying sunscreen within 20 min was shown to transmit lesser UV to the skin by 20–35%, compared to either a single application, or a reapplication after 2 h as is the current recommendation by both US FDA and the World Health Organisation (WHO) [85]. Diffey et al. suggest that the best time to reapply sunscreen is within 15–30 min after the first application, to achieve best performance [85]. Teramura et al. found a double application of 1 mg/cm^2 was found to be as efficacious as a single application of 2 mg/cm^2. Furthermore, there was no change in the final SPF obtained whether or not a time gap of 15 min was allowed between the two applications [86].

The two finger sunscreen rule, which was widely popularized on social media, was first suggested by Taylor and Diffey, who suggested that to achieve coverage of the head, neck, and face, a two finger length worth of sunscreen product must be used [87]. However, the head is not an area where sunscreen is usually used for those with hair coverage. A more practical option was suggested by Srinivas et al., who calculated the surface area of the face for males and females using a thread and suggested that 1 ml of sunscreen would be required for the female face and about 1.5 ml for the male face [88]. Taylor also recommended that it may be easier to apply one finger length's worth product on the face and neck and then apply the second finger's worth product within 30 min to maintain sunscreen efficacy [87].

Furthermore, application in two coats also increased the coverage significantly, with reduction of skip areas, as did spending adequate time on the application process [89, 90]. As a corollary to higher SPF sunscreens maintaining adequate protection even at lower application densities, lower SPF sunscreens also achieved higher SPF, at higher application volumes. An 8 SPF sunscreen was able to deliver ten times its SPF value when used at an application density of 2.5 mg/cm^2. At 2 mg/cm^2, the SPF achieved was 39.9, while an SPF 20 sunscreen was able to achieve 133.4 mg/cm^2 at a similar density of application [91].

Application density may also be a factor of reach. Areas that are difficult to reach, like the mid back, may be difficult to completely protect using sunscreens. Foam tip applicators and rollers have been tried to provide better sunscreen coverage over these difficult to reach areas [92]. Usage of sun protective clothing may be a simpler option.

Apart from density, consistency is also equally important. Intermittent use of sunscreen was shown to be less effective compared to daily sunscreen use, even if a product with higher SPF was used [93]. Aided by the recent availability of hybrid diffuse reflectance spectroscopy (HDRS), more research is now available to demonstrate the biostability or substantivity of sunscreens, by their presence on human skin.

Human behaviour can be positively influenced by increasing the level of awareness, and proper labelling statutes do play a role in influencing human behaviour. However, assumptions of consumer behaviour may not always be borne out in practice, as shown with this example. The recent FDA Deemed Rule and the Proposed Amendment, require the listing of active sunscreen ingredients in the principal display panel of the product. The intention is to help users be more aware of the ingredients in the product, and then make informed decisions to choose or reject the product. However, Tribby et al. assessed the practical utility of this step and concluded that active ingredients may not be the main reason for selection of a particular sunscreen by a user [94]. Still, consumers were recorded to spend a longer time viewing the principal front panel of a sunscreen product when the active ingredients were listed there and were more likely to read the usage instructions as well [95]. However, the recent survey in the USA, by Carrao et al., reaffirms our faith in awareness programmes, wherein the application density amongst 9000 participants was impressively high, compared to all of the data in the past. For the face, the average application density was 3 mg/cm^2, with a median of 1.78 mg/cm^2, while for the body, the application thickness was 1.52 mg/cm^2 on average, with a median of 1.35 mg/cm^2 [96].

12.3.2 Sunscreen Durability and the Need for Reapplication

Sunscreen durability may be the answer to several problems plaguing this essential health care intervention. Durable sunscreens reduce the need to reapply sunscreen, reduce the amount of sunscreen ingredients and the breakdown photoproducts thereof, released into the environment, and also reduce the possibility of systemic absorption since reapplications may be minimal to unnecessary.

A higher SPF sunscreen may be realistically better at providing sun protection, due to the inherent differences between the fluences of the light source used for SPF testing and the energy of natural sunlight. A 50 SPF sunscreen as labelled by standard testing may be expected to provide about 20 SPF in real-time conditions in natural sunlight [97]. However, data also exists to show that solar exposed sunscreen retained efficacy equivalent to the label claim [98]. The nature of the current SPF testing method and the inherent inconsistencies of the outcomes may play a role in explaining the variable outputs obtained.

To start with, the recommendation for using sunscreen every 2 h, every day, begs a closer look. The guideline was given out by the US FDA in its Proposed Amendment to the Final Monograph in 2007. In the earlier monographs, the recommendation noted on the label was to apply sunscreen liberally before sun exposure and to reapply after swimming or excessive sweating, in 1978, and in 1999, the recommendation was to reapply as needed, or after towel drying, swimming, or sweating. The revision in the 2007 notification changed the recommendation for sunscreens to be reapplied every 2 h, to avoid lowering the sun protection. This change was based on a single study of 67 beach goers who reported lesser sun burn when applying sunscreen at a frequency of every 1–2 h. No other research exists to support the claim that any less frequent sunscreen use is less effective [99, 100]. Also, the recommendations of the US FDA to reapply sunscreen every 2 h, solely related to UVB in terms of sunscreen SPF, do not take UVA considerations into account.

Today, several workers have recorded the durability of sunscreen in real life circumstances. Ruvolo et al. demonstrated the biostability of a single application of a 50 SPF sunscreen, for 6 h in people who did not perform any significant physical activity capable of producing sweating, with full retention of SPF. In the group where sweating was induced by physical activity, the SPF protection dropped by

40% to reach 30 SPF after 6 h of sweating. Furthermore, on reapplication SPF values increased to 100 and 150, after two and three applications, respectively [100].

After a single sunscreen application, Mette et al. found that both inorganic and organic sunscreens were able to provide 43% of their initial protective effect even after 8 h of a day that included staying in a hot environment, physical activity, and a bath. It is remarkable that after 8 h of using low SPF sunscreen (SPF 8), the drop in protection was only 55% and 58% for the inorganic and organic sunscreens, respectively. At 4 h, the loss of SPF was 38% for the inorganic sunscreen and 41% for the organic sunscreen. In this study, which aimed to closely simulate conditions over a day at a beach vacation, the duration of sun protection raises questions about the necessity for reapplication of sunscreen every 2 h [101].

Ouyang et al. demonstrated that even with application densities at half the recommended amount, sunscreen protection dropped only by 15–40% after 8 h of application which included 30 min of moderate exercise and 80 min of water exposure, both for high SPF and low SPF sunscreens. The higher SPF sunscreen of 70+ maintained SPF at 8 h, dropping only to 64, similar to the 15 SPF sunscreen which dropped to 13 SPF at the end of 8 h. For subjects that applied sunscreen at half the recommended density, the SPF values were at 26 and 7, for the high SPF and the low SPF sunscreen respectively [102].

Evaluating outdoor workers in a high UV index zone, it was found that a 50+ SPF sunscreen lost about 40% of its protection in 4 h [103]. However, in this study, in vivo SPF testing was not employed. Rather, facial fluorescence imaging outputs on skin brightness were digitally analysed, to arrive at the potential amount of sunscreen retained on the skin. The authors found that at 8 h, sunscreen was likely present on the skin at a density of 1.37 mg/cm^2, which suggests very good sunscreen durability, when an adequate amount is applied to start with. This amount of sunscreen is close to what is used for in vivo SPF testing and is higher than what is used for UVA-PF testing by the FDA standards. An in vivo testing using HDRS may have been able to provide better clarity on the SPF values of the retained sunscreen.

Using the same methodology as above with digital analysis of facial fluorescence readings, but in indoor workers, Rungananchai et al. noted the persistence in protection of 50+ SPF, protection grade of UVA (PA) +++ sunscreen was retained by 71.8% at the end of an 8 h workday [104]. At 8 h without physical activity, sun protection metrics dropped by only 25% for both organic and inorganic sunscreens [105].

Similarly, assessments of substantivity for water resistance and sweat resistance show that current sunscreen formulations lose very little protective ability after significant exposure to water and after sweating [106, 107]. Furthermore, it has been both shown that sunscreens accumulate on the skin surface and that there exists a depot effect which may increase systemic absorption when sunscreen is frequently reapplied [108, 109]. In face of the durability of sunscreens, the issue of systemic exposure can be reduced, since reapplication now, can be less frequent without losing effective protection.

With several studies available to show the durability of sunscreens on the skin based on in vivo testing, the statute to reapply sunscreen every 2 h needs revisiting.

Li et al. conclude that there is strong evidence to suggest that reapplication is not routinely necessary within an 8 h period. Reapplication may be needed within this period if the individual performs activities that may be related to sunscreen rub off or wash off, such as swimming, sweating or friction, Table 12.1 [110].

12.3.3 When to Reapply Sunscreen?

Based on the above discussion on sunscreen durability, it appears that a single, adequate application of a high SPF sunscreen will likely provide meaningful sun protection for 8 h. However, this needs to be validated for ultraviolet protection factor (UV-PF) as well. Furthermore, interindividual variations exist, for example, in terms of sweating or level of physical activity, as also the differences in product

Table 12.1 Studies demonstrating sunscreen durability

Author	Method	Base SPF	Test conditions	Outcome
Ruvolo et al. [100]	HDRS	50	Non-active group, sitting in an air-conditioning (AC) room at 22 °C	50 SPF at 6 h
		50	Wii® exercises for 20 min every hour in a 37.8 °C heated room	Retained 50 SPF at 2 h, 30 SPF at the end of 6 h
Bodekaer M et al. [101]	In vivo SPF testing	8	Simulation of a day at the beach, including a hot environment, physical activity, and a bath and toweling	Retention of 43% of SPF at the end of 8 h
Ou-Yang et al. [102]	In vivo SPF testing	70, 15	Application of two sunscreens at two different densities each, 2 and 1 mg/cm², for 8 h, including water exposure and exercise	70 SPF sunscreen, applied at 2 mg/cm² was found to give an SPF of 64 after 8 h
Kobwanthanakun et al. [103]	Facial Fluorescence Camera with Digital Image Analysis	50+	Coverage and sustainability of sunscreen applied on the face, over an 8 hour workday, among outdoor workers	31.63% reduction in mean sunscreen coverage at the end of 8 h
Korting et al. [106]	In vivo SPF testing	50+, 30, 25, 15	Substantivity after plain water and salt water exposure for 80 min, and sweating for ≥60 min	Marginal reduction of SPF, with >95% of SPF retention for the 50+ SPF sunscreen
Beyer et al. [105]	In vivo SPF testing	8	8 h, no physical activity	75% of baseline SPF retained

performance based on factors ranging from the filters used to the formulation stability and finally, differences in conditions of exposure. These decide the substantivity of a sunscreen, which is its resistance to removal by water or sweat, and the durability, which is the resistance to removal by wear [107].

The need for durable sunscreens arises because only 20–60% of sunscreen users reapply sunscreen despite data that suggests that sunscreen reapplication can significantly increase both the level and the durability of sun protection [100]. Reapplication seems to be more common when people are expected to stay outdoors in the sun, with added circumstances of sweating [111]. High SPF sunscreens which retain efficacy for up to 6–8 h may obviate the need for reapplication, while reducing overall sunscreen burden for the individual and the environment. Water resistance sunscreen formulations, specifically, are associated with good durability and substantivity. Ideally, the best case is to provide more information to the consumers based on the exact performance metrics used to judge the specific sunscreen product, which may be a difficult or even impractical exercise [107].

Alternatively, the need to reapply sunscreens can also be assessed at the consumer point of use. UVR stickers are useful to some extent in identifying the best time to reapply sunscreen. UVR detection stickers change colour on UV stimulation of photochromic molecules in dyes in the sticker. This reminds the user to reapply sunscreen. Dosimeters are more useful in research settings but may be impractical for daily use [112]. Use of UV cameras to identify sunscreen presence on the skin is widely publicized on social media and can be a very useful tool to guide coverage of sunscreen application. Using a UV camera, Pratt et al. identified that the eyelid and periorbital regions are missed during routine sunscreen application. While this method enables patient education directed towards more uniform coverage of sunscreen application, its reliability as a measure of sunscreen persistence on the skin is not clear [113]. UV imaging was not found to correlate meaningfully with sun protection, based on studies that employed HDRS [100].

Multispectral imaging can be a useful tool to help users achieve sunscreen coverage on sun-exposed areas and may work as interactive tools to increase awareness. Heatmaps generated by multispectral imaging were used to help users increase uniformity and coverage of sunscreen application. Participants were asked to apply sunscreen first, and then evaluate the coverage using the heatmap, and then reapply the product to achieve uniform cover. This resulted in an increase in sunscreen application density from 1.04 to 1.45 mg/cm^2, a 40% increase, which may then confer closer to optimal sun protection benefits, than an unguided application [114].

12.3.4 Should Sunscreen Be Used Everyday, Always?

Also, the case of daily sunscreen use has been recently contested by Diffey et al., at least for people living in latitudes at or above 45°North [97]. Assuming an acceptable daily dose of 0.5 standard erythemal dose (SED), Diffey et al. argue that the minimal UVR that reaches the skin during the colder winter months at latitudes above 45°North does not require sunscreen use. The recognition and avoidance of unnecessary sunscreen use was modelled to result in a 25% decrease in consumption, with advantages for users in terms of reduced systemic absorption and a lesser environmental burden for the planet. On the other hand, at latitudes closer to the equator, 30°North and lesser, sunscreens need to be applied daily, in cognizance of increased UVR in these geographic zones. The author exhorts that sunscreen use must be rational, balancing human health and environmental needs. Sunscreens are still recommended for use during summer, which accounts for 40% of the total sunscreen consumption according to Diffey's model. By reducing unnecessary sunscreen use, and by encouraging sun safety measures like seeking shade, and by using other photoprotective agents like clothing, it is possible to reduce sunscreen consumption by half.

12.3.5 Can Sunscreens Be Reapplied During Exercise? And After Sweating?

When using sunscreens labelled as sweat resistant, consumers have an apprehension if the sunscreen will be occlusive to prevent sweating and therefore cause increased perception of skin warmth. The concern is also related to whether there is an interference of thermoregulation with the use of sunscreens. Ou-Yang et al. studied the rates of exercise induced sweating with and without sunscreen application on a split face, split forearm model, and found no difference between the two sides, with regard to sweat rate or skin temperature. This implies that users can safely continue to use and/or reapply sunscreen when pursuing recreational activities that may be associated with some level of sweating [115].

12.3.6 When Is the Best Time to Start Using Sunscreens?

UVR has been established as a significant causative factor for photodamage of the skin, resulting in end points such as photocarcinogenesis, photo ageing, and pigmentation. Sunscreens have been demonstrated to have a significant impact on preventing or at least reducing, solar related ageing, and pigmentation. The impact of sunscreens in preventing skin cancer is considered beneficial, though the pathogenesis of cancer, the longer duration of observation required, and the human factor related to actual sunscreen usage, make it complex to establish an absolute quantum of benefit. Still, starting sunscreens early in life seems to be the best way at managing UV damage on skin. Diffey showed that the regular use of daily use, topical sun protection agents can reduce lifetime UV exposure [116]. The study found that an early start to using sun protection products was more impactful compared to the SPF and spectral profile of protection afforded by the sun care product or the seasonality of use. Harrison et al. noted that the use of ultraviolet protection factor (UPF) 30–50+ clothing in young children reduces melanoma risk, and this approach may be more sustainable and safe, as a sun protection practice [117].

In skin of colour, sunscreening agents are used largely from a pigmentation prevention perspective. The most commonly known pigmentary condition in SOC, other than postinflammatory hyperpigmentation (PIH) is melasma, which in an Indian study was found to arise in the 3rd decade and be exacerbated by hormonal triggers like the use of oral contraceptive pills (OCP) and pregnancy [118]. Advising sunscreen usage in early adult life, as suggested by Diffey et al., seems acceptable as a pigmentation mitigation measure.

Tanning occurs from very early life, as a normal physiological phenomenon, starting from the first summer of life, in areas where seasonal climates are experienced. Infants who were exposed to the summer sun, showed facultative skin pigmentation at levels comparable to that of adults, indicating that for vulnerable populations, protection against sun must be begun potentially early [119].

12.3.7 Do Sunscreens Take Time to Start Working?

It has been considered that physical sunscreens start working right away whereas chemical sunscreens require about 20–30 min to achieve maximum photoprotection performance. De Galvez et al. used UV photography techniques to map the time at which a sunscreen becomes fully functional on the skin, using the ISO 24443 sunscreen standard and found that this could be as early as 5 min [120]. Also post-sunscreen application, it is recommended to wait for 8–10 min, for the product to settle in, to reduce rub off when wearing clothes [76].

12.3.8 Is It Okay to Use a Moisturizer with Sunscreen?

While some sunscreen filters, typically inorganic minerals are known to cause some level of skin dryness, chemical filters usually are more moisturizing. Therefore, mineral sunscreens are more favoured by those with oily skin. However, it has become an informal standard of care to use multiple products in a morning routine, and to layer products one over another. Accordingly, and as per common belief, sunscreens are said to be required to layer over moisturizers, but specific scientific evidence is lacking. In 2013, Klushke et al., commented that using a cream or a lotion before sunscreen application, potentially reduced the water resistance of the sunscreen, probably by reducing the adhesion of the sunscreen to the skin [121]. For best performance, sunscreens must soak into the skin and stick well providing a layer of cover on the skin's surface, and therefore agents that prevent the sunscreen integration into the top layers of the stratum corneum, impair sunscreen efficacy [122]. Recently, de Galvez et al. used ultraviolet reflectance photography to conclude that using a moisturizing cream, either before or after using a sunscreen, did not affect sunscreen performance [123]. However, since most consumers are not aware and potentially can never become completely aware of the possible interactions of the moisturizers or other products they choose to use as layers before applying sunscreen, it may be more safe to assume that these agents may interfere with sunscreen efficacy. It may be good to avoid a moisturizer ahead of using sunscreen, at least where water exposure or sweating is anticipated.

On this note, use of a popular class of cosmetics, called moisturizers with SPF, have been known to be inferior to using standard sunscreens in terms of sun protection and skipped areas [124].

12.4 Sunscreens and the FFA Question

The question of whether UV filters contribute to or aggravate the development of frontal fibrosing alopecia (FFA) is a recent one. This discussion highlights the potential for a beneficial skin care agent to cause inadvertent side effects and is similar to the issues around systemic absorption in a few ways. Like the potential for systemic absorption, which is directly related to a depot effect of sunscreens with continued ingress into the skin on repeated application, persistence of UV filters, typically titanium dioxide, in the hair follicle microenvironment, is implicated in FFA [125]. Also, as a relatively new problem, the extent of impact is yet to be fully established, again drawing a parallel with systemic toxicity of sunscreens, such as the potential for endocrine disruption. FFA, much like systemic impact of sunscreens, is a multifactorial problem, which makes it difficult to apply a definite weightage to the contribution of UV screening chemicals.

As a topic that's relatively new to both clinician and consumer, this link between sunscreen use and FFA merits a detailed view. The section below details the evolution of the perceived link between FFA and sunscreen ingredients, and attempts to provide the user a snapshot of published research so far, with an aim to enable clinical decision making.

The earliest suggestion for a potential connection between sunscreens and FFA was raised by Aldoori et al. in 2016, analysing the personal care product use of women with FFA compared to age matched controls. The authors found an association between facial skin care products and FFA. Attention was drawn to the higher frequency of sunscreen usage in known cases of FFA, compared to the control group. Furthermore, the exposure to sunscreen chemicals in products not marketed as sunscreens, e.g., makeup and foundations, was highlighted to emphasize the potentially high exposure to this group of ingredients [126]. However, the methods used in this study to arrive at statistical significance were contested by Seegobin et al., who noted that the observations were not adjusted for age, which is an influencing factor in FFA [126], and by Dhana and team [126] who raised concerns about a selection bias for both cases and controls, though the methods called into question were subsequently defended by Aldoori et al. [127].

The controversial but highly clinically relevant linkage was further supported by the outcomes of a study by Kidambi et al., who explored the role of facial leave on products such as sunscreens and moisturizers, in men [128]. While the group found a temporal association between the use of leave on facial care products and FFA, they were unable to explain the loss of hair on noncontact sites such as the forearms, and the occipital scalp, and the link to mucosal lesions was unclear. Furthermore, not all subjects with FFA were found to have used sunscreens, disputing a potential causal role, though subjects with FFA who used sunscreens were found to have used these products at a higher frequency. The authors also contended that affluence, a factor known to have been linked to FFA, may have created some level of bias, since sunscreen use is also higher in more affluent groups. However, the reverse impact of sunscreen use as a construct of affluence, which then influences the occurrence of FFA, cannot be ignored. The use of moisturizers containing sunscreen agents in this study was highlighted by Strazzulla et al., as not many consumers are aware of sunscreen agents in such personal care products which may lead to under reporting [129].

It is possible that the increased exposure to UV filters, as has been implicated in these studies, may not be related just to the use of products marketed for skin care alone. Many hair care products, both rinse off and leave in, contain small amounts of UV filters to protect the product against photooxidation. This is particularly seen in products marketed as 'colour protect'. This forms a potential source of continuous exposure to UV filters, which may bypass the consumer's knowledge or attention, unless awareness promotes a careful perusal of the product label [130].

A temporal and localized association of using a sunscreen spray on the central part of the scalp, in a woman with lichen planus pigmentosus (LPP), and a strikingly similar instance of FFA occurring in areas of sunscreen use on the scalp, lends credence to the link between the underlying fibro genetic autoimmune pathology in FFA and sunscreen products [131, 132]. Moreno-Arrones et al., provided further support for the sunscreen link in FFA, through a large, multicenter case control study, evaluating 664 women and 106 men [132]. The study found a significant association between FFA and the use of facial sunscreen, with an odds ratio of 1.6, for women. The association was highly significant for men who used facial sunscreens with an odds ratio of 11.6. Other significant associations include exposure to hormones, either through pregnancy or medications, comorbid conditions like hypothyroidism, LPP, and rosacea. In contradiction, Panchaprateep et al. reported that sunscreens and cosmetics were not identified as potential causes in retrospective analysis of cases in a 10-year period. Here, the 'front puff' Thai hairstyle, associated with a significant element of traction was considered as a risk factor for FFA [133]. The Mayo Clinic also produced two studies, in one of which FFA was considered in subtype analysis in a cohort of patients with LPP and found no specific link between the use of sunscreens and disease course [134]. One of the studies, which was based on a survey, noted a higher than average use of sunscreens among those with FFA, but concluded that such daily, regular use of sunscreens and multiple other personal care products containing UV filters were unlikely to be associated with FFA [135]. The lack of an impact for sunscreens was further bolstered by data from Brazil which evaluated 451 matched pairs of cases and controls and found no relevant link between sunscreen use and FFA. However, meaningful associations were identified between hair straightening agents containing formalin, use of soaps purchased over-the-counter and facial moisturizer, and FFA. The mention of the facial moisturizer needs a little attention [136]. Recalling the above view of Stratzzulla et al., many skin care products contain smaller amounts of UV filters as product photoprotection agents. Even though the quantity of such additives may be much lesser than what is used in a sunscreen product, the long-term exposure of such leave on products may be significant over time [129]. Interestingly, the Brazilian study found the use of anti-residue/clarifying shampoos as negatively correlated with FFA, suggesting that some moiety left in contact with the skin, scalp, and/or hair follicles may drive some part of the pathogenesis of FFA [136]. Benzyl salicylate which is used in fragrance mixes for products including sunscreens has also been implicated in FFA. It is important to note that benzyl salicylate is also a component of products marketed as 'herbal' [137].

Leecharoen et al., explored the use of personal care products among Asian women and found that the use of sunscreens and moisturizers was higher in women with either patterned hair loss or FFA compared to controls. The use of moisturizer was higher in the FFA group compared to those with pattern hair loss (PHL) and the use of sunscreens was higher in the group with PHL as compared to those with FFA [138]. This study is interesting, as thus far, we have considered the potential for sunscreen agents in moisturizers to be related to the occurrence of FFA, even if unbeknownst to the consumer. However, the use of sunscreen products themselves, as in the group with PHL, was not associated with a higher incidence of FFA. As seen in the section on sunscreen ingredients, the nature and type of UV filters vary widely across chemical class. An elucidation of the exact ingredient may be needed to correctly arrive at a true association if one does exist. Factors as diverse as unspecified facial surgery have been associated with frontal alopecia. Sunscreen use prior to disease onset was identified as significant for frontal alopecia in this study [139].

With the pendulum swinging both ways, in terms of available data linking UV filters and FFA, a series of meta-analyses were published on the topic. In 2022, Maghfour et al., analysing nine reports of 1248 cases of FFA and 1259 controls, concluded that sunscreen use was associated with a 2.2 times higher likelihood to develop FFA, while the comparable risk for moisturizers was 2.09. The authors propose a few pathways by which sunscreens potentially play a role in the pathogenesis of FFA: immune mediated lichenoid reaction, hormone disruption, and interference with UV induced immunomodulation, oxidative damage, and an allergic contact pathway. Agents like benzophenone which are used in sunscreens but are present much more ubiquitously as product protectors in personal care products are likely to be involved. Hydantoin and quaternium-15 found in moisturizers and personal care products (PCPs) are also suspect [140]. The rising incidence of FFA in the last few years, closely mirroring the increase of UV filters, either as standalone sunscreen agents or in other facial care products like moisturizers, foundations, BB and CC creams, day creams, and other items of makeup, has been highlighted by Kepinska et al. [141]. Increased product retention due to age induced reduction in levels of sebum secretion may explain the predisposition of FFA to occur in perimenopausal and postmenopausal women [141]. Interestingly, as noted above, the use of a clarifying shampoo was associated with a lesser risk of FFA, as reported by Ramos et al. [136]. While a lesser frequency of hair washing is noted in individuals with FFA, this may be related to concerns of hair loss in such patients. This also points to the possibility of removal of extrinsic triggers with frequent hair washing as a protective factor, especially while using anti-residue shampoos.

Most of the reported data lack detailed information about the nature of the UV filters. However, considering the inclusion of personal care products where sunscreen filters are added for product stability, chemical filters are likely implicated. Oxybenzone is known both as the UV filter most associated with allergic and photoallergic contact dermatitis, and also as one of the most commonly added filters in personal care products. Octinoxate is equally known to be a widely used UV protecting product additive in PCPs. Independently, diethylamino hydroxybenzoyl hexyl benzoate (DHHB) and drometrizole trisiloxane have been reported to be associated with FFA. The presence of titanium particles in hair follicles, as evidence for triggering FFA, has been controversial [142]. Based on the observation of titanium nanoparticles in the hair follicles of those with FFA, eight times more commonly than in controls, a rationale for the avoidance of skin care, hair care, and make up-based containing these nanoparticles, exists [143]. Regardless of the exact extrinsic agent, increased exposure of individuals to multiple ingredients in personal care products may be a reason to explain the increase in the number of cases, female predominance, and more recently, a younger age to onset of clinical symptoms in FFA [144].

Most recently, Kam et al., in a metaanalysis spanning Cochrane, Pubmed, Embase, and Medline databases concluded that facial sunscreens, leave on facial products and facial moisturizers are associated with FFA, implicating UV protecting chemicals as likely environmental agents in the etiopathogenesis of the condition [145].

However, are sunscreens the cause or a bystander phenomenon? Higher levels of actinic damage are noted in involved sites in persons with FFA, indicating significant sun exposure. In that case, use of sunscreens may only reflect the sun exposure levels of the individuals rather than a causative role. Researchers found actinic damage to be more common in patients with FFA, than in those who did not, with sunscreen use being higher in those with actinic damage. Furthermore, among confirmed cases of FFA, trichoscopic and histopathological features were similar in those who used sunscreens and those who did not. The authors conclude that the more common use of sunscreens in those with FFA may be related to the actinic damage and not be a causative factor as presumed thus far [146].

Even as the ambiguity continues, it may be worth considering a cessation of contact with UV filters, as was shown by hair regrowth in FFA, on discontinuing sunscreen [147–149].

To conclude, at this juncture, a fair level of data still points to a significant role of UV filters in the development of FFA. While more information is required as to the exact culprits, it may be prudent to avoid sunscreens containing potentially implicated filters, as mentioned in this discussion above, for individuals diagnosed with FFA. Further elucidation of discrete ingredients may enable future formulations to avoid such moieties, should the evidence linking sunscreens and FFA strengthen further with more data.

12.5 Sunscreens for Special Groups

12.5.1 Pregnancy and Nursing Women

Chemical filters like benzophenones and some cinnamates have been shown to possess endocrine disrupting abilities, with potential impact on foetal exposure. Specifically, foetal exposure to benzophenone-3 (BP-3) was associated with an impact on testicular Leydig function in adult life in humans [150]. The newer generation chemical sunscreens with larger particle sizes are not expected to be systemically absorbed and may be eventually shown to be safe in pregnancy, but at the moment, there is scant data to declare these filters as safe in pregnancy or nursing.

In pregnancy and nursing, the US FDA approves only mineral sunscreens, zinc oxide and titanium dioxide [80]. Of these titanium dioxide nanoparticles have been implicated as having some level of impact on foetal development, in animal studies. Specifically, pregnancy may alter the reactivity of non-reactive or otherwise inert nanoparticles, leading to adverse biological outcomes [151]. Prenatal titanium nanoparticle exposure has been studied to impair development. However, with relevance to sunscreens, titanium dioxide from sunscreens is not expected to be absorbed systemically, and the route is more likely to be inhalational when sunscreen sprays containing TiO2 are used [152].

Zinc nanoparticles possess the broadest range of UV protection among sun filters currently available, and therefore are useful in pregnancy, where hormonal changes can precipitate the occurrence of pigmentary conditions such as melasma. Thus far, adverse effects due to the use of zinc sunscreens in terms of endocrine disruption potential have not been reported [151]. Though serious adverse effects may not be anticipated since topical and oral zinc has been safely used in multiple medical applications, it is necessary to rigorously assess the specific impact from nanomineral exposure.

Minor ingredients such as fragrances in formulations meant for this special group may contain endocrine disrupting substances and must be scrutinized in the same way as for active chemical filters.

12.5.2 Sunscreens in Children

Sunscreens are recommended after the age of 6 months. Prior to that, physical sun protection measures are recommended, including protective clothing, seeking shade, and the use of hats. For children, sunscreens without significant systemic absorption are considered better. The filters best suited to this purpose seem to be the mineral sunscreens, with zinc and titanium oxides, which have not been shown to have significant cutaneous penetration from topically applied formulations.

The systemic absorption of sunscreens has recently caught the attention of the world, after the work of Matta et al. [153]. However, the biological impact of such absorption, typically endocrine disruption in susceptible populations, while not expected to be huge, is not expected to be insignificant as well. Earlier, Janjua et al. noted that filters like oxybenzone, octinoxate, and enzacamene demonstrated transdermal penetration, systemic absorption, and were excreted in the urine. This study was done on young men and postmenopausal women, and the authors concluded that the systemic presence of the chemical filters may not be biologically significant based on the short-term study. However, they also raised a cautionary note about the potentially higher impact of such absorption and of the external endocrine disruption on prepubertal children, whose endogenous hormone production would be at a lower level. The larger body surface area to body weight ratio in younger children, and immature clearance systems not adequately developed to process and eliminate these filters, in ways similar to adults, necessitates the need for safer filters, with lesser chances of systemic absorption [154, 155].

In a recent Thai study, 85% of sunscreens marketed as suitable for children were found to contain at least one chemical filter, even though the presence of easily absorbed chemical filters with known endocrine disruption, such as benzophenone-3 (BP 3) and octinoxate, were less commonly found in sunscreens marketed for children [156]. Druml et al. noted that sunscreens marketed as for baby or babies mostly aligned with approved sunscreen recommendations, where oxybenzone was not present as an ingredient in most products. However, for sunscreens marketed as for children or kids or sports or active, endocrine disrupting chemical filters were identified in the ingredient list [157].

It may be safe to extend the same safety concerns as for pregnancy, nursing, and infancy to the period of childhood and adolescence considering their vulnerability from an endocrinological viewpoint, and similarly, adopt the same guidelines for safe sunscreen filters. Where a risk of skin cancer exists, or in the treatment of certain photoaggravated skin diseases, or when excessive exposure with potential chances of sunburn is anticipated, sunscreen use is mandatory. The benefit of routine and general use of sunscreens in children of SOC is unclear.

12.5.3 Sunscreens for Sensitive Skin

Asian skin is considered to be sensitive to chemical insults due to the unique proportion of skin surface lipids, natural moisturizing factors, compared to Caucasian/African-American skin types. Darker skin types are considered to have the least amount of ceramides. Asian skin, while having an equal amount of ceramides compared to Caucasian skin, and similar rates of transepidermal water loss (TEWL) was found to have the weakest barrier function, being more prone to spontaneous desquamation. This was attributable to differences in intercellular cohesion and levels of natural moisturizing factors in the stratum corneum. Along with a thinner stratum corneum, an increased density of eccrine glands which facilitate deeper penetration of applied topical agents may explain the predisposition of Asian skin types to skin sensitivity due to exogenous chemical insults [158].

Phadungsaksawasdi found the presence of sunscreen filters with known skin sensitization potential such as BP-3 in products marketed for sensitive skin. Bisoctrizole was found to be more common in sunscreens meant for sensitive skin [156].

12.5.4 Sunscreens for Those with Connective Tissue Disorders

Photosensitivity is a known feature of connective tissue disorders, and in recommending sunscreens for individuals with these autoimmune skin diseases, Keyes et al. suggested the use of inorganic sunscreens due to the least potential for allergenicity. At the minimum, UV filters with known propensity to cause photoallergic reactions like oxybenzone, octocrylene, octinoxate, and avobenzone, should be avoided in this set of people [48].

In conclusion, while sunscreens are an essential part of skin care, and an integral part of dermatologists' prescriptions, the way in which they are employed, need to be tailored to unique individual needs. Newer filters, improved formulations, robust guidelines, and ongoing feedback on the impact of sunscreens on the human body and the environment all promise to make the exploration of sunscreen science fascinating in the years to come.

12.6 Preface

This book is written for postgraduate students of dermatology and for undergraduate students with an interest in dermatology. It is also meant for practising dermatologists who are looking to upgrade practical knowledge on this key personal care product. The awareness of sunscreen use, at least in India, has been taken forward as much by dermatologists as has been by skin care influencers and beauty gurus.

To that understanding, this book has been specifically worked on for enhanced readability, even for those without an advanced medical background.

The flow of the content has been planned as a narrative, starting from an understanding of melanin, and its protective behaviour in skin of colour. We then move on to understanding the impact of light, across all of the solar domains, with particular emphasis on skin of colour, and stop to briefly explore the role of sunscreens in preventing skin cancer. The story continues on to the types and kinds of sunscreens, old and new, and concludes with understanding the clinical considerations around sunscreens, chapters of interest for practising clinicians, presented in crisp vignettes. Keeping in mind that this book will be used by postgraduates, brief reviews of the various filters, recent advances, and capsule summaries for quick reading and even quicker revisions are included.

References

1. Reichrath J, Lehmann B, Carlberg C, Varani J, Zouboulis CC. Vitamins as hormones. Horm Metab Res [Internet]. 2007 Feb [cited 2024 Mar 3];39(2):71–84. Available from: https://pubmed.ncbi.nlm.nih.gov/17326003/
2. Pryor Y, Lindo J. Deconstructing Eurocentrism in skin pigmentation research via the incorporation of diverse populations and theoretical perspectives. Evol Anthropol [Internet]. 2023 Aug 1 [cited 2024 Mar 28];32(4):195–205. Available from: https://pubmed.ncbi.nlm.nih.gov/37450551/
3. Sagarad S V., Sukhani N, Machanur B, Patil S. Effect of vitamin D on anginal episodes in vitamin D deficient patients with chronic stable angina on medical management. J Clin Diagn Res [Internet]. 2016 Aug 1 [cited 2024 Mar 28];10(8):OC24. Available from: https://www.ncbi.nlm.nih.gov/pmc/articles/PMC5028482/
4. Charoenngam N, Shirvani A, Reddy N, Vodopivec DM, Apovian CM, Holick MF. Association of vitamin D status with hospital morbidity and mortality in adult hospitalized patients with COVID-19. Endocr Pract [Internet]. 2021 Apr 1 [cited 2024 Mar 28];27(4):271–8. Available from: https://pubmed.ncbi.nlm.nih.gov/33705975/
5. Lucock MD, Jones PR, Veysey M, Thota R, Garg M, Furst J, et al. Biophysical evidence to support and extend the vitamin D-folate hypothesis as a paradigm for the evolution of human skin pigmentation. Am J Hum Biol [Internet]. 2022 Apr 1 [cited 2024 Mar 28];34(4). Available from: https://pubmed.ncbi.nlm.nih.gov/34418235/
6. Hanel A, Carlberg C. Skin colour and vitamin D: an update. Exp Dermatol [Internet]. 2020 Sep 1 [cited 2024 Mar 2];29(9):864–75. Available from: https://pubmed.ncbi.nlm.nih.gov/32621306/
7. Schagen SK, Zampeli VA, Makrantonaki E, Zouboulis CC. Discovering the link between nutrition and skin aging. Dermatoendocrinol [Internet]. 2012 Jul 7 [cited 2024 Mar 26];4(3):298. Available from: https://www.ncbi.nlm.nih.gov/pmc/articles/PMC3583891/
8. Reichrath J, Perez A, Müller SM, Chen TC, Kerber A, Bahmer FA, et al. Topical calcitriol (1,25-dihydroxyvitamin D3) treatment of psoriasis: an immunohistological evaluation. Acta Derm Venereol [Internet]. 1997 [cited 2024 Mar 28];77(4):268–72. Available from: https://pubmed.ncbi.nlm.nih.gov/9228216/
9. Furukawa JY, Martinez RM, Morocho-Jácome AL, Castillo-Gómez TS, Pereda-Contreras VJ, Rosado C, et al. Skin impacts from exposure to ultraviolet, visible, infrared, and artificial lights–a review. J Cosmet Laser Ther. 2021;23(1–2):1–7.

10. Retamoso VR, Feijóo LB, Vasquez Rubio DA, dos Santos LAFV, Vargas Barcelos AL, Piccoli J da CE. Black skin color but not VDR gene represent a risk factor for low serum levels of vitamin D in self-declared black individuals. Clin Nutr ESPEN [Internet]. 2023 Jun 1 [cited 2024 Mar 28];55:230–7. Available from: https://pubmed.ncbi.nlm.nih.gov/37202051/
11. Hassanein MM, Huri HZ, Baig K, Abduelkarem AR. Determinants and effects of vitamin D supplementation in postmenopausal women: a systematic review. Nutrients [Internet]. 2023 Feb 1 [cited 2024 Mar 28];15(3). Available from: https://pubmed.ncbi.nlm.nih.gov/36771392/
12. Dadda S, El Houate B, El Bouhali B. Multifactorial hypovitaminosis D among women in the South-East Oases of Morocco. Arch Osteoporos [Internet]. 2022 Dec 1 [cited 2024 Mar 28];18(1). Available from: https://pubmed.ncbi.nlm.nih.gov/36574180/
13. Borba VZC, Lazaretti-Castro M, Moreira S da S, De Almeida MCC, Moreira ED. Epidemiology of vitamin D (EpiVida)-a study of vitamin D status among healthy adults in Brazil. J Endocr Soc [Internet]. 2022 Jan 1 [cited 2024 Mar 28];7(1). Available from: https://pubmed.ncbi.nlm.nih.gov/36518902/
14. Islam MZ, Bhuiyan NH, Akhtaruzzaman M, Allardt CL, Fogelholm M. Vitamin D deficiency in Bangladesh: a review of prevalence, causes and recommendations for mitigation. Asia Pac J Clin Nutr [Internet]. 2022 Jun 1 [cited 2024 Mar 28];31(2):167–80. Available from: https://pubmed.ncbi.nlm.nih.gov/35766552/
15. Charoenngam N, Shirvani A, Holick MF. Vitamin D for skeletal and non-skeletal health: what we should know. J Clin Orthop Trauma [Internet]. 2019 Nov 1 [cited 2024 Mar 28];10(6):1082–93. Available from: https://pubmed.ncbi.nlm.nih.gov/31708633/
16. Libon F, Cavalier E, Nikkels AF. Skin color is relevant to vitamin D synthesis. Dermatology [Internet]. 2013 Nov [cited 2024 Mar 28];227(3):250–4. Available from: https://pubmed.ncbi.nlm.nih.gov/24134867/
17. Xiang F, Lucas R, De Gruijl F, Norval M. A systematic review of the influence of skin pigmentation on changes in the concentrations of vitamin D and 25-hydroxyvitamin D in plasma/serum following experimental UV irradiation. Photochem Photobiol Sci [Internet]. 2015 [cited 2024 Mar 28];14(12):2138–46. Available from: https://pubmed.ncbi.nlm.nih.gov/26548800/
18. MacLaughlin J, Holick MF. Aging decreases the capacity of human skin to produce vitamin D3. J Clin Invest [Internet]. 1985 [cited 2024 Mar 28];76(4):1536–8. Available from: https://pubmed.ncbi.nlm.nih.gov/2997282/
19. Divyalakshmi C, Golda J, Sukumaran P, Selvadurairaj S, Lourdhurajan R, Divyalakshmi C, et al. Vitamin D levels in non-users of sunscreen versus once-daily sunscreen users: a retrospective analysis from a cosmetic dermatology center in South India. Cosmoderma [Internet]. 2022 Feb 4 [cited 2024 Mar 28];2:10. Available from: https://cosmoderma.org/vitamin-d-levels-in-non-users-of-sunscreen-versus-once-daily-sunscreen-users-a-retrospective-analysis-from-a-cosmetic-dermatology-center-in-south-india/
20. Raymond-Lezman JR, Riskin SI. Benefits and risks of sun exposure to maintain adequate vitamin D levels. Cureus [Internet]. 2023 May 5 [cited 2024 Mar 28];15(5). Available from: https://www.ncbi.nlm.nih.gov/pmc/articles/PMC10239563/
21. Brunsgaard EK, Jensen J, Grossman D. Melanoma in skin of color: part II. Racial disparities, role of UV, and interventions for earlier detection. J Am Acad Dermatol [Internet]. 2023 Sep 1 [cited 2024 Mar 11];89(3):459–68. Available from: https://pubmed.ncbi.nlm.nih.gov/35533770/
22. Charoenngam N, Sriussadaporn S. Darker skin color measured by Von Luschan chromatic scale and increased sunlight exposure time are independently associated with decreased odds of vitamin D deficiency in Thai ambulatory patients. J Nutr Metab [Internet]. 2021 [cited 2024 Mar 29];2021. Available from: https://pubmed.ncbi.nlm.nih.gov/33728062/
23. Wille K, Richard A, Nieters A, Rohrmann S, Quack Lötscher K. Vitamin D and parathyroid hormone in the umbilical cord blood—correlation with light and dark maternal skin color. Food Sci Nutr [Internet]. 2022 Dec 1 [cited 2024 Mar 29];10(12):4201–8. Available from: https://pubmed.ncbi.nlm.nih.gov/36514767/

24. Öhlund I, Lind T, Hernell O, Silfverdal SA, Äkeson PK. Increased vitamin D intake differentiated according to skin color is needed to meet requirements in young Swedish children during winter: a double-blind randomized clinical trial. Am J Clin Nutr. 2017;106(1):105–12.
25. Jolliffe DA, Hanifa Y, Witt KD, Venton TR, Rowe M, Timms PM, et al. Environmental and genetic determinants of vitamin D status among older adults in London, UK. J Steroid Biochem Mol Biol [Internet]. 2016 Nov 1 [cited 2024 Mar 29];164:30–5. Available from: https://pubmed.ncbi.nlm.nih.gov/26776442/
26. Tugrul B, Demirdag HG, Hanli Sahin A. Vitamin D levels in children during winter and the relationship between sunscreen and sun protection behaviors. Dermatol Pract Concept [Internet]. 2023 Jul 31 [cited 2024 Mar 29];13(3):e2023190. Available from: https://pubmed.ncbi.nlm.nih.gov/37557131/
27. Tran V, Janda M, Lucas RM, McLeod DSA, Thompson BS, Waterhouse M, et al. Vitamin D and sun exposure: a community survey in Australia. Curr Oncol [Internet]. 2023 Feb 1 [cited 2024 Mar 29];30(2):2465–81. Available from: https://pubmed.ncbi.nlm.nih.gov/36826149/
28. (PDF) Cutaneous photoprotection: a review of the current status and evolving strategies [Internet]. [cited 2024 Mar 3]. Available from: https://www.researchgate.net/publication/340352263_Cutaneous_Photoprotection_A_Review_of_the_Current_Status_and_Evolving_Strategies
29. The effect of regular sunscreen use on vitamin D levels in an Australian population. Results of a randomized controlled trial—PubMed [Internet]. [cited 2024 Mar 29]. Available from: https://pubmed.ncbi.nlm.nih.gov/7726582/
30. Singh S, Jha B, Tiwary NK, Agrawal NK. Does using a high sun protection factor sunscreen on face, along with physical photoprotection advice, in patients with melasma, change serum vitamin D concentration in Indian conditions? A pragmatic pretest-posttest study. Indian J Dermatol Venereol Leprol [Internet]. 2019 May 1 [cited 2024 Mar 29];85(3):282–6. Available from: https://pubmed.ncbi.nlm.nih.gov/30409925/
31. Afarideh M, Sartori-Valinotti JC, Tollefson MM. Association of sun-protective behaviors with bone mineral density and osteoporotic bone fractures in us adults. JAMA Dermatol [Internet]. 2021 Dec 1 [cited 2024 Mar 29];157(12):1437–46. Available from: https://pubmed.ncbi.nlm.nih.gov/34705034/
32. Tsugawa N, Kuwabara A, Ogasawara H, Nishino M, Nakagawa K, Kamao M, et al. Vitamin D status in Japanese young women in 2016–2017 and 2020: seasonal variation and the effect of lifestyle including changes caused by the COVID-19 pandemic. J Nutr Sci Vitaminol (Tokyo) [Internet]. 2022 [cited 2024 Mar 29];68(3):172–80. Available from: https://pubmed.ncbi.nlm.nih.gov/35768248/
33. Libon F, Courtois J, Le Goff C, Lukas P, Fabregat-Cabello N, Seidel L, et al. Sunscreens block cutaneous vitamin D production with only a minimal effect on circulating 25-hydroxyvitamin D. Arch Osteoporos [Internet]. 2017 Dec 1 [cited 2024 Mar 29];12(1). Available from: https://pubmed.ncbi.nlm.nih.gov/28718005/
34. Layer thickness of SPF 30 sunscreen and formation of pre-vitamin D—PubMed [Internet]. [cited 2024 Mar 29]. Available from: https://pubmed.ncbi.nlm.nih.gov/26977044/
35. Faurschou A, Beyer DM, Schmedes A, Bogh MK, Philipsen PA, Wulf HC. The relation between sunscreen layer thickness and vitamin D production after ultraviolet B exposure: a randomized clinical trial. Br J Dermatol [Internet]. 2012 Aug [cited 2024 Mar 29];167(2):391–5. Available from: https://pubmed.ncbi.nlm.nih.gov/22512875/
36. Hoesl M, Dietz K, Röcken M, Berneburg M. Vitamin D levels of XP-patients under stringent sun-protection. Eur J Dermatol [Internet]. 2010 Jul [cited 2024 Mar 29];20(4):457–60. Available from: https://pubmed.ncbi.nlm.nih.gov/20494856/
37. Krieger JP, Cabaset S, Canonica C, Christoffel L, Richard A, Schröder T, et al. Prevalence and determinants of vitamin D deficiency in the third trimester of pregnancy: a multicentre study in Switzerland. Br J Nutr [Internet]. 2018 Feb 14 [cited 2024 Mar 29];119(3):299–309. Available from: https://pubmed.ncbi.nlm.nih.gov/29318983/

38. Bonilla C, Ness AR, Wills AK, Lawlor DA, Lewis SJ, Davey Smith G. Skin pigmentation, sun exposure and vitamin D levels in children of the Avon Longitudinal Study of Parents and Children. BMC Public Health [Internet]. 2014 Jun 12 [cited 2024 Mar 29];14(1). Available from: https://pubmed.ncbi.nlm.nih.gov/24924479/
39. Pereira LA, Luz FB, Carneiro CMMDO, Xavier ALR, Kanaan S, Miot HA. Evaluation of vitamin D plasma levels after mild exposure to the sun with photoprotection. An Bras Dermatol [Internet]. 2019 Jan 1 [cited 2024 Mar 29];94(1):56–61. Available from: https://pubmed.ncbi.nlm.nih.gov/30726465/
40. Passeron T, Bouillon R, Callender V, Cestari T, Diepgen TL, Green AC, et al. Sunscreen photoprotection and vitamin D status. Br J Dermatol [Internet]. 2019 Nov 1 [cited 2024 Mar 29];181(5):916–31. Available from: https://pubmed.ncbi.nlm.nih.gov/31069788/
41. Sarkar R, Ghunawat S, Narang I, Verma S, Garg VK, Dua R. Role of broad-spectrum sunscreen alone in the improvement of melasma area severity index (MASI) and Melasma Quality of Life Index in melasma. J Cosmet Dermatol [Internet]. 2019 Aug 1 [cited 2024 Mar 29];18(4):1066–73. Available from: https://pubmed.ncbi.nlm.nih.gov/31033184/
42. True photoallergy to sunscreens is rare despite popular belief—PubMed [Internet]. [cited 2024 Mar 29]. Available from: https://pubmed.ncbi.nlm.nih.gov/20646669/
43. Sunscreen allergy in Singapore—PubMed [Internet]. [cited 2024 Mar 29]. Available from: https://pubmed.ncbi.nlm.nih.gov/9471986/
44. Chuah SY, Leow YH, Goon ATJ, Theng CTS, Chong WS. Photopatch testing in Asians: a 5-year experience in Singapore. Photodermatol Photoimmunol Photomed [Internet]. 2013 Jun [cited 2024 Mar 29];29(3):116–20. Available from: https://pubmed.ncbi.nlm.nih.gov/23651271/
45. Lim SYD, Goon ATJ, Leow YH, Chong TYR, Tan EST, Cheng WNS. Photopatch testing in Singapore: a 10-year retrospective study. Photodermatol Photoimmunol Photomed [Internet]. 2023 Nov 1 [cited 2024 Mar 29];39(6):642–7. Available from: https://pubmed.ncbi.nlm.nih.gov/37749909/
46. Ludriksone L, Elsner P. Adverse reactions to sunscreens. Curr Probl Dermatol [Internet]. 2021 Oct 1 [cited 2024 Mar 29];55:223–35. Available from: https://pubmed.ncbi.nlm.nih.gov/34698020/
47. Ekstein SF, Hylwa S. Sunscreens: a review of UV filters and their allergic potential. dermatitis [Internet]. 2023 Jun 1 [cited 2024 Mar 11];34(3):176–90. Available from: https://pubmed.ncbi.nlm.nih.gov/36279254/
48. Keyes E, Werth VP, Brod B. Potential allergenicity of commonly sold high SPF broad spectrum sunscreens in the United States; from the perspective of patients with autoimmune skin disease. Int J Womens Dermatol [Internet]. 2019 Sep 1 [cited 2024 Mar 29];5(4):227. Available from: https://www.ncbi.nlm.nih.gov/pmc/articles/PMC6831754/
49. Rodríguez E, Valbuena MC, Rey M, Porras de Quintana L. Causal agents of photoallergic contact dermatitis diagnosed in the national institute of dermatology of Colombia. Photodermatol Photoimmunol Photomed [Internet]. 2006 Aug [cited 2024 Mar 29];22(4):189–92. Available from: https://pubmed.ncbi.nlm.nih.gov/16869867/
50. Valbuena Mesa MC, Hoyos Jiménez E V. Photopatch testing in Bogota (Colombia): 2011–2013. Contact Dermatitis [Internet]. 2016 Jan 1 [cited 2024 Mar 29];74(1):11–7. Available from: https://pubmed.ncbi.nlm.nih.gov/26086895/
51. Bryden AM, Moseley H, Ibbotson SH, Chowdhury MMU, Beck MH, Bourke J, et al. Photopatch testing of 1155 patients: results of the U.K. multicentre photopatch study group. Br J Dermatol [Internet]. 2006 Oct [cited 2024 Mar 29];155(4):737–47. Available from: https://pubmed.ncbi.nlm.nih.gov/16965423/
52. García Castro R, Velasco Tirado V, Alonso Sardón M, González de Arriba M. Standard photopatch test battery? Proposal based on current epidemiology and experience in our Skin Allergy Unit. Photodermatol Photoimmunol Photomed [Internet]. 2021 Sep 1 [cited 2024 Mar 29];37(5):449–53. Available from: https://pubmed.ncbi.nlm.nih.gov/33738844/

53. Chaiyabutr C, Sukakul T, Limphoka P, Kumpangsin T, Boonchai W. Photopatch testing in a tropical country, Thailand: 20 years' experience. Photodermatol Photoimmunol Photomed [Internet]. 2021 Jan 1 [cited 2024 Mar 29];37(1):28–33. Available from: https://pubmed.ncbi.nlm.nih.gov/32816407/
54. [Results and assessment of photopatch testing in Spain: towards a new standard set of photoallergens]—PubMed [Internet]. [cited 2024 Mar 29]. Available from: https://pubmed.ncbi.nlm.nih.gov/17397595/
55. Kerr AC, Ferguson J, Ibbotson SH, Dawe RS, Haylett AK, Rhodes LE, et al. A European multicentre photopatch test study. Br J Dermatol [Internet]. 2012 May [cited 2024 Mar 29];166(5):1002–9. Available from: https://pubmed.ncbi.nlm.nih.gov/22283432/
56. Subiabre-Ferrer D, Esteve-Martínez A, Blasco-Encinas R, Sierra-Talamantes C, Pérez-Ferriols A, Zaragoza-Ninet V. European photopatch test baseline series: a 3-year experience. Contact Dermatitis [Internet]. 2019 Jan 1 [cited 2024 Mar 29];80(1):5–8. Available from: https://pubmed.ncbi.nlm.nih.gov/30221361/
57. Codeço C, Alves PB, Figueiredo AC, Flor D, Gonçalo M. Shedding a light on the importance of photopatch testing: a 12-year experience in a dermatology unit. Contact Dermatitis [Internet]. 2023 Jun 1 [cited 2024 Mar 29];88(6):438–45. Available from: https://pubmed.ncbi.nlm.nih.gov/36807918/
58. Suzuki K, Futamura K, Sugiyama M, Matsunaga K, Yagami A. Allergic contact dermatitis caused by dimethicodiethylbenzalmalonate (polysilicone-15, Parsol SLX) and bis-ethylhexyloxyphenol methoxyphenyl triazine (Tinosorb S) in sunscreen cream. Contact Dermatitis [Internet]. 2022 Jul 1 [cited 2024 Mar 29];87(1):108–10. Available from: https://pubmed.ncbi.nlm.nih.gov/35306675/
59. Sarre ME, Guérin-Moreau M, Lepoittevin JP, Martin L, Avenel-Audran M. Allergic contact cheilitis caused by polysilicone-15 (Parsol® SLX) in a lipcare balm. Contact Dermatitis [Internet]. 2014 Feb [cited 2024 Mar 29];70(2):119–21. Available from: https://pubmed.ncbi.nlm.nih.gov/24450826/
60. Aerts O, Clinck B, Schramme M, Lambert J. Contact allergy caused by Tinosorb® M: let us not forget about xanthan gum. Contact Dermatitis [Internet]. 2015 Feb 1 [cited 2024 Mar 29];72(2):121–3. Available from: https://onlinelibrary.wiley.com/doi/full/10.1111/cod.12324
61. De Groot AC, Van Zuuren EJ, Hissink D. Contact allergy to Tinosorb® M: recommendations for diagnostic improvement. Contact Dermatitis [Internet]. 2014 [cited 2024 Mar 29];70(4):251–4. Available from: https://www.researchgate.net/publication/260802511_Contact_allergy_to_TinosorbR_M_Recommendations_for_diagnostic_improvement
62. Andrade P, Gonalo M, Figueiredo A. Allergic contact dermatitis to decyl glucoside in Tinosorb M. Contact Dermatitis [Internet]. 2010 Feb [cited 2024 Mar 29];62(2):119–20. Available from: https://pubmed.ncbi.nlm.nih.gov/20136897/
63. González-Pérez R, Trébol I, García-Río I, Arregui MA, Soloeta R. Allergic contact dermatitis from methylene-bis-benzotriazolyl tetramethylbutylphenol (Tinosorb M). Contact Dermatitis [Internet]. 2007 Feb [cited 2024 Mar 29];56(2):121. Available from: https://pubmed.ncbi.nlm.nih.gov/17244092/
64. Pereira N, Coutinho I, Andrade P, Gonçalo M. The UV filter tinosorb M, containing decyl glucoside, is a frequent cause of allergic contact dermatitis. Dermatitis [Internet]. 2013 Jan [cited 2024 Mar 29];24(1):41–3. Available from: https://pubmed.ncbi.nlm.nih.gov/23340401/
65. Liuti F, Borrego L. Contact dermatitis caused by Tinosorb® M: the importance of pach testing with pure methylene bis-benzotriazolyl tetramethylbutylphenol. Contact Dermatitis [Internet]. 2015 Sep 1 [cited 2024 Mar 29];73(3):192–3. Available from: https://pubmed.ncbi.nlm.nih.gov/25962512/
66. Hoffmann SS, Elberling J, Thyssen JP, Hansen KS, Johansen JD. Does aluminium in sunscreens cause dermatitis in children with aluminium contact allergy: a repeated open application test study. Contact Dermatitis [Internet]. 2022 Jan 1 [cited 2024 Mar 29];86(1):9–14. Available from: https://pubmed.ncbi.nlm.nih.gov/34536036/

67. Guenther J, Johnson H, Yu J De, Adler BL. Photoallergic contact dermatitis: no fun in the sun. Cutis [Internet]. 2022 Nov 1 [cited 2024 Mar 29];110(5). Available from: https://pubmed.ncbi.nlm.nih.gov/36638383/
68. Pastor-Nieto MA, Sánchez-Pedreño P, Martínez-Menchón T, Melgar-Molero V, Alcántara-Nicolás F, de la Cruz-Murie P. Allergic contact dermatitis caused by phenylethyl resorcinol, a skin-lightening agent contained in a sunscreen. Contact Dermatitis [Internet]. 2016 Oct 1 [cited 2024 Mar 29];75(4):250–3. Available from: https://pubmed.ncbi.nlm.nih.gov/27620125/
69. Boonchai W, Sathaworawong A, Wongpraparut C, Wanitphakdeedecha R. The sensitization potential of sunscreen after ablative fractional skin resurfacing using modified human repeated insult patch test. J Dermatolog Treat [Internet]. 2015 Sep 3 [cited 2024 Mar 29];26(5):485–8. Available from: https://pubmed.ncbi.nlm.nih.gov/25633273/
70. Wanitphakdeedecha R, Phuardchantuk R, Manuskiatti W. The use of sunscreen starting on the first day after ablative fractional skin resurfacing. J Eur Acad Dermatol Venereol [Internet]. 2014 Nov 1 [cited 2024 Mar 29];28(11):1522–8. Available from: https://pubmed.ncbi.nlm.nih.gov/24320057/
71. Rocholl M, Weinert P, Bielfeldt S, Laing S, Wilhelm KP, Ulrich C, et al. New methods for assessing secondary performance attributes of sunscreens suitable for professional outdoor work. J Occup Med Toxicol [Internet]. 2021 Dec 1 [cited 2024 Mar 29];16(1):1–11. Available from: https://occup-med.biomedcentral.com/articles/10.1186/s12995-021-00314-2
72. Diffey B. Sunscreens: expectation and realization. Photodermatol Photoimmunol Photomed [Internet]. 2009 [cited 2024 Mar 29];25(5):233–6. Available from: https://pubmed.ncbi.nlm.nih.gov/19747240/
73. Kim SM, Oh BH, Lee YW, Choe YB, Ahn KJ. The relation between the amount of sunscreen applied and the sun protection factor in Asian skin. J Am Acad Dermatol [Internet]. 2010 Feb [cited 2024 Mar 29];62(2):218–22. Available from: https://pubmed.ncbi.nlm.nih.gov/19962787/
74. Neale R, Williams G, Green A. Application patterns among participants randomized to daily sunscreen use in a skin cancer prevention trial. Arch Dermatol [Internet]. 2002 Oct 1 [cited 2024 Mar 29];138(10):1319–25. Available from: https://pubmed.ncbi.nlm.nih.gov/12374537/
75. Szepietowski JC, Nowicka D, Reich A, Melon M. Application of sunscreen preparations among young Polish people. J Cosmet Dermatol [Internet]. 2004 Apr [cited 2024 Mar 29];3(2):69–72. Available from: https://pubmed.ncbi.nlm.nih.gov/17147558/
76. Petersen B, Wulf HC. Application of sunscreen--theory and reality. Photodermatol Photoimmunol Photomed [Internet]. 2014 [cited 2024 Mar 29];30(2–3):96–101. Available from: https://pubmed.ncbi.nlm.nih.gov/24313722/
77. Schalka S, dos Reis VMS, Cucé LC. The influence of the amount of sunscreen applied and its sun protection factor (SPF): evaluation of two sunscreens including the same ingredients at different concentrations. Photodermatol Photoimmunol Photomed [Internet]. 2009 [cited 2024 Mar 29];25(4):175–80. Available from: https://pubmed.ncbi.nlm.nih.gov/19614894/
78. Faurschou A, Wulf HC. The relation between sun protection factor and amount of suncreen applied in vivo. Br J Dermatol [Internet]. 2007 Apr [cited 2024 Mar 29];156(4):716–9. Available from: https://pubmed.ncbi.nlm.nih.gov/17493070/
79. Ferrero L, Pissavini M, Doucet O. How a calculated model of sunscreen film geometry can explain in vitro and in vivo SPF variation. Photochem Photobiol Sci [Internet]. 2010 [cited 2024 Mar 22];9(4):540–51. Available from: https://pubmed.ncbi.nlm.nih.gov/20354649/
80. Federal Register:: Sunscreen drug products for over-the-counter human use [Internet]. [cited 2024 Mar 20]. Available from: https://www.federalregister.gov/documents/2019/02/26/2019-03019/sunscreen-drug-products-for-over-the-counter-human-use
81. Young AR, Boles J, Herzog B, Osterwalder U, Baschong W. A sunscreen's labeled sun protection factor may overestimate protection at temperate latitudes: a human in vivo study. J Invest Dermatol [Internet]. 2010 [cited 2024 Mar 11];130(10):2457–62. Available from: https://pubmed.ncbi.nlm.nih.gov/20535128/

82. Russak JE, Chen T, Appa Y, Rigel DS. A comparison of sunburn protection of high-sun protection factor (SPF) sunscreens: SPF 85 sunscreen is significantly more protective than SPF 50. J Am Acad Dermatol [Internet]. 2010 Feb [cited 2024 Mar 29];62(2):348–9. Available from: https://pubmed.ncbi.nlm.nih.gov/20115958/
83. Ou-Yang H, Stanfield J, Cole C, Appa Y, Rigel D. High sun-protection factor sunscreens (≥70) may provide ultraviolet protection above minimal recommended levels by adequately compensating for lower sunscreen user application amounts. J Am Acad Dermatol [Internet]. 2013 Sep [cited 2024 Mar 29];69(3):481–3. Available from: https://pubmed.ncbi.nlm.nih.gov/23957971/
84. Cole C, Appa Y, Ou-Yang H. A broad spectrum high-SPF photostable sunscreen with a high UVA-PF can protect against cellular damage at high UV exposure doses. Photodermatol Photoimmunol Photomed [Internet]. 2014 [cited 2024 Mar 11];30(4):212–9. Available from: https://pubmed.ncbi.nlm.nih.gov/24806442/
85. Diffey BL. When should sunscreen be reapplied? J Am Acad Dermatol [Internet]. 2001 [cited 2024 Mar 29];45(6):882–5. Available from: https://pubmed.ncbi.nlm.nih.gov/11712033/
86. Teramura T, Mizuno M, Asano H, Naito N, Arakane K, Miyachi Y. Relationship between sun-protection factor and application thickness in high-performance sunscreen: double application of sunscreen is recommended. Clin Exp Dermatol [Internet]. 2012 Dec [cited 2024 Mar 29];37(8):904–8. Available from: https://pubmed.ncbi.nlm.nih.gov/23050556/
87. Taylor S, Diffey B. Simple dosage guide for suncreams will help users. BMJ: Br Med J [Internet]. 2002 Jun 6 [cited 2024 Mar 29];324(7352):1526. Available from: https://www.ncbi.nlm.nih.gov/pmc/articles/PMC1123459/
88. Srinivas C, Lal S, Thirumoorthy M, Sundaram S, Karthick P. Sunscreen application: not less, not more. Indian J Dermatol Venereol Leprol [Internet]. 2006 Jul 1 [cited 2024 Mar 29];72(4):306. Available from: https://ijdvl.com/sunscreen-application-not-less-not-more/
89. Heerfordt IM, Torsnes LR, Philipsen PA, Wulf HC. Sunscreen use optimized by two consecutive applications. PLoS One [Internet]. 2018 Mar 1 [cited 2024 Mar 29];13(3). Available from: https://pubmed.ncbi.nlm.nih.gov/29590142/
90. Heerfordt IM, Torsnes LR, Philipsen PA, Wulf HC. Photoprotection by sunscreen depends on time spent on application. Photodermatol Photoimmunol Photomed [Internet]. 2018 Mar 1 [cited 2024 Mar 29];34(2):117–21. Available from: https://pubmed.ncbi.nlm.nih.gov/29235160/
91. Zastrow L, Groth N, Klein F, Kockott D, Lademann J, Renneberg R, et al. The missing link--light-induced (280-1,600 nm) free radical formation in human skin. Skin Pharmacol Physiol [Internet]. 2009 Jan [cited 2024 Mar 3];22(1):31–44. Available from: https://pubmed.ncbi.nlm.nih.gov/19122479/
92. Light JG, Frantz T, McNamara K, Bashyam AM, Feldman SR. Efficacy of Applicator Devices for Self-Application of Topicals to the Back. J Cutan Med Surg [Internet]. 2020 May 1 [cited 2024 Mar 29];24(3):249–52. Available from: https://pubmed.ncbi.nlm.nih.gov/32052653/
93. Phillips TJ, Bhawan J, Yaar M, Bello Y, LoPiccolo D, Nash JF. Effect of daily versus intermittent sunscreen application on solar simulated UV radiation-induced skin response in humans. J Am Acad Dermatol [Internet]. 2000 [cited 2024 Mar 29];43(4):610–8. Available from: https://pubmed.ncbi.nlm.nih.gov/11004615/
94. Tribby CP, Julian AK, Perna FM. Perceived usefulness and recall of sunscreen label information by consumers. JAMA Dermatol [Internet]. 2021 May 1 [cited 2024 Mar 29];157(5):573–6. Available from: https://pubmed.ncbi.nlm.nih.gov/33760056/
95. Lowry M, Julian AK, Tribby C, Perna F. Consumers pay attention to ingredients on the front of a label: an eye tracking study. Transl Behav Med [Internet]. 2023 Sep 28 [cited 2024 Mar 29];13(10):768–74. Available from: https://pubmed.ncbi.nlm.nih.gov/37335903/
96. Carrao AM, Coleman JC, Guo JJ, Kumari H. A novel online survey approach designed to measure consumer sunscreen application thickness—implications for estimating environmental emissions. Journal of Exposure Science & Environmental Epidemiology 2023

[Internet]. 2023 Oct 28 [cited 2024 Mar 29];1–8. Available from: https://www.nature.com/articles/s41370-023-00608-z

97. Diffey B. When should sunscreen be applied: the balance between health benefit and adverse consequences to humans and the environment. Int J Cosmet Sci [Internet]. 2023 Oct 1 [cited 2024 Mar 28];45 Suppl 1(S1):45–51. Available from: https://pubmed.ncbi.nlm.nih.gov/37799082/
98. The impact of natural sunlight exposure on the UVB-sun protection factor (UVB-SPF) and UVA protection factor (UVA-PF) of a UVA/UVB SPF 50 sunscreen—PubMed [Internet]. [cited 2024 Mar 29]. Available from: https://pubmed.ncbi.nlm.nih.gov/21283919/
99. Wright MW, Wright ST, Wagner RF. Mechanisms of sunscreen failure. J Am Acad Dermatol [Internet]. 2001 [cited 2024 Mar 29];44(5):781–4. Available from: https://pubmed.ncbi.nlm.nih.gov/11312424/
100. Ruvolo E, Aeschliman L, Cole C. Evaluation of sunscreen efficacy over time and re-application using hybrid diffuse reflectance spectroscopy. Photodermatol Photoimmunol Photomed [Internet]. 2020 May 1 [cited 2024 Mar 29];36(3):192–9. Available from: https://pubmed.ncbi.nlm.nih.gov/32027038/
101. Bodekær M, Faurschou A, Philipsen PA, Wulf HC. Sun protection factor persistence during a day with physical activity and bathing. Photodermatol Photoimmunol Photomed [Internet]. 2008 [cited 2024 Mar 29];24(6):296–300. Available from: https://pubmed.ncbi.nlm.nih.gov/19000186/
102. Realistic sunscreen durability: a randomized, double-blinded, controlled clinical study—PubMed [Internet]. [cited 2024 Mar 29]. Available from: https://pubmed.ncbi.nlm.nih.gov/29320597/
103. Kobwanthanakun W, Silpa-archa N, Wongpraparut C, Pruksaekanan C, Manuskiatti W. An evaluation of the course of facial sunscreen coverage and sustainability over an 8-hour work-day among outdoor workers. Health Sci Rep [Internet]. 2021 Sep 1 [cited 2024 Mar 29];4(3). Available from: https://pubmed.ncbi.nlm.nih.gov/34401526/
104. Rungananchai C, Silpa-archa N, Wongpraparut C, Suiwongsa B, Sangveraphunsiri V, Manuskiatti W. Sunscreen application to the face persists beyond 2 hours in indoor workers: an open-label trial. J Dermatolog Treat [Internet]. 2019 Jul 4 [cited 2024 Mar 29];30(5):483–6. Available from: https://pubmed.ncbi.nlm.nih.gov/30273065/
105. Beyer DM, Faurschou A, Philipsen PA, Hædersdal M, Wulf HC. Sun protection factor persistence on human skin during a day without physical activity or ultraviolet exposure. Photodermatol Photoimmunol Photomed [Internet]. 2010 Feb [cited 2024 Mar 29];26(1):22–7. Available from: https://pubmed.ncbi.nlm.nih.gov/20070835/
106. Korting HC, Schöllmann C. Resistance of liposomal sunscreen formulations against plain water as well as salt water exposure and perspiration. Skin Pharmacol Physiol [Internet]. 2011 Dec [cited 2024 Mar 29];24(1):36–43. Available from: https://pubmed.ncbi.nlm.nih.gov/20720455/
107. Poh Agin P. Water resistance and extended wear sunscreens. Dermatol Clin [Internet]. 2006 Jan [cited 2024 Mar 29];24(1):75–9. Available from: https://pubmed.ncbi.nlm.nih.gov/16311169/
108. Matta MK, Florian J, Zusterzeel R, Pilli NR, Patel V, Volpe DA, et al. Effect of sunscreen application on plasma concentration of sunscreen active ingredients: a randomized clinical trial. JAMA [Internet]. 2020 Jan 21 [cited 2024 Mar 27];323(3):256–67. Available from: https://jamanetwork.com/journals/jama/fullarticle/2759002
109. Bodekær M, Åkerström U, Wulf HC. Accumulation of sunscreen in human skin after daily applications: a study of sunscreens with different ultraviolet radiation filters. Photodermatol Photoimmunol Photomed [Internet]. 2012 Jun [cited 2024 Mar 29];28(3):127–32. Available from: https://pubmed.ncbi.nlm.nih.gov/22548393/
110. Li H, Colantonio S, Dawson A, Lin X, Beecker J. Sunscreen application, safety, and sun protection: the evidence. J Cutan Med Surg [Internet]. 2019 Jul 1 [cited 2024 Mar 28];23(4):357–69. Available from: https://pubmed.ncbi.nlm.nih.gov/31219707/

111. Norman KG, Loretz L, Kowcz A, Kaufman LE, Ruvolo E, Traudt M, et al. Application habits and practices of regular sunscreen users in the United States: results of an online survey. Food Chem Toxicol [Internet]. 2023 Nov 1 [cited 2024 Mar 29];181. Available from: https://pubmed.ncbi.nlm.nih.gov/37813178/
112. Morton SK, Harrison SL. Slip, slop, slap, slide, seek and sport: a systematic scoping review of sun protection in sport in Australasia. Curr Oncol [Internet]. 2022 Jan 1 [cited 2024 Mar 20];30(1):401–15. Available from: https://pubmed.ncbi.nlm.nih.gov/36661682/
113. Pratt H, Hassanin K, Troughton LD, Czanner G, Zheng Y, McCormick AG, et al. UV imaging reveals facial areas that are prone to skin cancer are disproportionately missed during sunscreen application. PLoS One [Internet]. 2017 Oct 1 [cited 2024 Mar 29];12(10). Available from: https://pubmed.ncbi.nlm.nih.gov/28968413/
114. Le Digabel J, Questel E, Lauze C, Carballido F, Josse G. In vivo evaluation of sunscreen application by multispectral imaging: a new tool for educating sunscreen users. Skin Res Technol [Internet]. 2023 Aug 1 [cited 2024 Mar 29];29(8). Available from: https://www.ncbi.nlm.nih.gov/pmc/articles/PMC10397373/
115. Ou-Yang H, Meyer K, Houser T, Grove G. Sunscreen formulations do not interfere with sweat cooling during exercise. Int J Cosmet Sci [Internet]. 2018 Feb 1 [cited 2024 Mar 29];40(1):87–92. Available from: https://pubmed.ncbi.nlm.nih.gov/29105107/
116. Diffey BL. The impact of topical photoprotectants intended for daily use on lifetime ultraviolet exposure. J Cosmet Dermatol [Internet]. 2011 Sep [cited 2024 Mar 13];10(3):245–50. Available from: https://pubmed.ncbi.nlm.nih.gov/21896139/
117. Harrison SL, Buettner PG, Nowak MJ. Sun-protective clothing worn regularly during early childhood reduces the number of new melanocytic nevi: the North Queensland sun-safe clothing cluster randomized controlled trial. Cancers (Basel) [Internet]. 2023 Mar 1 [cited 2024 Mar 29];15(6). Available from: https://pubmed.ncbi.nlm.nih.gov/36980647/
118. Achar A, Rathi SK. Melasma: a clinico-epidemiological study of 312 cases. Indian J Dermatol [Internet]. 2011 Jul [cited 2024 Mar 29];56(4):380. Available from: https://www.ncbi.nlm.nih.gov/pmc/articles/PMC3178998/
119. MacK MC, Tierney NK, Ruvolo E, Stamatas GN, Martin KM, Kollias N. Development of solar UVR-related pigmentation begins as early as the first summer of life. J Invest Dermatol [Internet]. 2010 [cited 2024 Mar 29];130(9):2335–8. Available from: https://pubmed.ncbi.nlm.nih.gov/20428184/
120. de Gálvez MV, Aguilera J, Buendía EA, Sánchez-Roldán C, Herrera-Ceballos E. Time required for a standard sunscreen to become effective following application: a UV photography study. J Eur Acad Dermatol Venereol. 2018;32(4):e123–4.
121. Kluschke F, Weigmann HJ, Schanzer S, Meinke M, Vergou T, Sterry W, et al. Gain or loss? Sunscreen efficiency after cosmetic pretreatment of the skin. Skin Pharmacol Physiol [Internet]. 2014 Jan [cited 2024 Mar 29];27(2):82–9. Available from: https://pubmed.ncbi.nlm.nih.gov/24052131/
122. Kluschke F, Patzelt A, Lademann J, Sterry W, Lange-Asschenfeldt B. Skin care. Sun care. a successful symbiosis? J Dtsch Dermatol Ges [Internet]. 2013 Oct [cited 2024 Mar 29];11(10):1020–1. Available from: https://pubmed.ncbi.nlm.nih.gov/23730932/
123. Gálvez MV de, Aguilera J, Leal M, Sánchez-Roldán C, Herrera-Ceballos E. Sunscreens effectiveness are not altered by concomitant use of moisturizing creams: an ultraviolet reflectance photography study. Photodermatol Photoimmunol Photomed [Internet]. 2022 May 1 [cited 2024 Mar 29];38(3):250–8. Available from: https://pubmed.ncbi.nlm.nih.gov/34674316/
124. Lourenco EAJ, Shaw L, Pratt H, Duffy GL, Czanner G, Zheng Y, et al. Application of SPF moisturisers is inferior to sunscreens in coverage of facial and eyelid regions. PLoS One [Internet]. 2019 Apr 1 [cited 2024 Mar 29];14(4). Available from: https://pubmed.ncbi.nlm.nih.gov/30943192/
125. Brunet-Possenti F, Deschamps L, Colboc H, Somogyi A, Medjoubi K, Bazin D, et al. Detection of titanium nanoparticles in the hair shafts of a patient with frontal fibrosing alopecia. J

Eur Acad Dermatol Venereol [Internet]. 2018 Dec 1 [cited 2024 Mar 29];32(12):e442–3. Available from: https://pubmed.ncbi.nlm.nih.gov/29578625/

126. Aldoori N, Dobson K, Holden CR, McDonagh AJ, Harries M, Messenger AG. Frontal fibrosing alopecia: possible association with leave-on facial skin care products and sunscreens; a questionnaire study. Br J Dermatol [Internet]. 2016 Oct 1 [cited 2024 Mar 29];175(4):762–7. Available from: https://pubmed.ncbi.nlm.nih.gov/26987767/
127. Aldoori N, Dobson K, Holden CR, McDonagh AJ, Harries M, Messenger AG. Frontal fibrosing alopecia: there is no statistically significant association with leave-on facial skin care products and sunscreens: reply from the authors. Br J Dermatol [Internet]. 2016 Dec 1 [cited 2024 Mar 29];175(6):1408–9. Available from: https://pubmed.ncbi.nlm.nih.gov/27619318/
128. Debroy Kidambi A, Dobson K, Holmes S, Carauna D, Del Marmol V, Vujovic A, et al. Frontal fibrosing alopecia in men: an association with facial moisturizers and sunscreens. Br J Dermatol [Internet]. 2017 Jul 1 [cited 2024 Mar 29];177(1):260–1. Available from: https://pubmed.ncbi.nlm.nih.gov/28112792/
129. Strazzulla LC, Avila L, Lo Sicco K, Shapiro J. Response to "Frontal fibrosing alopecia in men: an association with facial moisturizers and sunscreens." Br J Dermatol [Internet]. 2017 Jul 1 [cited 2024 Mar 29];177(1):323. Available from: https://pubmed.ncbi.nlm.nih.gov/28301047/
130. Callander J, Frost J, Stone N. Ultraviolet filters in hair-care products: a possible link with frontal fibrosing alopecia and lichen planopilaris. Clin Exp Dermatol [Internet]. 2018 Jan 1 [cited 2024 Mar 29];43(1):69–70. Available from: https://pubmed.ncbi.nlm.nih.gov/28994172/
131. Canavan TN, McClees SF, Duncan JR, Elewski BE. Lichen planopilaris in the setting of hair sunscreen spray. Skin Appendage Disord [Internet]. 2019 Feb 1 [cited 2024 Mar 29];5(2):108–10. Available from: https://pubmed.ncbi.nlm.nih.gov/30815445/
132. Moreno-Arrones OM, Saceda-Corralo D, Rodrigues-Barata AR, Castellanos-González M, Fernández-Pugnaire MA, Grimalt R, et al. Risk factors associated with frontal fibrosing alopecia: a multicentre case-control study. Clin Exp Dermatol [Internet]. 2019 Jun 1 [cited 2024 Mar 30];44(4):404–10. Available from: https://pubmed.ncbi.nlm.nih.gov/30259544/
133. Panchaprateep R, Ruxrungtham P, Chancheewa B, Asawanonda P. Clinical characteristics, trichoscopy, histopathology and treatment outcomes of frontal fibrosing alopecia in an Asian population: a retro-prospective cohort study. J Dermatol [Internet]. 2020 Nov 1 [cited 2024 Mar 30];47(11):1301–11. Available from: https://pubmed.ncbi.nlm.nih.gov/32710515/
134. Bole R, Wyles S, Larkin S, Imhof R, Torgerson RR. Lichen planopilaris in women: a survey-based study examining baseline hair characteristics and product use in 129 patients seen at Mayo Clinic. Int J Womens Dermatol [Internet]. 2019 Mar 1 [cited 2024 Mar 30];6(2):105–8. Available from: https://pubmed.ncbi.nlm.nih.gov/32258343/
135. Imhof RL, Larkin SC, Cantwell HM, Torgerson RR, Tolkachjov SN. The association of frontal fibrosing alopecia with skin and hair care products: a survey-based case series of 56 patients seen at the Mayo Clinic. J Am Acad Dermatol [Internet]. 2021 Feb 1 [cited 2024 Mar 30];84(2):532–4. Available from: https://pubmed.ncbi.nlm.nih.gov/32437720/
136. Ramos PM, Anzai A, Duque-Estrada B, Farias DC, Melo DF, Mulinari-Brenner F, et al. Risk factors for frontal fibrosing alopecia: a case-control study in a multiracial population. J Am Acad Dermatol. 2021;84(3):712–8.
137. Alagappan U, Tay YK, Lim SPR. Pigmented contact dermatitis secondary to benzyl salicylate. Acta Derm Venereol [Internet]. 2013 [cited 2024 Mar 30];93(5):590. Available from: https://pubmed.ncbi.nlm.nih.gov/23529141/
138. Leecharoen W, Thanomkitti K, Thuangtong R, Varothai S, Triwongwaranat D, Jiamton S, et al. Use of facial care products and frontal fibrosing alopecia: coincidence or true association? J Dermatol [Internet]. 2021 Oct 1 [cited 2024 Mar 30];48(10):1557–63. Available from: https://pubmed.ncbi.nlm.nih.gov/34264523/
139. Pham CT, Juhasz M, Ekelem C, Conic RRZ, Hashemi K, Csuka D, et al. The association of frontal alopecia with a history of facial and scalp surgical procedures. Skin Appendage

Disord [Internet]. 2022 Jan 1 [cited 2024 Mar 30];8(1):13–9. Available from: https://pubmed.ncbi.nlm.nih.gov/35118123/
140. Maghfour J, Ceresnie M, Olson J, Lim HW. The association between frontal fibrosing alopecia, sunscreen, and moisturizers: a systematic review and meta-analysis. J Am Acad Dermatol [Internet]. 2022 Aug 1 [cited 2024 Mar 30];87(2):395–6. Available from: https://pubmed.ncbi.nlm.nih.gov/35074440/
141. Kępińska K, Jałowska M, Bowszyc-Dmochowska M. Frontal fibrosing alopecia—a review and a practical guide for clinicians. Ann Agric Environ Med [Internet]. 2022 [cited 2024 Mar 30];29(2):169–84. Available from: https://pubmed.ncbi.nlm.nih.gov/35767748/
142. Abuav R, Shon W. Are sunscreen particles involved in frontal fibrosing alopecia?-a TEM-EDXS analysis on formalin-fixed paraffin-embedded alopecia biopsies (Pilot Study). Am J Dermatopathol [Internet]. 2022 Dec 1 [cited 2024 Mar 30];44(12):E135–6. Available from: https://pubmed.ncbi.nlm.nih.gov/36197059/
143. Lyakhovitsky A, Kartvelishvily E, Drousiotis T, Lyakhovitsky K, Baum S, Barzilai A. Hair shaft morphology, elemental composition, and nanoparticles in frontal fibrosing alopecia: a case-control study. Acta Derm Venereol [Internet]. 2021 Sep 1 [cited 2024 Mar 30];101(9). Available from: https://pubmed.ncbi.nlm.nih.gov/34396423/
144. Rosales Santillan M, Goldberg JB, Goldberg LJ. Exploring potential decreasing age of patients with frontal fibrosing alopecia. JAAD Int [Internet]. 2022 Dec 1 [cited 2024 Mar 30];9:28–9. Available from: https://pubmed.ncbi.nlm.nih.gov/36034744/
145. Kam O, Na S, Guo W, Tejeda CI, Kaufmann T. Frontal fibrosing alopecia and personal care product use: a systematic review and meta-analysis. Arch Dermatol Res [Internet]. 2023 Oct 1 [cited 2024 Mar 30];315(8):2313–31. Available from: https://pubmed.ncbi.nlm.nih.gov/37014396/
146. Porriño-Bustamante ML, Montero-Vílchez T, Pinedo-Moraleda FJ, Fernández-Flores Á, Fernández-Pugnaire MA, Arias-Santiago S. Frontal fibrosing alopecia and sunscreen use: a cross-sectional study of actinic damage. Acta Derm Venereol [Internet]. 2022 [cited 2024 Mar 30];102. Available from: https://pubmed.ncbi.nlm.nih.gov/35604235/
147. Cranwell WC, Sinclair R. Sunscreen and facial skincare products in frontal fibrosing alopecia: a case-control study. Br J Dermatol [Internet]. 2019 Apr 1 [cited 2024 Mar 30];180(4):943–4. Available from: https://pubmed.ncbi.nlm.nih.gov/30367472/
148. Cranwell WC, Sinclair R. Frontal fibrosing alopecia: regrowth following cessation of sunscreen on the forehead. Australas J Dermatol [Internet]. 2019 Feb 1 [cited 2024 Mar 30];60(1):60–1. Available from: https://pubmed.ncbi.nlm.nih.gov/29896853/
149. Gamret AC, Potluri VS, Krishnamurthy K, Fertig RM. Frontal fibrosing alopecia: efficacy of treatment modalities. Int J Womens Health [Internet]. 2019 Apr [cited 2024 Mar 30];11:273–85. Available from: https://pubmed.ncbi.nlm.nih.gov/31118828/
150. Holmboe SA, Scheutz Henriksen L, Frederiksen H, Andersson AM, Priskorn L, Jørgensen N, et al. Prenatal exposure to phenols and benzophenones in relation to markers of male reproductive function in adulthood. Front Endocrinol (Lausanne) [Internet]. 2022 Dec 9 [cited 2024 Mar 27];13. Available from: https://pubmed.ncbi.nlm.nih.gov/36568115/
151. Osmond MJ, McCall MJ. Zinc oxide nanoparticles in modern sunscreens: an analysis of potential exposure and hazard. Nanotoxicology [Internet]. 2010 Mar [cited 2024 Mar 30];4(1):15–41. Available from: https://pubmed.ncbi.nlm.nih.gov/20795900/
152. Wu Y, Chen L, Chen F, Zou H, Wang Z. A key moment for TiO2: prenatal exposure to TiO2 nanoparticles may inhibit the development of offspring. Ecotoxicol Environ Saf [Internet]. 2020 Oct 1 [cited 2024 Mar 30];202. Available from: https://pubmed.ncbi.nlm.nih.gov/32800246/
153. Matta MK, Zusterzeel R, Pilli NR, Patel V, Volpe DA, Florian J, et al. Effect of sunscreen application under maximal use conditions on plasma concentration of sunscreen active ingredients: a randomized clinical trial. JAMA [Internet]. 2019 Jun 4 [cited 2024 Mar 15];321(21):2082–91. Available from: https://pubmed.ncbi.nlm.nih.gov/31058986/

154. Janjua NR, Kongshoj B, Andersson AM, Wulf HC. Sunscreens in human plasma and urine after repeated whole-body topical application. J Eur Acad Dermatol Venereol [Internet]. 2008 Apr [cited 2024 Mar 30];22(4):456–61. Available from: https://pubmed.ncbi.nlm.nih.gov/18221342/
155. Janjua NR, Mogensen B, Andersson AM, Petersen JH, Henriksen M, Skakkebæk NE, et al. Systemic absorption of the sunscreens benzophenone-3, octyl-methoxycinnamate, and 3-(4-methyl-benzylidene) camphor after whole-body topical application and reproductive hormone levels in humans. J Invest Dermatol [Internet]. 2004 [cited 2024 Mar 30];123(1):57–61. Available from: https://pubmed.ncbi.nlm.nih.gov/15191542/
156. Phadungsaksawasdi P, Sirithanabadeekul P. Ultraviolet filters in sunscreen products labeled for use in children and for sensitive skin. Pediatr Dermatol [Internet]. 2020 Jul 1 [cited 2024 Mar 30];37(4):632–6. Available from: https://pubmed.ncbi.nlm.nih.gov/32323359/
157. Druml L, Ilyas AM, Ilyas EN. Sunscreen label marketing towards pediatric populations: guidance for navigating sunscreen choice. Curcus [Internet]. 2023 Oct 10 [cited 2024 Mar 30];15(10). Available from: https://pubmed.ncbi.nlm.nih.gov/37954729/
158. Rawlings A V. Ethnic skin types: are there differences in skin structure and function? Int J Cosmet Sci [Internet]. 2006 Apr [cited 2024 Mar 2];28(2):79–93. Available from: https://pubmed.ncbi.nlm.nih.gov/18492142/

MIX
Papier aus verantwortungsvollen Quellen
Paper from responsible sources
FSC® C105338

FSC
www.fsc.org

If you have any concerns about our products,
you can contact us on
ProductSafety@springernature.com

In case Publisher is established outside the EU,
the EU authorized representative is:
Springer Nature Customer Service Center GmbH
Europaplatz 3, 69115 Heidelberg, Germany

Printed by Libri Plureos GmbH
in Hamburg, Germany